Canadian Transcultural Nursing

ASSESSMENT AND INTERVENTION

Canadian Transcultural Nursing

Assessment and Intervention

RUTH ELAINE DAVIDHIZAR, DNS, RN, CS, FAAN

Dean and Professor,
Division of Nursing,
Bethel College,
Mishawaka, Indiana

JOYCE NEWMAN GIGER, EdD, RN, CS, FAAN

Professor, Graduate Studies,
University of Alabama at Birmingham,
School of Nursing,
Birmingham, Alabama

With 17 illustrations

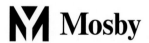 **Mosby**

St. Louis Baltimore Boston Carlsbad Chicago Naples New York Philadelphia Portland
London Madrid Mexico City Singapore Sydney Tokyo Toronto Wiesbaden

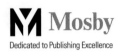

Mosby
Dedicated to Publishing Excellence

A Times Mirror
Company

Publisher **Sally Schrefer**
Editor **Michael S. Ledbetter**
Developmental Editor **Lisa P. Newton**
Project Manager **Dana Peick**
Production Editor **Dan Begley**
Manuscript Editor **Carl Masthay**
Design and Layout **Amy Buxton/E. Rohne Rudder**
Manufacturing Supervisor **Linda Ierardi**

Printed in the United States of America.
Composition by The Clarinda Company
Printing/binding by Maple-Vail Book Manufacturing Group
Cover by Pinnacle

Mosby, Inc.
11830 Westline Industrial Drive
St. Louis, Missouri 63146

Library of Congress Cataloging-in-Publication Data

Canadian transcultural nursing / [edited by] Joyce Newman Giger, Ruth
  Elaine Davidhizar
      p.   cm.
   Includes bibliographical references and index.
   ISBN 0-8151-4389-3 (alk. paper)
    1. Transcultural nursing—Canada.   I. Giger, Joyce Newman.
  II. Davidhizar, Ruth Elaine.
    [DNLM: 1. Transcultural Nursing—Canada.   2. Nursing Assessment.
  3. Cross-Cultural Comparison.   WY 107 C212 1998]
  RT86.S4C36   1998
  610.73'0971—dc21
  DNLM/DLC
  for Library of Congress   98-20114
                                              CIP

98 99 00 01 02 / 9 8 7 6 5 4 3 2 1

CONTRIBUTORS

Maggie Angnatok, RN
*Regional Nurse in Coastal
  Nursing Stations
Nain, Labrador*

Cynthia Baker, PhD, RN
*Associate Professor,
Faculty of Nursing,
University of New Brunswick,
Moncton, New Brunswick*

Mardi S. Bernard, BSN, RN
*Outreach Coordinator,
Rundle Elementary School,
Edmonton, Alberta*

John Howard Brunt, PhD, RN
*Assistant Professor, Faculty of
  Nursing,
University of Victoria,
Victoria, British Columbia*

Sandra C. DeLuca, PhDc, MEd,
  RN
*Nursing Education Division,
Fanshawe College,
London, Ontario*

Paula Didham, BSN, M.AD.Ed,
  RN, FNP
*Nursing Access Coordinator,
Western Memorial Regional
  Hospital School of Nursing
Nain, Labrador*

Nancy A. Edgecombe, MSN, RN
*Nursing Consultant,
Community Health Programs,
Department of Health and Social
  Services,
Government of the Northwest
  Territories*

Heather Jessup-Falcioni, MN, RN
*Assistant Professor, Alternate
  Stream,
School of Nursing,
Laurentian University of Sudbury
Val Caron, Ontario*

Katherine Jones, MSN, RN
*Ryerson School of Nursing,
Ryerson Polytechnic University,
Toronto, Ontario*

Mary Anne Krahn, BScN, RN
*Clinical Educator,
Children's Care at the London
  Health Sciences Centre,
London, Ontario*

Marjorie Elizabeth Linwood,
  BSN, RN
*Professor,
College of Graduate Studies and
  Research,
University of Saskatchewan,
Saskatoon, Saskatchewan*

Coleen Redskye, RN
*Community Nurse,
Forest and Kettle Point Reserve,
Sarnia, Ontario*

Mary Reidy, RN, BN, MEC
*Facultie of Science in Nursing,
Pavilion Margareti-d'Youville,
University of Montreal,
CP 6128, FUCC URFALEA
Montreal, Quebec*

JoLynn J. Reimer, RN, BSN, MA
*Instructor,
Calgary Conjoint Nursing
  Program,
University of Calgary & Mount
  Royal College,
Calgary, Alberta*

Josefina Estéban Richard, RN,
  MN, BN
*Assistant Cardiac Director,
Cardiac Prevention and
  Rehabilitation Research Center,
Dalhousie University;
Halifax, Nova Scotia*

Ruth Shearer, RN, MS, MSN
*Assistant Professor,
Bethel College,
Mishawaka, Indiana*

Marie-Elizabeth Taggart, PhD,
  RN
*Full Professor (Retired),
University of Montreal,
Montreal, Quebec*

Geraldine T. Thomas, PhD
*Associate Professor of Classics,
St. Mary's University,
Halifax, Nova Scotia*

Evelyn Voyageur, BscN, RN
*Nurse in Charge, Medical Services
  Branch,
First Nations Hospital,
Port Hardy, British Columbia*

Olive Yonge, PhD, Cpsych, RN
*Associate Dean, Undergraduate
  Programs,
Nursing Faculty,
University of Alberta,
Edmonton, Alberta*

Lucy Willis, BS, MA, EdD, RN
*Professor,
College of Graduate Studies and
  Research,
University of Saskatchewan,
Saskatoon, Saskatchewan*

TO OUR PARENTS
Lucille & Ralph Holderman
and the late Naomi Holderman
and the late Ionia Holmes Newman

TO OUR HUSBANDS
Ronald Davidhizar and Argusta Giger, Jr.

TO OUR MENTORS
Angela Barron McBride, PhD, RN, FAAN and
Richmond Calvin, EdD, Frances P. Dixon, BS

To the students of Bethel College, past, present, and future
and all nurses and students who seek a better way
to render culturally appropriate care.

FOREWORD

In June 1997, the Twenty-first Quadrennial Conference of the International Congress of Nursing (ICN) was held in the most multicultural of all cities: Vancouver, British Columbia. At that site, virtually all plenary speakers addressed the issues surrounding our increased multicultural societies and the globalization of nursing science. Yet few nursing texts are specifically written to cross national borders. It is exceedingly timely therefore that this edition of Giger and Davidhizar's very successful book *Transcultural Nursing: Assessment and Intervention* has been expanded to encompass Canadian health and social issues as well as highlighting 12 additional ethnic groups residing in Canada.

In their 1995 review of the state of the science, the American Academy of Nursing's Expert Panel on Cultural Diversity noted the paucity of literature linking transcultural nursing research with actual clinical practice. One of the strengths of the Davidhizar and Giger book is that it fosters thinking to construct these linkages. After a review synthesizing literature relevant to a specific ethnic group, each chapter author takes the next step in clinical proficiency by illustrating specific intervention strategies that might be used to foster specified patient outcomes for members of the targeted ethnic group.

Furthermore, the authors take care to guard against the ecological fallacy: assuming individual characteristics on the basis on generalized cultural norms. Cultural content is presented clearly with a considerable number of caveats regarding stereotyping individual cultural members.

Finally, we in the United States have much to learn from policies and interventions initiated in Canada. The Canadian government through its enactment of the Multiculturalism Act (1987), the Canada Health Act (1984), and the Charter of Human Rights and Freedom (1984) provides a unifying base of expectations of cultural competencies for health care providers. The rigorous Canadian cultural training programs such as that developed by Basanti Majumdar offers excellent models for application in the United States.

I anticipate that this edition will be reciprocally beneficial to readers in Canada and the United States. We have much to learn from each other.

Toni Tripp-Reimer, RN, PhD, FAAN
Professor of Nursing and Anthropology,
Associate Dean for Nursing Research,
The University of Iowa,
Iowa City, Iowa

PREFACE

The concept of transcultural nursing is relatively new to the nursing literature. In fact, it has been only in the last three decades that nurses have begun to develop an appreciation for the need to incorporate culturally appropriate clinical approaches into the daily routine of client care. Although nurses have begun to recognize the need for culturally appropriate clinical approaches, the literature on the subject is either scanty or does not provide a systematic method for comprehensive assessment and intervention. However, a good foundation in transcultural nursing is essential for the nurse because it can provide a conceptual framework for holistic client care in a variety of clinical settings and assist the nurse throughout a nursing career.

When we were challenged 10 years ago by the nursing students at Bethel College in Mishawaka, Indiana, United States, to develop a systematic approach to client assessment for use with individuals from diverse cultural backgrounds, we had no idea how profoundly important this topic would become for all health care providers. Canada is very similar to the United States and is rapidly becoming a multicultural, heterogeneous, pluralistic society. With changing demographics, it is imperative that nurses develop not only sensitivity, but also cultural competence to render safe, effective care to all clients.

When we were first challenged by the students at Bethel College, we discovered that the students had difficulty finding adequate literature to assist in planning for clients from diverse cultural backgrounds. We, like our students, had identified a similar need by virtue of our own diverse cultural backgrounds: one of us is African American and was raised in the South, and the other is White and was raised in an Eskimo setting in Alaska. Thus, in response to both a personal interest and the need identified by our students, we set about to synthesize a body of literature that would assist students in developing the theoretical knowledge necessary to provide culturally appropriate care. This effort culminated in our first American version and has been revised in a second edition and has also been translated into French.

With our second edition, which brought forth the first chapter on our Canadian neighbors, we began to realize that there was a pressing need for a textbook that described the people, their cultural heritage, and their unique experiences in the Canadian health care systems. We were delighted when Darlene Como and Loren Wilson (our former editors) asked us to write this book. It has been interesting getting to know some of the culturally diverse peoples of Canada through the eyes of our very knowledgeable Canadian chapter contributors.

While we are pleased that the literature has vastly improved since the initial release of the first American version of this text, there is still much work to be done in this area. Our new Canadian version, like its American cousin, is divided into two parts. The first part, which focuses on theory, includes an introduction and six chapters describing the six cultural phenomena that make up our transcultural conceptual theory of assessment. The six cultural phenomena that we have identified as being evidenced in all cultural groups are (1) communication, (2) space, (3) social organization, (4) time, (5) environmental control, and (6) biological variations. The chapters in Part One describe how these phenomena vary with application and utilization across cultures.

Part Two contains chapters by contributing authors in which the six cultural phenomena are systematically applied to the assessment and care of individuals in specific cultures. The cultures selected for inclusion represent those likely to be encountered by a nurse practicing in Canada.

We have chosen contributing authors with expertise and clinical backgrounds in the care of selected cultural groups. As in our American edition, many of our chapters were written by contributing authors who actually represent by ethnic heritage the cultural group described. Not only are unique and diverse cultures represented, but also the contributing authors actually span Canada from coast to coast.

We are pleased that our chapter contributors are nurses who have expertise and sensitivity in the cultural group and in the unique care strategies that a nurse should use in providing culturally appropriate and competent care.

Since publication of the first American edition, we have developed a quick reference, user-friendly assessment tool for use with clients in diverse clinical settings. Our model has either been cited, excerpted, or modified for inclusion in approximately 125 new nursing textbooks. Our model has shown great applicability across clinical disciplines. As such, the text has been included in the library of the Education Testing Service (ETS) as the only text of its kind to validate test items developed for the former RN-NCLEX and the current RN-CAT used in the United States.

This book was written primarily for all nurses and nursing students who are interested in developing a knowledge of transcultural concepts to apply to client-centered care. However, we believe that our new Canadian version also will be applicable across other disciplines, such as psychology, sociology, medicine, and anthropology, because it provides not only a nursing perspective, but also a historical and bioethnological approach to transcultural health care.

In our commitment to transcultural nursing, we have made every effort, through extensive research, to be as culturally sensitive as possible and not offend our readers or specific racial, cultural, ethnic, or religious groups. Despite our careful attention to detail to prevent his from happening, we realize that the presentation of literature and research findings are often interpreted differently by individuals. We apologize for any content that our readers may find to be of an insensitive nature and assure our readers that as nurse researchers, clinicians, and academicians we did our best to present only factual information.

ACKNOWLEDGMENTS

We would like to acknowledge and thank our former editor, Linda Duncan, whose vision in the future allowed this project to come to fruition. We would also like to thank Darlene Como, our former editor, who took up the challenge to continue this project. We would like to thank Loren Wilson, our former editor, who continued to challenge us to provide the best referenced text on this subject. We would like to thank our current editor, Michael Ledbetter, who has worked diligently to bring this project to fruition. A special thanks to Lisa Newton for being available for our many questions. We must also thank Dan Begley and Carl Masthay for their diligence in bringing the most culturally and linguistically accurate text to Canadian health care providers.

We would like to thank Dr. Clyde Root, director of Library Services, Bethel College, for the multitude of computer searches conducted on our behalf. A special recognition goes to the people who by their religious affiliation proved to be invaluable content experts in providing advice, counsel, and information on special religious groups. These individuals include Judy Mason, a member of the staff, University of Alabama at Birmingham, School of Nursing, whose expert advice on Jehovah's Witnesses proved to be invaluable. Similarly, we would like to thank Tamra Walters, a former baccalaureate nursing student at the University of Tulsa, Tulsa, Oklahoma, who read our first edition and graciously provided in-depth insight on the Church of Jesus Christ of Latter Day Saints (Mormons).

We wish to thank the many individuals who not only took the photos but also provided them for use in this textbook. We thank all the individuals who posed for these pictures. It goes without saying that we cannot begin to thank our chapter contributors. Thank you so much for believing in this project. Each of you has made invaluable contributions. Finally, we would like to thank each other for the unselfish sacrifice of more than 10 years of our time on this project and acknowledge the friendship and respect that has grown over the years. We believe that the diversity of our heritages (one African American and one White American) and our ability to complement each other is a testimonial to the achievement of racial, ethnic, and cultural harmony across the United States, Canada, and countries throughout the world in this century.

Ruth Elaine Davidhizar
Joyce Newman Giger

SPECIAL ACKNOWLEDGMENTS

A special acknowledgment is made to Dr. Joyce Newman Giger, my friend and colleague who was in 1996 diagnosed with a 4-year previously undiagnosed breast cancer. In 1997, Dr. Giger was diagnosed with what was thought to be terminal breast cancer or some other mysterious illness. I would like to take this opportunity to say the following:

Joyce: During the writing of this book you have struggled with endless diagnostic procedures, the traumatic misdiagnosis of a terminal illness, and then a series of changing diagnoses and recommended treatments as doctors sought to unravel inconsistent diagnostic reports. Through all of this, you maintained your steadfast faith in the goodness of God and your trust that his will would be done. Your hope in life and your knowledge that your life has a special plan not only saw us through this book, but will also see us through as we plan the next one. Just as you stood by me in support as I recovered from my automobile accident, I stand by you in support through the unchartered waters of your battle with the new mysterious disease and breast cancer. I hope for a new and challenging treatment for breast cancer in our lifetime. On your behalf and on behalf of your friends at Mosby, Inc., I dedicate this book to all the women of the world who are breast-cancer survivors. May each and every woman with breast cancer continue to rise to enjoy all the precious moments of life.

With Love, Ruth

CONTENTS

PART ONE

Framework for Cultural Assessment and Intervention Techniques

CHAPTER 1 Introduction to Transcultural Nursing

Theories of transcultural nursing with established clinical approaches to clients from varying cultures are relatively new. According to Madeleine Leininger (1987), founder of the field of transcultural nursing in the mid-1960s, the education of nursing students in this field is only now beginning to yield significant results. Today, nurses with a deeper appreciation of human life and values are developing cultural sensitivity for appropriate, individualized clinical approaches. Transcultural nursing concepts are being incorporated into the curricula for student nurses in the United States and Canada.

The Transcultural Nursing Society, founded in 1974, is promoting interest in transcultural concepts and the education of transcultural nurses at the graduate level (Giger and Davidhizar, 1990; Wenger, 1989). Since its inception, the society has promoted such efforts at annual transcultural nursing conferences in different worldwide locations. The Society also implemented the first certification plan in transcultural nursing. Through the efforts of the society, many nurses of the United States and Canada have received certification. Other international conferences such as those supported by the Rockefeller Foundation in October 1988 in Bellagio, Italy, have sought to promote international health care management. The society also publishes the *Transcultural Nursing Society Newsletter,* international nursing journals, the *International Journal of Nursing Studies,* and the *International Nursing Review.* Although the literature on patient approaches in culturally diverse situations is mushrooming and nurses are beginning to do transcultural research studies, relatively few theories on transcultural nursing up to now have provided a systematic method for comprehensive nursing assessment (Brink, 1990a, 1990b; Leininger, 1995, 1985a, 1985b; Spector, 1996; Tripp-Reimer, 1984a, 1984b; Tripp-Reimer

and Dougherty, 1985; Tripp-Reimer and Friedl, 1977).

CULTURE DEFINED

Culture is a patterned behavioral response that develops over time as a result of imprinting the mind through social and religious structures and intellectual and artistic manifestations. Culture is also the result of acquired mechanisms that may have innate influences but are primarily affected by internal and external environmental stimuli. Culture is shaped by values, beliefs, norms, and practices that are shared by members of the same cultural group. Culture guides our thinking, doing, and being and becomes patterned expressions of who we are. These patterned expressions are passed down from one generation to the next. Other definitions of culture have been offered by Leininger (1991, 1985a, 1985b), Spector (1996), and Andrews and Boyle (1996). According to Leininger (1991, 1985a, 1985b) culture is the values, beliefs, norms, and practices of a particular group that are learned and shared and that guide thinking, decisions, and actions in a patterned way. Spector (1996) contends that culture is a metacommunication system based on nonphysical traits such as values, beliefs, attitudes, customs, language, and behaviors that are shared by a group of people and are passed down from one generation to the next. According to Andrews and Boyle (1996), culture represents a unique way of perceiving, behaving, and evaluating the external environment and as such provides a blueprint for determining values, beliefs, and practices. Regardless of the definition chosen, the term "culture" implies a dynamic, ever-changing, active or passive process.

Cultural values are unique expressions of a particular culture that have been accepted as appropriate over time. They guide actions and decision making and facilitate self-worth and self-esteem.

Leininger (1985a) postulates that cultural values develop as a direct result of an individual's desirable or preferred way of acting or knowing something that is often sustained by a culture over time and that governs actions or decisions.

THE NEED FOR CANADIAN TRANSCULTURAL NURSING KNOWLEDGE

Canada is so large that it covers most of the northern part of the North American continent. Canada is bordered on the south by the United States, on the east by the Atlantic Ocean, on the west by the Pacific Ocean, and on the north by the Arctic Ocean. Canada is so vast that it encompasses 10 million square kilometers (3,852,000 square miles, of which 291,571 are freshwater). Canada is divided into 10 provinces and two territories (the Yukon and the Northwest Territories). The Atlantic provinces are Newfoundland, Nova Scotia, New Brunswick, and Prince Edward Island; the Central provinces are Quebec and Ontario; the prairie provinces are Manitoba, Saskatchewan, and Alberta; and the western province is British Columbia.

Ontario is the largest and most populous of the principally English-speaking provinces, whereas the Province of Quebec, mostly French speaking, is second in both population and industrial production. Ranging from 42 degrees to 83 degrees north latitude, the principal regions of Canada lie almost entirely within the North Temperate Zone, with only the northernmost portions of the territories inside the North Frigid Zone (The Catholic Encyclopedia, 1967; World Almanac, 1997).

It is believed that demography is destiny, demographic change is reality, and demographic sensitivity is imperative. In 1996, there were 30,286,600 people residing in Canada's 10 provinces and 2 territories (Statistics Canada, 1997). Although the number of people residing in Canada continues to increase, the country is rapidly becoming a multicultural, pluralistic society. In 1988, 1 in 6 Canadians reported being born outside Canada (Statistics Canada, 1990). It is projected that by the year 2000, approximately 1 in every 5 Canadians will represent an ethnic minority and that these groups will share over 100 different cultural and linguistic groups (Shareski, 1992). In fact, the ethnic origins of the population include British (25.3%), French (24.4%), German (3.6%), Italian (2.8%), Ukrainian (1.7%), other single origins (14.3%), and persons of multiple origins (27.9%) (Statistics Canada, 1990).

Canada is such a mosaic of faces and cultures that Canadians claim to have coined the term "multiculturalism." This concept is one in which people of diverse origins and communities remain free to preserve and enhance their own cultural heritage while participating in Canadian society as equal partners (Bailey and Bailey, 1995).

For 20,000 years, Canada (an Iroquian word meaning 'settlement') has been the domain of the descendants of the early Asians nomads who wandered across the Bering Straits land bridge from Siberia. By 9000 B.C., the nomads had spread throughout North and South America, creating cultures as varied as those of the Inuit in the Arctic north and the Aztecs and Incas of Mexico and Peru. There are three categories of aboriginal people that are specified under the terms of the Indian Act of 1982 (Health Canada, 1996). These three categories (Indians, Inuit, and Métis) are referred to collectively as "aboriginal people." However, many aboriginals of Indian descent prefer the term "First Nations" (Bailey and Bailey, 1995). Before contact with the Europeans, Canada's First Nations (Indian) population was estimated at 500,000. However, after exposure to the Europeans, the First Nations population was decimated by smallpox, scarlet fever, tuberculosis, and other diseases, and the census plunged to 102,000 by 1871 (The Royal Commission on Aboriginal People, 1995). Today the population is rebounding and is now estimated to be 2.8% of the total population of Canada, or approximately 870,000 individuals (Young, 1994; Indian and Northern Affairs, 1996). Native Canadians are the majority of only one jurisdiction—the Northwest Territories—where they account for 58% of the population. The Yukon has the second largest proportion of Native Canadians in its population, with 21% (Statistics Canada, 1989).

Of the Native peoples (the Indians, American Indians, aboriginal people), the largest group are divided into five main cultures with varying customs and languages. (1) The Eastern Woodland Indians (Iroquoian and most Algonquians [pronounced /al-GON-kee-uns/]) were renowned for their wigwams, not to be confused with tipis, in which (2) the nomadic Plains Indians (Blackfoot, Cree, Assiniboine [Stoney], and Dakota) lived. (3) The Plateau Indians (Athapaskans, Salish, and the Kutenai) live between the Rockies and the coastal mountain ranges of British Columbia. (4) The Northwest Coastal Indians (Tlingit and Haida) produce magnificent totem poles. The Subarctic Indians (the Déné, or Northern Athapaskans) live mainly in the forest and tundra belt. According to 1996 census data, 593,050 persons were registered as Indians. This number is disproportionately low because many Indians are not registered and therefore are not included into the official census count (Young, 1994; Indian and Northern Affairs, 1996).

According to the 1986 census data, Canada was home to 27,000 registered Inuit (Inuit or Eskimos) (Health and Welfare Canada, 1991). However it is suggested that a more accurate number of Inuit, because of a lack of registration, is 34,000 (Young, 1994). The Algonquian name "Eskimo" was long assumed to mean 'eaters of raw meat', but this name has been found to have been first applied to the Algonquian Micmacs of Gaspé Peninsula and properly means 'speaking the language of a foreign land' (Mailhot, 1978). The term "Inuit" means 'people' in the Inuit language. In Canada, the Eskimos are officially called "Inuit" by the Canadian government. However, the Eskimos of the Bering Sea region prefer, instead, to be called "Yupik," whereas Northslope Alaska Eskimos prefer "Inupiat," and the Mackenzie River Delta Eskimos prefer "Inuvialuit" (Damas, 1984). The Inuit live in the tundra and on the Arctic belt. For many centuries, the Inuit were in almost total isolation.

The third aboriginal group is the Métis. The Métis are the offspring of a French Canadian and an American Indian. Registered and unregistered Métis at the time of the 1986 census is estimated to be 130,000 (Statistics Canada, 1989; Young, 1994).

The first Europeans to visit Canada were the Vikings in the tenth century. Their settlement, dating from around A.D. 1000 was discovered in Newfoundland. The first successful European settlement in Canada was established in Nova Scotia in 1605. The first English settlements were created in Nova Scotia in 1624. As early as the first half of the seventeenth century, Germans settled near Quebec. Canada's first Black people came either as slaves or as refugees from slavery. In addition, thousands of American Blacks escaped from Southern plantations and made their way to Canada after slavery was abolished in Canada in 1793. The first Chinese arrived in 1858, and the first Ukrainians arrived in the 1870s. The Italians arrived in two huge waves. The first came between the turn of the century and 1914 and the second from 1950 to 1970. Immigration from Japan did not begin until 1967. As thousands of European immigrants settled into Canada in the early 1900s, health care was profoundly affected (Bradadat and Saydak, 1993). Immigrants who settled in ethnic communities tended to remain outside the mainstream Anglo-Saxon culture. They retained many of their own cultural values and beliefs, including traditional health care practices. For example, the group of Mennonites who immigrated from southern Russia brought their own midwives and lay healers (Dawson, 1936).

In any multicultural society, nurses need to be prepared to provide culturally appropriate care for each client regardless of that client's cultural background (Giger and Davidhizar, 1995). A nurse who does not recognize the value and importance of culturally appropriate care cannot possibly be an effective care agent in multicultural health care settings such as those found throughout Canada.

In light of the ever-changing demographics of Canada, it is imperative that the "Canadian Nursing Workforce 2000" rapidly adapt itself to a changing heterogeneous society. Providing culturally appropriate and thus competent care in the year 2000 and beyond will be a complex and difficult task for many nurses. In many professional health career programs such as nursing, medicine, and respiratory therapy, students are rarely taught culturally appropriate and competent care techniques. Thus, when these individuals encounter clients from culturally diverse backgrounds in the clinical setting, they are often unable to accurately assess and provide the kind of interventions that are culturally appropriate.

The burden of teaching nurses culturally competent care techniques will rest not only with the individual programs of practice development, but also with the health care agency itself. Regardless of who is responsible for this task, nurses must develop an understanding about culture and its relevance to competent care.

A nurse who does not recognize the value and importance of culturally appropriate care cannot possibly be an effective care agent in this changing demographic society. If nurses do not recognize that the intervention strategies planned for a Canadian Black client with diabetes are uniquely different from those planned for a Vietnamese Canadian, Italian Canadian, and so on, they cannot possibly hope to change the health-seeking behaviors or actively encourage the wellness behaviors of this client or any client. When nurses consider race, ethnicity, culture, and cultural heritage, they become more sensitive to clients. This is not to suggest that there is a cookbook approach to delivering care to clients by virtue of race, ethnicity, or culture. There is as much variation within certain races, cultural groups, or ethnic groups as there is across cultural groups. When the informed nurse considers the significance of culture, clients are approached with a more informed perspective.

The time to learn differing perspectives about culture is at hand. As professional health care providers, nurses will be asked to step forward to provide the leadership to ensure that all people have equal access to quality, culturally appropriate, and culturally competent health care. This task can be accomplished only through culturally diverse nursing care.

CULTURAL ASSESSMENT
Using nonnursing models

In a pluralistic society, nurse practitioners need to be prepared to provide culturally appropriate nursing care for each client, regardless of that client's cultural background. To provide culturally appropriate nursing care, nurses must understand specific factors that influence individual health and illness behaviors (Tripp-Reimer, Brink, and Saunders, 1984).

According to Affonso (1979), cultural assessment can give meaning to behaviors that might otherwise be judged negatively. If cultural behaviors are not appropriately identified, their significance will be confusing to the nurse.

Although transcultural nursing theories have appeared in the literature (Affonso, 1979; Leininger, 1985a, 1985b, 1991), adequate nursing assessment methods to accompany these theories have not been consistently provided. One of the most comprehensive tools used for nursing cultural assessment is the *Outline of Cultural Material* by Murdock et al. (1971); however, this tool was developed primarily for anthropologists who were concerned with ethnographic descriptions of cultural groups. Although the tool is well developed and contains 88 major categories, it was not designed for nurse practitioners and thus does not provide for systematic use of the nursing process. Another assessment tool is found in Brownlee's (1978) *Community, Culture, and Care: A Cross-Cultural Guide for Health Care Workers*. Brownlee's work is devoted to the process of practical assessment of a community, with specific attention given to health areas. The work deals with three aspects of assessment: what to find out, why it is important, and how to do it. Brownlee's assessment tool has been criticized as being too comprehensive, too difficult, and too detailed for use with individual clients. Although this tool was developed for use by health care practitioners, it is not exclusively a nursing assessment tool.

Using nursing-specific models

Transcultural nursing as defined by Leininger (1991) is a "humanistic and scientific area of formal study and practice which is focused upon differences and similarities among cultures with respect to human care, health (or well-being), and illness based upon the people's cultural values, beliefs, and practices." According to Leininger (1991), the ultimate goal of transcultural nursing is the use of relevant knowledge to provide culturally specific and culturally congruent nursing care to people. From this theoretical perspective, Leininger (1985a, 1985b) provides a comprehensive transcultural theory and assessment model. For over 30 years, this model has helped nurses discover and understand what health care means to various cultures. Leininger's sunrise model symbolizes the rising of the sun (care). The model depicts a full sun with four levels of foci. Within the circle in the upper portion of the model are components of the social structure and world-view factors that influence care and health through language and environment. These factors influence the folk, professional, and nursing systems or subsystems located in the lower half of the model. Also included in the model are levels of abstraction and analysis from which care can be studied at each level. Various cultural phenomena are studied from the micro-, middle-, and macro-perspectives (Leininger, 1985a, 1985b). Leininger's model has served as the prototype for the development of other culturally specific nursing models and tools (Bloch, 1983; Branch and Paxton, 1976; Orque, 1983; Rund and Krause, 1978).

An analysis of culturally specific models and tools

Tripp-Reimer, Brink, and Saunders (1984) analyzed selected culturally appropriate models and tools to determine if significant differences existed between the models. They concluded that most cultural assessment guides are similar because they all seek to identify major cultural domains that are important variables if culturally appropriate care is to be rendered. Nine culturally appropriate models or guides were analyzed, including Aamodt (1978), Bloch (1983), Branch and Paxton (1976), Brownlee (1978), Kay (1978), Leininger (1977), Orque (1983), Rund and Krause (1978), and Tripp-Reimer (1984b). In analyzing the models, Tripp-Reimer, Brink, and Saunders (1984) concluded that the same two limitations existed in each guide. The first limitation was the tendency to include too much cultural content, ultimately negating the "heart of the matter," which is the process itself. The second limitation was that it is often impossible to separate client-specific data from normative data.

Using nursing diagnoses

The relative significance of culturally appropriate health care cannot be appreciated if the nurse does not understand the value of culturally relevant nursing diagnoses. Geissler (1991) reports a study to de-

termine the applicability of the North American Nursing Diagnosis Association (NANDA) taxonomy as a culturally appropriate assessment tool for use with diverse populations. In the study, three nursing diagnoses were analyzed to validate their cultural appropriateness: (1) impaired verbal communication, (2) social isolation, and (3) noncompliance in culturally diverse situations. Participants in the study ($n = 245$ nurses) were experts in the field of transcultural nursing and were members of either the Transcultural Nursing Society or the American Nurses Association Council on Cultural Diversity (Geissler, 1991). Findings from this study also indicate that nursing diagnoses tend to (1) be client focused rather than provider focused and therefore do not acknowledge the existence of other culturally relevant viewpoints (such as those expressed by the provider); (2) be generalized and as a result having an increased likelihood, when applied in diverse cultural settings, for stereotyping and victimization because so-called non-Western medical models are believed to be "abnormal" and thus require necessary interventions; and (3) involve the mislabeling of phenomena, which in actuality arise as expressions of cultural dissonance rather than expressions of political, social, psychologic, or economic factors.

In the study reported by Geissler (1991), the NANDA nursing diagnosis, "impaired communication, verbal, related to cultural differences," is an excellent example of a client-oriented diagnosis that does not recognize linguistic cultural differences. The study concludes that the NANDA diagnosis of "impaired verbal communication" connotes that the client's verbal communication and ability to understand and use language is impaired in some way. This diagnosis does not consider the causative factors creating the impairment (Giger, Davidhizar, Evers, and Ingram, 1994). It is apparent that individuals who speak a different language from that used by health care providers or nurses may be very capable of both use and comprehension of a specific language when interacting with persons fluent in that language (Giger, Davidhizar, Evers, and Ingram, 1994). According to Geissler (1991), if the client in this situation is "verbally impaired," the nurse is equally impaired. Geissler also concludes that the

NANDA diagnosis of "impaired verbal communication" does not adequately address the issue of nonverbal communication, which was identified in the earlier nursing literature as an essential assessment factor (Giger and Davidhizar, 1990, 1991, 1995).

According to Geissler (1991), nursing diagnoses related to social isolation and noncompliance need further defining characteristics for use with culturally diverse populations. Rather than using the term "noncompliance," Geissler (1991) suggests that the term "nonadherence" may be more appropriate because this term may more accurately reflect behavior resulting from cultural dissonance than the other term does. At the same time, the use of "nonadherence" may remove the stigma of guilt experienced by the health care recipient who is inappropriately labeled "noncompliant."

GIGER AND DAVIDHIZAR'S TRANSCULTURAL ASSESSMENT MODEL

In response to the need for a practical assessment tool for evaluating cultural variables and their effects on health and illness behaviors, a transcultural assessment model that greatly minimizes the time needed to conduct a comprehensive assessment is offered in an effort to provide culturally competent care. The metaparadigm for the Giger and Davidhizar Transcultural Assessment Model includes (1) transcultural nursing and culturally diverse nursing, (2) culturally unique individuals, (3) culturally sensitive environments, and (4) health and health status based on culturally specific illness and wellness behaviors.

Transcultural nursing defined

In the context of Giger and Davidhizar's Transcultural Assessment Model (discussed later in this chapter) (1990, 1991, 1995), transcultural nursing is viewed as a culturally competent practice field that is client centered and research focused. Although transcultural nursing is viewed as client centered, it is important for nurses to remember that culture can and does influence how clients are viewed and the care that is rendered.

Every individual is culturally unique, and nurses are no exception to this premise. Nonetheless, nurses must use caution to avoid projecting on the client their own "cultural uniqueness" and "world views" if culturally appropriate care is to be provided. Nurses must carefully discern personal cultural beliefs and values to separate them from the client's beliefs and values. To deliver culturally sensitive care, the nurse must remember that each individual is unique and is a product of past experiences, beliefs, and values that have been learned and passed down from one generation to the next.

According to Stokes (1991), nursing as a profession is not "culturally free" but rather is "culturally determined." Nurses must recognize and understand this fact to avoid becoming grossly ethnocentric (Stokes, 1991). Since there is a contingent relationship between cultural determination and the delivery of culturally sensitive care, the transcultural nurse must be guided by acquired knowledge in the assessment, diagnosis, planning, implementation, and evaluation of the client's needs based on culturally relevant information. This ideology does not presuppose that all individuals within a specific cultural group will think and behave in a similar manner with relative predictability. The astute nurse must remember that there is as much diversity *within* a cultural group as there is *across* cultural groups. Nonetheless, the goal of transcultural nursing is the discovery of culturally relevant facts about the client to provide culturally appropriate and competent care.

Although transcultural nursing is becoming a highly specialized field of specially educated individuals, every nurse regardless of academic or experiential background must use transcultural knowledge to facilitate culturally appropriate care. Regardless of preparation in the field of transcultural nursing, every nurse who is entrusted with care of clients must make every effort to deliver culturally sensitive care that is free of inherent biases based on gender, race, or religion.

Culturally diverse nursing care

Culturally diverse nursing care refers to the variability in nursing approaches needed to provide culturally appropriate and competent care. By the year 2000 and beyond, it will be necessary for nurses to

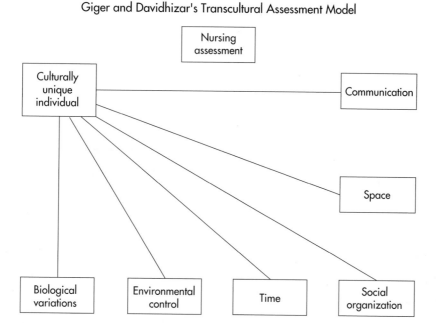

Figure 1-1 Application of cultural phenomena to nursing care and nursing practice.

utilize transcultural knowledge in a skillful and artful manner to render culturally appropriate and competent care to a rapidly changing, heterogeneous client population. Culturally diverse nursing care must take into account six cultural phenomena that vary with application and use yet are evident in all cultural groups: (1) communication, (2) space, (3) social organization, (4) time, (5) environmental control, and (6) biological variations (Figs. 1-1 and 1-2).

Culturally unique individuals

To provide culturally appropriate and competent care, it is important to remember that each individual is culturally unique and as such is a product of past experiences, cultural beliefs, and cultural norms. Cultural expressions become patterned responses and as such give each individual a unique identity. Although there is as much diversity within cultural and racial groups as there is across and among cultural and racial groups, knowledge of general baseline data relative to the specific cultural

group is an excellent starting point to provide culturally appropriate care.

Culturally sensitive environments

Culturally diverse health care can and should be rendered in a variety of clinical settings. Regardless of the level of care—primary, secondary, or tertiary—knowledge of culturally relevant information will assist the nurse in planning and implementing a treatment regimen that is unique for each client.

In response to the apparent lack of practical assessment tools available in nursing for evaluating cultural variables and their effects on health and illness behaviors, this text provides a systematic approach to evaluating the six essential cultural phenomena to assist the nurse in providing culturally appropriate nursing care (Fig. 1-1). Although the six cultural phenomena are evident in all cultural groups, they vary in application across cultures. Thus an individualized assessment of these areas is necessary when working with clients from diverse cultural groups (Fig. 1-2).

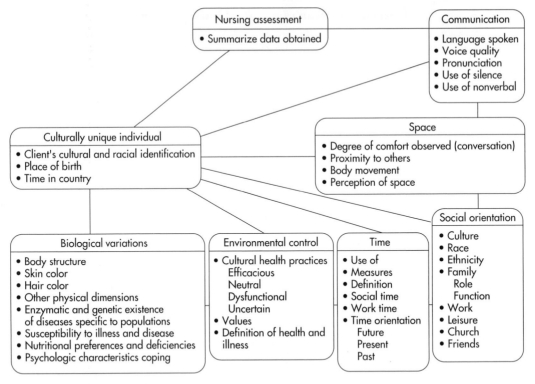

Figure 1-2 Giger and Davidhizar's transcultural assessment model.

DEVELOPMENT AND REFINEMENT OF THE GIGER AND DAVIDHIZAR TRANSCULTURAL ASSESSMENT MODEL
Clinical application

Since its introduction in 1991, the Giger and Davidhizar Transcultural Assessment Model has been applied to the care of clients in a variety of clinical specialties: the maternity client (Giger, Davidhizar, and Wieczorek, 1993), the operating room client (Bowen and Davidhizar, 1991), and the psychiatric client (Giger, Davidhizar, Evers, and Ingram, 1994).

In 1993, Spector illustrated the model's utility by combining it with the Cultural Heritage Model. The combination of these two models (Fig. 1-3), which appears in Potter and Perry's *Fundamentals of Nursing* text, is unique because it provides a holistic method of providing culturally competent care. In addition, using Giger and Davidhizar's six cultural phenomena, though in a different hierarchi-

cal arrangement, Spector (1996) created a unique quick reference guide for cultural assessment of people from a variety of racial and cultural groups (Table 1-1).

In 1993, Kozier, Erb, Blaise, Johnson, and Smith-Temple used the model to provide a mechanism by which cultural behaviors relevant to health assessment could easily be identified across cultural groups. Their work relative to Giger and Davidhizar's Transcultural Assessment Model is a compilation of basic culturally relevant information (Table 1-2). This work was further utilized in 1995 by Kozier, Erb, Blaise, and Williamson. In addition, in 1992, the editors at Éditions Lamarre translated the model into French for use by French and French-Canadian nurses.

In 1993, the National League for Nursing published *Nursing Management Skills: A Modular Self-Assessment Series, Module IV, Transcultural Nursing*

GIGER AND DAVIDHIZAR'S TRANSCULTURAL ASSESSMENT MODEL

CULTURALLY UNIQUE INDIVIDUAL

1. Place of birth
2. Cultural definition
   What is . . .
3. Race
   What is . . .
4. Length of time in country (if appropriate)

COMMUNICATION

1. Voice quality
   A. Strong, resonant
   B. Soft
   C. Average
   D. Shrill
2. Pronunciation and enunciation
   A. Clear
   B. Slurred
   C. Dialect (geographical)
3. Use of silence
   A. Infrequent
   B. Often
   C. Length
      (1) Brief
      (2) Moderate
      (3) Long
      (4) Not observed
4. Use of nonverbal
   A. Hand movement
   B. Eye movement
   C. Entire body movement
   D. Kinesics (gestures, expression, or stances)
5. Touch
   A. Startles or withdraws when touched
   B. Accepts touch without difficulty
   C. Touches others without difficulty
6. Ask these and similar questions:
   A. How do you get your point across to others?
   B. Do you like communicating with friends, family, and acquaintances?
   C. When asked a question, do you usually respond (in words or body movement, or both)?

D. If you have something important to discuss with your family, how would you approach them?

SPACE

1. Degree of comfort
   A. Moves when space invaded
   B. Does not move when space invaded
2. Distance in conversations
   A. 0 to 18 inches
   B. 18 inches to 3 feet
   C. 3 feet or more
3. Definition of space
   A. Describe degree of comfort with closeness when talking with or standing near others
   B. How do objects (e.g., furniture) in the environment affect your sense of space?
4. Ask these and similar questions:
   A. When you talk with family members, how close do you stand?
   B. When you communicate with coworkers and other acquaintances, how close do you stand?
   C. If a stranger touches you, how do you react or feel?
   D. If a loved one touches you, how do you react or feel?
   E. Are you comfortable with the distance between us now?

SOCIAL ORGANIZATION

1. Normal state of health
   A. Poor
   B. Fair
   C. Good
   D. Excellent
2. Marital status
3. Number of children
4. Parents living or deceased?
5. Ask these and similar questions:
   A. How do you define social activities?
   B. What are some activities that you enjoy?
   C. What are your hobbies, or what do you do when you have free time?

Figure 1-2, cont'd   For legend see page 10.

Continued

GIGER AND DAVIDHIZAR'S TRANSCULTURAL ASSESSMENT MODEL–cont'd

D. Do you believe in a Supreme Being?
E. How do you worship that Supreme Being?
F. What is your function (what do you do) in your family unit/system?
G. What is your role in your family unit/system (father, mother, child, advisor)?
H. When you were a child, what or who influenced you most?
I. What is/was your relationship with your siblings and parents?
J. What does work mean to you?
K. Describe your past, present, and future jobs.
L. What are your political views?
M. How have your political views influenced your attitude toward health and illness?

TIME

1. Orientation to time
   A. Past-oriented
   B. Present-oriented
   C. Future-oriented
2. View of time
   A. Social time
   B. Clock-oriented
3. Physiochemical reaction to time
   A. Sleeps at least 8 hours a night
   B. Goes to sleep and wakes on a consistent schedule
   C. Understands the importance of taking medication and other treatments on schedule
4. Ask these and similar questions:
   A. What kind of timepiece do you wear daily?
   B. If you have an appointment at 2 PM, what time is acceptable to arrive?
   C. If a nurse tells you that you will receive a medication in "about a half hour," realistically, how much time will you allow before calling the nurses' station?

ENVIRONMENTAL CONTROL

1. Locus-of-control
   A. Internal locus-of-control (believes that the power to affect change lies within)
   B. External locus-of-control (believes that fate, luck, and chance have a great deal to do with how things turn out)
2. Value orientation
   A. Believes in supernatural forces
   B. Relies on magic, witchcraft, and prayer to affect change
   C. Does not believe in supernatural forces
   D. Does not rely on magic, witchcraft, or prayer to affect change
3. Ask these and similar questions:
   A. How often do you have visitors at your home?
   B. Is it acceptable to you for visitors to drop in unexpectedly?
   C. Name some ways your parents or other persons treated your illnesses when you were a child.
   D. Have you or someone else in your immediate surroundings ever used a home remedy that made you sick?
   E. What home remedies have you used that worked? Will you use them in the future?
   F. What is your definition of "good health"?
   G. What is your definition of illness or "poor health"?

BIOLOGICAL VARIATIONS

1. Conduct a complete physical assessment noting:
   A. Body structure (small, medium, or large frame)
   B. Skin color
   C. Unusual skin discolorations
   D. Hair color and distribution
   E. Other visible physical characteristics (e.g., keloids, chloasma)
   F. Weight
   G. Height
   H. Check lab work for variances in hemoglobin, hematocrit, and sickle phenomena if Black or Mediterranean
2. Ask these and similar questions:
   A. What diseases or illnesses are common in your family?

Figure 1-2, cont'd For legend see p. 10.

GIGER AND DAVIDHIZAR'S TRANSCULTURAL ASSESSMENT MODEL–cont'd

B. Describe your family's typical behavior when a family member is ill.

C. How do you respond when you are angry?

D. Who (or what) usually helps you to cope during a difficult time?

E. What foods do you and your family like to eat?

F. Have you ever had any unusual cravings for:
   (1) White or red clay dirt?
   (2) Laundry starch?

G. When you were a child what types of foods did you eat?

H. What foods are family favorites or are considered traditional?

NURSING ASSESSMENT

1. Note whether the client has become culturally assimilated or observes own cultural practices.

2. Incorporate data into plan of nursing care:
   A. Encourage the client to discuss cultural differences; people from diverse cultures who hold different world views can enlighten nurses.
   B. Make efforts to accept and understand methods of communication.
   C. Respect the individual's personal need for space.
   D. Respect the rights of clients to honor and worship the Supreme Being of their choice.
   E. Identify a clerical or spiritual person to contact.

F. Determine whether spiritual practices have implications for health, life, and well-being (e.g., Jehovah's Witnesses may refuse blood and blood derivatives; an Orthodox Jew may eat only kosher food high in sodium and may not drink milk when meat is served).

G. Identify hobbies, especially when devising interventions for a short or extended convalescence or for rehabilitation.

H. Honor time and value orientations and differences in these areas. Allay anxiety and apprehension if adherence to time is necessary.

I. Provide privacy according to personal need and health status of the client (NOTE: the perception and reaction to pain may be culturally related).

J. Note cultural health practices.
   (1) Identify and encourage efficacious practices.
   (2) Identify and discourage dysfunctional practices.
   (3) Identify and determine whether neutral practices will have a long-term ill effect.

K. Note food preferences.
   (1) Make as many adjustments in diet as health status and long-term benefits will allow and that dietary department can provide.
   (2) Note dietary practices that may have serious implications for the client.

Figure 1-2, cont'd For legend see p. 10.

(Sheridan and Zimbler, 1993). Included in this publication are numerous articles on the application of the model in a variety of clinical situations to be used by nurses to learn and refine managerial skills. In 1994, the Nashville-based production company Envision, Inc., produced a half-inch VHS-format videotape titled *Cultural Diversity in Healthcare: A Different Point of View,*" utilizing Giger and Davidhizar's Transcultural Assessment Model as the overarching framework for the videotape. In addi-

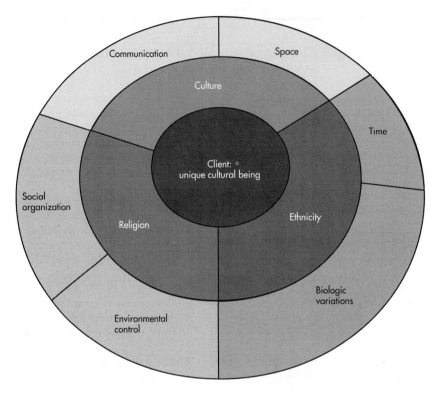

Figure 1-3   Model of the client within a culturally unique heritage and the cultural phenomena that have a great influence on nursing care. (From Potter PA, Perry AG: *Fundamentals of nursing,* ed 3, St. Louis, 1993, Mosby).

tion, the model continues to be refined with the development of a transcultural nursing assessment guide introduced in Bobak and Jensen's (1993) *Maternity and Gynecological Care* (Giger, Davidhizar, and Wieczoerek, 1993). Based on the numerous applications, adaptations, and citations of this model, it seems to provide a realistic model for collecting and analyzing data in an efficient, time-conscious manner.

In 1994, the fourth edition of Mosby's *Medical, Nursing, and Allied Health Dictionary* was published. Included in the new edition is the section "Guidelines for Relating to Patients from Different Cultures," which was excerpted from the work of Giger and Davidhizar.

Application to other disciplines

The model is broad enough in scope to be recognized for applicability by other health care profes-

sions, such as medical imaging, dentistry, education and training departments, and hospital administration (Davidhizar, Giger, and Dowd, 1997a). This model has had numerous applications in medical imaging: one a description of its use in dealing with diversity in radiology departments (Davidhizar, Dowd, and Giger, 1997b), one a proposal of its use in the theory base of the profession of radiography (Davidhizar, Dowd, and Giger, 1997a), and a third describing how to deal with cultural differences affecting pain response (Davidhizar, Dowd, and Giger, 1997c). Dental hygienists are also involved with clients from diverse cultures. "Transcultural patient assessment, a method of advancing dental care," published in *Dental Assistant* (Davidhizar and Giger, 1998, in press), illuminates how awareness of the behavior of clients in the dental office is often culturally motivated. The model is also described in journals that cross health care professionals such as

Table 1-1   Cross-cultural examples of cultural phenomena impacting on nursing care

Nations of origin	Communication	Space	Time orientation	Social organization	Environmental control	Biological variations
Asian China Hawaii Philippines Korea Japan Southeast Asia (Laos, Cambodia, Vietnam)	National language preference Dialects, written characters Use of silence Nonverbal and contextual cuing	Noncontact people	Present	Family; hierarchial structure, loyalty Devotion to tradition Many religions, including Taoism, Buddhism, Islam, and Christianity Community social organizations	Traditional health and illness beliefs Use of traditional medicines Traditional practitioners: Chinese doctors and herbalists	Liver cancer Stomach cancer Coccidioidomycosis Hypertension Lactose intolerance
African West Coast (as slaves) Many African countries West Indian Islands Dominican Republic Haiti Jamaica	National languages Dialect: Pidgin, Creole, Spanish, and French	Close personal space	Present over future	Family: many female, single parent Large, extended family networks Strong church affiliation within community Community social organizations	Traditional health and illness beliefs Folk medicine tradition Traditional healer: root worker	Sickle cell anemia Hypertension Cancer of the esophagus Stomach cancer Coccidioidomycosis Lactose intolerance
Europe Germany England Italy Ireland Other European countries	National languages Many learn English immediately	Noncontact people Aloof Distant Southern countries: closer contact and touch	Future over present	Nuclear families Extended families Judeo-Christian religions Community social organizations	Primary reliance on modern health care system Traditional health and illness beliefs Some remaining folk medicine traditions	Breast cancer Heart disease Diabetes mellitus Thalassemia
Native American 170 Native American tribes Aleuts Eskimos (Inuit)	Tribal languages Use of silence and body language	Space very important and has no boundaries	Present	Extremely family oriented Biological and extended families Children taught to respect traditions Community social organizations	Traditional health and illness beliefs Folk medicine tradition Traditional healer: medicine man	Accidents Heart disease Cirrhosis of the liver Diabetes mellitus
Hispanic countries Spain Cuba Mexico Central and South America	Spanish or Portuguese primary language	Tactile relationships Touch Handshakes Embracing Value physical presence	Present	Nuclear family Extended families *Compadrazgo:* godparents Community social organizations	Traditional health and illness beliefs Folk medicine tradition Traditional healers: *curandero, espiritista, partera, senora*	Diabetes mellitus Parasites Coccidioidomycosis Lactose intolerance

Compiled by Rachel Specter, RN, PhD. In Potter, P.A., & Perry, A.G. (1993). *Fundamentals of nursing: concepts, process, and practice* (ed. 3). St Louis: Mosby.

Table 1-2   Cultural behaviors relevant to health assessment

Cultural group	Cultural variations (Common belief/practice)	Nursing implications
African-Americans	Dialect and slang terms require careful communication to prevent error (i.e., "bad" may mean 'good').	Question the client's meaning or intent.
Mexican Americans	Eye behavior is important. An individual who looks at and admires a child without touching the child has given the child the "evil eye."	Always touch the child you are examining or admiring.
Native Americans	Eye contact is considered a sign of disrespect and is thus avoided.	Recognize that the client may be attentive and interested even though eye contact is avoided.
Appalachians	Eye contact is considered impolite or a sign of hostility. Verbal patter may be confusing.	Avoid excessive eye contact. Clarify statements.
American Eskimos	Body language is very important. The individual seldom disagrees publicly with others. Client may nod yes to be polite, even if not in agreement.	Monitor own body language closely as well as client's to detect meaning.
Jewish Americans	Orthodox Jews consider excess touching, particularly from members of the opposite sex, offensive.	Establish whether client is an Orthodox Jew and avoid excessive touch.
Chinese Americans	Individual may nod head to indicate yes or shake head to indicate no. Excessive eye contact indicates rudeness. Excessive touch is offensive.	Ask questions carefully and clarify responses. Avoid excessive eye contact and touch.
Filipino Americans	Offending people is to be avoided at all cost. Nonverbal behavior is very important.	Monitor nonverbal behaviors of self and client, being sensitive to physical and emotional discomfort or concerns of the client.
Haitian Americans	Touch is used in conversation. Direct eye contact is used to gain attention and respect during communication.	Use direct eye contact when communicating.
East Indian Hindu Americans	Women avoid eye contact as a sign of respect.	Be aware that men may view eye contact by women as offensive. Avoid eye contact.
Vietnamese Americans	Avoidance of eye contact is a sign of respect. The head is considered sacred; it is not polite to pat the head. An upturned palm is offensive in communication.	Limit eye contact. Touch the head only when mandated and explain clearly before proceeding to do so. Avoid hand gesturing.

From Kozier, B., Erb, G., Blaise, K., Johnson, S., & Smith-Temple, J. (1993). *Techniques in clinical nursing* (ed. 2). Menlo Park, Calif: Addison-Wesley.

Hospital Topics (Davidhizar and Giger, 1996), *Community Health Education and Promotion Manual* (Giger, Davidhizar, Johnson, and Poole, 1998, in press), and *Health Traveler* (Giger, Davidhizar, Johnson, and Poole, 1997). Application of the Giger and Davidhizar model to diverse clinical settings is quickly producing a way for staff across disciplines to understand cultural diversity and to learn techniques of culturally competent care.

Refinement through research

Refinement of the model is also being enhanced through research efforts of various individuals. For example, in 1992, a graduate student from the University of Kansas completed a master's thesis titled "Utilizing Giger and Davidhizar's Transcultural Assessment Model for the Cultural Assessment of Farm Families" (Daugherty, 1992). In 1993, a graduate student at Georgia Southern University at Statesboro conducted a research study on the health beliefs and self-care practices of hypertensive African-American women using Giger and Davidhizar's Transcultural Assessment Model as a theoretical framework to guide and evaluate research findings (Walthour, 1993). In addition to these master's theses, several doctoral dissertations have been completed using the model. In 1995, a group of interdisciplinary researchers (nursing, behavioral medicine, lipoprotein research, human genetics, preventive medicine, nutrition, biostatistics) at the University of Alabama at Birmingham and Emory University received $750,000 from the Uniformed Health Sciences, University of the Health Sciences, Tri-Services Nursing Military Research Group, Department of Defense, to identify behavioral risk-reduction strategies and chronic indicators for premenopausal African-American women with coronary heart disease or associated risk factors. The model served as the overarching theoretical framework to test its usefulness as an educational tool to enhance and promote compliance. The study is titled "Culturally Appropriate Behavioral Risk Reduction Strategies and Chronic Indicators and High Risk Factors for Prem-

enopausal African-American Women (25-45) with Coronary Heart Disease" (Giger and Strickland, 1995).

ORGANIZATION OF THE TEXT

In this book the six cultural phenomena (communication, space, social organization, time, environmental control, and biological variations) are presented in individual chapters with areas that a nurse must assess when working with clients from multicultural populations. In addition, these six phenomena are applied to the care and management of clients in 10 subcultural groups found in Canada. A comprehensive nursing assessment is necessary for both the nurse practitioner and the researcher to provide culturally appropriate nursing care.

References

Aamodt, A.M. (1978). The care component in a health and healing system. In Bauwens, E. (Ed.), *The anthropology of health.* St. Louis: Mosby.

Affonso, D. (1979). Framework for cultural assessment. In Clark, A.L. (Ed.), *Childbearing: a nursing perspective* (ed. 2) (pp. 107-119). Philadelphia: F.A. Davis.

Andrews, M., & Boyle, J. (1996). *Transcultural concepts in nursing care.* Glenview, Ill.: Scott, Foresman.

Bailey, E., & Bailey, R. (1995). *Discover Canada.* Oxford, England: Berlitz Publishing Co.

Bloch, B. (1983). Assessment guide for ethnic/cultural variations. In Orque, M.S. & Bloch, B. (Eds.), *Ethnic nursing care: a multi-cultural approach* (pp. 49-75). St. Louis: Mosby.

Bobak, I., & Jensen, M. (Eds.). (1993). *Maternity and gynecological care* (ed. 5). St. Louis: Mosby.

Bowen, M., & Davidhizar, R. (1991). Communication with the client OR. *Today's OR Nurse, 1,* 11-14.

Bradadat, I., & Saydak, M. (1993). Nursing on the Canadian Prairies, 1900-1930. *Nursing History Review, I,* 105-117.

Branch, M.F., & Paxton, P.P. (Eds.). (1976). *Providing safe nursing care for ethnic people of color.* Englewood Cliffs, N.J.: Prentice-Hall.

Brink, P.J. (1990). *Transcultural nursing: a book of readings.* Prospect Heights, Ill.: Waveland Press.

Brink, P.J. (1990). Cultural diversity in nursing: how much can we tolerate? In McClusky, J., & Grace, H., (Eds.), *Current issues in nursing* (ed. 3). St. Louis: Mosby.

Brownlee, A.T. (1978). *Community, culture, and care: a cross-cultural guide for health workers.* St. Louis: Mosby.

Damas, D. (1984). Arctic: handbook of North American Indians (volume 5). Washington, D.C.: Smithsonian Institution.

Daugherty, B. (1992). *Utilizing Giger and Davidhizar's transcultural assessment model for the cultural assessment of farm families.* Unpublished master's thesis, University of Kansas, Lawrence, Kansas.

Davidhizar, R., & Giger, J. (1998, in press). Transcultural patient assessment: A method of advancing dental care. *Dental Assistant.*

Davidhizar, R., & Giger, J. (1996). Reflections on the minority elderly in health care. *Hospital Topics, 74*(3), 20-24.

Davidhizar, R., Dowd, S., & Giger, J. (1997a). Managing a multicultural radiology staff. *Radiology Management, 19*(1), 50-55.

Davidhizar, R., Dowd, S., & Giger, J. (1997b). Model for cultural diversity in the radiology department. *Radiologic Technology, 68*(3), 233-238.

Davidhizar, R., Dowd, S., & Giger, J. (1997c). Cultural differences in pain management. *Radiologic Technology, 68*(4), 345-348.

Dawson, C. (1936). *Group settlement: ethnic communities in western Canada.* Toronto: Ethnic Communities in Western Canada.

Geissler, E.M. (1991). Transcultural nursing and nursing diagnosis. *Nursing and Health Care, 12*(4), 190-203.

Giger, J., Davidhizar, R., Johnson, J., & Poole, V. (1998, in press). *Community health education promotion manual.* Gaithersburg, Md.: Aspen Publishers.

Giger, J., Davidhizar, R., Johnson, J., & Poole, V. (1997). The changing faces of America: using cultural phenomena to improve care. *The Healthcare Traveler,* 4(4), 10-40.

Giger, J., & Davidhizar, R. (1995). *Transcultural nursing: assessment and intervention.* St. Louis: Mosby.

Giger, J., & Strickland, O. (1995). Behavioral risk reduction strategies for chronic indicators and high risk factors for premenopausal African-American women (25-45) with coronary heart disease, Grant number N95-019, Department of Defense, Uniformed Health Services, University of the Health Sciences, Tri-Service Nursing Research, Bethesda, Md.

Giger, J., Davidhizar, R., Evers, S., & Ingram, C. (1994). Cultural factors influencing mental health and mental illness. In Taylor, C. (Ed.), *Merness' essentials of psychiatric nursing* (ed. 14) (pp. 217-236). St. Louis: Mosby.

Giger, J. Davidhizar, R., & Wieczorek, S. (1993). Culture and ethnicity. In Bobak, I., & Jensen, M. (Eds.), *Maternity and gynecological care.* (ed. 5) (pp. 43-67). St. Louis: Mosby.

Giger, J., & Davidhizar, R. (1991). *Transcultural nursing: assessment and intervention.* St. Louis: Mosby.

Giger, J., & Davidhizar, R. (1990). Transcultural nursing assessment: a method for advancing practice. *Internaional Nursing Review, 37*(1), 199-203.

Health and Welfare Canada. (1991). *Health status of Canadian Indians and Inuits 1990.* Ottawa: Health and Welfare, Canada.

Indian and Northern Affairs, Canada. (1996). *Facts from stats.* (Issue No. 11, March-April). Ottawa: Information Quality and Research Directorate.

Kay, M. (1978). Clinical anthropology. In. Bauwens, E.E. (Ed.), *The anthropology of health* (pp. 3-11). St. Louis: Mosby.

Kozier, B., Erb, G., Blaise, K., Johnson, J., & Smith-Temple, J. (1993). *Techniques in clinical nursing* (ed. 2). Reading, Mass.: Addison-Wesley.

Kozier, B., Erb, G., Blaise, K., & Wilkinson, J. (1995). *Fundamentals of nursing* (ed. 2). Reading, Mass.: Addison-Wesley.

Lefever, D., & Davidhizar, R. (1995). American Eskimos. In Giger, J., & Davidhizar, R. (Eds.), *Transcultural nursing: assessment and intervention.* St. Louis: Mosby.

Leininger, M. (1977). Transcultural nursing and a proposed conceptual framework. In Leininger, M., (Ed.), *Transcultural nursing care of infants and children: proceedings from the first transcultural conference.* Salt Lake City: University of Utah.

Leininger, M. (1985a). *Qualitative research methods in nursing.* Orlando, Fla.: Grune & Stratton.

Leininger, M. (1985b). Transcultural care, diversity and universality: a theory of nursing. *Nursing and Health Care, 6*(4), 209-212.

Leininger, M. (1991). Transcultural nursing: the study and practice field. *Imprint, 38*(2), 55-66.

Mailhot, J. (1978). L'étymologie de "Esquimau" revue et corrigée. *Études Inuit—Inuit Studies, 2,* 59-69.

Mosby's medical, nursing, and allied health dictionary. (1994). (ed. 4). St. Louis: Mosby.

Murdock, G., et al. (1971). *Outline of cultural materials* (ed. 4). New Haven, Conn.: Human Relations Area Files.

Leninger, M. (1995). *Transcultural nursing.* New York: McGraw Hill Publishing Company.

Orque, M. (1983). Orque's ethnic/cultural: a framework for ethnic nursing care. In Orque, M.S. & Bloch, B. (Eds.), *Ethnic nursing care: a multi-cultural approach* (pp. 5-48). St. Louis: Mosby.

Rund, N., & Krause, L. (1978). Health attitudes and your health programs. In Bauwens E.E., (Ed.), *The anthropology of health* (pp. 73-78). St. Louis: Mosby.

Shareski, D. (1992). Beyond boundaries: cross-cultural care. *Nursing British Columbia, 25,* 10-12.

Sheridan, D., & Zimbler, E. (1993). *Nursing management skills: a modular self-assessment series, module IV, transcultural nursing.* New York: National League for Nursing.

Spector, R. (1996). *Cultural diversity in health and illness* (ed. 3). Norwalk, Conn.: Appleton & Lange.

Spector, R. (1993). Culture, ethnicity, and nursing. In Potter, P. & Perry, A., (Eds.), *Fundamentals of nursing: concepts, process, and practice* (ed. 3). St. Louis: Mosby.

Statistics Canada. (1989). *A data book on Canada's Aboriginal population from the 1986 census of Canada.* Ottawa: Statistics Canada, Aboriginal Peoples Output Program.

Statistics Canada. (1990). *Canada at a glance.* 1990 communication, Ottawa, Division of Statistics, Canada.

Statistics Canada. (1997). Population Canada, the provinces and territories. CANSIM, Matrices 6367-6379.

Stokes, G. (1991). A transcultural nurse is about. *Senior Nurse, 11*(1), 40-42.

The Catholic encyclopedia. (1967). New York: McGraw-Hill Publishing Company.

The Royal Commission on Aboriginal People. (1995). Ottawa: Minister of Indian Affairs and Northern Development.

Tripp-Reimer, T. (1984a). Research in cultural diversity. *Western Journal of Nursing Research, 6*(3), 353-355.

Tripp-Reimer, T. (1984b). Cultural assessment. In Bellack, J. & Banford, P., (Eds.), *Nursing assessment: a multidimensional approach* (pp. 226-246). Monterey, Calif.: Wadsworth.

Tripp-Reimer, T., Brink, P., & Saunders, J. (1984). Cultural assessment: content and process. *Nursing Outlook, 32*(2), 78-82.

Tripp-Reimer, T., & Dougherty, M.C. (1985). Cross-cultural nursing research. *Annual Review of Nursing Research, 3,* 77-104.

Tripp-Reimer, T., & Friedl, M. (1977). Appalachians: a neglected minority. *Nursing Clinics of North America, 12*(1), 41-54.

Walthour, E. (1993). *Health beliefs and self-care practices of hypertensive African-Americans.* Unpublished master's thesis, Georgia Southern University, Statesboro, Ga.

Wenger, F. (1989). President's address. *Transcultural Nursing Society Newsletter, 9*(1), 3.

World almanac. (1997). Mahwah, N.J.: World Almanac Books.

Young, T. (1994). *The health of Native Americans.* New York: Oxford University Press.

CHAPTER 2 — Communication

BEHAVIORAL OBJECTIVES

After reading this chapter, the nurse will be able to:

1. Describe the importance of communication as it relates to transcultural nursing assessment.
2. Delineate barriers to communication that hinder the development of a nurse-client relationship in transcultural settings.
3. Understand the importance of dialect, style, volume, use of touch, context of speech, and kinesics and their relationship to transcultural nursing assessment and care.
4. Describe appropriate nursing intervention techniques to develop positive communication in the nurse-client relationship.
5. Understand the significance of nonverbal communication and the use of silence and their relationship to transcultural nursing assessment and care.
6. Explain the significance of the structure and format of names in various cultural groups.
7. Explain the significance of variations in word meanings across and within various cultural and ethnic groups.

The word "communication" comes from the Latin verb *communicāre*, 'to make common, share, participate, or impart' (Guralnik, 1984). Communication, however, goes further than this definition implies and embraces the entire realm of human interaction and behavior. All behavior, whether verbal or nonverbal, in the presence of another individual is communication (Potter and Perry, 1993; Watzlawich, Beavin, and Jackson, 1967; Haber, 1997).

As the matrix of all thought and relationships among people, communication provides the means by which people connect. It establishes a sense of commonality with others and permits the sharing of information, signals, or messages in the form of ideas and feelings. Communication is a continuous process by which one person may affect another through written or oral language, gestures, facial expressions, body language, use of space, or other symbols.

Nurses have long recognized the importance of communication in the healing process (Reakes, 1997; Buckett, 1995). Communication is the core of most nursing curricula. Despite this, communication frequently presents barriers between nurses and clients, especially when the nurses and the clients are from different cultural backgrounds. If the nurse and the client do not speak the same language, or if communication styles and patterns differ, both the nurse and the client may feel alienated and helpless. A client who does not understand what is happening or who feels misunderstood may appear angry, noncompliant, or withdrawn. The physical healing process may be impaired. Nurses may also feel angry and helpless if their communication is not understood or if they cannot understand the client. Without the ability to communicate, care will be inadequate. Nurses need to have not only a working knowledge of communication with clients of the same culture, but also a thorough awareness of racial, cultural, and social factors that may affect communication with persons from other cultures. Health care settings must have an organizational climate for multiculturalism (Bruhn, 1996). Fielding and Llewelyn (1987) related that although communication skills are needed in nursing curricula, the more important issue is the broader understanding of the client from a cultural perspective.

Nurses must have an awareness of how an individual, though speaking the same language that the nurse does, may differ in communication patterns and understandings as a result of cultural orientation. Nurses must also have communication skills in relating to individuals who do not speak a familiar language (Kasch, 1984; Knowles, 1983; Taylor, Malone, and Kavanagh, 1997; Buttaglia, 1992). Most nurses generally assume that their perceptions and assessment of the client's health status are accurate and congruent with those of the client. Despite the client education process, however, there is evidence that discrepancies in perceptions persist. These discrepancies should be of particular concern to the nurse when providing transcultural nursing care because they may interfere with the provision of that care. Many factors obstruct quality client care, including poor communication, noncompliance with the treatment regimen, inadequate or unnecessary treatment, and ethical problems. All these factors combine to create discrepancies in the perceptions between the nurse and the client (Molzahn and Northcott, 1989; Andrews and Boyle, 1995).

COMMUNICATION AND CULTURE

Communication and culture are closely intertwined. Communication is the means by which culture is transmitted and preserved (Delgado, 1983). Culture influences how feelings are expressed and what verbal and nonverbal expressions are appropriate. Canadians are generally more likely to conceal feelings, and Canada is generally considered to have a low-touch Western culture, whereas a member of an Eastern culture may be open and loud with expressions of grief, anger, or joy and may use touch more (Hall, 1966; Thayer, 1988; Cheng and Barlas, 1992). Other cultural variables, such as the perception of time, bodily contact, and territorial rights, also influence communication. The cultural differences in contact can be quite dramatic. Sidney Jourard (1971) reported that when touch between pairs of people in coffee shops around the world was studied, there was more touch in certain cities. For example, it was reported that touch occurred as frequently as 180 times an hour between couples in San Juan, Puerto Rico, and 110 times an hour in Paris, France. In other cities there was less touch; specifically, touch occurred two times an hour between couples in Gainesville, Florida, and zero times an hour in London, England.

Cultural patterns of communication are embedded early and are found in childrearing practices. Gibson (1984) studied the playgrounds and beaches of Greece, the Soviet Union, and the United States and compared the frequency and nature of touch between caregivers and children ranging from 2 to 5 years of age. The analysis of data indicates that although rates of touching for retrieving or punishing the children were similar, rates of touching for soothing, holding, and play were dissimilar. American children were less likely to be touched than children from other cultures. The communication practices of persons in individual cultural groups affect the expression of ideas and feelings, decision making, and communication strategies. The communication of an individual reflects, determines, and consequently molds the culture (Hedlund, 1992; Kretch, Crutchfield, and Ballachey, 1962). In other words, a culture may be limited and molded by its communication practices. Sapir (1929) proposed that individuals are at the mercy of the particular language that has become the medium of expression of their society. Experiences are determined by language habits that predispose the individual to certain conceptions of the world and choices of interpretation.

Variations in communication may be limited to specific meanings for a few individuals in a small group, such as a family group. On the other hand, some communication patterns appear to be found in persons from a certain culture. In any case, the nurse must be cautious about assuming that a certain communication pattern can be generalized to all persons in a designated cultural group because communication patterns are often unique. In assessing the client, the nurse should keep in mind common cultural patterns and approach the client as an individual who should not be categorized because of cultural heritage.

LINGUISTICS

Since communication is a broad concept and encompasses all of human behavior, it has been conceptualized in many ways. One way is to consider the structure of communication, as in linguistics. The major focus on the structure of communication has been developed within the fields of ethnomethodology in sociology and linguistics in anthropology. Structure may be perceived as a form of language and the use of words and behaviors to construct messages. The role of ethnomethodologists is to consider the structure and effects of communication and to look at rules of communication and the consequences of breaking these rules. Ethnomethodologists not only have emphasized the study of the structure and rules of language, but also have studied the structure and rules of nonverbal communication (Sudnow, 1967). Linguistics is the area within anthropology concerned with the study of the structure of language. Linguistic patterns represent more than the use of grammatically nonequivalent words; these patterns can create real disparity in social treatment.

FUNCTIONS OF COMMUNICATION

Another way to think about communication is to consider what it achieves or accomplishes in human interaction. Consideration of the functions of communication refers to examining what the communication accomplishes rather than how the communication is structured. A relationship exists between communication structure and communication function in the sense that structure does affect function.

As a part of human interaction, communication discloses information or provides a specific message. Messages can be sent with no expectation of a response. Included in the disclosure of information may be an element of self-disclosure. Communication may or may not be intended as a method of self-disclosure or a means to provide information about the self or the individual's perception of self (Hedlund, 1992; Luft and Ingham, 1984). Perceptions of self include acts that describe the self and estimations of self-worth. In some situations self-awareness may be achieved through communication. This function of communication involves interaction with people. Through communication with others, an individual may become more aware of personal feelings.

PROCESS OF COMMUNICATION

Communication may be conceptualized as a process that includes a sender, a transmitting device, signals, a receiver, and feedback (Murray and Zentner, 1993). A sender attempts to relay a message, an idea, or information to another person or group through the use of signals or symbols. Many factors influence how the message is given and how it is received. For example, physical health, emotional well-being, the situation being discussed and the meaning it has, other distractions, knowledge of the matter being discussed, skill at communicating, and attitudes toward the other person, and the subject being discussed may all affect the communication that takes place (Box 2-1). In addition, personal needs and interests; background, including cultural, social, and philosophical values; the senses and their functional ability; personal tendency to make judgments and to be judgmental of others; the environment in which the communication takes place; and past experiences that relate or are related to the present situation can all affect the message that is received. The receiver then interprets the message. Feedback is given to the sender about the message, and more communication may occur. If no feedback is given, there may be no reciprocal interaction.

Although the process of communication is universal, nurses should be aware that styles and types of feedback may be unique to certain cultural groups. For example, before the assimilation of the Alaskan Inupiat into the American culture, the Alaskan Inupiat would indicate a message was received by blinking rather than making a verbal response (Davidhizar, 1988c). Nonverbal responses are also found in the Vietnamese. Vietnamese persons may smile, but the smile may not indicate understanding. A Vietnamese person may say yes simply to avoid confrontation or out of a desire to please. A smile may cover up disturbed feelings. Nodding, which nurses commonly interpret as understanding and compliance, may, for a Vietnamese individual, simply indicate respect for the person talking (Hoang and Erickson, 1982; Rocereto, 1981; Stauffer, 1989). The nurse may be surprised later when the Vietnamese client who smiled and nodded does not follow through with the instructions given.

VERBAL AND NONVERBAL COMMUNICATION

Another way to conceptualize communication is in terms of verbal and nonverbal behavior (Box 2-2). Communication first of all involves language or verbal communication, including vocabulary or repertoire of words and grammatical structure (Barkauskas, 1994).

Although Canada is officially and constitutionally a bilingual English- and French- speaking country,

the people nevertheless predominantly speak English. In 1986, of the number of persons who resided in Canada, 60.6% spoke English as their mother tongue, compared with 24.3% who spoke French as their native tongue (Statistics Canada, 1989). However, the French spoken in Canada is not, for the most part, the language of France. At times it can be nearly unintelligible to a Parisian. The local tongue of Quebec where most of the population is French is known as *Quebecois,* or *Joual,* but variations occur around the province (Lightbody and Smallman, 1994). Linguistics in Canada is further complicated by other languages such as German, Dutch, Polish, Hindi, Urdu, Icelandic, Ukrainian, Chinese, Korean, Vietnamese, Gujarati, Japanese, Arabic, Italian, Spanish, Creole, and more than 50 indigenous languages spoken by Aboriginal people who compose 2.8% of the population (Wardhaugh, 1993; Cheng and Barlas, 1992; Young, 1994; Statistics Canada, 1996).

In Canada, there are 11 aboriginal language families though some are in danger of extinction because of declining fluency of the younger generation of people (Web page on aboriginal peoples, 1995). Constitutional rights regarding language are carefully guarded by the Canadian Parliament. A commission on official languages is designated to carry out the numerous provisions of the 1969 Official Languages Act (updated in 1988). Although this act recognized English and French as equal official languages, it also guaranteed official-language status to minority languages in an effort to protect certain basic rights of all people when dealing with the federal government and its various agencies (Stevenson, 1993). Many immigrants use their mother tongues, as do some aboriginal communities though it is now only the older members who know the original indigenous languages.

It is important for the nurse to understand that because Canada is a multilingual country this fact may profoundly influence the ability of immigrants to assimilate into the mainstream. In many instances, immigrants in Quebec and elsewhere in Canada are faced with a choice of English monolingualism, French monolingualism, bilingualism in both official languages, or learning neither language (Chiswick and Miller, 1996). For many immigrants, the cost and benefits associated with learning one or more languages predetermines specifically what language will be learned or how many languages will be learned. Learning the official Canadian languages for many immigrants may mean better access to jobs and higher earnings. In a classic study, Lieberson (1970) noted that among immigrants who were neither English or French speaking, there was a clear tendency to adopt English as the spoken language. This is largely because many immigrants choose to locate to English-speaking regions of Canada. In contrast, many French immigrants and to a lesser extent Italian and Portuguese immigrants who speak French are more likely to live in French-speaking Quebec. Regardless of the country of origin, many immigrants who reside in Quebec speak only French or are English-French bilingual (Chiswick and Miller, 1996).

It is important to appreciate that, along with language, significant communication cues are received from voice quality, intonation, rhythm, and speed, as well as from the pronunciation used. Dialect may differ significantly among persons both across and within cultures. Silence during communication may itself be a significant part of the message.

Communication involves nonverbal messages, which include touch, facial expressions, eye behavior, body posture, and the use of space (Giger and Davidhizar, 1995, 1990a). Spatial behavior also affects communication and encompasses a variety of behaviors, including proximity to others or to objects in the environment and movement (see Chapter 3). Although nonverbal communication is powerful and honest, its importance and meaning vary among and within cultures; therefore it is essential that the nurse have an awareness and appreciation of the role that body language may have in the communication process. In addition, some communications combine nonverbal and verbal components in the message that is sent. Two examples of combination messages are warmth and humor.

Language, or verbal communication

Language is basic to communication. Without language the higher-order cognitive processes of thinking, reasoning, and generalizing cannot be attained. Words are tools or symbols used to express ideas and feelings or to identify or describe objects. Words shape experiences and influence cultural perceptions. Words convey interpretations and influence relationships (Murray and Zentner, 1993; Pirandello 1970; Talbot, 1996). Although words provide a special way of looking at the world, the same words often have different meanings for different individuals within cultural groups. In addition, word meanings change over time and in different situations. It is important to ascertain that the message is received and understood as the sender intended. As early as 1954, Sullivan emphasized the importance of ongoing validation in a therapeutic relationship to verify interpretations made on the behavior and words of another. Even today, this validation remains relevant in a nurse-client relationship in which many experiential, educational, and cultural differences are present. Smith and Cantrell (1988) reported a study comparing the effect of personal questions and physical distance on anxiety rates. Pulse rates were found to be higher when the investigator asked personal questions, regardless of the physical distance from subjects. Although the data from this study indicate that the most important part of a message may be verbal, the opposite has also been found to be true. Thus both verbal and nonverbal communication must be considered before a conclusion about the true meaning of a message can be determined.

To provide culturally appropriate nursing care, nurses must separate values based on their own cultural background from the values of the clients to whom care is given. Transcultural communication and understanding break down when caregivers project their own culturally specific values and behaviors onto the client. Thiederman (1986) has suggested that projection of values, as well as hindering care, may actually contribute to noncompliance.

Vocabulary

Even though people may speak the same language, establishing communication is often difficult because word meanings for both the sender and the receiver vary based on past experiences and learning. Words have both denotative and connotative meanings. A denotative meaning is one that is in general use by most persons who share a common language. A connotative meaning usually arises from a person's personal experience. For example, although all Americans are likely to share the same general denotative meaning for the word *pig*, depending on the occupation and cultural perception of the person, the connotation may be entirely different and may precipitate completely different reactions. The word *pig* will invoke either negative or positive reactions from certain people based on occupation and culture. For example, an Orthodox Jew's reactions will differ from those of a pig farmer. For an Orthodox Jew the word *pig* is synonymous with the word *unclean* or *unholy* and thus should be avoided. On the other hand, for a pig farmer the word *pig* implies a clean, wholesome means of making a living. Numerous conflicts resulting from differences in word meaning among various ethnic and racial groups are reported in the literature. Among her many famous cultural studies, Margaret Mead (1947) reported on

the different meanings that the word *compromise* carries for an Englishman and an American:

In Britain, the word "compromise" is a good word, and one may speak approvingly of any arrangement which has been a compromise, including, very often one in which the other side has gained more than fifty per cent of the points at issue. Where, in Britain, to compromise means to work out a good solution, in America it usually means to work out a bad one, a solution in which all the points of importance are lost.

Often people who have learned a language have learned the meaning for the word in only one context. For example, Díaz-Duque (1982) reported that a Hispanic person who was told he was going "to be discharged tomorrow" somehow interpreted this to mean he was going to develop "a discharge from below." Díaz-Duque also indicated that for Hispanics problems arise with cognates such as *constipation*, since for Hispanics this term generally refers to nasal congestion rather than intestinal constipation.

Although barriers exist when people speak the same language, more profound barriers are present when different languages are spoken. Each language has a whole set of unconscious assumptions about the world and life. Understanding differences in the meaning of words can provide insight into people of different cultures. For example, many English-speaking Americans are puzzled by what seems to be a different time orientation among Spanish people. An understanding of the meaning of the word *time* helps provide insight into this different orientation. In Spanish, time is defined as "passing"—a clock "passes time" or "moves"; whereas in English a clock "runs." If time is moving rapidly, as English usage declares, we must hurry. On the other hand, the Spanish definition allows for a more leisurely attitude (Randall-David, 1989). Such cultural understandings can provide insight into the reasons why Spanish individuals are often late for health care appointments.

Language reflects the dominant concerns and interests of a people, which can be noted in the number of words for certain things. Some classic studies have reported that certain cultures use many words to describe a particular object of importance. For example, Thomas (1937) explained that in the Arabic language there are about 6000 [*sic*] names for camels. Boas (1938) pointed out that the Canadian Inuit have 20 or so words for snow depending on consistency and texture. The language of a people is a key that unlocks their culture. A nurse who is familiar with the language of clients will have the best chance of gaining insight into their culture.

Although few White Canadians speak any words of an Indian or Inuit language, some words such as *igloo, parka, muskey,* and *kayak* are commonly used (Lightbody and Smallman, 1994). English Canadians have also added to the richness of the global English language with words such as *kerosene* (paraffin), *puck* (from ice hockey), *bushed* (exhausted), and *moose* from Anglicized Native Canadian words (Lightbody and Smallman, 1994). In British Columbia some expressions reflect the province's history; a word like *leaverite* meaning a 'worthless mineral' is a prospecting word derived from the phrase "Leave 'er right there."

Names

Names have a special psychological and cultural significance. All people have names, and in every culture naming a newborn is considered important. The considerations that go into the naming process vary greatly from culture to culture. For example, in Roman tradition there is a given name for boys; a family name, which is second; and a third name that specifies an extended family unit. The name Caius Julius Caesar illustrates the importance of tribal connections, as well as male chauvinism (Clemmens, 1988). In Roman times girls had only one name, the female version of the family name; for example, Caesar's sister was Julia, as was his aunt, father's sister, and so on. During the early Roman times women lacked individuality and thus in Roman society were not worth being named.

The Hebrew tradition has a patrilineal way of looking at names, that is, a given name and "son of." Mothers' names are not included. A spiritual and traditional continuity is evidenced in this system of naming. The Hebrew tradition can be seen today in Iceland, where all males have their given names, followed by their father's given name, ending in

"son." In contemporary Western society, as well, there are systems of naming. The most common one in the dominant culture in the United States is a patrilineal succession and one or more given names. In the United States the middle name is often one that relates to the family, such as the mother's maiden name.

The Russian system of naming provides a clue to the significance placed on relating son and father as well as daughter and father. The mother is left out (unless with some names in -*in*), with Russians habitually addressing each other by the individual's given name together with the patronymic. The family name is omitted. Spaniards and Latin Americans (or Hispanics) include women more than other cultures, with children carrying their father's name first and their mother's name second. The mother's name usually appears only on documents and for formal occasions because the addition of the mother's name makes the name quite long. Another variation is seen in the Dutch, who have the option of using both the husband's and the wife's family names jointly. Among the various cultures the most common theme of naming is pride in lineage (Clemmens, 1985, 1988).

Grammatical structure

Cultural differences are reflected in grammatical structure and the use and meaning of phrases. Canadian English as a whole has also developed its own distinctive idioms and expression. The most recognizable is the interrogative "eh?" which sometimes seems to appear at the end of almost every spoken sentence. In another example, for some Hispanic-American women having a stillborn child or a miscarriage do not equate with having a pregnancy. For some Hispanic-American women, a pregnancy is equated only with a successful live birth (Haffner, 1992). It is important for nurses to keep in mind that there is little validity in generalizations about the meaning of phrases by persons in varying cultures.

Length of sentence and speech forms may vary not only with culture, but also with social class. For example, Argyle (1992) noted that persons from the lower class commonly use short, simple sentences and are more direct than are persons with more education. Word choice, grammatical structure, speech fluency, and articulation provide cues to social status and class. Jargon is also a speech variation that may prove to be a barrier to communication. Nurses frequently have difficulty expressing things in simple jargon-free language (without medical terms) that clients can understand. On the other hand, a nurse who does not know the jargon used by the clients served may have a difficult time relating to them.

For some cultures, patterns of social amenities can create communication problems. Small talk, social chitchat, and discussion of mundane topics that may appear to "kill time" are necessary as preliminaries for more purposeful discussion. Yet the busy nurse seeking short, succinct answers to questions may be annoyed by the amount of anecdotal information that a Hispanic-American client gives. Many clients tend to add irrelevant material because it lessens embarrassment. They may be more comfortable if attention is not focused on their medical problem, and so they may intersperse actual symptoms with other biographical data. Cultural factors may also play a role in what seems to be verbal rambling. Patients who are used to folk healers believe that information on the weather, the environment, and eating habits are really important pieces of information for the health professional.

Voice qualities

Paralinguistics, or paralanguage, refers to something beyond the words themselves. Voice quality, which includes pitch and range, can add an important element to communication. The commonly used phrase, "Don't speak to me in that tone of voice," provides an indication of the significance of this aspect of the communication message.

The softer volume of Asian-American or Native speech may be interpreted by the nurse as shyness. On the other hand, the nurse's behavior may be viewed as loud and boisterous if the volume is loud and if there is a deliberate attempt to accent particular words. Sometimes people who speak softly, slowly, and without emphasis on particular words are viewed as "wishy-washy." When the nurse cannot hear what the client is saying, there is a tendency for the nurse to speak louder. It is important to remember that amplifying the volume does not necessarily equate with being understood or understanding (Spector, 1993). Nurses must remember that paralinguistic behavior is an important cultural consideration when assessing the client. The nurse can recognize this behavior by listening to nonword vocalizations such as sobbing, laughing, and grunting; tone of voice; and quality of voice.

The spoken English of the Atlantic provinces has inflections not heard in the west. The Ottawa Valley has a slightly different sound attributable mainly to the large numbers of Irish who settled there in the mid-1800s.

Intonation

Intonation is an important aspect of the communication message. When people say they feel "fine," they may mean they genuinely do or they do not feel fine but do not wish to discuss it. If said sarcastically, it may also mean they feel just the opposite of fine. There is often a latent or hidden meaning in what a person is saying, and intonation frequently provides the clue that is needed to interpret the true message.

Techniques of intonation vary among cultures. For example, Americans put commands in the form of suggestions and often as questions, whereas Arabic speech contains much emphasis and exaggeration (Argyle, 1992). Some cultures value indirectness and subtlety in speech and may be alienated by the frankness of Western health care professionals. Asian-Canadian clients, for example, may interpret this method of communication as rude, immature, and lacking finesse. On the other hand, health care professionals may label Asian-Canadian clients as evasive, fearful, and unable to confront problems (Sue, 1990).

Rhythm

Rhythm also varies from culture to culture; some people have a melodic rhythm to their verbal communication, whereas others appear to lack rhythm. Rhythm may also vary among persons within a culture. For example, some African-American ministers use a singsong rhythm to deliver fiery sermons.

Speed

Rate and volume of speech frequently provide a clue to an individual's mood. A depressed person will tend to talk slowly and quietly, whereas an aggressive, dominating person is more apt to talk rapidly and loudly.

Pronunciation

Canada inherited English primarily from the British settlers. Thus British English forms the basis of Canadian English. However, there are some pronunciation differences, for example, the British say "clark" for *clerk,* whereas Canadians say "clurk" (Lightbody and Smallman, 1994). Perhaps the best known difference between American and Canadian English is in the pronunciation of the last letter of the alphabet. Americans say zee; Canadians say zed. Although many non-North Americans, Canadians, and Americans may sound the same, there are real differences. Canadian pronunciation of *ou* is the most notable of these; words like *out* and *about* sound more like "oat" and "a boat" when spoken by Canadians.

"Ahs," "ers," and grunts also provide important dimensions to communication. Although hesitations may indicate a person who is unsure of self and is slow to make a commitment, for some cultures this can have the opposite meaning.

Silence

The meaning of silence varies among cultural groups. Silences may be thoughtful or may be blank and empty when the individual has nothing to say. A silence in a conversation may also indicate stubbornness and resistance, or apprehension or discomfort. Silence may be viewed by some cultural groups as extremely uncomfortable; therefore attempts may be made to fill every gap with conversation. Persons in other cultural groups value silence and view it as essential to understanding a person's needs. Many Native Canadians have this latter view of silence and so do some traditional Chinese and Japanese persons. Therefore, when one of these persons is speaking and suddenly stops, what may be implied is that the person wants the nurse to consider the content of what has been said before continuing. Other cultures may use silence in yet other ways. For example, English and Arabic persons use silence for privacy, whereas Russian, French, and Spanish persons may use silence to indicate agreement between parties. Some persons in Asian cultures may view silence as a sign of respect, particularly to an elder.

Nurses need to be aware of possible meanings of silence so that personal anxiety does not promote the silence to be interrupted prematurely or to be nontherapeutic. A nurse who understands the therapeutic value of silence can use this understanding to enhance care of clients from other cultures.

NONVERBAL COMMUNICATION

In his early and classic work, Hall (1966) suggested that 65% of the message received in communication is nonverbal. Through body language or motions (kinetic behavior), the person conveys what cannot or may not be said in words. For a message to be accurately interpreted, not only must words be translated, but also the meaning held by nuances, intonation patterns, and facial expressions. Just as verbal behavior may undo nonverbal behavior, nonverbal behavior may repeat, clarify, contradict, modify, emphasize, or regulate the flow of communication. Nonverbal behavior is less significant as an isolated behavior, but it does add to the whole communication message. To understand the client, the nurse may wish to validate impressions with other health team members because nonverbal behavior is often interpreted differently by different people. It is important for the nurse to be aware not only of the client's nonverbal behavior, but also of personal nonverbal behavior that may add to, undo, or contradict verbal communication (Reusch, 1961).

Touch

Touch, or tactile sensation, is a powerful form of communication that can be used to bridge distances between nurse and client (Davidhizar and Giger, 1988; Giger, Davidhizar, and Wieczorek, 1993; Giger and Davidhizar, 1995). Touch has many meanings (Box 2-3). It can connect people, provide affirmation, be reassuring, decrease loneliness, share warmth, provide stimulation, and increase self-concept. Being touched can be highly valued and

Box 2-3

MEANINGS OF TOUCH

Touch may:

1. Connect one individual with another both literally and figuratively by indicating availability
2. Provide affirmation and approval
3. Be reassuring by providing empathy, interest, encouragement, nurturance, caring, trust, concern, gentleness, and protection
4. Decrease loneliness by indicating a relationship with another
5. Share warmth, rapport, love, intimacy, excitement, and happiness
6. Provide stimulation by being a mode of sensation, perception, and experience
7. Increase self-concept
8. Communicate frustration, anger, aggression, or punishment
9. Invade personal space and privacy by physical and psychological assault or intrusion
10. Convey a negative type of relationship with another
11. Cause sexual arousal
12. Allow a person to perform a functional or professional role, such as a physician, barber, or tailor, and be devoid of personal message
13. Reflect cordiality, such as a handshake by business associates and among strangers and acquaintances

sought after. On the other hand, touch can also communicate frustration, anger, aggression, and punishment; invade personal space and privacy; and convey a negative (such as subservient) type of relationship with another. In certain situations touch can be disconcerting because it signals power. In a study reported by Thayer (1988), higher-status individuals were found to enjoy more liberties concerning touch than their lower-status associates. It is generally considered improper for individuals to put their hands on superiors.

Touching or lack of touch has cultural significance and symbolism and is a learned behavior. Cultural uses of touch vary. Each culture trains its children to develop different kinds of thresholds to tactile contacts and stimulation so that their organic, constitutional, and temperamental characteristics are accentuated or reduced. Some cultures are char-

acterized by a "do not touch me" way of life. These persons may view fondling and kissing as embarrassing. Some cultures include every possible variation on the theme of tactility. In some countries in North America, the dominant culture generally tolerates hugs and embraces among intimates and a pat on the shoulder as a gesture of camaraderie. The firm, hearty handshake is symbolic of good character and a sign of strength. In some Native Canadian groups, however, the hand is offered in some interpersonal interactions, but the expectation is different. Rather than a firm handshake, there is a light touch or grasp or even just a passing of hands. Some Native Canadians interpret vigorous handshaking as an aggressive action and are offended by a firm, lengthy handshake (Montagu, 1971).

Americans often give a lingering touch a sexual connotation. For some Americans, even casual touching is considered taboo and may be a result of residual Victorian sexual prudence (DeThomaso, 1971). Other cultures also consider touching taboo; the English and Germans carry untouchability further than Americans do. On the other hand, highly tactile cultures do exist, such as the Spanish, Italians, French, Jews, and South Americans (Montagu, 1971). However, generalizations about different national or ethnic groups in the area of touch can be problematic. For example, Shuter (1976) reported on studies of touch in Costa Rica, Columbia, and Panama. Findings from this study indicate that Latin Americans may be commonly highly contact-oriented individuals. Thayer (1988) also compared couples in Costa Rica, Columbia, and Panama and found that partners in Costa Rica were touched and held more often than partners in the other two countries.

Most cultures give touch different rules and meanings depending on the sex of the persons involved. Whitcher and Fisher (1979) reported that women in a hospital study had a strikingly positive reaction to being touched, with subsequent lowering of blood pressure and anxiety before surgery, whereas men found the same experience upsetting, with a subsequent increase in blood pressure and anxiety. Thayer (1988) reported on a study at the Kansas City International Airport in which it was found that women greeted women and men more physically, with lip kisses, embraces, and more kinds of touch and holding and for longer periods than did men. For men a more common greeting was to shake hands. Regardless of gender, some research has been reported showing that people who are most uncomfortable with touch are also uncomfortable with communicating through other means and have lower self-esteem (Thayer, 1988). Other studies have shown that people who touch more are less afraid and suspicious of other people's motives and intentions and have less anxiety and tension in their everyday lives. In some cultures leaning back, showing the palm of the hand, and fussing with the other person's collar may be perceived as possible courting behaviors because they may convey an invitation for closeness or affiliation. Touching behaviors such as reaching out during conversation to poke the other person in the chest may be viewed as domineering behavior. However, laughing while being poked may be a way to submit to and at the same time trivialize or eliminate the other person's aggressive intent (Scheflen, 1972).

In some cultures touch is considered magical and healing. For example, some Mexican and Native Americans view touch as symbolic of "undoing" an evil spell, as a means for prevention of harm, or as a means for healing (Montagu, 1971). On the other hand, Vietnamese Canadians may find touching shoulders with another to be anxiety producing because they believe that the soul can leave the body on physical contact and health problems may result (Rocereto, 1981). The Vietnamese regard the human head as the seat of life and therefore highly personal. Procedures that invade the surface or any orifice of the head can frighten the Vietnamese, who fear that these procedures could provide an escape for the essence of life (Muencke, 1983).

Nurses must be alert to the rules of touch for individuals encountered in the work role. Lane (1989) found that nurses perceive male clients as being less receptive to touch and closeness than their female counterparts, which could be attributed to the fact that males generally have a larger personal space than females. Thus it is believed that people generally maintain a greater distance from males (Insel, 1978; Sommer, 1959). Lane concluded that there may be a double standard concerning touch because of societal norms and expectations: male clients may be more receptive to touch than female nurses, but female nurses are perhaps more comfortable with the closeness and touch of female clients.

Although the rules of touch may be unspoken and unwritten, they are usually visible to the observer. A nurse should stay within the rules of touch that are culturally prescribed. It is essential that the nurse use touch judiciously and avoid forcing touch on anyone. Nurses must keep in mind that the message conveyed through touch depends on the attitude of the person involved and on the meaning of touch both to the person touching and to the person being touched. Generally the need for intimacy and touch is so strong that the satisfaction of that need is a greater influence on behavior than the fears about its inappropriateness (Johnson, 1965). A momentary and seemingly incidental touch can establish a positive, temporary bond between strangers, making them more compliant, helpful, positive, and giving. In all cases touch needs to be applied deliberatively, with empathy, and with close attention given to the person's particular needs. All cultural groups have rules, often unspoken, about who touches whom, when, and where. The astute nurse must be mindful of the client's reaction to touch to avoid being perceived as intrusive.

Facial expression

Facial expression is commonly used as a guide to a person's feelings. Research shows that generally in Americans, facial expression is used as a part of the communication message. A constant stare with immobile facial muscles indicates coldness. During fear, the eyes open wide, the eyebrows raise, and the mouth becomes tense with the lips drawn back. When a person is angry, the eyes become fixed in a hard stare with the upper lids lowered and the eyebrows drawn down. An angry person's lips are often tightly compressed. Eyes rolled upward may be related to tiredness or may show disapproval. Narrowed eyes, upper lip curled up, and a moving nose commonly signal disgust. A person who is embarrassed or self-conscious may turn the eyes away or down; have a flushed face; pretend to smile; rub the eyes, nose, or face; or twitch the hair or beard or mustache. A direct gaze with raised eyebrows shows surprise (Ekman and Friesen, 1975; Polhemus, 1978).

Facial expression also varies with culture. Italian, Jewish, African-American, and Spanish persons smile readily and use many facial expressions, along with gestures and words, to communicate feelings of happiness, pain, or displeasure. Irish, English, and Northern European persons tend to have less facial expression and are generally less responsive, especially to strangers. Facial expression can also be used to convey an opposite meaning of the one that is felt; for example, in the Orient, negative emotions may be concealed with a smile (Sue and Sue, 1990).

Eye movement

Research on eye movement has vastly increased as a result of the development of computer-based data collection and analysis routines. Eye movement-recording techniques provide a vast array of data to the researcher (Rayner, 1992; Shapiro, 1991; Grainger, 1992).

Eye movement is an important aspect of interpersonal communication. Generally during social interaction, most people look each other in the eye for short periods (Argyle and Dean, 1965; Davidhizar, 1988a). People use more eye contact while they are listening and may use glances of about 3 to 10 seconds. When glances are longer than this, anxiety is aroused.

Eye contact is an important tool in transcultural nursing assessment and is used both for observation and to initiate interaction. In the United States, the dominant culture (predominately Whites) value eye contact as symbolic of a positive self-concept, openness, interest in others, attentiveness, and honesty. Eye contact can communicate warmth and bridge interpersonal gaps between people. A nurse who wears glasses and wants to make a point may increase the intensity of eye contact by taking the glasses off. The removal of glasses has also been cited as a technique that can humanize an individual's face because barriers to eye contact are removed (Giger and Davidhizar, 1990b; Personal Report for the Executive, 1987).

Lack of eye contact may be interpreted as a sign of shyness, lack of interest, subordination, humility, guilt, embarrassment, low self-esteem, rudeness, thoughtfulness, or dishonesty. In social interaction the speaker glances away from the listener to indicate collecting thoughts or planning what is to be said. If contact is not resumed, disinterest may be interpreted. Pupil dilatation and constriction can also be a clue to anxiety level and positive response (Hess, 1965, 1975).

Most Mexican-Canadian and Black Canadian clients are comfortable with eye contact (Murray and Huelskoetter, 1991; Guruge and Donner, 1996). In contrast to this view, others have suggested that through a process of socialization in a "minority status" of relative powerlessness, some United States African Americans have learned to deliberately avoid eye contact with others (Giger, Davidhizar, Evers, and Ingram, 1994). In fact, in the United States avoidance of eye contact is sometimes considered rude, an indication of lack of attention, or a sign of mental illness (Bigham, 1964; Giger and Davidhizar, 1990b; Paynich, 1964). On the other hand, McKenzie and Chrisman (1977) reported that for some Filipinos eye contact that turns away is associated with the possibility of being a witch. Other groups who find eye contact difficult include some Oriental people and some Native Americans and Native Canadians who relate eye contact to impoliteness and an invasion of privacy. Many First Nations people, whether United States or Canadian, view eye contact as disrespectful because it is believed that "looking in an individual's eyes" is "looking into an individual's soul" (Henderson and Primeaux, 1981; McRae, 1994).

Persons in certain Indian cultures avoid eye contact with persons of a higher or lower socioeconomic class. The Vietnamese generally practice less eye contact (Giger and Davidhizar, 1990b; Rocereto, 1981), and prolonged eye contact is also avoided by some African Americans (Giger and Davidhizar, 1990b). In some Indian cultures eye contact is given a special sexual significance. Some Orthodox Jews also attribute a sexual significance to eye contact by an elderly man with a woman other than his wife (Sue and Sue, 1990). Some Appalachian people tend to avert their eyes because for them eye contact is related to hostility and aggressiveness (Tripp-Reimer and Friedl, 1977). Certain cultures place more focus on the eyes than others; for example, in India and Greece the use of the eyes is all important (Eibl-Eibesfelt, 1972).

Body posture

Communication is also affected by body posture. A nurse can bridge distance in an interaction by placing the forearms on the table, palms up. In Western culture, palms up can send a message of acquiescence even while disagreeing. However, the nurse should also recognize that palms up in other cultures may have a sexual implication. Therefore the decision to use this gesture should be weighed carefully.

Body posture can provide important messages about receptivity. In some Western cultures such as among White Canadians and Whites in the United States, the closer a listener's overall posturing matches the posture of the speaker, the higher the likelihood of receptivity. If the individuals' unconscious gestures are different, probably their perspectives on the matter at hand are also different. Matching body movements to those of another person can communicate a sense of solidarity even if solidarity is not present. Body posture can also communicate attitude toward a person. For example, among the dominate culture of Whites in the United States and in Canada, an attentive posture is indicated by leaning toward a person. Attentive posture is used toward people of higher stature and toward people who are liked (Mehrabian, 1968, 1981). An American man may indicate sexual attraction by placing his arms in front of his body with his legs closed. An American woman, on the other hand, indicates attraction by a more open posture, that is, arms down at the side (Hall, 1966). Physical pain is communicated by rigid muscles, flexed body, and cautious movements. Argyle and others (1970) reported that in England dominance is communicated when the dominant person stands or sits more erect than the compliant or submissive person. Knowledge of so-ciocultural heritage is essential in interpreting body language because various body parts are used differently in different cultures.

COMMUNICATIONS THAT COMBINE VERBAL AND NONVERBAL ELEMENTS

Some interpersonal communications combine both verbal and nonverbal elements. The communications of warmth and humor are two of these.

Warmth

Warmth is a quality or state that promotes feelings of friendship, well-being, or pleasure. Warmth can be communicated verbally ("You really laid still during the procedure, and that surely helped us to do it as quickly as possible") and may also be communicated nonverbally, as by a pat on the shoulder or a gentle smile.

Although warmth is also a matter of perception, communication that focuses on human needs is more likely to be related to warmth in the speaker. Statements that show respect, address the human need to be needed, and promote self-acceptance will usually be interpreted positively and can increase motivation, morale, and cooperation. Personal recognition and concern also communicate warmth. Verbal recognition (such as a "hello" on meeting) or a statement of genuine concern (such as "How are you feeling?") can convey interest and may facilitate a positive relationship between client and family and the nurse (Davidhizar, 1989).

The nurse's communication of warmth is an important and dynamic aspect of a therapeutic nurse-client relationship. If the client is from another culture and is having difficulty with understanding communication, the nurse's warmth may be vital to promoting a positive relationship.

Humor

Humor is a powerful component of verbal and nonverbal communication. Humor can create a bond of shared pleasure between people, decrease anxiety and tension, build relationships, promote problem solving and learning, provide motivation, and enable personal survival. As a healthy and constructive coping mechanism, humor can provide a discharge for aggressive feelings in a more or less acceptable way and can enable stressful situations to be managed (Davidhizar, 1988b). Humor that is therapeutic does not ridicule and rarely uses cynicism (Huckaby, 1987). Personality, culture, background, and levels of stress and pain may influence reactions to humor. When people are from a different culture, humor must be used in limited and well-thought-out situations because humor can be an obstacle to a relationship if it is misunderstood. The nurse must carefully assess the individual client and the situation to decide if humor is appropriate. Humor not only can improve communication when used appropriately, but may also affect the immune system by promoting the body's ability to combat such problems as cancer and diseases of the connective tissue such as arthritis and lupus (Simonton and Matthews-Simonton, 1978).

When the individual spoken with does not have a full grasp of the language and the nuances and puns that are often involved in humor, jokes and statements meant as humorous may not be understood or may be misinterpreted. It is also important for an individual who tries to speak in another language to be prepared to precipitate laughter. A statement meant to be serious may be perceived as comical. The ability to laugh at oneself and with others can ease the anxiety that may be present in an intercultural situation.

IMPLICATIONS FOR NURSING CARE
Guidelines for relating to patients from different cultures

Nurses commonly relate to clients in an interview setting. The nurse may also relate during the process of client care or at a more informal level on the hospital unit or in the clinic. Although cultural issues may cause the client to interpret the nurse's behavior from a unique perspective, adherence to the following guidelines will increase the likelihood that the nurse-client relationship will be positive (Box 2-4).

Assess personal beliefs of persons from different cultures Awareness of the nurse's personal beliefs is vital in relating to clients from diverse cultural back-

grounds (Carpio and Majumdar, 1991). A nurse working with a client from another background should carefully review personal beliefs and past experiences to determine conscious and unconscious attitudes. It is important for the nurse to set aside personal values, biases, ideas, and attitudes that are judgmental and may negatively affect care. Understanding cultural diversity occurs best through student or nurse exchange programs (Huttlinger and Keating, 1991). Leininger (1989) contends that "there is a major crisis in nursing in that most nurses are unprepared to function effectively with migrants and cultural strangers."

Assess communication variables from a cultural perspective To communicate with a client from another culture, it is essential to assess each client receiving care from a cultural perspective (College of Nurses of Ontario, 1990; Rosenbaum, 1991). A nurse who is reluctant to admit lack of understanding can significantly hinder the provision of adequate care (Burner, Cunningham, and Hattar, 1990). Each individual has a dominant culture and also belongs to a subculture. The cultural phenomenon of communication cannot be minimized when providing culturally appropriate nursing care. The nurse who understands differences in communication variables can attempt to transcend communication barriers to provide quality client care.

It is important to realize that cultural assessment does not require information on every aspect of a specific culture. However, data should elicit ethnic identity, including generation in Canada (that is, first or second generation). The beliefs of a first-generation immigrant, regardless of ethnic heritage, may differ from those of a second-generation person. Whenever possible, the client should be used as the primary informant because others, even though close to the client, may have different ideas and beliefs.

After a careful assessment of cultural factors that may enter into a relationship, the nurse must respond appropriately. For example, for Black Canadians and Mexican Canadians, who tend to value eye contact, it is important for the nurse to use eye contact (Kendall, 1996). On the other hand, when relating to Filipino Canadians, who are generally afraid

---

Box 2-4

GUIDELINES FOR RELATING TO PATIENTS FROM DIFFERENT CULTURES

1. Assess your personal beliefs surrounding persons from different cultures.
   - Review your personal beliefs and past experiences
   - Set aside any values, biases, ideas, and attitudes that are judgmental and may negatively affect care
2. Assess communication variables from a cultural perspective.
   - Determine the ethnic identity of the patient, including generation in America
   - Use the patient as a source of information when possible
   - Assess cultural factors that may affect your relationship with the patient and respond appropriately
3. Plan care based on the communicated needs and cultural background.
   - Learn as much as possible about the patient's cultural customs and beliefs
   - Encourage the patient to reveal cultural interpretation of health, illness, and health care
   - Be sensitive to the uniqueness of the patient
   - Identify sources of discrepancy between the patient's and your own concepts of health and illness
   - Communicate at the patient's personal level of functioning
   - Evaluate effectiveness of nursing actions and modify nursing care plan when necessary
4. Modify communication approaches to meet cultural needs.
   - Be attentive to signs of fear, anxiety, and confusion in the patient
   - Respond in a reassuring manner in keeping with the patient's cultural orientation
   - Be aware that in some cultural groups discussion concerning the patient with others may be offensive and may impede the nursing process
5. Understand that respect for the patient and communicated needs is central to the therapeutic relationship.
   - Communicate respect by using a kind and attentive approach
   - Learn how listening is communicated in the patient's culture
   - Use appropriate active listening techniques
   - Adopt an attitude of flexibility, respect, and interest to help bridge barriers imposed by culture
6. Communicate in a nonthreatening manner.
   - Conduct the interview in an unhurried manner
   - Follow acceptable social and cultural amenities
   - Ask general questions during the information-gathering stage
   - Be patient with a respondent who gives information that may seem unrelated to the patient's health problem
   - Develop a trusting relationship by listening carefully, allowing time, and giving the patient your full attention
7. Use validating techniques in communication.
   - Be alert for feedback that the patient is not understanding
   - Do not assume meaning is interpreted without distortion
8. Be considerate of reluctance to talk when the subject involves sexual matters.
   - Be aware that in some cultures sexual matters are not discussed freely with members of the opposite sex
9. Adopt special approaches when the patient speaks a different language.
   - Use a caring tone of voice and facial expression to help alleviate the patient's fears
   - Speak slowly and distinctly, but not loudly
   - Use gestures, pictures, and play acting to help the patient understand
   - Repeat the message in different ways if necessary
   - Be alert to words the patient seems to understand and use them frequently
   - Keep messages simple and repeat them frequently
   - Avoid using medical terms and abbreviations that the patient may not understand
   - Use an appropriate language dictionary
10. Use interpreters to improve communication.
    - Ask the interpreter to translate the message, not just the individual words
    - Obtain feedback to confirm understanding
    - Use an interpreter who is culturally sensitive

---

of eye contact, the nurse should avoid eye contact. When relating to Southeast Asians, it is important to remember that persons from this cultural background usually are very formal in language. It is essential that courtesy be shown by use of the family name or a title until one is given permission to address the client by a given name. Asians also use an indirect approach to obtaining information and so direct questions are not received well; it is considered rude, and the interviewer is not likely to receive the information sought (Hagen, 1988; Mattson, 1995; Stauffer, 1995).

Plan care based on the communicated needs and cultural background When planning care for persons from other cultures, care must be consistent with the lifestyle and unique needs of the client that have been communicated by the client to the nurse and mutually agreed on (Geissler, 1991; Grossman, 1996). To establish an appropriate plan, it is essential to improve personal knowledge about the customs and beliefs of the culture of the clients receiving care. The nurse should encourage the client to communicate cultural interpretations of health, illness, and health care. A client's perception of illness will affect not only communication, but also the care that is planned. Sensitivity to the uniqueness of each client is required if the nurse is to work effectively, particularly with clients from different cultures. This sensitivity can be gained only through appropriate communication techniques. Additionally, nurses who cannot communicate and correctly interpret cultural behavior will feel inadequate and helpless and quickly experience stress and burnout (Scholz, 1990).

O'Neil (1989) studied dissatisfaction of Inuit clients with care received by Western health-care providers. Findings from this study suggested that Western providers were strongly paternalistic and showed disregard for cultural factors. O'Neil also noted that failing to critique interactions, in light of the legacy of colonialism in health care for the Native people in Canada, provides a significant barrier to care. Chipperfield (1992) also found that respect was essential to client satisfaction. Further findings from this study noted that there were differences in perceptions of respect between elderly subjects of various cultural groups (Chipperfield, 1992). In another study, Browne (1995) interviewed Cree and Obijwa in northern Manitoba who were interacting with Western health care providers to develop insight concerning the nature of respect. These respondents noted that features of respect included values related to equality, inherent worth, uniqueness, and dignity of the individual (Browne, 1995). Therefore the nurse must evaluate the effectiveness of nursing actions with clients from diverse culture groups. It may

be necessary to modify the plan of care to provide an effective intervention based on communication needs and dissatisfaction with care provided. If treatment approaches reinforce the paternalism and power frequently exercised by health care providers in the past, different, alternative strategies that incorporate respectful interactions into nursing practice and that emphasize client autonomy in health care may be utilized (Egan, 1994).

It is important to remember that the best teachers in learning about culture are people themselves. Individuals must be communicated with at their personal level of functioning. Values and beliefs of persons from different cultures may affect the way care is delivered. Many cultures have similar idiosyncrasies that must be considered. Finally, it is important to evaluate the effectiveness of nursing actions with clients from diverse culture groups. It may be necessary to modify the plan of care to provide an effective intervention based on communicated needs.

Modify communication approaches to meet cultural needs A factor that commonly interferes with care delivery to a person from another culture is confusion and fear about the treatment process. The fact that a non-English-speaking or non-French-speaking client is ill and receiving treatment can interfere with the client's ability to communicate. The nurse must be attentive to signs of anxiety and respond in a reassuring manner in keeping with the person's cultural orientation.

Some cultures are primarily oral and do not rely on a written form of communication. In such a society, the spoken word holds greater meaning and power. For example, Hmongs are considered an oral cultural group. For these individuals, the formation of and acceptance in a social group is primarily dependent on the spoken word (Shadick, 1993). When interacting with individuals from an oral culture, the nurse must remember that if the teaching-learning process is to be effective, instruction must be oral.

When working with persons from diverse cultural backgrounds, the astute nurse must recognize that the communication process may be impeded by hesitancy to speak to Westerners about health concerns. Some Native Canadians are becoming more confident and willing to speak out about their personal needs. However, Hagey and Buller (1983) noted that the Ojibwa people traditionally avoided direct verbal questioning by health care workers and viewed it as a form of violation of dignity and inappropriate. Such questions could be met with complete silence and meaningless answers. For some Ojibwa, in response to a question, it would be entirely acceptable for an answer to be given in a few days or weeks. It is critical that the nurse serve as a client advocate to provide culturally sensitive care. It is also essential that the nurse learn to appreciate a value held by some Ojibwa that espouses deep-rooted ideals of noninterference, which may be found among some indigenous and ethnic groups (Grypma, 1993). Regardless of cultural background, listening is one of the most effective therapeutic techniques (Potter and Perry, 1993).

Understand that respect for the client and communicated needs is central to the therapeutic relationship The need to communicate respect for the client is a nursing concept that crosses all cultural boundaries. Regardless of the language spoken or the cultural orientation, communication is increased and interpersonal distance is reduced by the nurse whose approach focuses on individuals and their emotional and physical needs. Communication of respect is central to a focus on emotional needs. Respect for clients is communicated by a kind and attentive approach where the client is heard. Active listening techniques are used, such as encouraging clients to share thoughts and feelings by reflecting back what has been heard. The nurse should be attentive to how listening is communicated in the client's culture. For example, for some persons listening may be indicated by eye contact, whereas for others listening may mean having the listener turn a listening "ear." Predictions about what the client is trying to express may be made to encourage elaboration. Listening communicates genuine interest and caring. The feeling of being heard is powerful, reducing distance and drawing people together into positive interpersonal interactions. An attitude of flexibility, respect, and interest can bridge artificial barriers of distance imposed by culture and role.

Communicate in a nonthreatening manner The interview should be started in an unhurried manner with adherence to acceptable social and cultural amenities. It is usually wise to start with general social topics. During the information-gathering stage, general rather than specific questions should be asked. The interviewer should allow time for the respondent to give what appears to be unrelated information. For many persons a direct approach appears rude and uncaring. For example, persons of European background and Spanish individuals often value "small talk" and will not relate optimally to the nurse who talks only about illness-related matters. Many persons, specifically Oriental and Spanish-speaking persons, respond better to a nondirect approach with open-ended questions than to direct questions and answers (Giger and Davidhizar, 1990b).

When personal matters are discussed, it is important to allow time for the development of a relationship. For example, Native Canadians tend to be hesitant to discuss personal affairs quickly. For such individuals it is important to first develop trust, which may be difficult in an emergency where answers to questions are needed quickly. Because of this hesitancy on the part of Native Canadians to speak, it is especially important for the nurse to listen carefully and give the client full attention.

The appearances of being too busy, of not having time to listen, of not giving sufficient time for an answer, and of not really wanting to hear are equally effective in "cutting off" the client. Patients will be encouraged to talk by a nurse who "wants" to hear.

Use validating techniques in communication Although validating techniques are always important, they are especially important when the client is from a different culture. The nurse should be alert for feedback that the client is not understanding and should use restating and validating techniques such as, "Did I hear and understand you correctly?"

Even if an interpreter is used, the nurse should not assume that the meaning has been transmitted without some distortion. It is difficult to transmit exact meaning when both persons speak the same language and even more so when both persons do not.

Be considerate of reluctance to talk when the subject involves sexual matters Spanish clients and Canadian Indians, who tend to be hesitant to talk about sexually related matters, may talk more freely to a nurse of the same sex. When talking about sexual matters with a male child from certain cultures (such as Spanish, Pakistani, or Arabic), it is important to have the father rather than the mother present.

Adopt special approaches when the client speaks a different language A client who enters the health care system without being able to speak to the caregivers enters a frightening and frustrating world. Canada is home to over 100 different linguistic and cultural groups (Guruge and Doner, 1996). The number of cultures and languages that are found among the Canadian people contributes to problems in effective nurse-client communication as well as follow-up treatment (Gunderson, 1996). Public health programs have not adequately met the multicultural composition of the populations (Edwards and MacMillan, 1990). This is particularly true of the indigenous population where limited ability to speak, understand, and read English is a significant barrier to care, particularly for the older Native Canadians and those from rural areas or who live on a reserve (Red Horse, Johnson, and Weiner, 1989). Problems in communicating between caregivers and immigrants also exist and are often augmented because of the multilingual nature of these individuals. A few health promotion projects have been specifically targeted to multiethnic communities in Canadian cities. Rigorous evaluations of their influence have not yet been reported (Edwards and MacMillan, 1990; Jacobson, 1994). Translation of health information pamphlets from English to the language of the client from a differing cultural background has also been done but on a limited scale. For clients who do not speak English or French, even the most basic procedures such as registering at the emergency desk may seen as an insurmountable barrier. Without the availability of reciprocal two-way communication, the nurse must find creative alternative strategies to relate to the client at an effective level. A caring tone of voice and a caring facial expression are essential in alleviating the client's fear.

The nurse should guard against the common assumption that the client will understand better if the nurse talks loudly. If an interpreter is not available and the client seems to have some understanding of the language, speaking slowly and distinctly, using a lot of gestures, acting out, using pictures, and repeating the message several times in different ways may enable the client to understand what is being said. The nurse should be alert for words that the client seems to understand so that these words can be used more frequently. Messages should be kept simple and stated sentence by sentence, not paragraph by paragraph.

It is especially necessary to avoid using medical terms and jargon when speaking to a client with only partial understanding of the language. Abbreviations such as "TPR" and "BP" should be avoided. An individual usually first understands standard words and picks up slang expressions and professional terms at a much later stage of language acquisition.

The nurse should select a dictionary that has both the language the nurse speaks and the language the client speaks, such as a Spanish-English dictionary. In addition, standard nursing references such as *Taber's Cyclopedic Medical Dictionary* (Taber, 1993) and *Mosby's Medical, Nursing, and Allied Health Dictionary* (1997) have sections that give common medical statements and questions in several languages.

Use interpreters to improve communication Assessment tools are available for Spanish-speaking immigrants and refugee communities at minimal or no cost (Urrutia-Rojas and Aday, 1991). The nurse should be alert for the client who pretends to understand to please the caregiver and gain acceptance. This patient will usually say "yes" to all questions. When a client does not speak the nurse's language, an interpreter should be included who may be either a family member or a person from an agency or the community. The interpreter should be able to translate not only the literal meaning of the words, but also the nonverbal messages that accompany the communication. Interpreters who "act out" their message through intonation, facial expression, or gestures are more likely to be effective in getting the message across. Even when every effort is made to ensure effective translations, neither the nurse nor the interpreter can be completely sure that accurate communication has been accomplished; therefore obtaining feedback remains essential. Communication through a third party compounds the problem of sending a message clearly. Interpreters often face the difficulty of interpreting versus translating. Although a message may be translated into another language, helping another understand is much more complex and involves interpreting the message into understandable terms. An interpreter must have transcultural sensitivity, understand how to impart knowledge, and understand how to be a client advocate to represent the client's needs to the nurse. Interpreting with cultural sensitivity is much more complex than simply putting the words into another language (Díaz-Duque, 1982; Muencke, 1970; Putsch, 1985). Learning a second language is an important tool in lowering cultural barriers. A nurse who learns the language of the clients who are served will find that this profoundly affects communication (Stoltzfus, 1993). Boston (1993) conducted a study in Montreal of Italian immigrant families to determine if they had a perception of frustration with their caregivers because of language barriers. Findings from this study indicated that respondents expressed fear and helplessness about their treatment because of the language barriers. Even when an interpreter was provided, family members believed that their own deeper concerns and fears were not adequately communicated.

Case Study

A 35- to 37-year-old Black Canadian woman who has been recently diagnosed as having hypertension is admitted for a medical work-up. Her history reveals that she has recently moved from New Orleans to Quebec. The nurse is having difficulty communicating with the client because she not only speaks Black English but also has a heavy Southern drawl and tends to speak in pidgin English. Another factor complicating the development of the nurse-client relationship is that not only does the client not understand the hospital jargon and medical terms, but even word meanings for the nurse and the client vary. For example, when the nurse asks if the client likes her physician, she responds, "He's bad." Only later does the nurse discover that the client was speaking in an argot that is a special linguistic code for some Blacks. The client appears very fearful and anxious about being in the hospital. When questioning the client, the nurse finds that the fear and anxiety are related to the connotative and denotative meanings of the word "hospital." In this case the client believes that hospitals are associated with death and that she may not leave the hospital alive. When the nurse communicates with the client, she speaks very loudly and repeats the same words again and again.

STUDY QUESTIONS

1. Describe at least two problems encountered by the nurse when giving nursing care to persons who do not speak Canadian English as their primary language.
2. List at least three words that have been added to the English language by Canadians.
3. Describe four communication approaches that the nurse can use to give culturally appropriate care.
4. Describe approaches the nurse can use when relating to a client whose primary language is not Canadian English.
5. Describe at least two nonverbal indicators of anxiety the nurse may encounter when dealing with a client who does not speak Canadian English.
6. List at least two problems encountered by the nurse who assumes that speaking louder will improve communication.

References

Andrews, M.M., & Boyle, J.S. (1995). *Transcultural nursing*. Philadelphia: Lippincott-Raven.

Argyle, M. (1992). *The social psychology of everyday life*. New York: Routledge.

Argyle, M., & Dean, J. (1965). Eye-contact, distance, and affiliation. *Sociometry, 28*, 289-304.

Argyle, M., Salter, H., Nicholson, N., Williams, M., & Burgess, P. (1970). The communication of inferior and superior attitudes by verbal and nonverbal signals. *British Journal of Social and Clinical Psychology, 9*, 221-231.

Barkauskas, V.H. (1994). *Quick reference to cultural assessment*. St. Louis: Mosby.

Bigham, C. (1964). To communicate with Negro patients. *American Journal of Nursing, 64*(9), 113-115.

Boas, F. (Ed.). (1938). *General anthropology*. Boston: D.C. Heath.

Boston, P. (1993). Culture and cancer: The relevance of cultural orientation within cancer education programmes. *European Journal of Cancer Care, 2*, 72-76.

Browne, A. (1995). The meaning of respect: a first nation's perspective. *The Canadian Journal of Nursing Research, 27*(4), 95-109.

Bruhn, J. (1996). Creating an organizational climate for multiculturalism. *Health Care Supervisor, 14*(4), 10-16.

Buckett, H. (1995). Tales from the road. *Health Traveler, 3*(2), 48.

Burner, O., Cunningham, P., & Hattar, H. (1990). Managing a multicultural nurse staff in a multi-cultural environment. *Journal of Nursing Administration, 20*(6), 30-36.

Buttaglia, B. (1992). Skills for managing multicultural teams. *Cultural Diversity at Work, 4*(3), 4.

Carpio, B., & Majumdar, B. (1991, August). Putting culture into curricula. *The Canadian Nurse, 87*, 32-33.

Cheng, P., & Barlas, R. (1992). *Culture shock*. Portland, Oreg.: Graphic Arts Publishing Company.

Chipperfield, J.G. (1992). A longitudinal analysis of perceived respect among elders: changing perceptions for some ethnic groups. *Canadian Journal of Aging, 11*(1), 15-30.

Chiswick, B., & Miller, P. (1996). Language and earnings among immigrants in Canada: a survey. In Dunleep, H., & Wunnava, P. (Eds.), *Immigrants and immigration policy: individual skills, family ties, and group identities* (pp. 57-78). London: JAI Press.

Clemmens, E. (1985). An analyst looks at languages, cultures, and translations. *American Journal of Psychoanalysis, 45*(4), 310-321.

Clemmens, E. (1988). Some psychological functions of language. *American Journal of Psychoanalysis, 43*(4), 294-304.

College of Nurses of Ontario. (1990). *Standards of nursing practice for registered nurses and registered nursing assistants*. Toronto.

Davidhizar, R. (1988a). Distance in managerial encounters. *Today's OR Nurse, 10*(10), 23-29.

Davidhizar, R. (1988b). Humor—no nurse should be without it. *Today's OR Nurse, 10* (1), 18-20.

Davidhizar, R. (1988c). Personal communication, Mishawaka, Indiana.

Davidhizar, R. (1989). Developing managerial warmth. *Dimensions of Critical Care, 8*(1), 28-34.

Davidhizar, R., & Giger, J. (1988). Managerial touch. *Today's OR Nurse, 10*(7), 18-23.

Delgado, M. (1983). Hispanics and psychotherapeutic groups. *International Journal of Psychotherapy, 33*(4), 507-520.

DeThomaso, M. (1971). Touch power and the screen of loneliness. *Perspectives in Psychiatric Care, 9*(3), 112-117.

Díaz-Duque, O. (1982). Advice from an interpreter. *American Journal of Nursing, 82* (9), 1380-1381.

Edwards, N., & MacMillan, K. (1990, January/February). Tobacco use and ethnicity: the existing data gap. *Canadian Journal of Public Health, 81*, 32-37.

Egan, G. (1994). *The skilled helper: a problem-management approach to helping* (ed. 5). Pacific Grove, Calif.: Brooks/Cole.

Eibl-Eibesfelt, I. (1972). Similarities and differences between cultures in expressive movements. In Hinde, R.A, (Ed.), *Nonverbal communication* (pp. 297-312). Cambridge, England: Cambridge University Press.

Ekman, P., & Friesen, W.V. (1975). *Unmasking the face: a guide to recognizing emotions from facial clues*, Englewood Cliffs, N.J.: Prentice-Hall.

Fielding, R., & Llewelyn, S. (1987). Communication training in nursing may damage your health and enthusiasm: some warnings. *Journal of Advanced Nursing, 12*(3), 281-290.

Geissler, E. (1991). Transcultural nursing and nursing diagnosis. *Nursing and Health Care, 12*(4), 190-192.

Gibson, J. (1984, January). As they grow: 1 year olds. *Parents*, p. 128.

Giger, J., & Davidhizar, R. (1990a). Culture and space. *Advancing Clinical Care, 6*(6), 8-10.

Giger, J., & Davidhizar, R. (1990b). Transcultural nursing assessment: a method for advancing nursing practice. *International Nursing Review, 37*(1), 199-202.

Giger, J., & Davidhizar, R. (1995). *Transcultural nursing: assessment and intervention.* St. Louis: Mosby.

Giger, J., Davidhizar, R., Evers, S., Ingram, C. (1994). Cultural factors influencing mental health and mental illness. In Taylor, C. (Ed.), *Merness' essentials of psychiatric nursing* (pp. 214-238). St. Louis: Mosby.

Giger, J., Davidhizar, R., & Wieczorek, S. (1993). Culture and ethnicity. In Bobak I. & Jensen M., (Eds.), *Maternity and gynecological care* (ed. 5) (pp. 43-67). St. Louis: Mosby.

Grainger, R. (1992). Eye movements: a new psychotherapeutic tool. *American Journal of Nursing, 92*(5), 18.

Grossman, D. (1996). Cultural dimensions in home health care nursing. *American Journal of Nursing, 96*(7), 33-36.

Grypma, S. (1993, September). Culture shock. *The Canadian Nurse, 89,* 33-36.

Gunderson, J. (1996, April)). Progress in building communication link. *The Canadian Nurse, 92,* 9-10.

Guralnik, D. (Ed.). (1984). *Webster's new world dictionary* (ed. 3). New York: William Collins & World Publishing.

Guruge, S., & Donner, G. (1996, September). Transcultural nursing in Canada. *The Canadian Nurse, 92,* 34-39.

Haber, J. (1997). Therapeutic communication. In Haber, J., Krainovich-Miller, B., McMahon, A., & Price-Hoskins, P. (Eds.), *Comprehensive psychiatric nursing* (ed. 5) (pp. 122-142). St. Louis: Mosby.

Haffner, L. (1992). Translation is not enough: interpreting in a medical setting. *Western Journal of Medicine, 157*(3), 248-254.

Hagen, E. (1988, July 8). *Southeast Asians in the United States: an overview of belief systems, and the refugee experience.* Paper presented at the seminar Working with the Southeast Asian Health Consumer, St. Mary Medical Center, Long Beach, Calif.

Hagley, B., & Buller, E. (1983). Drumming and dancing: a new rhythm in nursing care. *The Canadian Nurse, 79*(4), 28-31.

Hall, E.T. (1966). *The silent language.* New York: Doubleday.

Hedlund, N. (1992). Communication. In Beck, C.K., Rawlins, R.P., & Williams, S. (Eds.), *Mental health-psychiatric nursing: a holistic life approach* (ed. 3). St. Louis: Mosby.

Henderson, G., & Primeaux, M. (1981). *Transcultural health care.* Don Mills, Ont.: Addison-Westley.

Hess, E.H. (1965). Attitude and pupil size. *Scientific American, 212,* 46-54.

Hess, E.H. (1975). The role of pupil size in communication. *Scientific American, 233*(5), 110-119.

Hoang, G., & Erickson, R. (1982). Guidelines for providing medical care to Southeast Asian refugees. *Journal of the American Medical Association, 248*(6), 710-714.

Huckaby, D. (1987). Take time to laugh. *Nursing, 87*(17), 81.

Huttlinger, K., & Keating, S. (1991). Understanding cultural diversity through a student exchange program. *Nurse Educator, 16*(5), 29-34.

Insel, P.M. (1978). *Too close for comfort: the psychology of crowding.* Englewood Cliffs, N.J.: Prentice Hall.

Jacobson, S. (1994). Native American health. *Annual Review of Nursing Research, 12,* 193-213.

Johnson, B. (1965). The meaning of touch in nursing. *Nursing Outlook, 13*(2), 59-60.

Jourard, S.M. (1971). *The transparent self.* New York: D. Van Nostrand-Reinhold.

Kasch, C. (1984). Interpersonal competence and communication in the delivery of nursing care. *Advances in Nursing Science, 62,* 71-88.

Kendall, J. (1996). Creating a culturally responsive psychotherapeutic environment for African American youths: a critical analysis. *Advances in Nursing Science, 18*(4), 11-28.

Knowles, R. (1983). Building rapport through neurolinguistic programming. *American Journal of Nursing, 83,* 1011-1014.

Kretch, D., Crutchfield, R., & Ballachey, E. (1962). *Individual in society.* New York: McGraw-Hill.

Lane, P. (1989). Nurse-client perceptions: the double standard of touch. *Issues in Mental Health Nursing, 10,* 1-13.

Lieberson, S. (1970). *Language and ethnic relations in Canada.* New York: John Wiley.

Lightbody, M., & Smallman, T. (1994). *Canada: a travel survival kit.* Oakland, Calif: Lonely Planet Publications.

Leininger, M. (1989). The transcultural nurse specialist: imperative in today's world. *Nursing and Health Care, 10,* 251-255.

Luft, J., & Ingham, H. (1984). The Johari window: a graphic model of awareness in interpersonal relations. In Luft, J. (Ed.), *Group processes: an introduction to group dynamics* (ed. 3). Palo Alto, Calif: National Press Books.

Mattson, S. (1995, May). Culturally sensitive perinatal care for Southeast Asians. *Journal of Obstetric and Gynecological Nursing, 24,* 335-338.

McKenzie, J., & Chrisman, N. (1977). Healing herbs, gods, and magic: folk health beliefs among Filipino-Americans. *Nursing Outlook, 25*(5), 326.

McRae, L. (1994). Cultural sensitivity in rehabilitation related to Native clients. *Canadian Journal of Rehabilitation, 7*(4), 251-256.

Mead, M. (1947). The application of anthropological technique to cross-national communication. *Transcultural New York Academy of Science, Series II, 9,* 4.

Mehrabian, A. (1968). The influence of attitudes from the posture, orientation, and distance of a communicator. *Journal of Consulting Clinical Psychology, 32,* 296-308.

Mehrabian, A. (1981). *Silent messages: implicit communication of emotion and attitude.* Belmont, Calif: Wadsworth.

Molzahn, A., & Northcott, H. (1989). The social bases of discrepancies in health/illness perceptions. *Journal of Advanced Nursing, 14*(2), 132-140.

Montagu, A. (1971). *Touching: the significance of the human skin.* New York: Columbia University Press.

Mosby's medical, nursing, and allied health dictionary. (1997). (ed. 5). St. Louis: Mosby.

Muencke, M. (1970). Overcoming the language barrier. *Nursing Outlook, 18*(4), 53-54.

Muencke, M. (1983). Caring for Southeast Asian refugee patients in the USA. *American Journal of Public Health, 74*(4), 431-438.

Murray, R., & Huelskoetter, N. (1991). *Psychiatric/mental health nursing: giving emotional care* (ed. 2). Norwalk, Conn.: Appleton & Lange.

Murray, R., & Zentner, J. (1993). *Nursing assessment and health promotion strategies through the life span* (ed. 5). Norwalk, Conn.: Appleton & Lange.

O Neil, J. (1989). The cultural and political context of patient dissatisfaction in cross-cultural clinical encounters: a Canadian Inuit study. *Medical Anthropology Quarterly, 3*(4), 325-344.

Paynich, M. (1964). Cultural barriers to nurse communication. *American Journal of Nursing, 64*(2), 87-90.

Personal Report for the Executive. (1987). New York: National Institute of Business Management.

Pirandello, L. (1970). Language and thought. *Perspectives in Psychiatric Care, 8*(5), 230.

Polhemus, T. (Ed.). (1978). *The body reader: social aspects of the human body.* New York: Pantheon Books.

Potter, R., & Perry, A. (1993). *Fundamentals of nursing: concepts, process, and practice* (ed. 3). St. Louis: Mosby.

Putsch, R. (1985). Cross-cultural communication. *Journal of the American Medical Association, 254,* 3347-3348.

Randall-David, E. (1989). *Strategies for working with culturally diverse communities and clients* [Brochure]. Washington, D.C.: U.S. Department of Health and Human Services.

Rayner, K. (1992). *Eye movements and visual cognition.* New York: Springer-Verlag.

Reakes, J. (1997). Communication. In Johnson, B. (Ed.), *Psychiatric-mental health nursing* (ed. 4). Philadelphia: Lippincott.

Red Horse, J., Johnson, T., & Weiner, D. (1989). Commentary: cultural perspectives on research among American Indians. *American Indian Culture and Research Journal, 13*(3), 267-271.

Reusch, J. (1961). *Therapeutic communication.* New York: W.W. Norton.

Rocereto, L. (1981). Selected health beliefs of Vietnamese refugees. *Journal of School Health, 51*(1), 63-64.

Rosenbaum, J. (1991, April). A cultural assessment guide. *The Canadian Nurse,* 32-33.

Sapir, E. (1929). The status of linguistics as a science. *Language, 5,* 207-214.

Scheflen, A. (1972). *Body language and social order.* Englewood Cliffs, N.J.: Prentice Hall.

Scholz, J. (1990). Cultural expressions affecting patient care. *Dimensions in Oncology Nursing, IV* (1), 16-20.

Shadick, K. (1993). Development of a transcultural health education program for the Hmong. *Clinical Nurse Specialist, 7*(2), 48-53.

Shapiro, F. (1991, May). Eye movement desensitization and reprocessing procedure: from EMD to EMD/R—a new treatment model for anxiety and related traumata. *The Behavioral Therapist,* pp. 133-135.

Shuter, R. (1976). Proxemics and tactility in Latin America. *Journal of Communication, 26*(3), 46-52.

Simonton, O.C., & Matthews-Simonton, S. (1978). *Getting well again.* Los Angeles: Jeremy P. Tarcher.

Smith, B., & Cantrell, P. (1988). Distance in nurse-patient encounters. *Journal of Psychosocial Nursing, 26*(2), 22-26.

Sommer, R. (1959). Studies in personal space. *Sociometry, 22,* 247-260.

Spector, R. (1993). Cultural, ethnicity, and nursing. In Potter, P. & Perry, A. (Eds.), *Fundamentals of nursing. concepts process, and practice* (ed. 3). St. Louis: Mosby.

Statistics Canada. (1989). *A data book on Canada's Ab-original population from the 1986 census of Canada.* Ottawa: Statistics Canada, Aboriginal Peoples Output Program.

Stauffer, R. (1989). Personal communication, Honolulu, Hawaii.

Stauffer, R. (1995). Vietnamese Americans. In Giger, J., & Davidhizar, R. (Eds.), *Transcultural nursing, assessment, and intervention* (ed. 2). St. Louis: Mosby.

Stevenson, G. (1993). Transport and communications. In *Canada* (pp. 50-75). New York: Facts on File, Inc.

Stoltzfus, V. (1993, May). Language and culture. *Goshen College Bulletin,* p. 32.

Sudnow, D. (1967). *Passing on.* Englewood Cliffs, N.J.: Prentice Hall.

Sue, D., & Sue, D. (1990). *Counseling the culturally different: theory and practice* (ed. 2). New York: John Wiley & Sons.

Sullivan, H. (1954). *The interpersonal theory of psychiatry.* New York: W.W. Norton.

Taber, C. (1993). *Taber's cyclopedic medical dictionary* (ed. 17). Philadelphia: F.A. Davis.

Talbot, L. (1996). The power of words. *Canadian Journal of Nursing Research, 28* (1).

Taylor, C., Malone, B., & Kavanagh, K. (1997). Sociocultural aspects of love. In Johnson, B. (Ed.), *Psychiatric-mental health nursing* (ed. 4). Philadelphia: Lippincott.

Thayer, S. (1988, March). Close encounters. *Psychology Today,* pp. 31-36.

Thiederman, S.B. (1986). Ethnocentrism: a barrier to effective health care. *Nurse Practitioner, 11*(8), 52-59.

Thomas, W. I. (1937). *Primitive behavior: an introduction to the social sciences.* New York: McGraw-Hill.

Tripp-Reimer, T., & Friedl, M. (1977). Appalachians: a neglected minority. *Nursing Outlook, 32*(2), 41-45.

Urrutia-Rojas, X., & Aday, L.A. (1991). A framework for community assessment: designing and conducting a survey in a Hispanic immigrant and refugee community. *Public Health Nursing, 8*(1), 20-26.

Wardhaugh, R. (1993). Language policy. In *Canada* (pp. 1-25). New York: Facts on File, Inc.

Watzlawich, P., Beavin, J., & Jackson, D. (1967). *Pragmatics of human communication.* New York: W.W. Norton.

Whitcher, S.J., & Fisher, J.D. (1979). Multidimensional reaction to therapeutic touch in hospital setting. *Journal of Personality, Sociology, and Psychology, 37*(1), 87-96.

Young, T. (1994). *The health of Native Americans.* New York: Oxford University Press.

CHAPTER 3　Space

BEHAVIORAL OBJECTIVES

After reading this chapter, the nurse will be able to:

1. Discuss factors related to distance and immediate receptors that influence spatial behavior.
2. Define the term "personal space" and relate its significance to care plan development for clients from varying cultures.
3. Explain how actions of the nurse may contribute to feelings of anxiety and loss of control for clients from transcultural backgrounds.
4. List actions the nurse can take to promote feelings of autonomy and self-worth when caring for clients from transcultural backgrounds.
5. Delineate the difference between tactile space and visual space and the relationship to transcultural nursing care.

Personal space is the area that surrounds a person's body; it includes the space and the objects within the space. Personal space is an extension of the body and is also referred to as outer space; inner space refers to the personal state of consciousness or awareness (Haber, 1997; Sommer, 1969). An individual's comfort level is related to personal space, and discomfort is experienced when personal space is invaded. Although personal space is an individual matter and varies with the situation, dimensions of the personal space comfort zone also vary from culture to culture.

Spatial behavior is an important consideration in measuring distance in relationships. Since spatial behavior is usually judged to be spontaneous and unintentional, individuals are typically more likely to trust the accuracy of actions rather than words as a reflection of true feelings. Although a large percentage of spatial behaviors are spontaneous and unintentional, communication in this domain can be managed to promote favorable and desired impressions. For example, a nurse may

choose to stand when greeting a client to show respect.

To understand human behavior, one must understand something of the nature of our receptor systems and how the information received by these systems is modified by culture. Since spatial behavior is a response to sensory stimulation in the internal and external environment, the phenomenon of space can be understood only as an integral part of the sensory systems, that is, sight, sound, touch, and smell. Spatial behavior encompasses a variety of behaviors, including proximity to others, objects in the environment, and movement.

PERCEPTION OF SPACE

Sensory apparatuses fall into two categories:

1. *Distance receptors* are those apparatuses that are concerned with the examination of distant objects. The sensory receptors for distance include the eyes, ears, and nose.
2. *Immediate receptors* are those apparatuses that are used to examine the world up close. Sensory receptors used to examine the world up close in-

clude touch, which is the sensation received from the skin membranes (Hall, 1969, 1977).

These two classifications can be broken down even further to facilitate the nurse's understanding of the phenomenon of space. For example, the skin is the chief organ of touch and is sensitive to heat gain and heat loss—both radiant heat and conducted heat are detected by the skin. Therefore the skin must be perceived as both an immediate and a distance receptor. In general, there is a relationship between the evolutionary age of the receptor system and the amount and quality of information it can convey to the central nervous system. Many psychologists estimate that the touch system is as old as life itself (Hall, 1966). Because the ability to respond to stimuli is based on touch, the response to touch is one of the basic criteria for the maintenance of life. In comparison, sight is believed to be the last and most specialized sense to be developed in humans. From an anthropological view, vision became more important than olfactory response when our primitive ancestors left the ground and took to trees in search of food and safety. Stereoscopic vision became essential for our primate ancestors because without it jumping from branch to branch was difficult and dangerous.

Distance receptors

Distance receptors include sensory apparatuses for visual, auditory, and olfactory perception. It is essential that the nurse understand the relationship between sight, touch, and smell and how the reaction to these stimuli can be modified by culture.

Visual and auditory perception As indicated earlier, vision was the last of the senses to evolve. However, it is by far the most complex. Seemingly, more data are fed to the nervous system through the eyes at a much greater rate than through the senses of touch or hearing. For example, the information that can be gathered by a blind person outdoors is limited to a circle of 20 to 100 feet because a blind person can perceive by way of auditory or olfactory stimuli only what is immediately surrounding him or her. However, with sight a person can see the stars if there is a clear sky at night. Even very talented blind persons are limited to an average speed of per-

ception of 2 to 3 miles an hour over familiar territory. In contrast, with sight a person has to fly faster than sound before additional visual aids are needed to avoid bumping into things. The amount of information that can be gathered by the eyes as contrasted to the ears cannot be precisely calculated. If such a calculation were possible, it would require not only a translation process but also the ability on the part of scientists to know precisely what to count. A general notion held by most scientists is that the relative complexities of the two systems, visual and auditory, can be obtained by comparison of the size of the nerves connecting the eyes and the ears to the centers of the brain (Brown, Leavitt, and Graham, 1977).

The optic nerve contains roughly 18 times as many neurons as the cochlear nerve; therefore one might assume that it transmits at least that much more information. The eyes may act as a defense mechanism because they normally alert us to danger; the eyes may be as much as a thousand times more effective than the ears in gathering information to protect us from harmful stimuli. The area that the unaided ear can effectively cover in the course of daily living is quite limited. The ear is very efficient but only up to a distance of 20 feet. At about 100 feet one-way vocal communication is possible but at a somewhat slower rate than at a conversational distance. Although two-way conversation is also possible at this distance, it is considerably altered. Beyond this distance the auditory cues begin to break down rapidly. The unaided eye, on the other hand, can gather an extraordinary amount of information within a 100-yard radius and is efficient for human interaction at up to a mile (Hall, 1969).

The impulses that activate the eyes and the ears differ in speed and quality. For example, at a temperature of 0° C (32° F) at sea level, sound waves can travel 1100 feet per second and be heard in frequencies of 50 to 1500 cycles per second (Hertz). On the other hand, light rays can travel 186,000 miles per second and thus are visible at a maximal frequency of 500 trillion per second at yellow-green (Hall, 1969).

Many complex and remarkable instruments have been invented to extend the eyes and ears. Radio and television have revolutionized the perception of space and shortened distances between people worldwide. During World War II, radio was relied on quite extensively to bring news from the occupied countries to parts of the free world. Perhaps one of the most famous broadcasts of this period was done by Tokyo Rose, whose broadcasts, which were reported to be untrue, influenced many people in the listening audience about the nature and direction of World War II. However, radio lacked the visual stimuli offered later by television, which filled in perception gaps left by radio. Television came of age in the 1960s, when for the first time, brighter, clearer, and bolder pictures were offered to viewers. The addition of color filled another perception gap and enhanced our receptor fields. For the first time in history, from their living rooms, the people of the United States could view their president doing the ordinary, the extraordinary, and the unusual. For example, the people of the United States were informed about the Cuban missile crisis by their President Kennedy on television. They were also able to see their president playing with his children in the Oval Office. In 1963, when President Kennedy was assassinated, nothing was left to the imagination of the people of the United States who were mesmerized by complete television coverage from assassination to burial. Because of television the nation and the world at large experienced grief still present today and mourned collectively. In 1997, when Princess Diana (formerly Her Royal Highness, Princess of Wales) was killed in a tragic automobile accident, it was estimated that more than 2 billion people mourned throughout the world collectively through the modern medium of television. It is believed that her legend, though admirable, was largely created and captured imaginatively by the media.

In summary, visual space has an entirely different character from that of auditory space. The overriding quality that differentiates visual space from auditory space is that visual information tends to be less ambiguous and more focused than auditory information is. Therefore visual information is less subject to external manipulation than auditory information is. One major exception to this rule is the blind person who has learned to understand selectively the high range of audio frequencies, which can assist in locating objects within a familiar or unfamiliar room. For example, a blind person may know where the door is in a room by the relationship of the sound that comes from that direction.

Even today it is not known what effects the incongruencies between auditory and visual space have on individuals. Some data indicate that auditory space may be a factor in performance. J.W. Black, a phonetician, demonstrated that the size and reverberation (vibrations of external sounds) of a room can affect an individual's reading rate. In a classic study, Black (1950) found that people read more slowly in larger rooms, where the reverberation time, or circulation of sound, is slower than in smaller rooms. Hall (1966, 1969) interviewed subjects in regard to the slowing of reverberation time in a larger room. Among the interviewees was a gifted English architect who improved the performance of a malfunctioning committee by simply blending the auditory and visual worlds of the conference chamber where the committee met. The complaint the architect had received was that the chairman was inadequate and was about to be replaced. However, the architect had reason to believe that the difficulties encountered by this committee were caused by more problems in the environment than just the chairman. In this situation the meeting room was next to a busy street where traffic noises were intensified by reverberations from the hard walls and rugless floors inside the building and particularly in the meeting room. The architect was able to readjust the room by adding an acoustic ceiling, carpet, and soundproof walls. Once interferences were reduced, the chairman was able to conduct the meeting without undue strain, and complaints about the chairman ceased.

People who are brought up in different cultures learn unknowingly to screen out various information and to sort information into relevant or irrelevant categories, and once set, these perceptual patterns remain stable throughout life. For example, Japanese people screen visually in a variety of ways and are more perceptive to visual stimuli. Japanese people are therefore perfectly content with paper walls as acoustic screens. A Westerner who finds himself in a Japanese inn where a party is going on next door may be in for a new sensory experience, since only paper-thin walls separate each room. In contrast, German and Dutch people depend on double doors and thick walls to screen out sound and may have difficulty if they must rely on their own powers of concentration to screen out sound. If two rooms are the same size and one screens out sound and the other one does not, a sensitive German or Dutch person who is trying to concentrate will feel less intruded on in the former than in the latter and thus less crowded (Hall, 1966, 1969).

Olfactory perception Some cultures place more importance on olfactory perceptions than others do. For example, Hall (1966, 1969) found Americans culturally underdeveloped in the use of the olfactory apparatus. Hall (1966) contended that the deprivations of the olfactory stimulus are a result of the extensive use of deodorants and the suppression of odors in public places, which has resulted in a land of olfactory blandness and sameness that is difficult to duplicate anywhere else in the world.

People in Canada and the United States are continuously bombarded with commercials for room deodorizers, antiperspirants, mouthwashes, carpet deodorizers, and so on. All these factors result in bland, undifferentiated spaces and deprive many people in Canada and the United States of the richness and variety of life. For example, if one is cooking with garlic, a room deodorizer may be used during the cooking process, causing the garlic smell to be eliminated. It is this type of behavior on the part of Canadian and United States people that obscures memories. It is believed that smells evoke much deeper memories than either vision or sound; when the sound or the sight of what has happened has passed, the memory of the smell lingers on. Even today many Canadian and United States citizens equate certain holidays, such as Christmas, with certain smells. For example, since Christmas is traditionally equated with the smell of baked goods, holly, pine, and fruit, today many people in Canada and the United States try to reproduce these smells at Christmas. An individual who has an artificial Christmas tree may buy a pine-scented spray to create the effects of a fresh tree. Another old-fashioned scent for many Canadian and United States citizens

is country potpourri, which has now been simulated in aerosol cans for easy dispensing. A new car can be simulated by a car spray that smells like new leather. Soap may be purchased to recreate a desired feeling; for example, the soap mother used at home may create a feeling of hominess. Smells may also create a negative reaction. For example, an individual who washes with lye soap may be thought to have body odor because the smell is unusually strong and medicinal. A medicinal smell is perceived by most persons in Canada and the United States to be appropriate for a hospital room but not in a non–health care setting.

Odor is perhaps one of the most basic methods of communication. It is primarily chemical in nature and is therefore referred to in a chemical sense. The olfactory sense has diverse functions and not only differentiates individuals, but also makes it possible to identify the emotional state of others. Even an infant can learn to identify his or her parents through the sense of smell. Although the young infant has not learned to see and discriminate patterns well, the infant can distinguish identity through the olfactory sense.

In a hospital setting an employee who has an unpleasant odor creates a real management dilemma. The supervisor may counsel and even reprimand the employee for poor hygiene. Employees who have the smell of alcohol may be sent home. It is important that the nurse appreciate that odors may be pathological, as in certain diabetic states, or the result of certain mouthwashes or soaps. If a client has an unpleasant odor, the nurse should first assess whether some pathological condition is present, such as an inflammatory process. In a psychiatric hospital, a client's odor could be associated with a condition such as schizophrenia, and although there is some thought that such an odor may be pathological, it is more likely to be related to a lack of motivation for self-care skills.

Immediate receptors

Immediate receptors are those that examine the world up close and include tactile stimuli received by way of the skin membranes. It is important that the nurse appreciate the effect culture may have on an individual's reaction to these stimuli and how these stimuli can be modified by cultural influences.

Skin membranes Human beings receive a tremendous amount of information from the distance receptors, which include the eyes, ears, and nose. Because of the vast amount of information that is received from the distance receptors, few people think of the skin as a major sense organ. However, if we humans lacked the ability to perceive heat and cold, we would soon perish. Without the ability to perceive heat and cold or to react appropriately to these stimuli, we would freeze in the winter and become overheated in the summer. The skin, as a major sense organ, is so grossly overlooked that even some of its subtle sensing and communicating qualities are overlooked. Nerves called "proprioceptors" keep us informed as to exactly what is happening as we work our muscles. These nerves provide the feedback that enables us to move our bodies smoothly; thus they occupy a key position in kinesthetic space perception. The body also has another set of nerves called "exteroceptors," which are located in the skin and convey the sensations of heat, cold, touch, and pain to the central nervous system. In light of the fact that two different systems of nerves are employed in the perception of space, kinesthetic space is considered qualitatively different from thermal space. However, nurses must remember that these two systems work together and that they are mutually reinforcing most of the time.

It has been only in modern scientific times that some remarkable thermal characteristics of the skin have been discovered. The capacity of the skin for emitting and detecting radiant or infrared heat is extraordinarily high. One might assume that because the capacity of the skin to emit and detect radiant or infrared heat is so highly developed, it was important to survival in the past and most certainly had a significant function in early human beings. Although the discovery of the thermal characteristics of the skin has occurred only within recent times, the importance of the skin as an immediate receptor should not be overlooked by the nurse.

Humans are well equipped to send and receive messages concerning emotional states based on changes in skin temperature. Skin temperature can give very important clues to the emotional state of the individual. A common indicator of embarrassment or anger in fair-skinned individuals is blushing. However, dark-skinned people also blush. Therefore blushing cannot be perceived as simply a matter of change in skin coloration. The nurse must carefully observe dark-skinned persons when looking for changes in emotional state such as embarrassment or anger by observing a swelling of regions of the forehead. The additional blood to these areas will raise the temperature, and these areas will appear flushed. Therefore, even if there is no significant change in color to these areas in dark-skinned individuals, these areas will appear warm to the touch.

Many novel instruments have been developed to make it possible to study heat emission. These instruments should make it possible to study the thermal details of interpersonal communication, an area not previously accessible to direct observation. Thermographic devices (infrared detaching devices and cameras) that were originally developed for satellites and homing missiles have been developed for recording subvisual phenomena. Photographs taken in the dark using radiant heat of the human body have shown that an inflamed area of the body actually emits more heat than the surrounding areas do. Diagnosis of cancer is also possible with thermographic devices that measure blocked circulation of blood. Thermographic devices have been useful in health care delivery because skin color does not affect the amount of heat delivered; dark skin does not emit more or less heat than light skin does. Thus the observable phenomenon in all individuals regarding heat emission is the blood supply in a given area of the body.

Increased heat on the surface is detected in three ways:

1. Thermal detectors in the skin, particularly if two individuals are close enough to each other.
2. Intensified olfactory interactions, which are augmented when skin temperature rises. Perfumes or body or face lotions may be smelled at a greater distance when the body temperature is increased.
3. Visual examination, which can give clues to an increase or decrease in body temperature. For ex-

ample, an individual who is pale may have a decrease in body temperature, whereas a person who appears flushed may have an increase in body temperature.

Certain individuals or racial groups are more aware of subtle changes in skin temperature. In addition, some persons accentuate or take advantage of this medium of communication. For example, an individual knowledgeable about variations in skin temperature according to location may apply perfume to certain parts of the body. The phenomenon of crowding is a chain reaction set in motion when there is not enough space to dissipate the heat within a crowd and the heat becomes more intense. A hot crowd will require more room than a cool crowd if they are to maintain the same degree of comfort and lack of involvement. It is important for the nurse to remember that when thermal spaces overlap and people can smell each other, they become more involved and may even be under the chemical influences of each other's emotions. Some individuals by virtue of cultural heritage have trouble with the phenomenon of crowding. These individuals are more likely to be unable to sit in a chair soon after someone else has vacated it. An example of this phenomenon is often given by sailors on submarines who are forced to participate in "hot bunking," the practice of sharing a bunk as soon as someone gets out of it. It is not understood why one's own heat is not objectionable whereas a stranger's may be. It may be attributable in part to the fact that humans have a great sensitivity to small differences; therefore individuals respond negatively to a heat pattern that is not familiar (Hall, 1966, 1969).

Body-heat regulation lies deep in the brain and is controlled by the hypothalamus. Culture affects attitudes in regard to the perception of skin-temperature changes. Human beings exert little or no conscious control over the heat system of the body. Many cultural groups tend to stress phenomena that can be controlled and deny those that cannot. In other words, because some individuals by virtue of their cultural heritage have been taught to ignore certain uncontrollable stimuli, they experience body heat as a highly personal stimulus. Body heat is therefore linked to intimacy as well as to the

experiences of childhood. An adult who as a child was used to close personal contact with parents and other loved ones may have a pleasant association when in a crowded environment where heat and warmth are radiated. On the other hand, an adult who was subjected to discomfort in close relationships or who was not exposed to closeness as a child may experience a great deal of difficulty and anxiety when in a close environment, such as an overcrowded bus.

A person born in a heavily populated country where closeness was necessitated by overcrowding may experience conscious discomfort in moving to another locality where closeness is not the norm. On the other hand, persons born in thinly populated countries may have a conscious feeling of overcrowding in a country where closeness is the norm. For example, a tourist from Canada visiting a country such as Hong Kong, Jamaica, or China, all of which are extremely overpopulated, may quickly react to the experience of closeness and associate the country with unpleasantness. This experience is not limited to different cultures but may also be noted when a rural person visits an urban setting, such as a Canadian from Red Lake, Ontario, visiting Quebec City.

The English language is full of expressions that relate to skin sensation and body temperature changes. For example, it is not uncommon in the United States and Canada to hear individuals say that another person made them hot under the collar, gave them a cold stare, involved them in a heated argument, or warmed them up. These expressions may be more than just a figure of speech; they may be a way of recognizing the changes in body temperature that occur both personally and in other people. Thus these common experiences have been incorporated into the language in the United States and Canada.

Relationship between tactile space and visual space

Touch and visual spatial experiences are so interwoven with one another that they cannot be separated easily. Young children and infants learn to reach, grasp, fondle, and mouth everything in the environment. Teaching children the relationship between tactile and visual space is a difficult task that requires many years of training for children to subordinate the world of touch to the visual world. Visual and tactile space can be distinguished by the fact that tactile space separates the viewer from the object, whereas visual space separates objects from each other. As early as 1945, Michael Baliant described two different perceptual worlds: sight oriented and touch oriented. According to Baliant, the touch-oriented world is both immediate and friendlier than the sight-oriented world, in which space is friendly but filled with dangerous and unpredictable objects, namely, people. Using Baliant's definition of tactile space, it is difficult to conceive that designers and engineers have failed to grasp in all of their scientific research the deep significance of touch, particularly active touch (actually contacting others or objects). Individuals incorporate both tactile and visual stimuli in relating to the world. For example, although automakers tend to rely heavily on visual perception when designing a particular automobile, they are also concerned with tactile perception, as evidenced by their giving attention to such things such as luxury upholstery, automatic windows, doors, gas cap locks, ornate trimmings, and carpeting. In response to these stimuli, prospective buyers touch both the car's interior and exterior before making a purchase.

Some objects in the environment are appraised and appreciated almost entirely by touch, even when these objects are visually presented, such as objects made from wood, cloth, or ceramics. The Japanese are very conscious of the significance of texture. Emphasis is placed on the smoothness of the item being crafted. It may be perceived that it requires more time to make a smooth-textured item than a rough-textured item and that the time spent on the crafted item is related to the care and concern of the craftsman. The objects that are produced by Japanese people may be perceived as being made by caring craftsmen.

Touch is the most personal of all the sensations. Touch is sometimes described as the most important sense because it confirms the reality perceived through the other senses (Montagu, 1971). Touch is central to the human communication process and is often used to communicate messages. Beyond general communication, touch is associated with breaking down the distance between individuals. Most people associate life's most intimate moments with touch. For example, during lovemaking or in a loving relationship, touch takes on a private and special meaning. Nurses have long appreciated touch as an important component of the nurse-client interaction (Clement, 1987; Giger, Davidhizar, Johnson, and Poole, 1997). Nurses face the challenge of developing trust, creating a humanistic and responsive atmosphere, and effectively exchanging information in a system energized by high technology and concern for cost effectiveness. Most nursing literature focuses on touch as a communication behavior and describes using touch to communicate caring (Geldard, 1960; Leininger, 1977; Mintz, 1969; Montagu, 1971), the physiological and psychological dynamics of touch (Davidhizar and Giger, 1989; Giger and Davidhizar, 1995; Spector, 1996; Goodykoontz, 1980; Hedlund and Jeffrey, 1992; Heidt, 1981; Krieger, 1975; Lynch, 1978; West, 1981), and the components of touch behavior. Research also supports the belief that using touch appropriately with clients can result in positive physiological and psychological responses (Day, 1973; Seaman, 1982; Ujhely, 1979). Nurses need to be aware of the characteristics of touch and how they can affect the entire communication process.

In contrast to tactile space is the phenomenon of visual space. To understand visual space, the nurse must understand that no persons see exactly the same thing when actively using their eyes in a natural situation; people do not relate to the world around them in exactly the same way. For example, different persons will visually notice different objects because of perceptual differences (Davidhizar, Dowd, and Giger, 1997). It is important for the nurse to recognize these differences and at the same time be able to translate from one perceptual world to another. The distance between the perceptual worlds of two persons of the same culture may be considerably less than the distance between the perceptual worlds of two persons of different cultures. There is significant evidence that people brought up in different cultures live in different perceptual worlds. North Americans tend to have a more linear perceptual field. This difference is demonstrated in art and architectural design. North American artists prefer designs that are linear, whereas Chinese and Japanese artists prefer depth and maintaining constancy in a design.

SPATIAL BEHAVIOR

Spatial behavior is often described in nursing literature in relation to the universal need for territoriality (Allekian, 1973; Davidhizar, 1988; Hayter, 1981; Hedlund and Jeffrey, 1992; Oland, 1978; Reakes, 1997; Brant, 1983). People by nature are territorial. Territoriality refers to a state characterized by possessiveness, control, and authority over an area of physical space. If the need for territoriality is to be met, the person must be in control of some space and must be able to establish rules for that space. The need for territoriality cannot be fully met unless individuals can defend their space against invasion or misuse by others (Roberts, 1978). Hayter (1981) has suggested three important aspects of territoriality to consider when planning nursing care: a physical space of one's own, a personal space, and the territory of expertise or role. One can also relate territoriality needs to spatial behaviors of or proximity to others, to objects in the environment, and to body movement or position. Territoriality serves to achieve diverse functions for individuals, including meeting needs for security, privacy, autonomy, and self-identity. A variety of factors may influence needs for territoriality, including culture, age, sex, and health status. It is important for the nurse to understand the effect such variables may have on spatial behavior.

Proximity to others

Proxemics is the term for the study of human use and perception of social and personal space (Hall, 1974). Physical distancing varies with setting and is culturally learned (Murray and Huelskoetter, 1991). Generally, in Western culture there are three primary dimensions of space: the intimate zone (0 to 18 inches), the personal zone (18 inches to 3 feet), and the social or public zone (3 to 6 feet) (Hall, 1966). The intimate zone may be used for comforting, pro-

tecting, and counseling and is reserved for people who feel close. The personal zone usually is maintained with friends or in some counseling interactions. Touch can occur in the intimate and personal zones. The social zone is normally used when impersonal business is conducted or with people who are working together. Sensory involvement and communication are often less intense in the social zone. Wide variations to these general dimensions do occur and are often influenced by cultural background (Giger and Davidhizar, 1990, 1995). Montagu (1971) has suggested that child-rearing practices affecting sleep behavior may have an effect on the use of space, especially as it determines acceptable interaction distance. He reported on varying cultural approaches apparently related to family group sleeping arrangements and the Western middle-class practice of separating the child from parents for sleep. According to Oland (1978), the Western practice of putting small children in a room of their own, which separates them from other family members, may enculturate children to desire isolation and separation and cause or facilitate a desire for more extensive territory.

Among the Inuit and northern Indians of Canada, the practice of separate bedrooms varies dramatically because living quarters are often small, with all persons sleeping in the same room (Brucke, Maloney, Pothaar, and Baumgart, 1988; Lefever and Davidhizar, 1995; Young, 1988; Giger and Davidhizar, 1995). For these individuals, proximity to others in small living quarters is often a necessity for survival because staying inside with the body heat of others may be necessary to avoid freezing in the frigid arctic temperatures (Lefever and Davidhizar, 1995). The need for space also varies for many Southeast Asian immigrants who have come to Canada as refugees. These individuals are also accustomed to living in crowded living situations. Therefore, for some Southeast-Asian Canadians, spacious living accommodations may cause discomfort (Van Esterik, 1980; Stauffer, 1995).

Spatial needs and the desire for a certain proximity to certain people continue throughout life and have been studied in the elderly. In nursing homes, elderly clients may have certain chairs identified as theirs and become upset when a stranger sits in their chair or in the seat nearby that is reserved for a special friend. Moving from household to household to stay with children on a rotating basis, rather than being viewed as a pleasant variation, is also likely to be upsetting. Since the elderly are more likely to experience separation from others through the death of a spouse and the moving away of offspring, their spatial needs may appear to change; that is, they may withdraw or may reach out more for others (Ittelson, Proshansky, Rivlin, and Winkel, 1974).

Interpersonal messages are communicated not only by body proximity but also by the location and availability of the nurse during the day. A client who knows that the nurse will answer when the call bell is pressed feels differently from the client who does not understand how the call bell works or believes that it is an imposition to ask for help and waits for the nurse to ask what can be done (Schuster and Ashburn, 1986).

Individuals have different requirements for sensory stimulation. Either overstimulation, as by crowding, or understimulation, as by isolation, may cause an untoward reaction. For example, in times of disaster overstimulation induced by crowding can be so extreme that it can result in insanity or death. In this example, a person is perceived as being in a little black box and unable to move about freely, and such a perception causes the person to jostle, push, and shove. How the individual responds to jostling and therefore to the enclosed space depends on how he or she feels about being touched by strangers. It is this constant touching and being touched that may result in widespread panic and "freezing" in disaster situations (Hall, 1966).

An enclosed space requirement can also be overstimulating. For example, a client who must remain in a hospital room in bed and in isolation for a lengthy period can be overstimulated because of the spatial limits presented by the boundaries, including bed rest and the four walls of the room. Nursing interventions for this client include opening curtains, calling by intercom frequently to check on the client, and stopping by to see the client as often as possible. A client in isolation can suffer from understimulation in regard to tactile stimulation. The few people who do enter the room may hesitate to touch the client out of fear of contracting the illness. One of the greatest problems expressed by clients with acquired immunodeficiency syndrome (AIDS) is the isolation they experience because of physical distancing from others. Family members afraid of catching AIDS may hesitate to touch, hug, or kiss the AIDS victim. Caregivers also may show their fear by standing a greater distance from the client, wearing gloves, and having less frequent encounters with the client (Zook and Davidhizar, 1989).

The strong link between curing, the major focus of health care, and caring by health care practitioners has been emphasized by Leininger (1977), who cites touch as one of the special constructs of the caring process. As a therapeutic element of human interaction, touch can help the nurse to show caring.

Cultural implications Watson (1980) noted that although there are variations in spatial requirements from individual to individual, persons in the same cultural group tend to act similarly. For example, nomads do not seem to desire a permanent territory but are content with establishing a temporary territory and then moving on. Because individuals are usually not consciously aware of their personal space requirements, they frequently have difficulty understanding a different cultural pattern. What may be considered an act of friendliness by one person (such as standing close to another person) may be perceived by the other as a threatening invasion of personal space. A person who wishes to maintain distance will indicate this by body language. Clients who step back, do not face the nurse directly, or pull their chair back from the nurse are sending messages indicating additional space requirements. The nurse's responsiveness to the client's spatial requirements is an important factor in the client's emotional comfort. It is important that the nurse be cognizant of the effects of culture on the client's spatial needs and use sensitivity in responding to the client's need for personal territory. Subtle cultural variations in the use of nonverbal signals often lead to misunderstanding; thus, to meet the client needs, it is essential that the nurse have knowledge of cultural variations in spatial requirements.

Nurses and clients from the population groups of Native Americans, Appalachians, Japanese Americans, and Mexican Americans often find a comfortable position between the personal and social distance (Tripp-Reimer and Lively, 1993). Watson (1980) studied cultural differences in the use of personal space. He compiled a range of space by nationality and found that persons in the United States, Canadians, and the British require the most personal space, whereas Latin Americans, Japanese, and Arabic persons need the least. These latter groups seemingly have a much higher tolerance for crowding in public spaces than do some other cultural groups, such as North Americans and northern Europeans, but they also appear to be more concerned about their own requirements for the space they live in. In particular, the Japanese tend to devote more time and attention to the proper organization of their living space for perception by all the senses (Hall, 1966). Asians are generally more sensitive to personal space and are more likely to feel comfortable conversing from a distance of 5 or 6 feet. Maintaining distance in relationships for some Asian Canadians is an indication of respect. Therefore it important to remember to avoid invading the personal space of these individuals. Some West Indians maintain little space between friends when communicating. For some West Indians, an outsider is expected to maintain some distance when interacting (Carson and Arnold, 1996).

A White Canadian female nurse from a nontactile culture may experience discomfort when a male client from a tactile culture, such as the Latin, African, or Indonesian culture, stands in the intimate zone while describing symptoms (Rawlins, Williams, and Beck, 1993; Tripp-Reimer and Friedl, 1977). Touching between persons of the same sex, including men, is more common among Arabic or South Vietnamese persons than it is among Americans. In the United States this kind of familiarity may be considered a homosexual pass (Hall, 1966). Hall and Whyte (1990) note that a handshake in Latin America, particularly between two men, is seen as cold and impersonal. For some Latins, the *doble abrazo,* in which two men embrace by placing their arms around each other's shoulders, is the accepted form of greeting. On the other hand, touching the shoulders of a Japanese man is seen as a humiliation and an unpardonable breach of traditional etiquette. Argyle and Dean (1965) reported that members of primitive societies in Africa and Indonesia also came close and maintained body contact during conversation.

In the Thai and Vietnamese cultures, the head is sacred and patting the head of a small child is considered offensive (Stauffer, 1995). For these individuals the head is considered to be the "seat of life." When the head is touched, it is believed that the spirit leaves through this channel. Therefore when the head needs to be touched for medical reasons, it is important to explain the reason and to ask permission from the adults (Carson and Arnold, 1996; Randall-David, 1989).

In Western culture a person who stands at a slight angle to another person indicates body position of readiness to communicate. A desire to exclude a third person can be shown by two persons who face each other directly and have ongoing eye contact. Rejection is also communicated by a person who stands at a right angle to another (Scheflen, 1972). The position of the toes can create distance by communicating rank. A person who feels subordinate will usually stand with the toes inward, whereas a person who feels superior will stand with the toes facing out (Personal Report for the Executive, 1987). A comparison of the movie shown in the United States *Three Men and a Baby* and the French comedy on which it was based, *Three Men and a Cradle,* illustrates the differences in responses in the two cultures. In the French version when the natural father returns to the two bachelors who have been inconvenienced by the care of the baby, icy silence occurs. The two men sit stiffly in their chairs and refuse to answer their friend's questions or even acknowledge his presence. In the version seen in the United States, when the natural father returns, he is pummeled and a loud scene occurs (Grosvenor, 1989).

Territoriality influences relationships between people. Some German people tend to need a larger space and are less flexible in their spatial behavior than some American, French, and Arabic people. Differences in spatial patterns between persons in different cultures apply not only to their body proximity, but also to such behavior as changing geographic location. For example, Germans often live in the same house their entire lives, Americans tend to change houses approximately every 5 years, and nomads are content with temporary territories rather than permanent ones. According to Evans and Howard (1973), some Puerto Ricans and African Americans may have different perspectives about space. Some African Americans have more eye contact when they speak, have greater body activity, and have a closer personal space (Sue and Sue, 1990). However, as indicated in Chapter 2, some African Canadians have been socialized through a long history of hostile, punitive interactions with Whites to avoid direct eye contact. This behavior may also influence personal space zones (Giger, Davidhizar, Evers, and Ingram, 1994; Giger and Davidhizar, 1995).

Objects in the environment

Objects in the environment offer additional dimensions to communication and can provide both positive and negative qualifiers to verbal communication. Easily movable chairs in a waiting room or office can be pulled together to provide physical closeness or separated to provide distance. Positioning chairs at a 90-degree angle can communicate a cooperative stance, whereas a side-by-side arrangement of chairs can decrease communication. Discomfort and consequently emotional distance can be created by uncomfortable furniture. The nurse's position during the conversation (such as sitting behind a desk or leaning against the corner of the desk looking down on the client seated at a lower level) can also promote the perception of psychological distance. The nurse must be aware of the effect culture may play on the client's reaction to objects in the environment and should respond in a way that client comfort will be increased (Pearlin, 1982). The nurse dealing with Native Canadians should appreciate the value Native Canadians place on objects they possess. These individuals tend to highly value generosity and a sense of sharing: "What is mine is here for all." For some of these people, only what is needed for the present is taken and used. This can be

a problem for the Native Canadian who is diabetic because if food is available, it will be shared with anyone, regardless of the special health needs (McRae, 1994).

Cleanliness in the environment may also be a significant factor in creating a healthy and comfortable milieu. Comfortable air conditioning in a client waiting room on a hot day can facilitate a client's ease and decrease anxiety. On the other hand, when the air conditioning is absent or malfunctioning on a hospital ward on a hot day, client and staff anxiety can escalate.

When the nurse is interacting with Native Canadians from rural settings, it is important to be aware that their lifestyle may be substandard by the nurse's standards. For some Native Canadians, living standards are substandard, and homes are often poorly heated, have no indoor plumbing, have unsafe water supplies, and lack telephones. A lack of vehicles and poor roads limit accessibility to facilities for food, clothing, and health service for many of these people. The environment can be profoundly important when ongoing health care is needed to monitor a chronic illness or to prevent recurrence of an acute illness (McRae, 1994).

Structural boundaries The term "personal boundaries" is sometimes used to describe the use of structural boundaries in the environment. A boundary separates a person from others and also helps define a person's space. Fences, doors, curtains, walls, desks, chairs, and other objects may create boundaries between persons (Scott, 1988). The purpose of a boundary is to facilitate individuation or separation from the environment. Developmentally, this concept begins at approximately 6 months of age. Mahler, Pine, and Bergman (1975) described an infant's first attempts at separation or individuation as consisting of behaviors such as pulling at the parent's hair, ears, or nose and pushing the body away from the parent to get a better look at him or her. At 7 to 8 months of age the infant begins to differentiate self from the parent. The child may examine the parent's jewelry or glasses and is anxious around others. These crucial developmental steps are indicative of the child's beginning formation of boundary, which continues throughout the toddler stage. By 3 years of age the toddler has a fairly stable sense of identity and self-boundaries.

Doors, walls, glass panels, and waist-high partitions serve as structural boundaries for nurses' territories in health care settings. Doors, curtains, and furniture arrangements may define client territories. Structural boundaries can help the individual adapt to both internal and external stresses. On the other hand, when structural boundaries are violated, anxiety may increase. The nurse needs to assess whether the client has rigid or flexible boundaries. If a client has open boundaries, less anxiety will be encountered in interactions with health professionals, who may violate personal boundaries. If the client has rigid boundaries, the nurse should guard against approaches that may be perceived as threatening.

The use of restraints with agitated clients involves physical invasion of both intimate space and body boundaries. Patients who resist restraints and become aggressive and combative may be viewed as resisting this personal invasion.

Just as individuals can be described by personal boundaries that determine comfort levels in relation to others, territoriality also describes an interpersonal phenomenon in the environment. As indicated earlier, territoriality is a state characterized by possessiveness, control, and authority over an area of physical space (Hayter, 1981). For the need for territoriality to be met fully, the person must be in control of some space, be able to establish rules for that space, and be able to defend it against invasion or misuse by others. In addition, the person's right to do things in the space must be acknowledged by others (Roberts, 1978). For example, a hospitalized client needs not only a personal sleeping area, but also a place to put and arrange personal belongings without fear that they will be bothered by others. There should also be freedom to do things in the personal space, such as taking a nap.

Nursing staff also have professional territorial imperatives. Nurses' stations and lounges may be designated as staff territory. When a psychiatric unit is renovated and staff are asked by administration to move from a locked nursing station concept to an open nursing station concept wherein clients may come to an open half wall to interact openly with staff who may be inside, staff may find this very intrusive of "their" territory and object to this invasion of their space. Nursing staff may also fear personal assault (Croker and Cummings, 1995; Roberts, 1991; Roberts, 1989). Staff needs for territory must be considered when unit staff and clients' areas are designed. Restricting certain staff from certain hospital areas (such as the mailroom or the copy machine room) may be seen as punitive and dehumanizing. Thus it is essential that explanations given for this restriction be clearly understood to avoid paranoid interpretations of this action.

Cultural implications Color is a phenomenon with cultural implications. In many North American cultures, warm colors such as yellow, red, and orange tend to stimulate creative and happy responses. In some Asian countries, white is associated with a funeral. In many African countries, red symbolizes witchcraft and death (Carson and Arnold, 1996). In some North Americans countries such as Canada and the United States, good mental health is often associated with the ability to coordinate the color of one's wardrobe (Ramirez, 1991). In contrast, in some countries in Africa, the Caribbean, and the South Pacific, bright, multiple colors are the accepted norm of dress (Carson and Arnold, 1996). Leff and Isaacs (1981) noted that a scarf tied around the forehead may not "indicate royalty" or schizophrenia but may be a cultural response by a West Indian to a headache. In Western culture, cool colors such as blue, green, and gray tend to encourage meditation and deliberation and thus may have a dampening effect on communication. The nurse should plan color in the environment to be therapeutic in an effort to enhance communication (Bartholet, 1968; Mufford, 1992).

Body movement or position

Body movement or position can also communicate a message to others. This concept has been well documented by the pioneering work of Efron (1941), Birdwhistell (1970), Scheflen (1972), Ekman and Friesen (1975), and Ekman (1985) and by recent reviews of the state of the art in this field (Bull, 1983; Davis, 1975; Davis and Skupien, 1982;

Hickson and Stacks, 1985; Wolfgang, 1984; Leathers, 1992). This information has also been applied to counseling and psychotherapeutic techniques through the work of Moreno (1946); Gendlin (1969); Steere (1982); Marcus (1985); and Perls, Hefferline, and Goodman (1983), all of whom made body movement and awareness central aspects of their therapeutic approach. Thus a broad body of knowledge supports the premise that through body movement a person may convey what is not verbalized.

It is well known that body movements may be of particular importance during periods of stress. Expressions of self through movement are learned before speech; therefore, when stress is experienced, a person may revert to a form of expression used at an earlier level. Attention to body movement can facilitate understanding of a person experiencing stress. There are endless expressions of body movement, such as finger pointing, head nodding, smiles, slaps on the back, head and general body movements, and even body sounds, including belching, knuckle cracking, and laughing. A seemingly insignificant act such as how a door bell is rung may bear the stamp of an individual's personality as well as emotional state. For example, the door bell may be rung loudly, impatiently, repetitively, tentatively, feebly, or aggressively (Bendich, 1988).

The nurse must also consider the effect of slow versus fast movements (Newman, 1976). In an emergency rapid movements are essential. On the other hand, a young child in the hospital for the first time may be frightened by a health professional who enters the room quickly, approaches the child rapidly, and picks the child up. In another situation an agitated psychiatric client who is approached slowly and with a quiet voice may be calmed by the slow movements of the nurse, which are seen as reassuring.

Nurses are also exploring movement as a therapeutic medium, such as movement therapy for the aged (Goldberg and Fitzpatrick, 1980; Stevenson, 1989), movement therapy after inactivity or infection (Folta, 1989; Kasper, 1989), dance and movement therapy, and exercise to music. It has been believed that movement therapy can provide a way to communicate when the ability to communicate feelings is limited. Movement therapy has also been used for relaxation and to provide relief of blocked emotion.

Body motions, or kinetic behaviors, can be categorized as follows (Knapp and Hall, 1992):

1. *Emblems.* Nonverbal actions that have a verbal translation into a word, phrase, or symbol. This includes sign language used in the operating room or the gesture of thumb and forefinger to form a circle to say "A-OK" in the United States or to indicate an obscenity in Brazil.
2. *Affect displays.* Facial expressions such as a frown, smile, or lips pulled down at the corners.
3. *Illustrations.* Nonverbal acts accompanying speech. Examples of this include an upturned thumb to indicate a ride is desired or pointing a finger to indicate a direction.
4. *Adapters.* Nonverbal behavior that modifies or adds to what is being said. For example, folded arms may indicate disgust or that a person is feeling closed to others; a wave may be used as a friendly greeting; leg swinging and finger tapping may indicate anxiety.
5. *Regulators.* Movements that maintain interaction and provide feedback. Head nods or changing gaze can indicate that it is the other person's turn to talk. A head nod can also indicate listening.

Cultural implications Body movement is also related to culture. For example, in the United States, head nodding is common, whereas in Africa the torso is frequently moved (Eibl-Eibesfeldt, 1972). Gestures are used by Americans and British to denote activity and by Italian or Jewish persons to emphasize words (Bigham, 1964). In some cultures, certain actions are not considered proper with strangers, such as touching, standing close to, or looking directly at a person. Some cultures give certain body movements a sexual interpretation. In the Western culture, stroking the hair, adjusting the clothes, or changing position to accent maleness or femaleness may have or be given a sexual connotation (Scheflen, 1972). Although a kiss is often given a sexual connotation in the United States, the Japanese kiss to show deference to superiors (Sue and Sue, 1990).

IMPLICATIONS FOR NURSING CARE

It is important for the nurse to remember that territoriality, or the need for space, serves four functions: security, privacy, autonomy, and self-identity (Oland, 1978). The nurse needs an understanding of cultural diversity and culturally appropriate behaviors in relation to these functions (Carson and Arnold, 1996; England, 1986). Security includes actual safety from harm and gives the person a feeling of being safe. The nurse must also remember that if a client is in a place where a feeling of control is experienced, the client will feel safer, less threatened, and less anxious (Giger and Davidhizar, 1995). People generally tend to feel safer in their own territory because it is arranged and equipped in a familiar manner. In addition, most people believe that there is a degree of predictability associated with being in one's own personal space and that this degree of predictability is hard to achieve elsewhere. Nurses must also remember that the anxiety level of a client is increased when the client is hospitalized. However, the same client may experience a decrease in anxiety if the client is allowed to return home, even if still sick. Some terminally ill clients request to go home because of the feeling of security experienced in one's own personal space.

In addition to security, personal space provides privacy and at the same time protected communication. Most people believe that it is not necessary to be on guard or to keep up pretenses—to be themselves—in the security of one's personal space. The fulfillment of the desire to be oneself contributes to feelings of decreased anxiety and promotes relaxation. Many people may complain of feeling tense and tired after a long day at work but may experience relaxation and ease of tension as soon as they get home. Two factors that contribute to these feelings are that (1) activities at home are different from those at work and (2) people experience more relaxation in their personal space (Hayter, 1981). If it becomes necessary to transfer a client from one room to another or from one floor to another, the nurse should remember that the client may experience increased anxiety because of a sense of loss of security and privacy (Smith, 1976). This feeling of loss of security and privacy can also be related to nursing practice. For example, a nurse manager who returns from vacation to find office furniture rearranged may feel unsettled until the furniture is returned to a familiar arrangement. The nurse should keep in mind that clients may already be experiencing feelings of anxiety that are related to the reasons for seeking health care. Additional anxiety invoked by issues involving territoriality can be minimized by the nurse who develops an understanding of another person's culture and its implications for territoriality or interpersonal space.

Another important aspect of territoriality for nurses is the function of autonomy. Autonomy is the means by which a person can control what happens. In personal territory a person may feel free to ask questions, resist suggested actions, hold out for those things that are most important personally, and share personal feelings. A client, on the other hand, is out of personal territory and lacks control. Therefore it is important for the nurse to determine if the client has an adequate understanding of the treatment regimen and is not submitting to treatment merely because of a lack of control of territory. Statements to the client that maximize feelings of control, such as, "How do you want to arrange the room?" or "Are you concerned about your treatment? We can walk down the hall to the visiting room, where it is private, to discuss your feelings," should promote feelings of security and autonomy for the client. Feelings of autonomy are also evidenced in nursing practice. For example, when a nurse manager needs to counsel an employee, the manager's control will be maximized if the counseling occurs in the manager's office. On the other hand, if the manager is viewed as too controlling, the manager may intentionally select a more neutral territory for the counseling, such as a conference room.

It is essential to remember that having personal space promotes self-identity by affording opportunities for self-expression and that personal well-being is often related to the critical distance a person keeps from others (Wilson and Kneisl, 1995; Reakes, 1997; Giger, Davidhizar, Johnson, and Poole, 1997). Another way to define self-identity in relation to personal space is to view self-identity as a mode of individuality. The personal space over which a person has jurisdiction often becomes a personal extension of self and a reflection of characteristics, personality, and interest. A nurse may communicate warmth and reduce feelings of anxiety by moving close to a client. On the other hand, rapidly moving toward an anxious client may dramatically increase the client's anxiety. People have a need to organize and arrange personal space so that it maximizes functioning and at the same time meets needs. For example, when a person purchases a new home, it becomes essential for that home to take on the person's identity. This is evidenced by the desire of the new occupants to change such items as the wallpaper, colors of the walls, carpet, lighting fixtures, and draperies. Regardless of whether these items are new, each person has a need for self-expression or individuality. When clients set out personal pictures of their family and other personal items from home and wear their own sleepwear, self-identity is enhanced. Therefore changing items to reflect this individuality becomes an essential aspect of personal security and autonomy.

Case Study

Mr. Bernhard Wolfgang, a 56-year-old German immigrant who works as an engineer, is admitted with chest pain and shortness of breath. Mr. Wolfgang is admitted to the coronary care unit to rule out myocardial infarction. Immediately after admission Mr. Wolfgang's wife comes to the coronary care unit with personal items such as family portraits, some roses from the client's garden, and some personal clothing. However, since the coronary care unit is restricted in space, personal items are not allowed, and the wife is instructed to take the items home.

On admission, Mr. Wolfgang's vital signs are stable, and his color is good. He reports that the chest pain is not debilitating and is more or less an occasional dull ache. After 2 days the diagnosis of myocardial infarction is confirmed, and Mr. Wolfgang remains restricted to bed but is transferred to a semiprivate room in the coronary care step-down unit. After admission to the coronary care step-down unit, the nurse notices that Mr. Wolfgang is anxious, somewhat withdrawn, and unable to express his needs and feelings.

STUDY QUESTIONS

1. When assessing Mr. Wolfgang, the nurse should realize that some German people have specific needs that are related to territoriality and space. Name at least two factors that affect some Germans and their spatial behavior.
2. List ways the nurse could enable Mr. Wolfgang to meet his needs for privacy and autonomy while in a semiprivate room.
3. Identify markers that would indicate Mr. Wolfgang's need for the establishment of a temporary territorial space.
4. Identify ways in which illness and hospitalization could threaten Mr. Wolfgang's personal sense of territoriality.
5. Identify factors present in a coronary care unit that could negatively affect spatial behavior.
6. List two factors related to perceptual and visual stimuli that adversely affect some German clients.
7. List ways the nurse could control perceptual and verbal stimuli that may affect Mr. Wolfgang.

References

Allekian, C.E. (1973). Intrusions of territory and personal space. *Nursing Research, 22,* 236-241.

Argyle, M., & Dean, J. (1965). Eye-contact, distance, and affiliation. *Sociometry, 28,* 289-304.

Baliant, M. (1945). Friendly expanses—hard empty spaces. *International Journal of Psychoanalysis, 4,* 38-46.

Bartholet, M. (1968). Effects of color on dynamics of patient care. *Nursing Outlook, 6*(10), 51-53.

Bendich, S. (1988). Appreciating bodily phenomena in verbally oriented psychotherapy sessions. *Issues in Mental Health Nursing, 9,* 1-7.

Bigham, C. (1964). To communicate with Negro patients. *American Journal of Nursing, 64*(9), 113-115.

Birdwhistell, R.L. (1970). *Kinesics and context.* Philadelphia: University of Pennsylvania Press.

Black, J.W. (1950). The effect of room characteristics on vocalizations and rate. *Journal of Acoustical Society in America, 22,* 174-176.

Brant, C. (1983). *Native ethics and rules of behaviour.* London, Ont.: University of Western Ontario.

Brown, J.W., Leavitt, L., & Graham, F. (1977). Response to auditory stimuli in six- and nine-week-old infants. *Developmental Psychobiology, 10,* 255-266.

Brucke, S., Maloney, R., Pothaar, D., & Baumgart, A. (1988). *Four views of childbearing and child health care: northern Indians, urban natives, urban Euro-Canadians and nurses.* A report for the National Health Research Development Program, Health and Welfare Canada, Ottawa.

Bull, P. (1983). *Body movement and interpersonal communication.* New York: John Wiley & Sons.

Carson, V., & Arnold, E. (1996). *Mental health nursing: the nurse-patient journey.* Philadelphia: W.B. Saunders Co.

Clement, J. (1987). Touch. *Association of Operation Room Nurses, 45*(6), 1429-1439.

Croker, K., & Cummings, A. (1995). Nurses reactions to physical assault by their patients. *Canadian Journal of Nursing Research, 27*(2), 81-93.

Davidhizar, R. (1988). Distance in managerial encounters. *Today's OR Nurse, 10*(10), 23-30.

Davidhizar, R., & Giger, J. (1989). Managerial touch. *Today's OR Nurse, 10*(7), 18-25.

Davidhizar, R., Dowd, S., & Giger, J. (1997). Model for cultural diversity in the radiology department. *Radiology Technology, 68*(3), 233-240.

Davis, M. (1975). *Towards understanding the intrinsic body movement.* New York: Ayer.

Davis, M., & Skupien, J. (1982). *Body movement and nonverbal communication: an annotated bibliography, 1971-1981.* Bloomington: Indiana University Press.

Day, F. (1973). The patient's perception of touch. In Anderson, E.H., Bergerson, B.S., Duffey, M., Lohr, M., & Rose, M.H. (Eds.), *Current concepts in clinical nursing* (vol. 4, pp. 266-275). St. Louis: Mosby.

Dodd, C. (1987). *Dynamics of intercultural communication.* Dubuque, Iowa: W.C. Brown.

Efron, D. (1941). *Gesture and environment.* New York: King's Crown Press.

Eibl-Eibesfeldt, I. (1972). Similarities and differences between cultures in expressive movements. In Hinde, R.A. (Ed.), *Nonverbal communication* (pp. 297-312). Cambridge, England: Cambridge University Press.

Ekman, P. (1985). *Telling lies.* New York: W.W. Norton.

Ekman, P., & Friesen, W.V. (1975). *Unmasking the face.* Englewood Cliffs, N.J.: Prentice-Hall.

England, J. (1986). Cross-cultural health care. *Canada's Mental Health, 34*(4), 13-15.

Evans, G.W., & Howard, R.B. (1973). Personal space. *Psychological Bulletin, 80,* 335-344.

Folta, A. (1989). *Exercise and functional capacity after myocardial infarction.* Paper presented at the 13th Annual Midwest Nursing Research Society Conference, Cincinnati, Ohio.

Geldard, F. (1960). Some neglected possibilities of communication. *Science, 131,* 1583-1588.

Gendlin, E.T. (1969). Focusing. *American Journal of Psychotherapy, 1,* 1-18.

Giger, J., & Davidhizar, R. (1990). Culture and space. *Advancing Critical Care, 5*(8), 8-11.

Giger, J., & Davidhizar, R. (1995). *Transcultural nursing: assessment and intervention.* St. Louis: Mosby.

Giger, J., Davidhizar, R., Johnson, J., & Poole, V. (1997). The changing face of America. *Health Care Traveler, 4*(4), 11-17.

Goldberg, W., & Fitzpatrick, J. (1980). Movement therapy with the aged. *Nursing Research, 29,* 339-346.

Goodykoontz, L. (1980). Touch: dynamic aspect of nursing care. *Journal of Nursing Care, 13,* 16-18.

Grosvenor, G.M. (1989, July). Vive la différence [President's editorial]. *National Geographic,* p. 15.

Haber, J. (1997). Therapeutic communication. In Haber, J., Krainovich-Miller, B., McMahon, A., & Price-Hoskins, P. (Eds.), *Comprehensive psychiatric nursing* (ed. 5). St. Louis: Mosby.

Hall, E., & Whyte, W. (1990). Interpersonal communication: a guide to men of action. In Brink, P.J. (Ed.), *Transcultural nursing: a book of readings.* Prospect Heights, Ill.: Waveland Press.

Hall, E.T. (1977). *Beyond culture.* Garden City, N.Y.: Anchor.

Hall, E.T. (1974). Proxemics. In Weitz S., (Ed.), *Nonverbal communication* (pp. 205- 229). New York: Oxford Press.

Hall, E.T. (1969). *The hidden dimension.* New York: Doubleday.

Hall, E.T. (1966). *The silent language*. Westport, Conn.: Greenwood Press.

Hayter, J. (1981). Territoriality as a universal need. *Journal of Advanced Nursing, 6*, 79-85.

Hedlund, N., & Jeffrey, F. (1993). Therapeutic communication. In Rawlins, R., Williams, S., & Beck, C. (Eds.), *Mental health-psychiatric nursing* (ed. 3) (pp. 65-91). St. Louis: Mosby.

Heidt, P. (1981). Effect of therapeutic touch on anxiety level of hospitalized patients. *Nursing Research, 30*, 32-37.

Hickson, M.L., & Stacks, D.W. (1985). *Nonverbal communication studies and applications*. Dubuque, Iowa: W.C. Brown.

Ittelson, W., Proshansky, H., Rivlin, I., & Winkel, H. (1974). *An introduction to environmental psychology*. New York: Holt, Rinehart, & Winston.

Kasper, C. (1989, April 3). *Exercise-induced degeneration of skeletal muscle following inactivity*. Paper presented at the 13th Annual Midwest Nursing Research Society Conference, Cincinnati, Ohio.

Knapp, M., & Hall, J. (1992). *Nonverbal communication in human interaction* (ed. 3). New York: Holt, Rinehart, & Winston.

Kreiger, D. (1975). Therapeutic touch: the imprimatur of nursing. *American Journal of Nursing, 75*, 785-787.

Leathers, D.B. (1992). *Successful nonverbal communication principles and applications* (ed. 2). New York: Macmillan.

Lefever, D., & Davidhizar, R. (1995). Eskimos. In *Transcultural nursing: assessment and intervention*. St. Louis: Mosby.

Leff, J., & Isaacs, A. (1981). *Psychiatric examination in clinical practice*. St. Louis: Mosby.

Leininger, M. (1977, December). Caring: the essence of central focus of nursing. *Nursing Research*, Report I, p. 2.

Lynch, J. (1978). The simple act of touching. *Nursing, 78*(8), 32-36.

Mahler, M., Pine, F., & Bergman, A. (1975). *The psychological birth of the human infant*. New York: Basic Books.

Marcus, N. (1985). Utilization of nonverbal expressive behavior in cognitive therapy. *American Journal of Psychotherapy, 39*(4), 467-478.

McRae, L. (1994). Cultural sensitivity in rehabilitation related to native clients. *Canadian Journal of Rehabilitation, 7*(4), 251-256.

Mintz, E. (1969). On the rationale of touch in psychotherapy. *Psychotherapy: theory, research, and practice, 6*(4), 232-234.

Montagu, A. (1971). *The significance of the human skin*. New York: Columbia University Press.

Moreno, J.L. (1946). *Psychodrama* (vol. 1). New York: Beacon House.

Mufford, C. (1992). A cure of many colors. *New Physician, 10*, 14-19.

Murray, R., & Huelskoetter, M. (1991). *Psychiatric-mental health nursing* (ed. 3). Norwalk, Conn.: Appleton & Lange.

Newman, M. (1976). Movement therapy and the experience of time. *Nursing Research, 25*, 273-279.

Oland, L. (1978). The need for territoriality. In Yura, H. &. Walsh, M.B, (Eds.), *Human needs and the nursing process* (pp. 97-140). New York: Appleton-Century-Crofts.

Pearlin, L. (1982). The social context of stress. In Goldberger, L. & Breznitz, S., (Eds.), *Handbook of stress* (pp. 367-379). New York: Free Press.

Perls, F.S., Hefferline, R., & Goodman, P. (1983). *Gestalt therapy*. New York: Dell.

Personal Report for the Executive. (1987, July 15). New York: National Institute of Business Management.

Ramirez, M. (1991). *Psychotherapy and counseling with minorities*. New York: Pergamon Press.

Randall-David, E. (1989). Strategies for working with culturally diverse communities and clients [Brochure]. Washington, D.C.: U. S. Department of Health and Human Services.

Rawlins, R., Williams, S., & Beck, C. (1993). *Mental health-psychiatric nursing* (ed. 3). St. Louis: Mosby.

Reakes, J. (1997). Communication. In Johnson. B. (Ed.), *Psychiatric-mental health nursing* (ed. 4). Philadelphia: J.B. Lippincott.

Roberts, S. (1989). *The effects of assault on nurses who have been physically assaulted by their clients*. Unpublished master's thesis, University of Toronto, Toronto, Ontario.

Roberts, S. (1991). Nurse abuse: a taboo topic. *Canadian Nurse, 87*, 23-25.

Roberts, S.L. (1978). *Behavioral concepts and nursing throughout the life span*. Englewood Cliffs, N.J.: Prentice-Hall.

Schleflen, A. (1972). *Body language and social order*. Englewood Cliffs, N.J.: Prentice-Hall.

Schuster, C., & Ashburn, S. (1986). *The process of human development: a holistic approach* (ed. 2). Boston: Little, Brown.

Scott, A. (1988). Human interaction and personal boundaries. *Journal of Psychosocial Nursing, 26*(8), 23-28.

Seaman, L. (1982). Affective nursing touch. *Geriatric Nursing, 3,* 162-164.

Sideleau, B. (1992). Space and time. In Haber, J., Leach-McMahon, A., Price-Hoskins, P., & Sideleau, B. (Eds.), *Comprehensive psychiatric nursing.* St. Louis: Mosby.

Smith, M. (1976). Patient responses to being transferred during hospitalization. *Nursing Research, 25,* 192-196.

Sommer, R. (1969). *Personal space: the behavioral basis of design.* Englewood Cliffs, N.J.: Prentice-Hall.

Spector, R. (1996). *Cultural diversity in health care* (ed. 4). Stamford, Conn.: Appleton & Lange.

Stauffer, R. (1995). Vietnamese Americans. In Giger, J. & Davidhizar, R. (Eds.), *Transcultural nursing: assessment and intervention.* St. Louis: Mosby.

Steere, D.A. (1982). *Bodily expressions in psychotherapy.* New York: Brunner/Mazel.

Stevenson, J. (1989. April 3). *Exercise in frail elders: findings and methodological issues.* Paper presented at the 13th Annual Midwest Nursing Research Society Conference, Cincinnati, Ohio.

Sue, D., & Sue, D. (1990). *Counseling the culturally different: theory and practice* (ed. 2). New York: John Wiley & Sons.

Tripp-Reimer, T., & Friedl, M. (1977). Applachians: a neglected minority. *Nursing Clinics of North America, 12*(41), 41-54.

Tripp-Reimer, T., & Lively, S. (1993). Cultural considerations in mental health-psychiatric nursing. In Rawlins, R., Williams, S., & Beck, C., (Eds.), *Mental health-psychiatric nursing* (ed. 3). St. Louis: Mosby.

Ujhely, G. (1979). Touch: reflections and perceptions. *Nursing Forum, 18*(1), 18-32.

Van Esterik, P. (1980). Cultural factors affecting adjustment of Southeast Asian refugees. In Tepper E., (Ed.) *Southeast Asian exodus: from tradition to resettlement* (pp. 151-172). Ottawa: The Canadian Asian Studies Association.

Watson, O.M. (1980). *Proxemic behavior: a cross-cultural study.* The Hague, The Netherlands: Mouton.

West, B. (1981). Understanding endorphins: our natural pain relief system. *Nursing 81*(11), 50-53.

Wilson, H., & Kneisl, C. (1995). *Psychiatric nursing* (ed. 5). Reading, Mass.: Addison-Wesley.

Wolfgang, A. (Ed.) (1984). *Nonverbal behavior: perspectives, applications, and intercultural insights.* Lewiston, N.Y.: C.J. Hogrete.

Young, T. (1988). *Health care and cultural change: the Indian experience in the central subarctic.* Toronto: University of Toronto Press.

Zook, R., & Davidhizar, R. (1989). Caring for the psychiatric inpatient with AIDS. *Perspectives in Psychiatric Nursing Care, 25*(2), 3-8.

CHAPTER 4

Social Organization

BEHAVIORAL OBJECTIVES

After reading this chapter, the nurse will be able to:
1. Describe how cultural behavior is acquired in a social setting.
2. Define selected terms unique to the concept of social organization, such as culture bound, ethnocentrism, homogeneity, bicultural, biracial, ethnicity, race, ethnic people of color, minority, and stereotyping.
3. Describe significant social organization groups.
4. Define family groups, including nuclear, nuclear dyad, extended, alternative, blended, single parent, and special forms of family groups.
5. List at least two primary goals inherent to the Canadian culture in regard to the family as a unit.
6. Describe the significant influence that religion may have on the way individuals relate to health care practitioners.

Cultural behavior, or how one acts in certain situations, is socially acquired, not genetically inherited. Patterns of cultural behavior are learned through a process called "enculturation" (also referred to as "socialization"), which involves acquiring knowledge and internalizing values. Most people achieve competence in their own culture through enculturation. Children learn to behave culturally by watching adults and making inferences about the rules for behavior (Nolt, 1992). Patterns of cultural behavior are important to the nurse because they provide explanations for behavior related to life events. Life events that are significant transculturally include birth, death, puberty, childbearing, childrearing, illness, and disease. Children learn certain beliefs, values, and attitudes about these life events, and the learned behavior that results persists throughout the entire life span unless necessity or forced adaptation compels the learning of different ways. It is important for the nurse to recognize the value of social organizations and their relationship to physiological and psychological growth and maturation (Murray and Huelskoetter, 1991).

CULTURE AS A TOTALITY

Most anthropologists believe that to understand culture and the meaning assigned to culture-specific behavior, one must view culture in the total social context. The concept of holism requires that human behavior not be isolated from the context in which it occurs. Therefore culture must be viewed and analyzed as a totality—a functional, integrated whole whose parts are interrelated and yet interdependent. The components of culture, such as political, economic, religion, kinship, and health systems, perform separate functions but nevertheless mesh to form an operating whole. Culture is more than the sum of its parts (Goldsby, 1977; Henderson and Primeaux, 1981). Because Canada has chosen to have its people of diverse origins and communities remain free to preserve and enhance their own cultural heritage, Canadians claim to have coined the term "multiculturalism" (Bailey and Bailey, 1995; World Almanac, 1997). Most Canadians view multiculturalism in a fundamentally different way from the focus in the United States where there has been an emphasis on achieving homogeneity.

Being culture bound

As children grow and learn a specific culture, they are to some extent imprisoned without knowing it. Some anthropologists have referred to this existence as being culture bound. In this context the term "culture bound" describes a person living within a certain reality that is considered the "reality." Most people have learned ways to interpret their world based on enculturation. Thus, although certain interpretations are understandable and persuasive to persons brought up to share the same frame of reference, other people may not share these interpretations and therefore may make little sense out of the context. Nurses are also culturally bound within the profession because they are likely to bring a unique scientific approach, the nursing process, to the determination and resolution of health problems. Many nurses are likely to consider the nursing process the best and only means of meeting the needs of all clients regardless of their cultural heritage. However, clients may view this modern scientific approach differently, believing that the nursing process meets their needs in some ways but not in others. The nursing process may not take into consideration alternative health services, such as folk remedies, holistic health care, and spiritual interventions. In these cultures, medicine is often practiced in unscientific ways based on the Western viewpoint. Therefore desirable outcomes for treatment may occur independently of medical and health care interventions.

Traditionally, Canadian nurses have been socialized to believe that modern Western medicine is the answer to all of humanity's health needs. Most illnesses have been attributed to a biological cause (Grpyma, 1993). More recently, Canadians and Canadian nurses in particular have been moving toward a more harmonious relationship with nature in which there is a growing sensitivity to the environment. Traditional attitudes toward disease are being reassessed. Today, more attention is being given to the concept of the individual as an organic whole both in treating Native Canadians and Canadian immigrants. Nursing leaders in Canada are calling for a change in nursing paradigms from scientific to holistic (Grpyma, 1993; Thompson, 1993; McRae, 1994; Guruge and Donner, 1996).

Ethnocentrism For the most part, people look at the world from their own particular cultural viewpoint. Ethnocentrism is the perception that one's own way is best. Even in the nursing profession, there is a tendency to lean toward ethnocentrism. Nurses must remain cognizant of the fact that their ways are not necessarily the best and that other people's ideas are not "ignorant" or "inferior." Nurses must remember that the ideas of lay individuals may be valid for them and, more importantly, will influence their health care behavior and consequently their health status (Giger and Davidhizar, 1995). Somewhat in contrast to the term "ethnocentrism" is the word "ethnic," which relates to races or to large groups of people classed according to common traits or customs. In populations throughout the world, people are bound by common ties, elements, life patterns, and basic beliefs germane to their particular country of origin.

In general, the medical paradigm used in the Western culture views health, illness, and dying as biophysical realities. However, the meaning a nurse places on life can affect relationships with clients. For example, if the nurse believes there is no relationship between illness and evil, this may be at conflict with the client who believes that illness is a punishment from God or the work of spirits (Gregory, 1988; Grpyma, 1993). On the hand, some Puerto Ricans believe that sickness and suffering is a result of one's evil deeds, whereas many Ugandans believe that an infant's illness or death is the result of a neighbor's curse (Grpyma, 1993).

Homogeneity It is difficult to find a homogeneous culture in Canada. If a homogeneous culture did exist in Canada, all individuals would share the same attitudes, interests, and goals—a phenomenon referred to as "ethnic collectivity." People who are reared in ethnic collectivity share a bond that includes common origins, a sense of identity, and a shared standard for behavior. These values are often acquired from experiences that are perceived to be cultural norms and that determine the thoughts and behaviors of individual members (Harwood, 1981; Saunders, 1954). The ultimate consequences of enculturation are carried over to health care and become an important influence on activities relative to health and illness behaviors.

In Canada, where there is emphasis on multiculturalism, homogeneity across cultures tends to receive little emphasis. It is important to note that even among ethnic groups there is intraethnic variation in health behaviors (Franks and Faux, 1990; Thompson, 1986, 1987; Kelly, 1993). For example, intraethnic variations are seen in the concept of mental illness (Guttmacher and Elinson, 1972; Berry, 1988; Beiser, Barwick, Berry, et al., 1988; Sands and Berry, 1993), in cultural definitions of health and illness, in skepticism about medical care and consequently the use or lack of use of health care services (Berkanovic and Reeder, 1973; Spector 1996; Prilleltensky, 1993), and finally in the willingness of the individual to assume a dependent role when ill (Suchman, 1964; Indian and Inuit Nurses of Canada, 1983).

In recent history, immigration to Canada has increased dramatically. Until the end of World War II, the greater proportion of immigrants to Canada came from Great Britain and the United States with the smaller proportion having come from other European countries. In contrast, since the 1960s, the proportion of immigrants from these countries has decreased, while the number of immigrants arriving from other countries such as Asia, India, Africa, the Caribbean, Central America, and South America has increased. Included among these newcomers are refugees born in countries such as Vietnam, Somalia, El Salvador, Cambodia, and Laos. It has been estimated that between 25,000 and 35,000 new immigrant children 19 years of age and under have been arriving each year (Hicks, LaLonde, and Pepler, 1993). For these children and their families, there are significant changes in environment, community, and interpersonal affiliations. For many individuals, immigration creates tremendous upheavals, multiple losses including fragmentation of kinship groups, difficulty adjusting to school, and changing values, which may contribute to stress and mental distress (Hicks, LaLonde, and Pepler, 1993). It is also important to understand that when immigrants have settled in a region where there is no similar

ethnocultural group, a greater number of stressors are experienced (Baker, Arseneault, and Gallant, 1994).

Bicultural The term "bicultural" is used to describe a person who crosses two cultures, lifestyles, and sets of values. To understand biculturalism, the nurse must understand the differences in meaning of ethnicity, race, biracial, and minority.

Ethnicity Ethnicity is frequently and perhaps erroneously used to mean "race," but the term "ethnicity" includes more than the biological identification. Ethnicity in its broadest sense refers to groups whose members share a common social and cultural heritage passed on to each successive generation. The most important characteristic of ethnicity is that members of an ethnic group feel a sense of identity.

The formulation of the Aboriginal Nurses Association of Canada (ANAC) is evidence of an effort among aboriginal nurses to foster a sense of identity among nurses of aboriginal ancestry, as well as among the Native Canadian and Inuit people. The founders of this organization share a common vision that is grounded in their unique perspective as aboriginal caregivers to aboriginal people. Today, a professional organization of Registered Nurses of Canadian Indian Ancestry provides a way for aboriginal nurses to work together toward common goals and purposes (Aboriginal Nurses Association of Canada, 1995).

Race In contrast to the term "ethnicity" is the term "race," which is related to biological history. Members of a particular race share distinguishing physical features such as skin color, bone structure, or blood group. Ethnic and racial groups can and do overlap because in many cases the biological and cultural similarities reinforce one another (Bullough and Bullough, 1982). A more precise definition of race is a breeding population that primarily mates within itself (Giger, Davidhizar, and Wieczorek, 1994). It is important to understand that there are very few races that still mate largely within their own group. There are some pure-blooded lineages found in certain parts of the world. For example, in the United States, some of the descendants of West Africans are of a "pure-blooded lineage" and live along the Georgia and South Carolina seacoasts. These people have protected their lineage because they have refused to intermarry. These individuals are known as the Gullah people, who have not only their own lineage but also their own distinct form of the English language (Wolfram and Clark, 1971). It is important for the nurse to remember that, regardless of race, all people have a cultural heritage that makes them ethnic (Giger, Davidhizar, and Wieczorek, 1994).

Biracial When an individual crosses between two racial and cultural groups, the individual is considered "biracial." To be both biracial and bicultural often creates an almost insurmountable dilemma for some persons. Physical attributes such as color, shape of eyes, or hair may have a profound effect on acceptance of the "biracial" individual by others. One problem associated with biracialism is the inability of the individual to identify or find acceptance in any one of the biologically related racial groups (Giger, Davidhizar, Evers, and Ingram, 1994). It is the total exclusion and the sense of not belonging to either of the racial or cultural groups that often creates the dilemma. For example, an African-American who is an "octoroon," a person with one-eighth African-American blood, may have difficulty being accepted as African American because of the lightness of the skin. Furthermore, this same person might be ostracized by some Whites because of the "blackness of the blood lineage." Some refer to the offspring of a French Canadian and an American Indian as a "Métis" (Bailey and Bailey, 1995). For some people of color, there is a perception that the belief held by Whites in America is that "color is the difference that makes the differences" (Giger, Johnson, Davidhizar, and Fishman, 1993).

Minority A minority can consist of a particular racial, religious, or occupational group that constitutes less than a numerical majority of the population. Using this definition for the term "minority," it is obvious that all types of people can belong to various kinds of minorities (Bullough and Bullough, 1982). Often a group is designated minority because of its lack of power, assumed inferior traits, or supposedly undesirable characteristics. In any society, cultural groups can be arranged in a hierarchical power structure. Dominant groups are considered to be powerful, whereas those in minority groups are considered inferior and lacking in power.

Surprisingly the term "minority" may not be synonymous with numbers. For example, until recently, the ruling class in South Africa (only 2% of the population) were White (Gary, 1991). In the United States, people of color (African Americans, Latin Americans, Asian Americans) are considered minorities. However, when the population of the world is considered in its aggregate, it is obvious that people of color are in the majority.

Gender is another example of how the term "minority" is used erroneously. Females in the United States compose a larger numerical percentage (51%) than males do (49%) but are considered to be in the minority because of their underrepresentation in high-level managerial positions in the workplace. In fact, 95% of all top managerial jobs in the corporate structure in the United States are held by White males (U.S. Department of Commerce, Bureau of Census, 1991).

The significance of the term "minority" cannot be underemphasized. The central defining characteristic of any minority group, according to Gary (1991), is its relative powerlessness and inability to chart its own course to a better way of life.

Ethnic minority The term "ethnic minority" is often used because it is less offensive to people of color than other terms are. Supposedly it takes into account ethnicity, race, and the relative status of the groups of persons included in the category. Were it not for the use of the word "minority," perhaps this terminological usage would be less culturally offensive to some groups of people (that is, ethnic people of color). According to Gary (1991), use of the term "people of color" might be the preferable option, particularly in situations where sensitivity to racial preferences needs to be heightened.

Stereotyping Stereotyping is the assumption that all people in a similar cultural, racial, or ethnic group are alike and share the same values and beliefs. For example, stereotyping occurs when a Canadian Inuit nurse is assigned to care for a Canadian Inuit client simply because of ethnicity and race. It is stereotypical when the assumption is made that all Canadian Inuit are alike, and therefore the Canadian Inuit nurse is more likely to be more sensitive to the needs of the Canadian Inuit client. Race and ethnicity do not, in and of themselves, make us "resident experts" on the belief and value systems of other individuals. Whether we engage in stereotyping as a result of scientifically proved research-based data or because of past associations and experiences, stereotyping can ultimately lead to faulty data gathering and faulty interpretation.

Role of gender and cultural significance

In traditional Chinese society, women have held subordinate roles to men, a belief that dates back to the first millennium B.C. (Mo, 1992). Traditional Chinese believe that the universe developed from two complementary opposites: *yīn* (Mandarin) or *yam* (Cantonese) for the female and *yáng* (Mandarin) or *yeūng* (Cantonese) for the male. For some traditional Chinese Americans, *yīn* represents the 'dark, cold, wet, passive, weak, feminine' aspect of humankind. In stark contrast, *yáng* represents the 'bright, hot, dry, active, strong, masculine' aspect of humankind (Mo, 1992). In traditional societies, there are "written" and "unwritten" roles that dictate behavior of girls and women (Strickland and Giger, 1994).

Although some countries in North America are highly evolved technologically, traditional beliefs about the role of women in society still exist throughout many regions of Canada. Peitchinis (1989) noted that discrimination exists for women in the workplace because women are viewed as having a higher absentee rate than their male counterparts have. For many women, this creates a barrier to entrance to the workplace and even more importantly places a "glass ceiling" for advancement that their male counterparts need not overcome (O'Brien, 1992). On the other hand, although women tend to be an oppressed group in the workplace, numerous studies have indicated that they have access to benefits such as child-care leaves, alternative working arrangements, child-care arrangements, and special brief leaves to deal with family problems not available to men (Hyland, 1990; Sussman, 1990; York, 1991).

The Canadian Mental Health Association (1987) noted that the majority of Canadian women are solely responsible for the major aspect of domestic tasks, and this fact undoubtedly compounds workplace stress. However, research on working women and stress also suggests that working women generally experience better overall health than women who work at home do (McDaniel, 1993). Nonetheless, McDaniel (1993) noted that it is important that health promotion programs related to physical health and fitness should be present in the workplace and in programs.

Pilowsky (1993) observes that immigrant women experience discrimination in the workplace, unequal employment opportunities, language difficulties, and housing problems that are of greater magnitude than those of Canadian-born women. Of the number of chemically dependent people in Canada, women make up one third to one half of the population (Mann House Corp., 1989). Women who live in rural and isolated areas are particularly vulnerable because they face problems with isolation and lack of treatment resources (Holmstrom, 1990). Researchers in Canada and the United States have also found that the prevalence of alcohol use among young adults and college students is high with 81% to 87% percent reporting use within the preceding year (Hindmarsh, Gliksman, and Newton-Taylor, 1993). Further findings from this study suggest that 12.8% of female nursing students engaged in binge drinking, reporting an attitude that "getting drunk is cool" (Faulkner, Ratner, Johnson, Bottorff, and Unsworth, 1996).

SOCIAL ORGANIZATION GROUPS AS SYSTEMS

Social organizations are structured into a variety of groups, including family, religious, ethnic, racial, tribal, kinship, clan, and other special interest groups. Groups are dependent on particular persons and are more affected by changes in members than other systems are. In most groups, except for racial and ethnic groups, the members may come and go. Thus the formation and the disintegration of groups are more likely to occur during the members' lifetimes than are the formation and the disintegration of other systems.

According to the general systems theory, social organization groups are characterized by a steady state and a sense of balance or equilibrium that is maintained even as the group changes. Most groups form, grow, and reach a state of maturity. Social organization groups begin with a variety of elements that include individuals with unique personalities, needs, ideas, potentials, and limits. In the course of development of the group, a pattern of behavior and a set of norms, beliefs, and values evolve. As the group strives toward maturity, parts become differentiated, and each member assumes special functions.

Family groups

One group of paramount concern for the nurse when working with persons transculturally is the family. Regardless of cultural background, the family is a basic unit of society. From a sociological perspective the family may be defined as a social unit that interacts with the larger society in which it exists. The discipline of economics may define the family in terms of how it works together to meet material needs. From a psychological perspective the family may be defined as a basic unit for personality development and the development of subgroup relationships such as parent-child relationships. Still another definition is offered from a biological perspective, which is a conceptualization of the family as a unit with the biological function of perpetuating the species.

The most predominant family system in Canada is the nuclear family, which is defined as a group consisting of parents (or a parent) and their non-adult children living in a single household. A similar definition views the family as a cluster of people whose relationship is stipulated by law in terms of marriage and descent and whose precise membership varies according to the circumstances.

A broader conceptualization of the term "family" is the view of the family as a relationship community of two or more persons in which individuals may come from the same or different kinship groups. Mauksch (1974) views the family as a basic human unit with generic properties, including the coexist-

ence of more than one human being involved in a continuous, presumably permanent, sharing of living facilities, a perception of reciprocal obligations, a sense of commonality, and a perception of certain obligations toward others. These varying definitions of the family range from viewing the family as having one structure exclusively to perceiving the family as a household unit representative of various types of family structures.

Types of family structures

Traditional nuclear family. According to Virginia Satir (1983), the traditional nuclear family consists of one man and one woman of the same race, religion, and age who are of sound mind and body and who marry during their early or middle twenties, are faithful to the other for life, have and raise their own children, retire, and finally die. This definition appears narrow; however, it has maintained popularity over the years and is still seen by many persons as the most desirable family form. Today a more current definition of the nuclear family allows for more variation. This newer definition defines the nuclear family as a family of two generations formed by a married woman and man with their children by birth or adoption (Govaets, 1987). Within this particular family form, as within all identified family forms, the assigned roles and functions performed by each member vary. One example is a common family structure that has the father working outside the home and the mother working at home taking care of the children and household tasks. However, today the traditional nuclear family often finds both mother and father working outside the home. Thus childrearing and childcare may be shared by both parents as well as by others outside the family such as a day care center.

In the mid-1960s, most Canadian families fit the traditional model with the male breadwinner and a female homemaker. In 1988, only 16% of Canadian families reflected this simple division of family roles (Townson, 1988). In 1990, more than 12% of all families in Canada were headed by single women, whereas slightly more than 2% were headed by single men (Ram, 1990). Of the number of people in the Canadian workforce, 55.9% are female (*Canadian Almanac*, 1993). Because a greater number of women are an integral part of the Canadian work force, many children are left without dependable childcare. In fact, 60% of Canadian children between 6 and 14 years of age are without dependable day care, and 68% of those below 6 years of age are also without dependable day care (Ram, 1990).

Nuclear dyad family. The nuclear dyad family consists of one generation and is made up of a married couple without children. There are numerous reasons why this particular family remains childless: the family may have chosen not to have children, they may not be able to have children or to adopt them, or the children may have died. In some cultures this family form is frequently thought of as a beginning point for the formation of the family. However, in other cultures the nuclear dyad family is considered a part of the mainstream of the social organization of the family. The number of nuclear dyad families continues to grow and survive as a functioning unit throughout the world.

Extended family. The extended family is multigenerational and includes all relatives by birth, marriage, or adoption. The family group is made up of grandparents, aunts, uncles, nieces, nephews, cousins, brothers, sisters, and in-laws. In today's society there is a tendency for children to leave the homes and communities of their parents, which has resulted in a separation of the nuclear family from the extended family.

Alternative family. The alternative family consists of adults of a single generation or a combination of adults and children who live together without social sanction of marriage. The alternative family is often either a communal arrangement—composed of roommates who might be either homosexual or heterosexual—or a love relationship between a man and a woman.

Single-parent family. The single-parent family consists of two generations and is made up of a mother or a father and children by birth or adoption. The reasons for a single-parent family include electing to be a single parent, divorce, death, separation, or abandonment. The prevalence of the single-parent family is increasing because of factors such as divorce and the acceptability of being a single parent (Zinn and Eitzen, 1987).

Reconstituted or blended family. The reconstituted or blended family is a family that is formed by "put-together parts" of previously existing families with the intention of forming a new nuclear family (Satir, 1983). The blended family, like the traditional nuclear family, is two generational. However, the blended family differs in form and may be made up of a single person who marries a person with children, or a man and a woman, both of whom have children, who marry. This family form may also yield biological children; thus there may be a composition of "yours," "mine," and "ours" in the family. The blended family can become very complicated because of the composition and blending of family members, which may include step-brothers, step-sisters, step-parents, and step-grandparents.

Special forms of families: gay families and communal families. In some cultures an even wider array of family forms occurs, particularly if ideas about marriage and the requirement that the nuclear family is essential to family definition are disregarded. These groups do function as families and therefore must be recognized. These special forms of families may be either one generational or multigenerational. Two or more adults constitute these special family forms, and they may or may not be of the same sex.

A commune is a group of people that intertwines husband-wife, parent-child, and brother-sister types of relationships of individuals who have elected to live together in one household or in closely adjoining structures. Family members in a commune must express a feeling of commitment to others in the group. Assigned family roles, as well as responsibilities, are divided among the members of the group. Generally there are specific rules and expectations for each member of the group. A commune may be formed when people have a common goal such as a religious, philosophical, or political goal, or a common need such as an economic, social, or physical need. Examples of communes include Israeli kibbutzim, religious cults, retirement homes for the elderly, and households where couples share resources.

Some gay households consist of two persons and generally function as a nuclear dyad. Other gay households may consist of more members, such as a commune. Today, perhaps as a result of the gay rights movement, homosexual couples have openly taken up residence together. Nevertheless, many members of society continue to be nonaccepting of this particular family form. Thus it remains difficult for the gay couple to either adopt children or be given custody of children when a gay partner is divorced.

Characteristics of a family system According to the general systems theory, a system is a group of interrelated parts or units that form a whole. When the general systems theory is applied to the family, the individual family members are those units that make up the identifiable family system. These parts or units act as one or more subsystems within the larger system. Within the family system, the subsystems refer to the way in which the members align themselves with one another. For example, in the family system the parents may be of one subsystem, whereas the children may be of another subsystem. At the same time, males and females of the family system may be of two other subsystems. A subsystem may consist of any number of members who are linked by some common factor. Within the family system, membership in a particular subsystem may be determined by generational considerations, sexual identity, areas of interest, or a specifically designated function. Individual family members may belong to several different subsystems. Family members also belong to external systems, such as the community system, the school system, and career systems. Subsystems may be constructed to ensure that important functions within the family system are carried out to maintain the overall family structure.

Fawcett (1975) studied the family as a living open system and thus viewed family nursing as an emerging conceptual framework for nursing care. Nurses have cared for families for years; however, it is only recently that nurse researchers have begun to study the family as a whole (Murphy, 1986). Nursing studies in family health are increasing, such as qualitative studies in family health by Campbell (1989), Phipps (1989), and Breitmayer, Gallo, Knafl, and Zoeller (1989).

Family as a behavioral system. The family is conceptualized as a behavioral system with unique properties inherent to the system. A close interrelationship exists between the psychosocial functioning of the family as a group and the emotional adaptation of individual family members. A distinguishable link exists between disorders of family living and disorders of family members. This link can best be understood in the context of systems theory. Systems theory is an orientation whereby people are recognized and defined by who they are in the context of their relationship with family, friends, and the society in which they live. Family systems theories were developed in the 1950s on both the east and west coasts of the United States. On the West Coast a group of people that included Jackson, Haley, and their associates in Palo Alto, California, explored the notions of communication theory and homeostasis applied to the family with a schizophrenic member (Bateson, Jackson, Haley, and Weakland, 1968; Satir, 1983). On the East Coast, in Washington, D.C., Bowen (1994) conceptualized a family systems theory based on a biological systems model. In Philadelphia, Minuchin (1974) used a systems model in his research with families with psychosomatic disorders.

Lewis, Beavers, Gossett, and Phillips (1976) and Caplan (1975) explored both disturbed families and healthy families from a systems perspective. A system is a whole that consists of more than the sum of its parts; a system can be divided into subsystems, but the subsystems are not representative pieces of the whole. To study the family from a cultural perspective, one must understand the basic characteristics of a family system and of a living system. Today in nursing the family nursing process is the same whether the focus is on the family as the client or the family as the environment. Therefore the nursing process used in family nursing is the same as that used with individuals, that is, assessment, nursing diagnosis, planning, intervention, and evaluation. According to Friedman (1986), the only distinguishable difference is that both the individual and the family receive care simultaneously. There are some inherent underlying assumptions germane to the family approach to the nursing process, including the beliefs that all individuals must be viewed within their family context, that families have an influence on individuals, and that individuals have an influence on families. Grossman (1995) notes that although family-focused health care has been present in community care in Canada it is imperative to strengthen nursing expertise in ambulatory services in hospitals not only to provide continuity for the client but also to improve coordination of family care.

Independent units. All systems have basic units that make functioning possible. Within the structure of the family system, the basic interdependent units are the individual family members. As with any open system, change within one family member affects the entire family system. For example, when one family member becomes physically or emotionally ill, the entire family system is changed in some way. Additional alterations in the family system occur because of the changing composition of family membership as a result of events such as birth, divorce, death, hospitalization, leaving home for college, or marriage. All these variables, whether positive or negative, may bring about disruption and disequilibrium in the family system. All family systems have dynamic characteristics that must be used when disruption or disequilibrium occurs if the family system is to be permitted to return to equilibrium as matter, energy, and information are exchanged (Lewis, 1979).

Environment. As with all open systems there is an internal and external environment that controls the direction of growth of the family system. The internal environment involves the social and physical factors within the family boundaries, the quality of which is reflected by such factors as (1) marital relationship, (2) location of power, (3) closeness of family members, (4) communication, (5) problem-solving abilities, (6) free expression of feelings, (7) ability to deal with loss, (8) family values, (9) degree of intimacy, and (10) autonomy of family members. Within the family system, the external environment involves the social and physical world outside of the family, such as church, neighbors, extended family, school, friends, work, health care system, political systems, and recreation.

Boundaries. Within the family system the "boundary" is the imaginary line or area of demarcation that keeps the family system separate and unique

from its external environment. As with all open systems, energy, in the form of information, material goods, and feeling states, passes among family members and the external environment. Openness and closeness in a family system are governed by the degree of information or energy that is exchanged and the nature of the boundaries. Information coming into the family system provides the family with information about the environment and about family functioning. If the family accepts the information, it may be used to formulate and respond to the environment, to assist the family in coping with disequilibrium, or to rejuvenate the family. Energy coming into the family can also be stored until needed. Finally, energy or information coming into the family can be rejected or ignored (Satir, 1983).

As with all open systems, the amount of energy or information that enters and leaves the system must be balanced within certain limits to maintain a steady state of functioning or homeostasis if proper adaptation of the system is to occur. Any system can become dysfunctional if the system is allowed to become too open or too closed. No truly closed systems exist, except in a theoretical sense. On the other hand, if a family system were totally open, the family system would probably lose its identity as a system separate from other systems to which family members belong. Therefore the family members might suffer from alienation, rootlessness, and a lack of belonging. The opposite extreme, or a theoretically closed family system, would consist of boundaries that were very rigid, and thus family members would become enmeshed, fixed, and unable to move out, grow, or change.

Communication within the family system The verbal and nonverbal interaction among family members is called "communication." Factors that contribute to the family member's patterns of communication include (1) the pattern of members acknowledging each other's verbal and nonverbal messages, (2) the degree of responsibility taken by each member for expressing individual feelings, thoughts, and reactions in a constructive way, (3) the extent to which the family encourages a clear exchange of words, (4) the extent to which family members are allowed to talk for themselves, and (5) the patterns of spontaneous talking. Bonding among family members occurs as a result of the form of communication patterns that exist.

Roles in the family Family member roles are patterns of wants, goals, beliefs, feelings, attitudes, and actions that family members have for themselves and others in the family. Roles are both assigned and acquired, and they specify what individuals do in the family. Although they are usually dependent on social class and cultural norms, roles are dynamic and change in response to factors both within the family and without. Roles are reciprocal and complement roles taken by other family members. Family equilibrium is dependent on how well roles in the family are balanced and reciprocated (Duvall and Miller, 1984; Friedman, 1986).

The way in which a family member assumes a particular role is influenced by various factors, including temperament, height, weight, gender, birth order, age, and health status. Certain roles, however, depend solely on the gender of the family member. Females can be sister, daughter, wife, mother, or girlfriend, whereas males can be brother, son, father, husband, or boyfriend. Other roles, such as breadwinner, homemaker, cook, handyman, or gardener, are performance roles and depend on the person's ability to perform a certain task. In contrast to performance roles are emotional roles, such as leader, nurturer, scapegoat, caretaker, jester, arbitrator, or martyr, which may be adopted at certain times as a means of adjusting to the demands of a family system, to an extended family crisis such as a long-term family illness, or to long-term family conflict. The functions of emotional roles are to reduce conflict among family members and to promote temporary adaptation among family members. However, consistent use of emotional roles may serve to impair adaptation, thus hindering the growth of the family. An example of this is when one family member, perhaps the oldest child, assumes the role of family caretaker by supporting other members and arbitrating disputes. The role may take on negative characteristics in this instance because the family caretaker may appear outwardly strong and capable but inwardly have unrealistic feelings, such as "I can't fail," or "I can't be weak." In this emotional role this person may function under pressure to be perfect but at the same time have feelings of self-doubt and fear. It is important for the nurse to remember that roles have a significant influence on individual adjustment.

Family organization To understand family organization, it is important for the nurse to remember that structuring of both functions and goals must be addressed. It is also important for the nurse to remember that most families are dynamic, endlessly adaptable, and continuously evolving in both structure and function. The functional ability of a family depends in part on the individual needs and wants of the members. If the nurse is unable to assist family members in meeting needs within the family structure, pain may be felt and confusion may exist. The nurse must keep in mind that, in the American culture, families are expected to be self-perpetuating and at the same time be the primary system for the transfer of social values and norms.

In the Canadian culture two primary goals are inherent to the family: (1) the encouragement and nurturance of each individual and (2) the production of autonomous, healthy children (O'Brien, 1992). Marital partners are expected to be supportive and protective of each other. Both the husband and the wife are expected to share a sense of meaning and emotional closeness within the boundaries of their relationship, thus fostering the goal of personality development. In families in which supportive relationships do not exist, the achievement of the first goal (the encouragement and nurturance of each individual) is not attainable. The second goal of the family includes encouraging children to develop their own identity and individuality by allowing them to develop ideals, feelings, and life directions. At the same time, children are encouraged to sense both similarities to and differences from others and to be able to initiate activities based on this information (Lewis, 1979). Factors that must be addressed to determine the degree to which the family will accomplish these two primary goals include the patterns of relationship and adaptive mechanisms that are present. There are many reasons why some families fail to accomplish these two primary goals, including psychiatric disturbance among family

---

Box 4-1

LEVELS OF FAMILY FUNCTIONING

LEAST ABSTRACT:

Level I: Family functions and activities

Level II: Intrafamilial interactions

Level III: Interpersonal relationships

MOST ABSTRACT:

Level IV: The family system

Level I deals with family affairs and functions. Included in this level are tangible, pragmatic activities that are either observable or easily identified; more important, these are things that family members are most comfortable in discussing. Four categories of family functioning have been identified in Level I:

1. **Activities of family living.** Families are expected to provide physical safety and economic resources. Included in this category is the ability of family members to obtain such necessities as food, clothing, shelter, and health care.

2. **Ability of the family members to assist one another.** Included in this category is the family's ability to assist one another in developing emotionally and intellectually and at the same time attaining a personal as well as family identity.

3. **Reproduction, socialization, and release of children.** Included in this category are functioning goals that would allow the family to become closely aligned, thereby allowing the transmission of subcultural roles and values.

4. **Integration between the family, its culture, and society.** Included in this category is the ability of the family to use external environmental resources for support and feedback.

Level II basically deals with communication and various interactions between family members, including what is said, how it is said, patterns of communication over time, the ability of each family member to communicate, and the quality of communication skills. Also included in this level is the transfer of information from family member to family member.

Level III deals with the way family members interact in relationships that occur within the family constellation. The dimensions of closeness and power, and the degree of empathy, support, and commitment that exist among family members are important. How the family functions in regard to decision making and problem solving is included in this level.

Level IV deals with the concepts of the family system, as well as how the family functions as a system. Level IV is the most abstract level of family functioning. It encompasses the concepts of wholeness, openness or closedness, homeostasis, and rules.

Data from Schneider, R. (1980, June). *Conceptual scheme of family organization and function.* Paper presented at a St. Louis University Medical Center conference, St. Louis, Missouri.

members, incomplete maturation of children, and disintegration of the family system. When adaptive mechanisms are used by the family, internal equilibrium may result. These adaptive mechanisms are dependent on (1) the level of communication skills within the family; (2) the individual contributions of each family member to the family welfare; (3) the mutual respect and love within the family; (4) the type, kind, and amount of stressors encountered; (5) the response pattern to stressors encountered in the internal and external environment; and (6) the support or resources available and the opportunity to participate in support systems (Ackerman, 1984; Black, 1991). For example, a family that has an alcoholic father may not be able to accomplish goals because this problem may result in psychiatric disturbances in the wife and children, and ultimately the

family system may disintegrate. The reasons for the disintegration of this family include not only the individual psychiatric disturbances but also accompanying difficulties such as incomplete maturation of children and adult members, financial instability, inability to adapt successfully to stressors, and more importantly the inability of each family member to perceive the family unit as caring and loving (Brown, 1986).

Levels of functioning. Four levels of family functioning that have been identified form a continuum in increasingly abstract levels (Box 4-1): (I) family functions and activities, (II) intrafamilial interactions, (III) interpersonal relationships, and (IV) the family system (Averaswald, 1973).

To understand the family from a cultural perspective, it is essential that the nurse recognize that family relationships are stronger among some ethnic or cultural groups than among others. However, the importance of socioeconomic class cannot be overlooked. According to Casavantes (1976), a pattern of strong family relationships exists particularly among poor people, who have few resources and must rely on the support of the family kinship network to meet physical and emotional needs. Middle- or upper-class people often have resources that extend beyond the extended family and are therefore able to avail themselves of physical and emotional support within the community. It is often believed that when people do not have money or other available resources for recreation and social activities in the community, they tend to spend more time together and depend on the family group for recreational and social outlets.

Regardless of socioeconomic class, families must organize and structure themselves. Structure refers to the organization of the family and includes the type of family, such as nuclear or extended. The value system of the family dictates the roles assigned in the family, communication patterns within the family, and power distribution within the family (Friedman, 1986; Scheflen and Scheflen, 1972). The basic beliefs about humankind, nature, the supernatural (fate), time, and family relationships constitute a family's value system. Value systems are often clustered by socioeconomic status or ethnic groups. For example, families from lower socioeconomic groups tend to have a present-time orientation and view themselves as being subjugated to the environment or the supernatural (fate). Often the family relationships are disrupted by desertion of a spouse or by the early emancipation of the children because of severe economic difficulties. These families have been able to survive and adapt by taking in other extended family members' children; for example, a grandmother may provide direct assistance by raising her son's or daughter's children. In these families power is usually authoritarian or not exerted at all.

Although the living conditions of many Native Canadians, especially those living in rural settings in the north, is often substandard because of poor economic status, there is nonetheless a strong sense of family identity (McRae, 1994). Some cultural theoreticians postulate that "to be poor in the Indian world is to be without relatives" (Henderson and Primeaux, 1981). In the Native Canadian population, all blood relatives are considered to be a part of the family. The extended family may include three generations living in one household as well as extending in a horizontal manner to include relatives from both sides of the family. First cousins are often treated as brothers and sisters with uncles and aunts as grandparents (Henderson and Primeaux, 1981).

Middle- and upper-class families in Canada for the most part espouse the Protestant work ethic values, which dictate the importance of working and planning for the future. These values encompass the belief that although man is somewhat evil, his behavior is changeable by hard work. In the middle- and upper-class family structure, financial stability and success are viewed as rewards for hard work. Within these classes, family relationships center around the nuclear family, socialization occurs with work-related or neighborhood friends, and power may be more egalitarian than in the lower-class family. Power tends to become more male dominated as the economic level of a family rises. Middle- and upper-class families often see themselves as able to control or have mastery over their environment (O'Brien, 1992).

The nurse must keep in mind that these statements on structure and organization of a family by class are broad generalizations of social class values and in themselves cannot account for cultural differences. For example, many ethnic groups, such as the Newfoundland Inuit family, regardless of socioeconomic status, place great importance on extended family relationships rather than on the individualism valued by White, Protestant, middle-class Canadians. A family with a good income but with a time orientation in the present, such as that commonly found among persons in the lower socioeconomic class, may fail to recognize the importance of saving money and thus may always struggle financially. To understand whether a family system organizes itself around a family unit, such as the extended family, or tends to be a more individualistic system, such as the nuclear family, the nurse must assess the family as a group. The Canadian family is composed of diverse multicultural populations and is defined by three criteria: kinship, function, and location.

Kinship. In the first criterion, kinship, there are three dyads that imply the existence of or location for the individual within the family structure: husband-father, wife-mother, or child-sibling. There are several conventional forms of family structures that are composed of these positions, including the nuclear family and the stem family. The nuclear family, which was discussed earlier, may consist of a husband, a wife, and their nonadult children and is based on all three dyads, with their marital, parental, and sibling elements. Whereas the nuclear family is restricted to a depth of two generations, the stem family encompasses three generations: grandparents, parents, and children.

Function. The second criterion, function, describes the purpose, goals, and philosophy of the family organization. Family function is defined as the expected action of an individual in a given role. In a description of family organization, the term "function" is used to depict family roles and the assigned tasks for those roles. Every family has unit functions that must be performed to maintain the integrity of the family unit and to meet the needs of the family. If individual family members' needs and societal expectations are to be met, the functioning role of the family must be clearly delineated. In family systems with two or more individuals, the family members have unit functional responsibilities related to their social positions. Depending on the position within the family structure, an individual may function in a variety of roles such as breadwinner, homemaker, companion, health motivator, or sexual partner. It is important for the nurse to remember that the maintenance of the family system is dependent on these various roles. Some cultural groups function in traditional ways in which the family is viewed as a holistic functioning unit. Other cultural groups may function as a disaggregate unit, meaning that the family does not function as a unit but members function independently.

Murray, Meili, and Zentner (1993) have described one approach to examining family functions in relation to the family's physical, affectional, and social properties. Physical functions include providing food, clothing, and shelter; protecting against danger; and providing health care. Affectional functions include meeting emotional needs. Social functions include providing social togetherness, fostering self-esteem, and supporting creativity and initiative. Another approach to examining family functions is the view of the family from a task-oriented perspective (Sussman, 1971). Tasks include socialization of children, strengthening competency of family members in relation to their adjustments within organizations, appropriate use of social organizations, providing an environment that fosters the development of identities and affectional behavior, and creating a satisfying, emotionally healthy environment essential to the family's well-being. Adaptation is essential to the family's ability to carry out functions and tasks and to meet the changing needs of society and other social systems, such as political, health-illness systems.

Location. Family location is also a significant criterion for understanding the family. Brod and La-Due (1989) and Jacobson (1994) discussed the variations that occurred among values of Canadian Cree families when families were evaluated in urban versus rural settings. Brod and LaDue (1989) found that when some Canadian Cree moved from rural to urban settings, there was an erosion of values emphasizing "mutual aid" and a contrasting increase in individualism, materialism, and secularism. When urban Canadian Cree are compared with their rural counterparts, it appears that urban Native Canadian Cree may view their counterparts as lacking the toughness and sophistication needed to make headway in a dominant urban culture. Despite the variations that occur with location changes, geographical separation does not mean a severing of kinship ties, according to Martin (1980); rather, geographical separation may serve to strengthen the emotional bonds between relatives.

Religious groups

According to many sociologists, religion is a social phenomenon (Carroll, Johnson, and Marty, 1979), which implies an interactive relationship with the other social units that constitute a society. However, many persons, particularly those with religious convictions, tend to think of religion in an entirely different way. For some people religion is seen in the context of a person's communion with the supernatural, and religious experiences fall outside ordinary experiences, whereas other people view religion as an expression of an instinctual reaction to cosmic forces (Johnstone, 1988). Another world view of religion depicts religion as an explicit set of messages from a deity. For the most part, all these beliefs tend to deemphasize, ignore, and perhaps even reject the sociological dimensions of religion. Nevertheless, whether it is being considered in general, in regard to a particular religious family such as Christianity or Buddhism, or in regard to a very specific religious group such as Baptists, religion is believed to interact with other social institutions and forces in society and to follow and illustrate sociological principles and laws. In other words, regardless of what religion is or is not, it is a social phenomenon and as such is in a continual reciprocal, interactive relationship with other social phenomena.

In 1996, in Canada, about 75% of the population represented three main Christian churches: Roman Catholic (15,015,889 members with 128,390 affiliated with the Ukrainian Rite church, compared with 14,887,499 affiliated with the Latin Rite Church), United (785,726 members); and Anglican (771,615 members). Other Christian churches include the Orthodox (120,000 members), Baptist (132,000 members), Christian Reformed (86,000 members), the Church of the Latter-Day Saints (126,000 members), Lutheran (85,000 members), Lutheran Council of Canada (284,507), Mennonite (120,000 members), Pentecostals (231,420 members), Presbyterians (152,685 members), Seventh-day Adventists (44,283), and Friends (no membership given). Numerous other religious denominations are represented including the Bahi'i faith (24,000 members), Buddhism (no membership given), Islam (350,000 Muslims), Judaism (340,000 Jews), and Sikhism (250,000 Sikhs) (Europa World Year Book, 1996).

Regardless of its definition, be it theological or sociological, many different kinds of groups are based on religion. Generally, religious structures fall into two basic types: the church type and the withdrawal-group type. The church type of structure is broadly based and represents the normative spiritual values of a society that most people adhere to by virtue of their membership in the society, such as Hinduism in India or Catholicism in Spain. For the most part, membership in certain societies dictates the faith that the person should belong to if that person has not made a conscious, deliberate choice to adhere to something else. The church type of structure is generally a comprehensive system that allows for individual variations and in practice does not make extremely rigorous demands on its members. In Canada, the church structure is encompassed within a number of major denominations. This denominational structure is in sharp contrast with the church structure in other countries, such as India or Spain, where most of the people belong to one faith and one church. In some countries, particularly Canada, individual churches are often closely identified with an ethnic group rather than with a social class, and churches thrive more or less as a means of asserting ethnic identity. For example, the Black church, regardless of denominational faith, has become synonymous with the Black life experience. The Amish people, on the other hand, subscribe to one denominational belief; however, the belief is synonymous with the Amish life experience.

The second type of religious structure is the withdrawal group, which expresses the beliefs of those for whom personal commitment and experience are more important than the family and the community functions of religion (Ellwood, 1995). Withdrawal groups meet the needs of those who believe that the faith or lack of faith by the majority is not for them. Persons involved in withdrawal groups define themselves by making a separate choice. These groups include the Amish or Jehovah's Witnesses, which tend to represent a more intense or unbending commitment than that held by the average person adhering to a religion. These groups may be called "sects." Groups that combine separation with syncretism and new ideas and place emphasis on mystical experience are often referred to as "cults." However, the word "cult" is often used in Western society with caution because it has acquired a negative connotation. In some religious groups such as the Church of the Latter-day Saints (Mormons), Muslims, Jehovah's Witnesses, Seventh-Day Adventists, Buddhists, or Hindus, as well as that of the Gypsy culture, the extended social organization of the religion is considered more important than membership in the individual family. It is essential to remember that although this view is held by some theological scholars (Ellwood, 1995) many members of these religious groups do not necessarily share this belief. For example, in the Church of the Latter-day Saints (the Mormon Church), children are taught at a very young age that families are eternal. In this sense, the family is viewed as a stable cohesive group bonded by love and as such is one of the most important units on earth today (Walters, 1994). Two groups that may have particular significance for the nurse are Jehovah's Witnesses and Seventh-Day Adventists.

Jehovah's Witnesses The founder of the Watchtower Bible and Tract Society, which is the legal corporation now used by Jehovah's Witnesses, was Charles Taze Russell. The name "Jehovah's Witness" was taken in Columbus, Ohio, in 1931 in an attempt to differentiate between the Watchtower Tract Society and the true followers of Russell, who were represented by the Dawn Bible Students and the Layman's Home Missionary Movement. From 1876 to 1879 Russell served as pastor of the Bible class that he organized in Pittsburgh, Pennsylvania, and was also the assistant editor of a small monthly magazine in Rochester, New York. However, he resigned from the editorial position in 1879 when controversy arose over his counterarguments on the "Atonement of Christ." In 1879 he founded the magazine *Herald of the Morning,* which developed into the magazine that is distributed today titled *The Watchtower Announcing Jehovah's Kingdom.* This magazine has grown from a circulation of 6000 to 20.9 million per month and is published in 125 languages. Today there is another Watchtower periodical titled *Awake,* which has a circulation of 18.3 million issues twice a month and is published in 81 languages (Jehovah's Witnesses 1997 Yearbook, 1997).

In 1884 Russell incorporated Zion's Watchtower Tract Society in Pittsburgh, which published a series of seven books. Russell himself actually wrote six of these books. The seventh volume, *The Finished Mystery,* caused a split in the group that culminated in a clean division. The larger portion of the group followed Joseph Franklin Rutherford, whereas the smaller portion remained by itself and subsequently became known as the Dawn Bible Students Association. Under Rutherford's leadership the Watchtower Bible Society began to attack the doctrines of organized religion. This group eventually became known as the present-day Jehovah's Witnesses and has branches in 232 lands and islands of the sea, with 5.6 million members. There are 1379 Jehovah's Witness congregations in Canada with a membership of 114,272 (Jehovah's Witnesses 1997 Yearbook, 1997). The Canadian headquarters are located in Halton Hills, Ontario.

Modern-day Jehovah's Witnesses still await the Millennium. They regard Christ as a creature who will come to destroy the forces of evil at Armageddon, and they teach that sinners who are not saved will perish, whereas the faithful will enter into the Kingdom of Joy and Happiness. Because they believe in the Second Coming of the Kingdom, they undertake no military services. They also hold the belief that the institutions of government are under the control of Satan. It is this belief that has been the basis for some of the persecution they have undergone over the years. One view of this group is that Jehovah's Witnesses are peaceful but somewhat fanatical and that they know their Bible backward and forward (Smart, 1984). Some theologians believe that this religion appeals to persons of very modest education (Smart, 1984). The Jehovah's Witness faith is based on the doctrines presented in Box 4-2.

Implications for nursing care. There are many implications for nursing care for the nurse who provides culturally appropriate nursing care to a Jehovah's Witness. The paramount concern for the nurse is that Jehovah's Witnesses are opposed to homologous blood transfusions (blood obtained from a blood bank or through donations). However, many but not all Jehovah's Witnesses will submit to certain types of autologous blood transfusions (autotransfusion). Whether autologous blood transfusions will be accepted by a Jehovah's Witness depends on the type of autologous transfusion. Jehovah's Witnesses hold the view that "God's determination is that blood represents life and thus is sacred" (Watch-

---

Box 4-2

BELIEFS OF JEHOVAH'S WITNESSES

---

1. Jehovah's Witnesses believe that there is one solitary Being from all eternity and that that Being is Jehovah God, the creator and preserver of the universe in all things that are visible and invisible.
2. Jehovah's Witnesses do not believe in the Holy Trinity of three Gods in one—God the Father, God the Son, and God the Holy Ghost—who are equal in power, substance, and eternity (Watchtower Bible and Tract Society, 1953). Rather, they believe that Satan is the originator of the Trinity doctrine and that this doctrine is just another of Satan's attempts to keep people from learning the truth about Jehovah and his Son, Christ Jesus, which is that there is no Trinity (Watchtower Bible and Tract Society, 1953).
3. Jehovah's Witnesses believe that there is only one God and that he is greater than his Son. They believe that the Son, the firstborn and only begotten, was sent by God but is not God himself and is not equal with God.
4. On the subject of the Virgin Birth, Jehovah's Witnesses believe that Jehovah God took the perfect life of his only begotten Son and transferred it from heaven to the womb of the unmarried virgin, Mary. They believe that Jesus's birth was not an incarnation but that he was emptied of all things heavenly and spiritual. This was a miracle in the sense that Jesus was born a man (and was flesh) instead of a spirit-human hybrid (Martin, 1985).
5. Jehovah's Witnesses believe that the human life that Jesus Christ laid down in sacrifice must be viewed as exactly equal to the life that Adam forfeited for all of his offspring. Thus Jesus' life must be viewed as a perfect human life, no more and no less (Watchtower Bible and Tra ct Society, 1955).
6. Jehovah's Witnesses believe that immortality is a reward for faithfulness and that it does not come automatically to a human at birth (Watchtower Bible and Tract Society, 1953).
7. On the subject of the Resurrection of Christ, Jehovah's Witnesses believe that Christ was raised from the dead, not as a human creature, but as a Spirit (Watchtower Bible and Tract Society, 1953).
8. Jehovah's Witnesses believe that Christ Jesus will return again, not as a human, but as a glorious spirit. National flags or symbols of the sovereign power of a nation are forbidden by Exodus 20:2-6. Thus those who believe and ascribe salvation only to God may not salute a national emblem without violating Jehovah's commandments against idolatry (Watchtower Bible & Tract Society, 1953).
9. Jehovah's Witnesses believe that the hell mentioned in the Bible is mankind's common grave and that even an honest child can understand it. Thus the doctrine of a burning hell where the wicked are tortured after death cannot be true.
10. Jehovah's Witnesses believe that man is a combination of two things: dust of the ground and breath of life. The combining of these two things produces a living soul, or a creature called man.
11. Jehovah's Witnesses believe that the undefeatable purpose of Jehovah God is to establish a righteous kingdom in these last days and that this purpose has already been fulfilled.
12. Jehovah's Witnesses believe that the Levitical commandments given by God to Moses included the commandment that no one in the House of David should eat blood or he would be cut off from the people.

---

tower, 1989). They believe that it is God's commandment that no human should sustain life by taking blood. Jehovah's Witnesses believe that if blood is taken from a creature and not used for sacrifice it should be disposed of and covered with dust. This belief clearly rules out autologous transfusions, whereby blood is precollected from the client for future use and is stored as either whole blood or as packed cells (Watchtower, 1989). In receiving this type of transfusion, it is believed that stored blood is no longer a part of the person. In refusing this type of autologous transfusion, Jehovah's Witnesses cite God's law: "You should pour it upon the ground as

water" (Deuteronomy 12:24). Yet, there are certain types of autologous transfusions that some Jehovah's Witnesses will accept. One type of autologous transfusion that might be acceptable is blood retrieved through induced hemodilution at the start of surgery (blood that is directed to storage bags outside the client's body). It is essential to remember that some Jehovah's Witnesses believe that if the autotransfusion is halted in any way, the acceptability of the procedure to the client would be questionable. Although this type of autologous transfusion might be acceptable, others such as blood collected from a wound by aspiration, pumped through a filter or a centrifuge to remove debris and clots, and then given back to the client would not be an acceptable alternative (Watchtower, 1989). In addition, some Jehovah's Witnesses will permit the use of certain blood volume expanders. Many Jehovah's Witnesses carry a card with the types of blood volume expanders permitted. The nurse should ask the client for this card or, if the client is unconscious, examine the client's personal belongings to find this extremely important card. When autologous blood transfusions or blood volume expanders are not plausible alternatives, many physicians look to alternatives to and during major surgery that are acceptable to Jehovah's Witnesses, including colloid or colloid replacement fluids, electrocautery, hypotensive anesthesia, or hypothermia. It is important for the nurse to remember that persons who subscribe to this belief are likely to refuse to have any surgical or medical interventions that will require a homologous blood transfusion. Even in the face of ominous danger and with the impending threat of loss of life, a Jehovah's Witness will refuse treatment for self and family members if a homologous transfusion is the only plausible blood-replacement option available. There have been many legal battles waged in the courts in regard to minor children and the parents' refusal to allow surgical or medical interventions. The consensus of the court in some countries such as the Supreme Court in the United States has been that a person of adult majority age has the right to refuse treatment but not to withhold treatment from a minor child.

A second concern for the nurse is in regard to the refusal of Jehovah's Witnesses to eat certain foods to which blood has been added, such as certain sausages and lunch meats. The nurse must take extra care to ensure that blood has not been added to foods that are served to Jehovah's Witnesses. Because Jehovah's Witnesses are pacifists and conscientious objectors, the nurse must take extra care to avoid raising such issues during interaction. In general, topics related to politics, government rule, or the like, should be avoided. Since Jehovah's Witnesses do not observe any national holidays or ceremonies, including Christmas, the nurse should avoid any attempts to involve the client in preparations for such celebrations.

Seventh-Day Adventists The Seventh-Day Adventist religion sprang from the "Great Second Advent Awakening," which shocked the religious world just before the middle of the nineteenth century. During this period reemphasis on the second advent of Jesus Christ was rampant in England and in Europe. It was not long before many of the Old World views and prophetic interpretations crossed the Atlantic and began to penetrate American theological circles (Martin, 1992). The American Seventh-Day Adventist group began in upper New York (Ellwood, 1995).

The first leader of the Seventh-Day Adventists was William Miller, a Baptist minister from Lower Hampton, New York. The Seventh-Day Adventist religion is based largely on the apocalyptic books of Daniel and Revelation. Many of the early students of the Seventh-Day Adventist religion, following the chronology of Archbishop Ussher, interpreted the 2300 days of Daniel as 2300 years, and thus they concluded that Christ would come back in about the year 1843. In 1818 Miller taught many of his followers that in about 25 years (1843) Jesus Christ would come again. Miller and his associates pinpointed October 22, 1843, as the specific final date on which Jesus Christ would return for his saints, visit judgment on sin, and establish the Kingdom of God on earth. Many theologians disagreed with Miller's contentions because they believed that Miller was teaching in contradiction to the word of God. According to biblical scripture, "the day and hour knoweth no man, no, not the angels of heaven but God alone" (Matthew 24:36). Because of Miller's early teaching, the first group of Seventh-Day Adventists were called "Millerites." However, the mistake of setting an exact date for Christ's Second Coming led to failure for the first Seventh-Day Adventist movement in the United States.

The modern Seventh-Day Adventist movement is based on the prophecy of Ellen G. White. White made an early assertion about Miller's prophecy that supported the prophecy and gave a date that she considered to be correct: October 22, 1844. Despite this failure in prediction, the group has grown and been active in evangelism. Today Seventh-Day Adventists believe Christ will return again very soon and that Christians have an obligation to keep some

---

Box 4-3

BELIEFS OF SEVENTH-DAY ADVENTISTS

1. *Inspiration and authority of the scriptures.* Seventh-Day Adventists believe that the scriptures of both the Old Testament and the New Testament were inspired by God and constitute the very word of God. They hold the Protestant position that the Bible is the sole root of the faith and practice of Christians.
2. *The nature of Christ.* Christ, called the "Second Adam," is pure and holy and connected with God and beloved by God. Seventh-Day Adventists believe that Christ is God and that he has existed with God for all eternity (Martin, 1985).
3. *The Atonement.* Seventh-Day Adventists do not believe that Christ made partial or incomplete sacrificial atonement on the cross. The all-sufficient sacrifice of Jesus was completed on the cross at Calvary.
4. *The Resurrection.* Seventh-Day Adventists believe that Jesus rose from the grave, ascended literally and bodily into heaven, and serves before God. They believe there will be a resurrection of both the just and the unjust. For the just, this resurrection will take place at the Second Coming of Christ, whereas the resurrection of the unjust will take place 1000 years later, at the close of the Millennium (Revelation 20:5-10).
5. *The Second Coming.* Seventh-Day Adventists believe that Jesus Christ will assuredly come the second time and that his second advent will be visible, audible, and personal.
6. *The plan of salvation.* Seventh-Day Adventists believe that one must be born again and fully accepted by the Lord. They believe there is nothing an individual can ever do that will merit the salvation of God. Salvation is by grace (Roman 3:20).
7. *The spiritual nature of man.* Seventh-Day Adventists believe that man rests in the tomb until the resurrection of the just, when the righteous will be called forth by Christ

(Revelation 20:4-5). It is at this point that the just will enter into everlasting life in their eternal home in the Kingdom of Glory.

8. *Punishment of the wicked.* Seventh-Day Adventists reject the doctrine of eternal torment because everlasting life is a gift from God (Romans 6:23). The wicked do not possess this and therefore shall not have eternal life (John 3:36).
9. *Sanctuary and investigative judgment.* Seventh-Day Adventists believe that the acceptance of Christ at conversion does not seal a person's destiny; rather, it determines his life's work after conversion. Man's record is closed when he comes to the end of his days; he is responsible for his influences during life and is likewise responsible for his evil influences after he is dead.
10. *Scapegoat teaching.* Seventh-Day Adventists repudiate the idea that Satan is the sin bearer.
11. *The Sabbath and the Mark of the Beast.* This doctrine is based on the Bible as interpreted by Seventh-Day Adventists and not according to Ellen White's writings. Seventh-Day Adventists do not believe that keeping the Sabbath is a means of keeping salvation or willing merit before God. They believe that man is saved only by grace.
12. *The question of unclean food.* Seventh-Day Adventists refrain from eating certain foods, not because of the laws of Moses but because it is a Christian duty to preserve the body in the best of health for the service and glory of God (I Corinthians 3:16).
13. *The "remnant church."* Seventh-Day Adventists believe that God has a precious remnant, a multitude of earnest and sincere individuals, in every church. The majority of God's children are scattered throughout the world and may practice their religion on Sunday.

---

of the laws of Moses, which includes worship on Saturday, the old Sabbath. Thirteen issues on doctrine that give direction for living and that are upheld by the Seventh-Day Adventist Church are presented in Box 4-3.

The Seventh-day Adventist Church of Canada is part of the Worldwide Seventh-day Adventist Church with headquarters in Washington, D.C.. In Canada, the Seventh-day Adventist Church was organized in 1901 and reorganized in 1932 (Hill,

1995). There are 44,283 Seventh-day Adventists in 330 churches throughout Canada (Europa World Yearbook, 1996). The Canadian headquarters are in Oshawa, Ontario (Bedell, 1994).

Implications for nursing care. The religious doctrines of Seventh-Day Adventists teach that the body is a temple of God and thus should be kept healthy. Persons who subscribe to this faith may avoid such items as seafood, meat, caffeine, alcohol, drugs, and tobacco in all forms. To provide culturally appropriate nursing care to a Seventh-Day Adventist, the nurse must have a knowledge and understanding of the religious doctrines of the Seventh-Day Adventist Church. A Seventh-Day Adventist may refuse surgical intervention on a Friday evening or Saturday morning or afternoon because the client may interpret such an intervention as being in direct conflict with religious doctrines. This same client may also refuse other medical interventions that might normally take place at these times, such as respiratory or physical therapy.

The religious doctrine in regard to unclean foods may cause some clients to refuse to eat certain foods with shells, such as lobster or crab; scavenger fish, such as catfish; or certain meats. This refusal to eat certain foods high in iodine or protein may cause these clients to have iodine and protein deficiencies; thus it is important for the nurse to teach these clients that iodine and protein substitutes are necessary in the diet. Some specialty shops that have Seventh-Day Adventist clientele stock a variety of protein substitutes for meats. These substitutes are often made from vegetables such as soybeans and may take the place of meats such as ground beef. These substitutes should be encouraged, particularly when they appear to be free of preservatives.

The nurse and the nurse manager should also be aware that a colleague who is a Seventh-Day Adventist may refuse to accept assignments on Friday evenings or Saturday during the day because the Sabbath begins on Friday at dusk and extends to Saturday at dusk. It is important for the nurse who is a Seventh-Day Adventist to ascertain at the time of employment whether working on Friday evenings or Saturday during the day is a requirement of the job. On the other hand, it is also important for the nurse manager to include staff in making nondiscriminatory policies in this regard. Inclusion of staff in policy making may serve to minimize implementation difficulties.

Ethnic groups in relation to family

Canadian Indians The Canadian Indian population is divided into 608 bands (Indian and Northern Affairs, 1996). A band is a formally recognized group covering all parts of Canada, except the high Arctic. Nearly 6 of 10 registered Indians, 347,919, live on reserves—areas of land set aside through treaties or the Indian Act for their sole use and benefit (Indian and Northern Affairs, 1996). Some Indian people have managed to maintain a separate identity and culture despite numerous attempts to assimilate them into the White man's world. In the nineteenth century many Indian children were taken from their families and placed in boarding schools where they were forbidden to speak their own language or practice Native traditions. The social costs of this cultural disturbance were high, with excessively high drop-out rates from school, alcohol abuse, and disproportionate numbers of Indians in jail. Today the federal government is leading rehabilitation efforts. Indian language, culture, and history programs are flourishing, and traditional beliefs and practices are being encouraged (Young, 1994). In 1990, of the 671 Indian communities identified by the Medical Service Branch, 5.1% were remote isolated (with no road access, scheduled flights, and minimal telephone or radio services), 13.8% are isolated (with no road service, but have scheduled flights and adequate access to telephone services), 14.2% were semi-isolated (with road access to physician services at a distance greater than 90 km) and 66.9% were nonisolated (with physician services less than 90 km) (Health and Welfare Canada, 1991). Providing culturally appropriate nursing care is complicated because bands of Indians may have their own language and religion, and belief system practices differ significantly among groups as well as among members of the same band (Vogel, 1990).

The Canadian Indian family is generally composed of extended family members who generally encompass several households. Through various religious ceremonies other individuals can become the same as a parent in the family network. In some Canadian Indian bands, grandparents are viewed as the family leaders, and respect for individuals increases with age. Also in some Canadian Indian bands, the family is viewed as important, particularly in periods of crises, when family members are expected to serve as sources of support and security. It is important for the nurse to remember that because some Native Canadians tend to place great emphasis on the extended family as a unit, the opinions and ideas of the family members should be solicited when one is giving culturally appropriate nursing care. Although physicians and hospitals may be available to Canadian Indians residing in nonisolated and semi-isolated localities, traditional healing ceremonies may still be held in high regard by some families, and it may be important to incorporate old ways to treat illness for a treatment plan to be effective.

Special interest groups Self-help or mutual aid groups appear to be an important health prevention phenomenon across Canada (Todres and Hagarty, 1993). In 1987, a report from Health and Welfare Canada suggested that there were roughly a half-million self-help groups with several million members across North America. In 1991, it was estimated that 420,000 people were members of a self-help or mutual aid group (Gottlieb and Peters, 1991). In Canada, 8 of 10 provinces have clearinghouse operations (Todres and Hagarty, 1993). Public, federal, and provincial dollars have assisted in funding the clearinghouses, which provide a range of services including compiling information, providing information and referral, technical assistance and consultation, skill development, community support and development, community education, and research.

There is a wealth of information in the Canadian nursing literature concerning the involvement of nurses in self-help groups. For example, Pirie and Smith (1992) reported a premenstrual syndrome (PMS) support group in Toronto in which they provided drug-free education and support for responding to PMS symptoms. Morris, Clarke, Bingham (1989) in Ontario reported it as a source of assistance for the family and friends who try to assist the approximately one in 100 Canadians who are afflicted with schizophrenia.

IMPLICATIONS FOR NURSING CARE

When nurses provide care to clients from a sociocultural background other than their own, they must have an awareness of and a sensitivity to the client's sociocultural background, including knowledge of family structure and organization, religious values and beliefs, and how ethnicity and culture relate to role and role assignment within group settings (Lynam, 1991). Any social organization or group can be viewed as the environment in which the client strives for health. The approach to nursing care depends on the situation. The nurse must remember that if even one family member (other than the client), regardless of culture and ethnic heritage, is receptive to nursing care, it is realistic and practical to view the family as an environment. Friedman (1986) contends that nursing care must be directed to the family as a whole as well as to the individual family member. The nurse must therefore view the family as having two separate entities, the first being the family as an environment and the second being the family as the client. Both approaches to client care can be useful when the nurse attempts to provide culturally appropriate nursing care.

If the family is viewed as an environment, the primary focus of nursing care is the health and development of individual family members within a very specific environment. In this context it is important for the nurse to assess the extent to which the family provides the individual basic needs of each person. It is also essential that the nurse remember that individual needs vary depending on developmental level and the current situation. The nurse should be cognizant of the fact that families provide more than just the physical necessities; the ability of the family to help the client meet psychosociological needs is paramount.

When families are viewed as an environment, it is extremely important for the nurse to recognize that other family members may also need intervention. For example, when a child is hospitalized, the parents may feel anxiety and stress; therefore intervention with them is just as important as intervention with the hospitalized child.

When families are viewed as clients, it is important to assess crucial factors that are germane to family structure and organization. For example, if a hypertensive client is admitted to a hospital unit, it is crucial that the nurse assess several factors related to the family, including the following:

1. The family's current dietary patterns
2. The family's desire as well as resources for changing the dietary patterns
3. The family's knowledge about hypertension and its effects on the body
4. The family's capabilities to support a hypertensive family member
5. The family's ability to cope with and manage stress and anxiety

Whether the family is viewed as an environment or as the client, it is essential to incorporate cultural concepts when developing the nursing plan of care. The nursing process is used regardless of whether the family is viewed as an environment or as the client. The delineations or differences that occur in the nursing process are the result of cultural variables and beliefs that are germane to a particular ethnic or cultural group. Therefore it is essential that the nurse incorporate cultural beliefs and concerns shared by family members into the plan of care.

It is estimated that there are only 40 to 50 aboriginal physicians practicing in Canada today (representing approximately 0.1% of all physicians) and further that there are only 300 aboriginal registered nurses (representing approximately 0.1% of nurses). Increasing the number of aboriginal caregivers is one way to enhance the provision of culturally appropriate care (Royal Commission of Aboriginal Peoples, 1995). In August of 1995, the government of Canada launched a process to negotiate practical arrangements with First Nations people to make self-government a reality. Although self-government already exists within the Canadian Constitution, a new partnership between aboriginal peoples and the federal government will implement this right and promote increased aboriginal leadership (First Nations in Canada, 1995).

Case Study

Susie Chung, a 24-year-old Chinese Canadian, is admitted with right, lower-quadrant abdominal pain. Within a few hours Miss Chung is taken to surgery for an appendectomy. When she returns to the floor, her vital signs remain stable. The nurse notes that even though Miss Chung is rapidly recovering, her immediate and extended family appear to hover about her. The nurse also notes that it is very difficult to administer nursing care because of the number of family members who are keeping a constant vigil.

STUDY QUESTIONS

1. List at least three social organization factors that influence the interactions between members of the same ethnic group or members of varying ethnic groups.
2. List at least two social organization factors that contribute to the development of cultural behavior.
3. Explain the role that religion may play for Susie Chung in regard to sociopsychological adaptation to her illness.
4. List at least three nursing interventions that may serve to minimize the confusion caused by the large number of family members who
   are keeping constant vigil in Susie Chung's room.
5. List at least two reasons why the family members of Susie Chung have congregated in the hospital room.
6. List at least three factors that would support Susie Chung's family being defined as a behavioral system.
7. List at least two imaginary and two real boundaries that would be found within Susie Chung's family structure.
8. List at least two roles that Susie Chung may take on in a social context within her family structure.

References

Aboriginal Nurses Association of Canada. (1995). *Aboriginal Nurses Association of Canada Handbook 1975-1995.* Ottawa: Indian and Inuit Health Careers Program.

Ackerman, N. (1984). *The theory of family systems.* New York: Gardner Press.

Averaswald, E. (1973). Families, change and the ecological perspective. In Ferber, A. (Ed.), *The book of family therapy.* Boston: Houghton Mifflin.

Bailey, E., & Bailey, R. (1995). *Discover Canada.* Oxford, England: Berlitz Publishing Co.

Baker, C., Arseneault, A., & Gallant, G. (1994). Resettlement without the support of an ethnocultural community. *Journal of Advanced Nursing, 20*(6), 1064-1072.

Bateson, G., Jackson, D., Haley, J., & Weakland, J. (1968). Toward a theory of schizophrenia. In Jackson, D.D. (Ed.), *Communication, family and marriage.* Palo Alto, Calif: Science & Behavior Books.

Bedell, K. (1994). *Yearbook of American and Canadian churches.* Nashville: Abingdon Press.

Beiser, M., Barwick, C., Berry J.W., et al. (1988). *After the door has been opened: mental health issues affecting immigration and refugees.* A report of the Canadian Task Force on Mental Health Issues affecting Immigrants and Refugees. Ottawa: Ministry of Multiculturalism and Citizenship and Health and Welfare.

Berkanovic, E., & Reeder, L.G. (1973). Ethnic, economic and social psychological factors in the source of medical care. *Social Problems, 21,* 246-259.

Berry, J. (1988). Acculturation and psychological adaptation: a conceptual overview. In Berry, J.W., & Annis, R.C. (Eds.), *Ethnic psychology: research and practice with immigrants, refugees, native peoples, ethnic groups and sojourners.* Amsterdam: Swets & Zeitlinger.

Black, C. (1991). *It will never happen to me.* Denver: MAC Publishing.

Bowen, M. (1994). *Family therapy in clinical practice.* Northvale, N.J.: Jason Aronson.

Breitmayer, B., Gallo, A., Knafl, K., & Zoeller, L. (1989, April 3). *Correlates of social competence among children with a chronic illness.* Paper presented at the 13th Annual Midwest Nursing Research Society Conference, Cincinnati, Ohio.

Brod, R., & LaDue, R. (1989). Political mobilization and conflict among western urban and reservation service programs. *American Indian Culture and Research Journal, 13*(3), 171-214.

Brown, S. (1986). Children with an alcoholic parent. In Estes, N., & Heinemann, M. (Eds.), *Alcoholism: development, consequences, and interventions* (ed. 3) (pp. 207-220). St. Louis: Mosby.

Bullough, V.L., & Bullough, B. (1982). *Health care for the other Americans.* East Norwalk, Conn.: Appleton-Century-Crofts.

Campbell, J. (1989, April 3). *Self-care agency in battered women.* Paper presented at the 13th Annual Midwest Nursing Research Society Conference, Cincinnati, Ohio.

Canadian Almanac. (1993). Canadian Almanac and Directory (ed. 46). Detroit: Gale Research.

Canadian Mental Health Association. (1987). *Women and mental health in Canada: strategies for change.* Toronto: Women and Mental Health Coalition, Canadian Mental Health Association.

Caplan, G. (1975). The family as a support system. In Caplan, G., & Killilea, M. (Eds.), *Support systems and mutual help: multidisciplinary exploration.* New York: Grune & Stratton.

Carroll, J., Johnson, D., & Marty, M. (1979). *Religion in America: 1950 to present.* New York: Harper & Row.

Casavantes, E. (1976). Pride and prejudice: a Mexican American dilemma. In Hernandez, C.A., Haug, M.J., & Wagner, N.N. (Eds.), *Chicanos: social and psychological perspectives* (ed. 2) (pp. 9-14). St. Louis: Mosby.

Deuteronomy 12:24. (1984). *New world translation of the holy scriptures* (p. 201). New York: Watchtower Bible and Tract Society of New York, Inc., International Bible Student Association.

Duvall, E., & Miller, B. (1984). *Marriage and family development* (ed. 6). East Norwalk, Conn.: Appleton-Century-Crofts.

Ellwood, R. (1995). *Many peoples, many faiths* (ed. 5). Englewood Cliffs, N.J.: Prentice Hall.

Europa World Yearbook (vol. 1). (1996). Rochester, Kent: Staples Printers Rochester Limited.

Faulkner, D., Ratner, P., Johnson, J., Bottorff, J., & Unsworth, E. (1996). Drinking the bamboo dry: alcohol use by nursing students. *The Canadian Nurse, 92,* 22-24.

Fawcett, J. (1975). The family as a living open system: an emerging conceptual framework for nursing. *International Nursing Review, 22,* 113.

First Nations in Canada. (1995). *Progress in the 1980s and 1990s.* CMA Webspinners.

Franks, F., & Faux, S. (1990). Depression, stress, mastery, and social resources in four ethnocultural women's groups. *Research in Nursing and Health, 13,* 283-292.

Friedman, M.M. (1986). *Family nursing: theory and assessment.* East Norwalk, Conn.: Appleton-Century-Crofts.

Gary, F. (1991). Sociocultural diversity and mental health nursing. In Gary, F., & Kavanaugh, C. (Eds.), *Psychiatric nursing* (pp. 138-163). Philadelphia: J.B. Lippincott.

Giger, J., Davidhizar, R., Evers, S., & Ingram, C. (1994). Cultural factors influencing mental health and mental illness. In Taylor, C. (Ed.), *Mereness' essentials of psychiatric nursing* (ed. 14) (pp. 215-238). St. Louis: Mosby.

Giger, J., Davidhizar, R., & Wieczorek, S. (1994). Transcultural nursing: have we gone too far or not far enough? In Strickland, O., & Fishman, D. (Eds.), *Nursing in a diverse society.* New York: Delmar Publications.

Giger, J., & Davidhizar, R. (1995). *Transcultural nursing: assessment and intervention.* St. Louis: Mosby.

Giger, J., Johnson, J., Davidhizar, R., & Fishman, D. (1993). Strategies for building a supportive faculty. *Nursing and Health Care, 14*(3), 144-159.

Goldsby, R.A. (1977). *Race and races* (ed. 2). New York: MacMillan.

Gottlieb, B., & Peters, L. (1991). A national demographic portrait of mutual aid participants in Canada. *American Journal of Community Psychology, 19,* 651-666.

Govaets, K. (1987). Cultural and socioeconomic dimensions in mental health nursing. In Norris, J., Kunes-Connell, N., Stockhard, S., Ehrhart, P.M., & Newton, G.R. (Eds.), *Mental health-psychiatric nursing: a continuum of care.* New York: John Wiley & Sons.

Gregory, D. (1988). Nursing practice in native communities. In Baumgart, A. & Larson, J. (Eds.), *Canadian nursing faces the future.* Toronto: Mosby.

Grossman, M. (1995). Family nursing in tertiary care: history or the promise of things to come? *Canadian Journal of Nursing Research, 27*(2), 3-5.

Grpyma, S. (1993, September). Culture shock. *The Canadian Nurse, 89,* 33-37.

Guruge, S., & Donner, G. (1996, September). Transcultural nursing in Canada. *The Canadian Nurse, 92,* 34-39.

Guttmacher, S., & Elinson, J. (1972). Ethnos-religious variation in perception of illness: the use of illness as an explanation for deviant behavior. *Social Science Medicine, 5,* 117-125.

Harwood, A. (Ed.). (1981). *Ethnicity and medical care.* Cambridge, Mass.: Harvard University Press.

Health and Welfare Canada (1987). *Mutual aid as a mechanism for health promotion and disease prevention.* Ottawa: Minister of Supply and Services.

Health and Welfare Canada (1991). *Health status of Canadian Indians and Inuit, 1990.* Ottawa: Minister of Supply and Services.

Henderson, G., & Primeaux, M. (1981). *Transcultural health care.* Reading, Mass.: Addison-Wesley.

Hicks, R., LaLonde, R., & Pepler, D. (1993). Psychosocial considerations in the mental health of immigrant and refugee children. *Canadian Journal of Community Mental Health, 12*(2), 71-87.

Hindmarsh, K., Gliksman, L., & Newton-Taylor, B. (1993). Alcohol and other drug use by pharmacy students in Canadian universities. *Canadian Pharmaceutical Journal, 126,* 358.

Holmstrom, C. (1990, April, May). Women and substance abuse. *Canadian Journal of Psychiatric Nursing, 22,* 6-10.

Hyland, S. (1990, September). Helping employees with family care. *Monthly Labour Review,* 22-26.

Indian and Inuit Nurses of Canada. (1983, September 27-29). National Conference, Brantford, Ontario.

Indian and Northern Affairs, Canada. (1996). *Facts from stats* (No. 11, March-April). Ottawa: Information Quality and Research Directorate.

Jacobson, S. (1994). Native American Health. *Annual Review of Nursing Research, 12,* 192-213.

Jehovah's Witnesses 1997 Yearbook. (1997). New York: Watchtower Bible and Tract Society.

Johnstone, R. (1988). *Religion in society* (ed. 3). Englewood Cliffs, N.J.: Prentice Hall.

Kelly, K. (1993). Volunteer work and settlement: a study of Chinese immigrant women. *Canadian Journal of Community Mental Health, 12*(2), 31-44.

Lewis, H. (1979). *How's your family?* New York: Brunner/Mazel.

Lewis, J.M., Beavers, W.R., Gossett, J.T., & Phillips, V.A. (1976). *No single thread: psychological health in family systems.* New York: Brunner/Mazel.

Lynam, J. (1991). Taking culture into account: a challenging prospect for cardiovascular nursing. *Canadian Journal of Cardiovascular Nursing, 2*(3), 10-15.

Mann House Corp. (1989). Drive straight home: fact sheet.

Martin, E.P. (1980). *The Black extended family.* Chicago: University of Chicago Press.

Martin, W. (1992). *The kingdom of the cults.* Minneapolis: Bethany House.

Mauksch, H. (1974). A social science basis for conceptualizing family health. *Social Science Medicine, 8,* 521.

McDaniel, S. (1993). Challenges to mental health promotion among working women in Canada. *Canadian Journal of Community Mental Health, 12*(1), 201-210.

McRae, L. (1994). Cultural sensitivity in rehabilitation related to native clients. *Canadian Journal of Rehabilitation, 7*(4), 251-256.

Minuchin, S. (1974). *Families and family therapy.* Cambridge, Mass.: Harvard University Press.

Mo, B. (1992). Modesty, sexuality, and breast health in Chinese American women. *The Western Journal of Medicine, 157,* 260-264.

Morris, R., Clarke, M., & Bingham, B. (1989, July August, September). Schizophrenia and the family. *Canadian Journal of Psychiatric Nursing,* 17-18.

Murphy, S. (1986). Family study and nursing research. *Image: Journal of Nursing Scholarship, 18*(4), 170.

Murray, R., & Huelskoetter, M. (1991). *Psychiatric mental health nursing.* Norwalk, Conn.: Appleton & Lange.

Murray, R., Meili, P., & Zentner, J. (1993). The family—basic unit for the developing person. In Murray, R., & Zentner, J. (Eds.), *Nursing concepts for health promotion* (ed. 5). Englewood Cliffs, N.J.: Prentice Hall.

Nolt, S. (1992). *A history of the Amish.* Intercourse, Pa.: Good Books.

O'Brien, S. (1992). Gender bias in family benefit provision. *Canadian Journal of Community Mental Health, 11*(2), 163-186.

Phipps, S. (1989, April 3). *A phenomenological study of males' experience with infertility.* Paper presented at the 13th Annual Midwest Nursing Research Society Conference, Cincinnati, Ohio.

Peitchinis, S. (1989). *Employment standards handbook.* Toronto: McClelland Stewart.

Pilowsky, J. (1993). The courage to leave: an exploration of Spanish-speaking women victims of spousal abuse. *Canadian Journal of Community Mental Health, 12*(2), 15-27.

Pirie, M., & Smith, L. (1992). Coping with PMS. *The Canadian Nurse, 88,* 23-24.

Prilleltensky, I. (1993). The immigration experience of Latin American families: research and action on perceived risk and protective factors. *Canadian Journal of Community Health Nursing, 12*(2), 101-116.

Ram, B. (1990). *New trends in the family: demographic facts and features.* Ottawa: Minister of Supply and Services.

Royal Commission on Aboriginal Peoples. (1995, June 16). *Looking forward, looking back.* CMA Webspinners.

Sands, E., & Berry, J. (1993). Acculturation and mental health among Greek-Canadians in Toronto. *Canadian Journal of Community Mental Health, 12*(2), 117-124.

Satir, V. (1983). *Conjoint family therapy* (ed. 3). Palo Alto, Calif.: Science & Behavior Books.

Saunders, L. (1954). *Cultural differences and medical care.* New York: Russell Sage Foundation.

Scheflen, A.E., & Scheflen, A. (1972). *Body language and the social order.* Englewood Cliffs, N.J.: Prentice-Hall.

Smart, N. (1984). *The religious experience of mankind* (ed. 3). New York: Charles Scribner's Sons.

Spector, R. (1996). *Cultural diversity in health care* (ed. 4). Stamford, Conn.: Appleton & Lange.

Strickland, O., & Giger, J. (1994). Women's health in the decade of the woman. In Strickland, O. & Fishman, D. (Eds.), *Nursing issues and ethics* (pp. 362-399). Albany, N.Y.: Delmar Publishing Company.

Suchman, E.A. (1964). Sociomedical variations among ethnic groups. *American Journal of Sociology, 70,* 319-331.

Sussman, H. (1990, Summer). Are we talking revolution? *Human Resource Development Journal,* 1-3.

Sussman, M.B. (1971, July). Family systems in the 1970s: analysis, politics, and programs. *Annals of American Academy of Political Social Science, 396,* 40-56.

Thompson, K. (1993). Self-governed health. *The Canadian Nurse, 89,* 29-32.

Thompson, P. (1986). *Health education for immigrant women: a manual and resource guide.* Vancouver: Orientation Adjustment Services for Immigrants Society.

Thompson, P. (1987). Health promotion with immigrant women: a model of success. *The Canadian Nurse, 83,* 20-24.

Todres, R., & Hagarty, S. (1993). An evaluation of a self-help clearinghouse: awareness, knowledge, and utilization. *Canadian Journal of Community Mental Health, 12*(1), 211-224.

Townson, M. (1988). *Leave for employees with family responsibilities.* Ottawa: Ministry of Labour, Government of Canada.

U.S. Department of Commerce. (1991, March). Bureau of Census, the Black population, P20-464. Washington, D.C.: U.S. Government Printing Office.

Vogel, V.J. (1990). *American Indian Medicine.* Norman: University of Oklahoma Press.

Walters, T. (1994, January). Personal communication to J.N. Giger, Salt Lake City, Utah.

Watchtower. (1989, March 1). Questions from readers. *Watchtower,* 30-31.

Watchtower Bible and Tract Society. (1953). *Let God be true* (rev. ed.). New York: The society.

Watchtower Bible and Tract Society. (1955). *You may survive Armageddon into God's new world.* New York: The society.

Wolfram, W.A., & Clark, H. (Eds.). (1971). *Black-white speech relationships.* Washington, D.C.: Center for Applied Linguistics.

World Almanac. (1997). Mahwah, N.J.: World Almanac Books.

York, C. (1991). The labour movement s role in parental leave and child care. In Shibley-Hide, J. & Essex, M. (Eds.), *Parental leave and child care: setting a research and policy agency.* Philadelphia: Temple University Press.

Young, T. (1994). *The health of Native Americans.* New York: Oxford University Press.

Zinn, M., & Eitzen, D. (1987). *Diversity in American families.* New York: Harper & Row.

CHAPTER 5 Time

BEHAVIORAL OBJECTIVES

After reading this chapter, the nurse will be able to:

1. Postulate an adequate definition for the term "time" in relation to transcultural nursing care.
2. Understand the significant role that culture plays in the understanding and perception of time.
3. Understand the significant role that the developmental process plays in the understanding and perception of time.
4. Understand the significance of the measurement of time and the relationship to transcultural nursing care.
5. Differentiate the terms "social time" and "clock time."
6. Describe the world view of clock time and social time.
7. Define the three broad areas of the structure of social time: temporal patterns, temporal orientation, and temporal perspectives.

Since the beginning of life on earth, time has been the greatest mystery of all. The mystery of time becomes evident as soon as thought is given to the concept. Our experience with time continuously leads us into puzzles and paradoxes. According to Wessman and Gorman (1977), it is through an awareness and conception of time that the products of the human mind, that is, time itself, seem to possess an existence apart from time's passage, which is perceived as personal and inexorable. We measure time, and time measures us. It is this intimate and personal yet aloof and detached character that constitutes the paradox of human time.

CONCEPT OF TIME

The concept of the passage of time is very familiar to most people regardless of cultural heritage. The days and nights come and go, and with each passing day and night humankind grows older. In the highly mechanized world of today there are numerous clocks and watches that ceaselessly tick away time

and determine the schedules by which hundreds of millions of people live. Thus it would seem that the concept of the passage of time should be second nature to humankind and thoroughly understood by all people (Giger and Davidhizar, 1995, Spector, 1996).

However, developing an awareness of the concept of time is not a simple phenomenon but a gradual process (Hymovich and Chamberlin, 1980). Most people, regardless of cultural heritage, remember a time when their perception of the passage of time was altered. Such occasions might have been during times of boredom or highly emotional and stressful events. During these events time might have seemed to have passed very slowly, or it might have seemed to have passed all too quickly. It must be remembered that a sense of time is not innate but is developed early as a result of everyday experiences that are common to all people. Thus a sense of time results from learning. It becomes a part of human nature before one is conscious of its presence. Even infants perceive the essence of time. Infants are fed on demand or according to a strict timetable and experience the succession of day by night. Thus infants are exposed to regular rhythmic changes that are reflected in rhythmic changes in bodily conditions, including being sated, awake, or asleep. Thus one phenomenon about time is that it is associated with rhythm and change.

Infants grow, develop, and begin to move through crawling. The speed with which crawling occurs determines the time it takes to get from one place to another. Thus even this simple task makes individuals aware that time is associated with speed and velocity, which is the second phenomenon about time. As individuals grow older, speech is learned by listening to stories that begin with "once upon a time." It is through these storytelling sessions that children learn that things did happen before they were born; thus time is associated with history and goes backward as well as forward with the succession of events. As the growth and development of the child continues, an awareness of punctuality is developed. Children may be punished for being slow or late, and regardless of their reaction to it, the punishment contributes to the formation of character and the development of the understanding of time. Thus the third phenomenon about time is that it is associated with social behavior (Sideleau, 1992).

The child begins to become conscious of time and asks questions such as, "Where was I before I was born?" "What did God do before He created the world?" "What will happen to me after I die?" Such questions lead to an understanding that time is associated with philosophy and religion. Children are taught to read time on a clock, and as they grow to adulthood, they learn that the clock is ubiquitous and that life is governed by the clock. Thus there is an erroneous identification of time with the clock. Through questioning, individuals begin to contemplate existence on earth and to develop an understanding that time is associated with something external over which there is no control and that appears absolute (Elton, 1975; Sideleau, 1992).

Developing an understanding of the definition of time by looking at the developmental process is clearly too simple. The development of the awareness of time is directly influenced by earlier ideas and prejudices that are mostly unconscious. However, because it is the nature of humankind to have a questioning frame of mind, ideas and prejudices may become conscious.

Other considerations concerning time include the question of whether time is concrete or abstract. Time is perceived as real in the sense of being concrete and having direct effects, or it is regarded as not real in the sense of being abstract. The mathematical and physical sciences adopt the view that time is an abstract dimension with only a locational or reference function (McGrath and Kelly, 1986). On the other hand, the biological sciences adopt the view that time is an essential ingredient in many life and behavioral processes such as gestation, healing, and metamorphosis. This difference in conceptualization of time may be related to an obvious difference between the physical and biological sciences and how each treats the concept of entropy. For the physical sciences entropy, or randomness, continuously increases over time, whereas the biological sciences see organization, structure, and information residing within the organism and in the organism's relation to its environment as increasing over time (Giger and Davidhizar, 1995).

MEASUREMENT OF TIME

Time has two distinct, though related, meanings. The first meaning is that of duration, which is the passage of an interval of time. The second meaning is that of specified instances, or points in time. These two meanings are related because a point in time is identified as being the end of a time interval that starts at an arbitrary or fixed reference point, such as the founding of Rome or the birth of Christ. Thus if one asks the question, "What is the time?" and the answer given is, "It is 10:00 A.M.," this answer refers to a point in time. At the same time, the answer refers to a time interval because it indicates the time from a certain reference point, which in this case is midnight the previous night (Elton, 1975; Sideleau, 1992). The two meanings are quite different and must not be confused with each other. Measuring devices are meant to determine intervals of time, and clocks and watches are designed to read direct points in time. Clocks and watches therefore have to be standardized against a standard clock. The purpose of a standard clock is to measure accurately the interval up to the present time. This phenomenon goes back to one universal standard clock against which all standard clocks are calibrated.

The purpose of a universal standard clock is to define operational time in terms of both interval and point in time (Landes, 1983). The purpose of measuring devices is to define time; however, people need to have intuitive ideas about time to specify the properties of the instrument. Measuring devices of a phenomenon such as time are more accurate than measuring devices of some other phenomena. For example, if an individual wanted to measure the weight of a person, this weight could be defined operationally as a point or reading on a scale. Thus a good scale would give accurate weight, just as any good clock would give accurate time. On the other hand, if an individual wanted to define a person's intelligence quotient (IQ) as the score obtained on an intelligence test but there was no general agreement about what constituted intelligence and what constituted a good intelligence test, the scores would not be as relevant or as meaningful as the weight or time measures.

Throughout the history of humankind there have been two obvious standards of time: the day and the year. The day is a remarkably easy period of time to recognize because of the experience of daylight and darkness, which result from the earth's spinning on its axis. The year is also easy to recognize because of the passage of the seasons, which are caused by the tilting of the earth's axis. Thus a day is the period of time for one complete revolution of the earth about its axis, whereas a year is the time taken for the earth to move one complete revolution around the sun, which takes just under 365.25 days. Therefore it is completely natural that we choose to mark the passage of time by first marking the days and then marking the years. Time measurement during the day has been divided into hours, and the hours in turn have been divided by 60 to give minutes. The minutes have been divided by 60 to give seconds.

Very early in the history of civilization the middle of each day was determined as the point when the sun was at its highest point during the day. This point was defined as noon, and clocks were made to read 12 when it occurred. Thus, if it is noon in one place, it is midnight at the opposite side of the earth but different times at other places on the earth. To understand how time varies, the earth must be viewed as a circle that passes through both the North and South poles.

Traditionally in science, Greenwich Observatory in Greenwich, London, has been taken to have 0 degrees of longitude; all other places on earth are given as so many degrees east or west of Greenwich. Therefore one half of the earth's surface has a longitude of up to 180 degrees east of Greenwich, whereas the other half has a longitude of up to 180 degrees west of Greenwich. The times of all places east of Greenwich are ahead of that of Greenwich, and the times of all places west of Greenwich lag behind that of Greenwich. For example, if an individual started from Greenwich and traveled eastward to a longitude of 45 degrees, the time would be 3 hours ahead of Greenwich time. The converse is that if an individual started at Greenwich and traveled westward to a longitude of 180 degrees, the time would be 12 hours behind that of Greenwich. In simpler terms, if it were 2 A.M. on Sunday morning at Greenwich, it would be 2 P.M. on Sunday at a longitude 180 degrees east of Greenwich and 2 P.M. on Saturday at a longitude 180 degrees west of Greenwich (Elton, 1975).

This phenomenon of time presents some interesting effects on persons who travel great distances. For example, it is possible for an international traveler to have two birthdays; that is, if a person crosses the international date line traveling eastward at 2 A.M. Sunday morning, at which point it suddenly becomes 2 A.M. Saturday, that person has Saturday all over again and thus is able to celebrate the birthday again. If this same international traveler who is about to celebrate a birthday on Saturday leaves from the point of origin at 2 A.M. on Saturday but crosses the international date line westward, the traveler suddenly finds that it is 2 A.M. Sunday morning and apparently has missed almost the entire day of Saturday and the birthday (Elton, 1975).

Clocks

According to historians and philosophers, the earliest clocks were undoubtedly sundials of various kinds, which were probably followed by devices that used the regular flow of a substance such as water, oil, or sand, or the steady combustion of oil or candles. The earliest clocks have been dated back to 1600 B.C. in Egypt and were used throughout classical times and the Middle Ages.

The thirteenth century saw the invention of a rhythmic motion clock, which was a saw-toothed crown wheel. However, the most important development in clock construction occurred with the introduction of the pendulum, which was first discovered by Galileo in 1581. Galileo discovered that a swinging pendulum would readily tick away a unit of time by a specific number of swings and that even if the swings gradually died, the unit of time would remain relatively unaffected. Thus, for the first time in history, time was measured more accurately.

Tropical years

An important distinction that has been made by scientists is the difference between a calendar year and a tropical year. According to scientists, a calendar year consists of 365 days, whereas a tropical year consists of 365.242199 solar days (the word "tropical" in this instance has nothing to do with a hot climate). The difference between these two numbers (tropical year and calendar year) is the reason for the necessity of leap years. Time that is based on the length of a tropical year is called "ephemeris time." One tropical year is defined in terms of having 31,556,925.9747 seconds. Today atomic clocks have replaced the old, outdated pendulum-and-weight and gravity-driven clocks. Atomic clocks are so accurate that in due course scientists speculate that the difference between atomic time and ephemeris time will become very apparent. In fact, atomic clocks are said to be 10 million times more accurate than any other clock on earth and are never more than 1 billionth of a second off. Atomic clocks are considered to be so accurate that the exact second of an event can be obtained at the time of the event.

Solar time

Solar time is perhaps the earliest way that time was measured (Dossey, 1982). Solar time takes into consideration a primary point, 12:00 noon, which is precisely the point at which the sun passes directly overhead (vertically above the meridian). The time between successive crossings of the sun directly over the same meridian is called a "solar day." However, this measurement of time is not without its problems. When days are measured in this way, they turn out to be not exactly constant. A solar day varies slightly in length throughout the year because of the orbiting of the earth around the sun.

The concept of solar time has many implications for nurses who work at extreme southern or northern points of the earth, as at the North Pole or South Pole. A nurse working in the northernmost part of Canada may find Indians operating on "Indian time" because the sun remains up during most of the summer and down during much of the winter. Activities requiring daylight can therefore be done anytime during a 24-hour period. Staying up much of the night and sleeping in the daytime is consistent with an orientation to do what feels right at whatever is the present time. On the other hand, "White man's time" is more future oriented and adheres to clocks and schedules rather than to the sun (Wuest, 1992; England, 1986; Lefever and Davidhizar, 1995; Young, 1988). Generally White men who have not grown up in the northernmost part of Canada but have relocated to this area tend to work during familiar working hours and to sleep during familiar sleeping hours. However, this pattern may not necessarily correlate with the same time orientation for others who are native to the northernmost part of Canada.

Calendar

Inventing a simple yet efficient calendar has presented difficulties since the invention of the first calendar. Scientists believe that these difficulties lie in the fact that the three obvious periods are attributable to the rotation of the earth about the sun. These three revolutional periods are not related simply one to the other. In fact, they have obvious differences. For example, 1 tropical year equals 365.224 solar days, and 1 month is considered to be the observed time between one full moon and the next, or 29.5306 solar days.

Throughout history we have measured time by counting the months and the calendar years and combining the two. However, this combination of months and years has proved to be most confusing. Even if we ignored the moon, there would still be the problem of the solar year not being a whole number of days, though this problem has conceivably been dealt with by the system of leap years. With so many different civilizations contributing to the development of the calendar, it is no wonder that we are left with a complicated system that children and even adults, regardless of ethnic or cultural heritage, find difficult to remember or understand. Many of the significant events linked with the calendar can be traced to specific persons in history such as Julius Caesar, who decreed that months should alternately have 30 and 31 days except for February (which at that time was the last month of the Roman calendar). Historians believe that all would have been well with the calendar if Julius Caesar had not decided to call the fifth month Julius in his honor. The problem began when Augustus followed Julius Caesar and also wanted a month. He promptly chose the month that followed Julius and named it Augustus. However, he very soon realized that his month was shorter than Caesar's month and promptly took a day from February, added it to his month, and readjusted the rest of the year. The result was that there were 3 long months in succession, that is June, July, and August. Even today, because of the vanity of Emperor Augustus, children continue to chant "Thirty days hath September."

According to the earlier decree by Julius Caesar, September would have been an alternate month with 31 days if August had been given 30 days as originally planned (Elton, 1975). Although there have been attempts over the last 50 years to standardize the calendar by international agreement through the League of Nations and the United Nations, these attempts have uniformly failed. For example, the day that is considered the beginning of the New Year in the United States is January 1, but the beginning of the New Year differs in many countries.

SOCIAL TIME VERSUS CLOCK TIME

The word "time" immediately presents an image of a clock or calendar. However, the term "social time" is not equivalent with clock time. Social time refers to patterns and orientations that relate to social processes and to the conceptualization and ordering of social life. For centuries, many of the great thinkers of the universe have recognized and argued that social time must be distinguished from clock time. As early as 1910, Henri Bergson insisted that the homogeneous time of newtonian physics was not the time that revealed the essence of humankind. On the other hand, Phillip Bock (1964), an anthropologist, showed that an Indian wake could be meaningfully analyzed in terms of "gathering time," "prayer time," "singing time," "intermission time," and "meal time." None of these times has a particular relationship to clock time. They all simply imply the passage of the mourner from one time to another by consensual feelings rather than by the clock.

According to some sociologists, certain kinds of psychological disorders may be viewed in terms of the individual living wholly in the present, the implication being that the past and the future are completely severed from the consciousness. The difference therefore between social time and clock time is that the former is a more inclusive concept whereas the latter may or may not be. Hoppe and Heller (1974) conducted a study on Mexican Americans and proposed that Mexican Americans have a present-time orientation that may possibly account for the tendency to be late for appointments. It is believed that present-time orientation, particularly in high-risk settings such as mental health facilities, may result in a crisis approach rather than a preventive one. For example, a client who has an immediate need at home may be late for appointments at the clinic or hospital, or may miss them altogether. The nurse should also keep in mind that clients with a present-time orientation may be reluctant to leave an appointment simply because the time is up.

This same lack of correlation between social time and clock time can be seen in mystical beliefs. According to mystical thought, magic can be employed to negate the temporal order that infers causality. For example, an Indian warrior who is wounded by an arrow may attend to his pain by hanging the arrow up where it is cool or by applying ointment to the arrow. What the Indian warrior is attempting to do is to reverse the clock time, that is, wrench the present back into the past to alter the course of events. For people who have mystical beliefs, temporal intervals are not simple, homogeneous series; rather, they contain an inherent quality and meaning or an essence and efficacy of their own (Cassirer, 1955). Therefore the objectivity represented by clock time is unknown to a person with mystical beliefs.

Many sociologists believe that people who lack or minimize clock time also lack regularity or temporal measurement. The natural and social phenomena may dictate regularity and measurement. Ariotti (1995) provides several examples of natural events that have been used to time human activities: (1) The arrival of the cranes in ancient Greece marked the time for planting. (2) The return of the swallow marked the time for the end of pruning. (3) The South African Bushmen notice the rising of Sirius and Canopus and are able to depict the progress of winter across the night sky by the movement of these celestial bodies across the night sky.

Archeologists have been able to piece together the history of humankind by measuring the passage of time, using the method of geologists. This measure of time is based on rates of deposits to and erosion of natural early elements. An example of this kind of measurement is tree-ring chronology, or dechronology (Weyer, 1961).

World view of social time versus clock time

People throughout the world view social time and clock time differently (Giger and Davidhizar, 1995; Davidhizar, Dowd, and Giger, 1997). For example, Sorokin (1964) noted that the division of time by weeks reflects social conditions rather than mechanical newtonian divisions. Most societies have some kind of week, but the weeks vary in length from 3 to 16 or more days. In most cases weeks are a reflection of the cycle of market activities. The Khasi people have an 8-day week because they hold market every eighth day. The Khasi people have named the days of the week after the places where the principal markets occur (Sorokin, 1964).

Some cultural groups exhibit a social time that not only is different from clock time, but is actually scornful of clock time. For example, there are peasants in Algeria who live with a total indifference to the passage of clock time and who despise haste in human affairs. These peasants have no notion of exact appointment times; they lack exact times for eating meals; and they have labeled the clock as "the devil's mill" (Thompson, 1967). Some Amish keep "slow time." When those around them adjust their time to go from "daylight saving time" to "standard time," the Amish set clocks one-half hour ahead (Randall-David, 1989; Gingerich, 1972; Wenger, 1991; Nolt, 1992). This has important implications for the nurse in trying to emphasize the importance of keeping medical appointments.

Despite the way people in various cultures view clock time as opposed to social time, the nurse must remember that clock time should not be regarded as unimportant or irrelevant (Giger and Davidhizar, 1995). Although for some people in some cultural groups there is no necessary correlation of clock time and social time, clock time does not take on paramount importance in a social context as it does in the modern Western world, where the watch or the clock can become something of a tyrant. In Jonathan Swift's *Gulliver's Travels,* Gulliver never did anything without looking at his watch, which he called his oracle. He said that his watch pointed out the time for every action of his life. Because of Gulliver's obsession with his watch, the Lilliputians concluded that the watch was Gulliver's god.

Aside from literature, many actual examples of human obsessive behavior in regard to clock time can be found. Lebhar (1958) wrote that he was exactly 43 years old and had probably only 227,760 hours to live, and he proceeded to detail how he would maximize the use of those remaining hours of his life. He concluded that if he reduced his sleep time from 8 hours to 6 hours, the 2 hours a day saved from sleeping would amount to 18,980 hours over a period of 26 years. If this savings were converted into 18-hour days, which is the equivalent of about 2 years and 11 months, he could virtually lengthen his remaining years by 2 years and 11 months. This example illustrates how human life can be turned into a lengthy succession of minutes and hours, with the individual's existence reduced to a compulsive and frantic effort to avoid waste.

Gilles and Faulkner (1978) conducted a study of the role of time in television news work. They found that time is a major factor in the production of unscheduled "hard" news. The definition for "hard" news refers to events such as fires, homicides, and accidents, which have a certain urgency to them. They summarized the findings of their research in three propositions. In the first proposition they concluded that the news value of an event is directly proportional to the time invested in covering it. An event may turn out to be relatively minor in the sense of not involving the trauma or shock value that was anticipated, but this factor was not considered when a film crew invested time in the event, and the story is likely to be used in the evening news program anyway. They found in the second proposition that what is considered news by the news crew depends on when it happens and how long it lasts. Although viewers tend to believe that what they see on the evening news is a compilation of the universal news events for that particular day, what is telecast each evening is actually a compilation of news events that the news crew was able to learn about, get a story line on, capture on film, and then process and edit the film. The researchers found in the third proposition that bias in the news reflects occupational assumptions and temporal constraints more than it does the political or social views of the news crew. More important than political and social biases are the assumptions that the news crew makes about what will make good news on television and the severe time constraints on those persons assigned to locate film and write about events in time for the evening news program. The researchers concluded that because of deadline pressures it is inevitable that events are reduced to surface actions and that the visuals seen each evening are of only the most dramatic events.

In today's modern technological society, clock time is of paramount importance. However, we must remember that even in a modern society the clock may be a relatively peripheral part of social life. Not all people in a modern technological society function under the inevitable tyranny of the clock.

In a survey of a representative sample of the French population, approximately 21% of the respondents indicated a belief that there was no urgency about being punctual and also stated that they had not experienced the feeling of wasting time (Stoetzel, 1953). It is the perception of some people in some cultural groups that there is little correlation between being punctual and wasting time (Hein, 1980). Hein further postulated that assumptions and definitions in regard to time are determined by culture and cultural variables and are reflected in interactions with others, personal views concerning punctuality, use or waste of time, and value and respect for time or a lack thereof. Waiting is a cultural counterpart to time because a particular behavior, person, or event is anticipated within a particular time frame. Waiting may have a meaning similar to that of time for some African-American clients. The nurse may schedule an appointment for an African-American client and wait for the client to arrive for the appointment. However, the client may not arrive for several hours, or perhaps even a few days, because of other important issues that in the client's mind took precedence over the appointment. Although the nurse viewed this time as waiting and therefore wasting time, the client for whom the appointment was made was not wasting time (Randall-David, 1989).

In some cultures, for example, among some persons of Asian origin, time is viewed as flexible, and so there is no need to hurry or be punctual except in extremely important cases. Asians may spend hours getting to know people and view predetermined abrupt endings as rude (Stauffer, 1995). Nonetheless, the nurse should emphasize the importance of keeping scheduled appointments. Hispanics or Latinos as well often have difficulty with scheduled appointments. In fact, Hispanics or Latinos are sometimes attributed by others as being on "Latin time." However, this is sometimes explained by Hispanics as the result of consideration for others who were not ready to leave for the appointment (Ruiz, 1981; Ruiz and Padella, 1977; Hoppe and Heller, 1974).

In the Canadian nursing profession, many nurses

have related professionalism and success in their career to a sense of precision about clock time. For example, in many health care facilities, a medication error is considered to occur when a medication is not given within 30 minutes of the prescribed time, even when the medication is given daily and is not a time-released medication. Thus the nurse must complete a medication error form for not giving a routine daily medication such as a vitamin or a laxative, which is neither time released nor urgent.

Most agencies relate medication errors to disciplinary action and dismissal. In some facilities the nurse is expected to complete all morning or evening care in a precise time frame even though many clients may not operate in the same time sphere as the facility schedule for client care. For example, a client may become upset when the night nurse refuses to help the client to shower at 3 A.M. because showering is a stated day-shift activity. In this case the client may be used to starting the day at 3 A.M. and may be unwilling to wait until 7 A.M. to do so. Another example concerns early morning vital signs, which may be taken by the night nurse to facilitate a timely assessment of the client's condition for the physician who makes early-morning rounds. The client may be annoyed at being awakened for such a brief procedure and then instructed by the nurse to return to sleep.

According to Zerubavel's (1979) analysis of the temporal order of the hospital, any unit of clock time is equal to any other unit whether one is talking about minutes, hours, days, or weeks. However, Zerubavel concluded that different days mean quite different things to different people. Because people perceive days differently, it is important to remember that some days are more or less desirable for some people. For example, some health care personnel may perceive the fact of working two weekends in succession as unfair. Similarly, evening or night duty is usually considered less desirable than day duty. Thus it is important for hospital administrators to understand the necessity for fairness in scheduling. Some hospitals have a policy that all personnel are expected to work their share of the less desirable times. In other hospitals, the staff are paid differentials for working what is perceived as the less desirable times, that is, evenings, nights, weekends, and holidays.

STRUCTURE OF SOCIAL TIME

The structure of social time is a complex phenomenon. To understand the structure of social time, three broad areas of social time must be analyzed: temporal pattern, temporal orientation, and temporal perspective.

Temporal pattern

Hawley (1986) identified the temporal pattern of social time as one of the most important aspects of ecological organization. He concluded that there are five basic elements in the temporal pattern of any social phenomenon: periodicity, tempo, timing, duration, and sequence.

Periodicity Periodicity refers to the various rhythms of social life and is characterized by activities related to both the needs and the activities of people. For example, every community has a functional routine that is supposedly peculiar to that community, such as the search for food, shelter, and mates, which occurs more or less with regular periodicity. People also have transcendental needs that are pursued with regular periodicity. For example, people may attend church weekly in pursuit of satisfying transcendental needs. Even physical functions of the body occur in a periodic manner. There are cyclical variations in physiological functions of the body, such as body temperature, blood pressure, and pulse.

Nelkin (1970) studied the behavior patterns of migrant workers and found several daily, weekly, and seasonal rhythms that were germane to their existence. Nelkin concluded that these migrant workers seemed to alternate between compact time and diffuse time. Migrant time was seen to be very present oriented, irrational, and highly personal. Nelkin concluded that migrant time was in sharp contrast to the typical time perception, which was future oriented, rational, and impersonal. Findings from the study indicate that social time for the migrants differed because it was a series of disconnected periods rather than a continuous and predictable process, which in part accounted for maladaptive behaviors such as excessive drinking, gambling, volatile social relationships, and apathy.

Periodicity is also considered important at the managerial level. An important aspect of managerial life concerns the periodicity of meetings. For example, it is inappropriate for managers of a volunteer organization to plan frequent meetings for the membership. It is believed that a volunteer organization can engage in systematic self-destruction and ensure itself of a high turnover of membership if the body seeks to gather its members too often. These organizations must justify their demands on the members' time and at the same time create the novelty necessary to maintain the interest of the membership. In contrast to this are nonvoluntary groups, such as those that are part of a job assignment. For example, in nursing administration regular meetings are necessary as part of the required management structure and are not usually planned with the intent of being novel and interesting. Because the management structure requires regular meetings, the meetings are planned regardless of specific agenda items.

Periodicities are also noted at the individual level. It is believed that when people are able to control their own work patterns (periodicity), satisfaction and productivity are maximized (Strauss, 1963). Some individuals spontaneously choose to alternate bouts of intense work with periods of idleness.

It is important for the manager to realize that productivity is cyclic and that equal periods of productivity cannot always be maintained. For example, after a period in which a nursing care unit experiences high client acuity necessitating an extremely heavy work load for the staff, employees will need to recover with a period of less intense pressure. It is unwise to follow a period of high acute work with another assignment that requires major time on the task. However, some work environments by their very nature cannot provide for individual periodicity. For example, industrial workers often must work at a continuous rhythmic pace, such as that seen on an automobile assembly line (Giger and Davidhizar, 1995).

To understand periodicity, the nurse must remember that it is an important aspect of human life and the first aspect of the temporal pattern. Period-

icity therefore refers to the recurrence of a social phenomenon with some kind of regularity that can be measured by clock time or by comparing the social phenomenon with other social phenomena.

Tempo Tempo is the second aspect of the temporal pattern and refers to rate (Morgenstern, 1960). Tempo may refer to the frequency of activities in some unit of social time or to the rate of change of some phenomenon. An example of this is the industrialization of the United States, which differs from that of Russia and China because of different rates (Gioscia, 1970). In a study done by the Southern Illinois University Foundation (Veterans World Project, 1972) it was suggested that one major problem among Vietnam veterans resulted from the rapidity with which they were brought home. The study concluded that the sudden transition from combat back to the United States by way of jet flights required a psychological adjustment that was often quite traumatic for these veterans.

Tempo also includes perceived rapidity of time and experience and the rapidity of various modes of social life, such as urban versus rural and work versus leisure. For example, the tempo of life in a large city such as Quebec City is much different from the tempo of life in a small rural prairie town. Thus a person who relocates may have difficulty adjusting to the different tempo (Giger and Davidhizar, 1995).

Tempo has many important consequences at the individual level because control of the tempo of one's work seems to be important for a healthy self-concept (Kohn, 1977). The tempo of change in social order appears to be related to emotional health; thus the more rapid the change, the greater is the stress of the individual. This thought became the theme of Alvin Toffler (1970), who coined the term "future shock"—the psychological disruptions that result from experiencing too much change in too short a time. An example of this is noted with Japanese people, who traditionally have had to change their culture and society at a very rapid pace. The very rapid tempo of the deliberate transformation of the Meiji era in Japan produced considerable stress for the Japanese people. Some historians have concluded that the 1878 revolution of Japan did save Japan from Western domination, but the generations that followed experienced the brunt of the hectic rate of change and suffered extraordinary mental agonies as a result of these forced changes (Pyle, 1969).

Timing Timing is the third element in the temporal pattern and is referred to as "synchronization." Timing involves the adjustment of various social units and processes with each other. The necessity for synchronization has led to the emphasis on clock time in modern society. Timing can be a crucial factor in the initiation of planned social changes and is of obvious importance in numerous social contexts, such as industrial processes, military campaigns, and political campaigns. A presidential candidate who supports a particular view that is not popular or timely may lose an election but may win at a later time when the view becomes popular or another view emerges. For example, Richard Nixon ran for president of the United States in 1960 and lost. Eight years later he ran for president again at the height of the Vietnam War, and since the issue of the war was a timely one, he campaigned on this issue and won. Success is related to being at the right place at the right time with popular ideas.

Another example of the importance of timing is provided by research data on institutionalized disturbed children. These children, because of their psychological limitations, can be permitted to engage in activities such as competitive sports for only limited amounts of time. The restrictions on time are necessary because the process of the game and the psychological processes can mesh for only limited periods of time before the two processes begin to conflict and lead to destructive behavior (Doob, 1970).

Some researchers have concluded that one of the most serious problems of the modern American family is the difficulty of synchronizing family life because of the diverse activities in which each member is engaged. Another difficulty that has emerged over the years lies in the efforts of rural immigrants to adjust to the stringent demands of industrial life. Some researchers have suggested that habitual functioning of these rural immigrants must be synchronized with the industrial process and that such synchronization disallows the individual's self-actualization.

Duration Duration is the fourth element of the temporal pattern and has been the concern of psychologists more than it has been the concern of sociologists. The psychological concern of duration is related to the duration of which the individual is conscious or to what has been referred to as the "spacious present." According to the classic early work of James (1890), one of the early writers in the field of social psychology, longer or shorter periods are conceived symbolically by adding to or dividing the vaguely bound unit that is the spacious present.

Duration has significance beyond the psychological level, however. Some noted sociologists have set forth a number of laws that relate to duration and behavior in organizations (Parkinson, 1970). Parkinson developed the laws of triviality and delay. The law of triviality states that the amount of time spent on any item in the agenda of an organizational meeting is inversely proportional to the money involved with that item. People may quibble far more about an item costing $50 than about an item costing $10,000. For example, in professional staff meetings at a state psychiatric hospital, an inordinate amount of time was spent discussing the purchase of a 75-cent plastic receptacle for holding clients' personal items such as toothbrushes and soap. A year later, when some plastic lids were missing, several meetings were devoted to developing a strategic nursing procedure for safeguarding these "valuable plastic receptacles." The policy developed to safeguard these receptacles mandated that the staff send a written requisition to the director of nursing, who in turn was required to write a written justification for replacement of the receptacle or the lid (Giger and Davidhizar, 1995). The law of delay asserts that delay is the deadliest form of denial. In addition, duration is perceived as a useful variable.

Researchers continue to investigate the effects of various phenomena such as perceived importance of time, anxiety, and boredom on the perception of time. For example, researchers have concluded that morale may be improved among workers if time is subjectively made to pass more quickly and if there are several methods whereby the apparent length of a period of time can be manipulated (Meade, 1960).

Sequence Sequence is the fifth element of the temporal pattern and is derived from the fact that there are activities requiring order. An obvious evidence of the utility of sequence is the measuring of values. For example, work before play is an ordering of activities that reflects a valuing hierarchy. In a classic 1946 study, Friedman measured values relating to physical activities, theoretic-scientific interests, and esthetic interests and found that subjects made similar choices on both time and money scales. Friedman concluded that when cost and time are equalized, similar preferential orderings are made for various activities.

In modern Canadian society time is indeed money. It is conceivable, however, that the sequential ordering of activities may reflect necessity rather than values as an industrial process. It is also possible that conflict may arise over whether the sequence actually does represent necessity rather than values. Generally this kind of conflict is more common in organizational settings in which disputes arise over the necessity of sequential orderings that are demanded by bureaucratic rules.

Finally, sequential ordering may reflect habit. Rituals of primitive societies are ordered in accordance with custom. Modern rituals also fall into this category, even though some are more appropriately viewed as reflections of values. For example, the ritual of a man removing his hat before entering a room or elevator is a habitual sequence. However, the ritual of the same man removing his hat before the national anthem is played is a sequence demanded by values.

Temporal orientation

Temporal orientation refers to the ordering of past, present, and future and to the fact that individuals and groups may be differentiated according to whether behavior is primarily related to the past, present, or future. Psychologists and sociologists, however, have raised objections to this particular ordering. One objection is that past, present, and future are perceived to make up an organic whole that cannot be separated (Cassirer, 1955; Sideleau, 1992).

A second objection involves variations in the ordering of past, present, and future among various groups. For example, the argument is made that an actor's orientation to a situation always contains an "expectancy aspect," which implies that all orientations are to a future state of a situation as well as to the present. However, this may be true only in a limited sense because actors generally do not anticipate their demise in the situation. It is also untrue that orientation to the future is a universal and inherent aspect of all social action (Giger and Davidhizar, 1995).

Future orientation refers to the fact that the future is a dominant factor in present behavior, and as such this kind of orientation is by no means universal. For example, the Navajo Indians' view of time does not include the expectancy aspect. In years past, efforts to get the Navajo Indians to engage in range control and soil conservation programs were extremely frustrating for government employees because the Navajos simply do not have a view of temporality that would lead them to act on the basis of an expected future (Hall and William, 1960). For the Navajo people the only real time, like the only real space, is that which is here and now (Iverson, 1992). For some Navajo Indians there is little reality of the future; thus the promise of future benefits is not worth thinking about (Hall and William, 1960). It is important for the nurse to remember that the way in which a society, group, or individual orders the past, present, or future will be consequential for behavior.

Kluckhohn and Strodtbeck (1961) have argued that the knowledge of rank ordering of these three modes can tell much about a social unit and the direction of change for that unit. Some Americans have typically placed a dominant emphasis on the future, which does not imply that they ignore either the past or the present. Although there are some undesirable connotations for the label "old fashioned," few Americans express total contentment with the present state of affairs. According to Kluckhohn and Strodtbeck, American values change easily as long as the change does not contradict what is perceived as the American way of life. There is a direct relationship between the extended future orientation and the amount of change. However, the change perceived is not expected to be the kind that threatens the existing order.

Generally speaking, resistance to change should be expected where there is a past orientation. Thus it should be expected that serious problems would arise in efforts to industrialize a society where a future orientation was lacking. For example, in a classic 1953 study, Ritzenthaler found that among the Chippewa Indians, who traditionally lack any concern for the future, there were serious problems when attempts were made to industrialize their work. Ritzenthaler also noted that the Chippewa Indians quit work as soon as they had sufficient money for immediate needs.

Temporal orientations are not immutable; they can change, and along with change come various behavioral changes. Therefore a shift of orientation to the present may have significant consequences in several contexts (Ketchum, 1951). For example, in a crowd situation the orientation may be drawn to the present, wherein some of the typical behaviors of crowds may manifest themselves as overreacting behaviors, such as struggling at a department store sale, racing to the exit doors in a fire, or panic in an airplane during turbulence. Similarly, in a marriage or relationship where the partners perceive the relationship to be of uncertain duration, they may begin to act in accordance with feelings rather than stable values. For example, one of the partners may transfer joint banking accounts and charge card accounts to individual status. In other words, when situations are structured so that people function in a present orientation that lacks future and past orientations, a variety of self-destructive and self-limiting behaviors may result.

Whenever a change is anticipated, orientation to the change may be resisted by individuals or groups, and serious consequences generally follow. The intermingling of traditional orientation, which is somewhat past oriented, with the pressures manifested by modernization, which may be somewhat present or future oriented, may cause societal agony. For example, many problems arose in a factory in Cantal, Guatemala, because the management refused to be sensitive to market variations or to the problem of obsolete equipment (Nash, 1967). Worse situations occurred in Iran, which is a past-oriented society. In past-oriented societies the past is of primary importance and the future of minimal significance. In Iran businessmen invested considerable sums of money in factories without any real plan on how to use these factories (Hall and William, 1960).

Temporal orientation is an important variable in societal behavior and is also significant at the societal level. Some psychological studies indicate that temporal orientation may be directly related to various kinds of emotional disorders, such as alcoholism, and to certain kinds of deviant behaviors, such as juvenile delinquency.

Temporal perspective

Temporal perspective refers to the image of past, present, and future that prevails in a society, a social group, or individuals. The rank ordering of past, present, and future is of significance, yet it is insignificant in gaining an adequate understanding of social time. For example, if a particular group is future oriented, that is, it ranks the future highest in its hierarchy of values, its behavior will depend largely on the way it perceives the future. If people in a society perceive that they may be extinct in the future, efforts may be made to ensure survival. The converse of this is that if people in a society perceive that they do not have a future (for example, they will be destroyed in a nuclear holocaust), they may adopt a present orientation, desiring to live life now to its fullest. An excellent example of this is found with the dying client's perception of time. For the dying client, living in the present is very important; however, the nurse should recognize other realms of time perception. The nurse should ascertain precisely how the client views the past, present, and future because these views may assist the nurse in helping the client cope with death and the challenges faced in the process (Maguire, 1984). An image of the future functions to direct present behavior in accordance with specific values, and some sociologists view a society as being magnetically pulled toward a future fulfillment of their own image of the future, as well as being pushed from behind by their past (Polick, 1973).

A future orientation to illness, disease, and health care is essential to preventive medicine. Actions are taken in the present to safeguard the future, particularly regarding certain disease conditions, such as using condoms to prevent AIDS, practicing safe sex, adhering to a diet to prevent elevated cholesterol or blood glucose levels, not driving while under the influence of alcohol, and using seat belts.

TIME AND HUMAN INTERACTION

Up to this point an effort has been made to create an awareness that social time arises out of interaction. Regardless of the cultural heritage of an individual or group, there is no kind of time that is natural to humans. Instead, time is a result of the structuring and functioning of social order. When a particular temporality emerges, it tends to persist and to influence subsequent interaction. Various cultural groups construct systems of time that have diverse meanings and therefore diverse consequences on social interactions (Giger and Davidhizar, 1995). The most fundamental differences in the meaning of time occur when cultural groups measure time predominantly by either social events or the clock.

Hanson (1988) noted that even when many Indians move into the urban setting and have seemingly assimilated into the White culture, their values and attitudes remain the same. However, other researchers have noted that time-orientation values may differ for a cultural group depending on location. For example, Burke, Kisilevsky, and Maloney (1989) noted that time orientation varied significantly for Canadian urban and northern rural Indian groups. They also concluded that generalization of time orientation among Indian groups is not warranted. Time orientation may also vary within a cultural group related to the presence of health concerns, real or anticipated (Schilder, 1981; Nojima, Oda, Nishii, et al., 1987).

Cultural groups that measure time predominantly by social events construct time according to the activities of the group. Conversely, cultural groups that measure time by the clock schedule activities according to the clock. In this regard, time is perceived basically as qualitative for those who measure time by social life and activities and as quantitative for those who measure time by the clock. When measured by social activities, time has significance only in terms of the activities that are occurring. When time is measured by the clock, it has significance only in terms of money, which is perceived to be a scarce commodity, and all activities that take place do so in the shadow of the clock.

There are few cultural groups or societies that could be characterized as bound exclusively by the clock or as wholly independent of any constraints of temporality. How a group perceives time, nevertheless, has implications for interactions. For example, the Balinese people have a detemporalizing concept of time (Geertz, 1973). For these people social time includes a calendar with a complex system of periodicities. According to Geertz, this is called a "premutational calendar" because it contains 10 different cycles of days ranging in length from 1 to 10 days. Although this is a complex system, it nevertheless serves various religious and practical purposes; it identifies nearly all the holidays and temple celebrations and at the same time guides the individual in daily activities. According to Geertz, the structure of this complex system allows and disallows certain activities on certain days. For example, certain days are good or bad for building a house, starting a business enterprise, moving from one location to another, going on a trip, harvesting and planting crops.

In contrast to the belief of the Balinese people is the belief held by some Canadians that time is money and therefore a scarce commodity. Thus human interactions are controlled in accordance with some notion of the appropriate amount of time for a particular situation. For example, some Canadians distinguish the amount of time that can rightfully be consumed by strangers from that which can be given to friends and relatives. Weigert (1981) concluded that interaction time is a measure of the meaning of the relationship between two persons. In the event that two casual acquaintances meet somewhere, it is unlikely that they will take more than a few minutes to express recognition or perhaps exchange a pleasantry or two; therefore the interaction time for such a meeting is limited. The converse of this is that if two good friends meet and one of the friends attempts to limit the interaction, the other friend may feel rejected. Therefore the violator is expected to account for the behavior, and if this accounting is not forthcoming, the friendship may be severely strained. A single logical conclusion is that interaction can be evaluated in terms of time consumption.

In Canada, methods to save time or to use time more effectively are in high demand. Numerous books, articles, workshops, tapes, and seminars imply that most Americans value time but at the same time do not believe they use it wisely. Many busy professionals feel torn between wise use of time and taking time for interpersonal relationships with fellow workers or friends. For example, a dilemma may arise when a person is busy and a coworker drops in and asks, "Do you have a minute?" If time is considered money, then a minute is costly. Since this worker values time, a reply of yes, may be viewed as costly and thus unjustifiable. On the other hand, a reply of no may be perceived by the other person as a lack of sensitivity, coldness, and a lack of interest. Therefore much of the advice given by time efficiency experts can do much to depersonalize human interactions. An individual who follows the advice of these experts to the letter may have far more hours in which to accomplish tasks but at the same time may have fewer friends and fewer intimate relationships (Giger and Davidhizar, 1995).

Drucker (1966) called the executive a captive because everyone can move in on an executive's time and, generally speaking, everybody does. An executive's time is often preempted by matters that are important to other people; therefore the executive has little or no time for self. A nurse manager who is responsive to others may find that there is little time to do paperwork in the office and thus may take a lot of paperwork home. A nurse manager's personal priorities are often modified when employees present "more urgent" problems.

CULTURAL PERCEPTIONS OF TIME

Appreciating cultural differences regarding time is important for the nurse in relating to both peers and clients. When people of different cultures interact, as is frequently the case in health care settings, there is a great potential for misunderstanding. If nurses are to avoid misreading issues that involve time perceptions, they must have an understanding of how

other persons in different cultures view time (Tripp-Reimer and Lively, 1993).

Campinha-Bacote (1997) compared time orientation among certain groups in relation to future-time and present-time orientation:

Dominant American	Future over present
African Black	Present over future
Puerto Rican American	Present over future
Mexican American	Present
Chinese American	Past over Present
Native American	Present

Individuals with future-oriented perceptions

Many Canadians are future oriented, placing hope in a better tomorrow (Grypma, 1993; Thompson and McDonald, 1989). Value is placed on planning, youth, and the prolongation of life. For example, some Canadians tend to defer gratification of personal pleasure until some future objective has been met, such as advanced education. Thus they will delay starting families, purchasing homes, buying an expensive car, or investing money until they have prepared for a profession through advanced education and so forth. Another noted difference among future-oriented persons is that these individuals tend to structure time rigidly. For these people, adhering to a time-structured schedule is a way of life, regardless of whether the schedule involves work or leisure. For the nurse who works with future-oriented individuals, it is important to talk about events in relation to the future and to adhere to the schedule for planned events in a timely and precise manner.

Individuals with present-oriented perceptions

Some ethnic and cultural groups in Canada are present oriented. Such individuals are preoccupied with immediate problems and actions rather than with anticipatory approaches to problems. In relation to health care, present-oriented individuals are not likely to be involved in preventive care; however, they will seek out emergency care in acute care facilities (Grypma, 1993; Guruge and Donner, 1996). Grypma (1993) notes that after a prenatal class was set up for some Canadian Indian women residing on a reservation and although these individuals had preregistered for the class and confirmed their appointment, they did not keep the appointment. The reason given by these women for not attending the class was a sudden weather shift and the low tide, which provided optimal conditions for picking abalone at islands nearby. For these women, the present-oriented need for food took precedence over planning for the future event of having a baby (Thompson and McDonald, 1989). It is important for the nurse to avoid labeling individuals who are present oriented and who may be late or absent for health appointments as lazy, disrespectful, or lacking interest in maintaining optimal health. Another explanation of individuals with present-time orientation is that they tend to react to time in a linear fashion. Because they perceive time as being on a straight plane, they believe that a present moment spent on a particular task or with a particular individual cannot be regained: "We will never have this moment again," or "We must do it now because we'll pass this way only once." This idea is in contrast to the thoughts held by persons with circular-time orientation, who say, "I'll get back with you," or "We can do it later." The implication of these latter statements is that both persons will be around and the essence of the moment can be relived (Giger and Davidhizar, 1995).

Many Canadian Indians and Inuit believe that only what is needed for the day should be used and nature will continue to provide for future needs (McRae, 1994). Atcheson (1987) noted that health and therefore life is a spiritual experience for Indians and the gifts of the Great Spirit should never be abused. Some Canadian Indians and Inuit believe that the person who gives the most to others should be respected. This is also in keeping with the notion of being present oriented. Many Canadian Indians and Inuit have been taught to live in the present and not be concerned with the future. Therefore they share what they have today (McRae, 1994; Hugey and Buller, 1983; Young, Ingram, and Swartz, 1990).

A common belief shared by some Canadian Blacks and Mexican Canadians is that time is flexible and events will begin when they arrive. For Canadian Blacks this belief has been translated through the years as a perception of time wherein lateness of 30 minutes to an hour is acceptable. Mbiti (1990) traced this perception of time back to West Africa, where the concept of time was elastic and encompassed events that had already taken place as well as those that would occur immediately.

It is important for the nurse to remember that time perception may also be related to socioeconomic status. For example, although some Canadians Blacks and Mexican Canadians can be characterized as present-oriented individuals, others have been assimilated into the dominant culture and are very time conscious and take pride in punctuality. These Canadian Blacks and Mexican Canadians are more likely to be future oriented and therefore are more likely to save and plan for important events. They are also likely to be well educated and to hold professional positions. This may not always be the case because some individuals may not be well educated or hold professional positions yet may value time and have future hopes for themselves and their children. According to Poussaint and Atkinson (1970), these individuals are more likely to encourage their children to seek higher education and to begin saving for the future.

Time perception may also be related to religious orientation. Some Inuit, Canadian Indians, Mexican Canadians, and Canadian Blacks hold strong religious beliefs, and this aspect of their concept of time is therefore very future oriented. These individuals, who may come from all socioeconomic and educational levels, have in common the belief that life on earth, with all of its pain and suffering, is bearable only because of the chance for future happiness after death. Such individuals, according to Smith (1976), may plan future activities related to their deaths; for example, they may plan their funeral, including their eulogy; purchase a grave plot; make a will; and otherwise prepare to die. Such individuals may also threaten heirs with disinheritance and talk about what the heirs will do with their hard-earned money.

Levine and Wolff (1985), with the assistance of

colleagues Laurie West and Harry Reis, compared the time sense of male and female students in Niteroi, Brazil, with similar students at California State University at Fresno. A total of 91 Brazilian students and 107 students from California were surveyed. The universities selected in Brazil and California were similar in academic quality and size, and the cities in which they were located were secondary metropolitan centers with populations of approximately 350,000. The researchers asked students about their perception of time in several situations, including what they considered late or early for a hypothetical lunch appointment with a friend. According to the data, the average Brazilian student defined lateness for the hypothetical lunch as 33 minutes after the scheduled lunchtime, whereas the Fresno students defined lateness for the hypothetical lunch as 19 minutes after the scheduled lunchtime. The Brazilian students allowed an average of 54 minutes before they considered someone early for an appointment, whereas the Fresno students drew the line for earliness at 24 minutes. When the Brazilian students were asked to give typical reasons for lateness, they were less likely to attribute it to a lack of caring than their North American counterparts were. Instead, the Brazilian students pointed to unforeseen circumstances that an individual could not control without prior knowledge. In addition, the Brazilian students appeared less inclined to feel personally responsible for their own lateness. The question that comes to mind for the nurse is, "Are Brazilians more flexible in their concepts of time and punctuality?" Another question for the nurse to consider is, "If Brazilians are more flexible in their concepts of time and punctuality, how does this relate to the stereotypical picture of the fatalistic and irresponsible temperament associated with Latins?" This example illustrates the need for nurses to guard against formulating stereotyped images of persons from other cultures. Instead, the nurse must have an understanding of cultural variables that differ among cultures, such as the variation in viewing time.

Levine and Wolff (1985) found similar differences in how students from North America and Brazil

characterize people who are late for appointments. In the survey, the Brazilian students indicated that a person who is consistently late is probably a person who is more successful than one who is consistently on time. These students seemed to accept the premise that someone of great stature is expected to arrive late; therefore a lack of punctuality is a badge of success. In contrast, according to the North American students, persons who arrive late for scheduled appointments, rush in late to meetings, turn in assignments late, or fail to notify others when they find they are going to be late are generally unorganized, have trouble with priorities, are inconsiderate, and thus will fail to advance professionally and will be less successful. Popular literature in the United States on creating a successful business and professional image espouses the need for continued punctuality.

PHYSICOCHEMICAL INFLUENCES IN RELATION TO TIME

Research on biological rhythms has found that internal body rhythms fluctuate within a 24-hour period. Biological capacities for some individuals are on a low ebb in the daytime, whereas for others they are at a high level during the day (Biological Rhythms, 1970; Yogman, Lester, and Hoffman, 1983; Ziac, 1984). Research has shown that the time of day in which medication is given influences its effectiveness and its side effects; drugs may be more potent when biological capacities are at a low ebb. However, it is important for the nurse to remember that although drugs might be more potent with low biological capacities, the treatment may be less therapeutic. Health care professionals often fail to take into account the client's biological rhythms when scheduling surgical procedures and diagnostic tests. For example, surgical interventions should be avoided when a client's biological capacities are low. Persons who are at a low ebb of biological functioning may be at greater risk for an exaggerated response to anesthesia or may be less able to respond to blood loss than those at normal functioning (Bremmer, Vitiello, and Prinz, 1983; Sideleau, 1992). Evidence also exists that diagnostic tests and treatments may be tolerated better by certain clients when they are timed according to biological rhythms. Hormones and other homeostatic physiological mechanisms fluctuate in the body in a rhythmic way. The timing of the collection of blood and urine samples is important and influences the interpretation of the information obtained.

Physicochemical levels are also related to age. Children have a higher metabolic rate than adults do, and such a rate tends to make time appear to move more slowly for children. On the other hand, older individuals have a slower metabolic rate, which results in time appearing to move more quickly.

Body rhythms may influence waking at a preselected time. Waking, however, is also a conditioned response. Body systems, including the nervous and endocrine systems, are the result not only of internal biological rhythms, but also of psychological phenomena, such as the time or date of previous traumatic events.

Psychological phenomena can greatly influence the client's time perception. For example, according to Sideleau (1992), individuals with psychiatric problems can manifest several types of time impairments, including the following:

1. Perception as related to rate and flow of time, that is, a sense that time passes too quickly or too slowly.
2. Failure to recognize finite division of time, which is manifested by confusion related to the inability to distinguish night from day.
3. Attention or inattention to time, that is, adhering too rigidly to schedules or the complete disregard for the value of time constraints or schedules.

It is important for the nurse to discern carefully whether the client's time perception is attributable to cultural phenomena or to some biochemical or psychological manifestation. For example, drug abusers tend to have an altered sense of time. If a hallucinogenic or excitatory drug is being used, the individual may experience temporal contraction and spatial expansion. For these individuals the distortion in time is so profound that they

often arrive early for appointments (Sideleau, 1992). In stark contrast, individuals who are influenced by the effects of tranquilizers experience time expansion and space contraction. These individuals are more likely to arrive late for an appointment. Although all these phenomena can be experienced by clients who have a biochemical imbalance or a psychological disorder, the nurse must carefully determine if the faulty perception is caused by the disorder or by a cultural phenomenon (Giger, Davidhizar, Evers, and Ingram, 1994; Giger, Davidhizar, Johnson, and Poole, 1997).

IMPLICATIONS FOR NURSING CARE

It is important for the nurse to be cognizant of the fact that time is perceived differently by some individuals from diverse ethnic, cultural, age, and socioeconomic groups (Gaglione, 1988). Accepting that there are different ways of perceiving time is the first step to increasing tolerance for time-related cultural behaviors.

The nurse should appreciate the breath of factors that affect perception of time. For example, Carter, Green, Green, and Dufour (1994) noted that homeless individuals are very present-time oriented. This can significantly affect follow-up care and compliance with treatment recommendations. On the other hand, certain illnesses may affect time perception. Individuals with schizophrenia tend to be present oriented and have a limited ability to focus on the future. This can significantly affect adjustment to the hospital and community living situations (Suto and Frank, 1994). Chronic illness may affect perception of time for the future. For some individuals, hope is important for an orientation to the future (Alberto, 1990).

The nurse who gains an understanding of time as a cultural variable with a significant effect on clients and ultimately on client care must also gain an understanding of how time is managed to give quality client care. A general attitude shared by health care professionals is that time is irreplaceable and irreversible and that to waste time is to waste life. Moreover, there is no such thing as a lack of time; regardless of the way individuals spend time, it goes at the same pace (Salmond, 1986). That is, each individual has 168 hours to live per week, no more and no less. As health care needs have changed over the years, so have the demands that are placed on nurses. Nurses are constantly being challenged to work in a more time-efficient manner, causing high levels of stress. Some nurses maintain that they are losing control and lack personal satisfaction and thus are becoming burned out. However, it is important for the nurse to remember that one way to remain in control and to have personal satisfaction as opposed to burnout is to adopt an efficient system of time management. Getting organized and precisely articulating priorities is related to job satisfaction (Feldman, Monicken, and Crowley, 1983; MacStavic, 1978; McNiff, 1984). Nurses have long known the importance of working smarter rather than longer or harder (Barros, 1983).

Conflicts between nurses and physicians are sometimes complicated by differences in time perception. Nurses tend to operate on an hourly time sense with adherence to rigid schedules to complete client care assignments. Physicians tend to measure time with the client not in actual time spent with the client, which often is quite brief, but in the duration of the illness or its treatment. Physicians are less likely to schedule time strictly and often appear not to appreciate the nurse's sense of time (Sheard, 1980; Young and Hayne, 1988).

Lest the nurse stereotype all persons in Canada as valuing timeliness, it must be emphasized that time and punctuality vary considerably from place to place and region to region. Each region and even each city has its own rhythm and rules. Words such as "now" and "later" can convey vastly different meanings. "Now" and "later" may also be interpreted differently by persons from different ethnic or cultural groups. For some African Americans "now" may not really imply immediately; rather, "now" may mean 'soon,' and so it could be hours before an action is taken. For the same African American "later" may not really imply within a few hours but "when you get around to it" (Mbiti, 1990). In contrast, for some future-oriented Canadians "now" means 'immediately,' and thus action is expected at once. For these same persons "later" means within a few hours. For Americans who travel abroad, major differences encountered, surpassed only by language problems, are the contrasting paces of life and the punctuality differences of people from other countries. These differences can also be noted in the United States when one travels from region to region. For example, in the South, regardless of whether the area is rural or urban, the general pace of life is slow and laid back and punctuality is not of paramount importance; thus people from this region may be stereotyped as "country folks." In contrast, in a large metropolitan area such as New York, the pace of life is associated with more rapid activity, such as walking fast, talking fast, and making decisions quickly. Time differences are also seen in various agencies and among various health professionals. For example, the nurse may find that a more rapid pace is required in a particular hospital setting. The pace may also vary in different clinical disciplines. Duties may differ, and the pace may be more accelerated in high-risk areas such as the intensive care unit, coronary care unit, emergency room, operating room, and psychiatric unit. On the other hand, these areas also experience "slow time" or "down time" when the census is low (Giger and Davidhizar, 1995).

When caring for clients who may have present-oriented time perceptions, such as some Black Canadians, some Canadians from Puerto Rico, some Canadian Indians, some Mexican Canadians, and some Chinese Canadians, the nurse must remember that it is necessary to avoid adhering to time as a fixed resource (an example would be rigid schedules for nursing care procedures such as baths, medications, and meals). In this case the nurse may find that the standards of the institution regarding time and the time orientation of the client may be in conflict with each other. Again, it is important for the nurse to remember that such individuals may perceive time as flexible and that what is happening now is more important than what is going to happen in the future. Therefore the nurse must be able to adapt client care within a range of time rather than by fixed hours.

Case Study

Miss Susie Jones is a 37-year-old Black Canadian client who has been coming to the hospital's outpatient clinic because she is a brittle diabetic. Miss Jones's diabetes was diagnosed 6 months previously; however, the diabetes remains uncontrolled by insulin. The client was put on a regimen of 40 units of lente insulin with 5 units of regular insulin at 7 A.M. and at 4 P.M. When Miss Jones comes to the clinic today, she relates to the nurse that she had an episode of "blacking out," or an "insulin reaction," because she forgot to eat after taking her morning insulin. This morning, as frequently in the past, Miss Jones is at least 1 hour late for her scheduled appointment. The following questions relate to variable time and its significance in relation to Susie Jones.

STUDY QUESTIONS

1. List at least two things in relation to the perception of time and culture that may be contributing factors in Susie Jones's tardiness for appointments.

2. List at least two things that the nurse could suggest to Susie Jones that would assist her in being on time for future clinic appointments.

3. List at least two factors about time that contribute to Susie Jones's noncompliance to the medical regimen.

4. Identify ways that the nurse could assist Susie Jones in developing an understanding about time and its relationship to important medications such as insulin.

5. Identify a contributing factor to the insulin reaction that was described to the nurse by Susie Jones.

References

Alberto, J. (1990). *A test of a model of the relationships between time orientation, perception of threat, hope, and self-care behaviors of persons with chronic obstructive pulmonary disease.* Doctoral dissertation, Indiana University School of Nursing, Bloomington, Indiana.

Ariotti, P.E. (1995). The concept of time in Western antiquity. In Fraser, J.T. & Lawrence, N. (Eds.), *The study of time* (vol. 3) (pp. 69-80). New York: Springer-Verlag.

Atcheson, J. (1987). *Traditional health beliefs and compliance in Native American tuberculosis patients.* Unpublished master's thesis, McMaster University, Hamilton, Ohio.

Barros, A. (1983, August). Time management: learn to work smarter, not longer. *Medical Laboratory Observer,* pp. 107- 111.

Biological rhythms in psychiatry and medicine. (1970). Chevy Chase, Md., U.S. Department of Health, Education, and Welfare, National Institute of Mental Health.

Bock, P. (1964). Social structure and language structure. *Southwestern Journal of Anthropology, 20,* 393-403.

Bremmer, W.J., Vitiello, M.V., & Prinz, P.N. (1983). Loss of circadian rhythmicity in blood testosterone levels with aging in normal man. *Journal of Clinical Endocrinology and Metabolism, 56*(6), 1278-1281.

Burke, S., Kisilevsky, B., & Maloney, R. (1989). Time orientations of Indian mothers and white nurses. *The Canadian Journal of Nursing Research, 21*(4), 5-20.

Campinha-Bacota, J. (1997). Understanding the influence of culture. In Haber, J., Krainovich-Miller, B., McMahon, A., & Hoskins, P. (Eds.), *Comprehensive psychiatric nursing* (ed. 5) (pp. 76-90). St. Louis: Mosby.

Carter, K., Green, R., Green, L., & Dufour, L. (1994). Health needs of homeless clients accessing nursing care at a free clinic. *Journal of Community Health Nursing, 11*(3), 139-147.

Cassirer, E. (1955). *An essay on man.* New York: Bantam Books.

Davidhizar, R., Dowd, S., & Giger, J. (1997). Model for cultural diversity in the radiology department. *Radiology Technology, 68*(3), 233-240.

Doob, L. (1970). *Patterning of time.* New Haven, Conn.: Yale University Press.

Dossey, L. (1982). *Space, time, and medicine*. Boulder, Colo.: Shambhala Publications.

Drucker, P. (1966). *The effective executive*. New York: Harper & Row.

Elton, L. (1975). *Time and man*. New York: Pergamon Press.

England, J. (1986). Cross-cultural health care. *Canada's Mental Health, 34*(4), 13-15.

Feldman, E., Monicken, L., & Crowley, M. (1983). The systems approach to prioritizing. *Nursing Administration Quarterly, 7*(2), 57-62.

Gaglione, B. (1988). *Cognitive orientations of three healthy retired American men*. Doctoral dissertation, Rutgers—The State University of New Jersey, New Brunswick, N.J.

Geertz, C. (1977). *The interpretation of cultures*. New York: Basic Books.

Gilles, R., & Faulkner, R. (1978). Time and television news work: task temporalization in the assembly of unscheduled events. *Sociological Quarterly, 19*, 89-102.

Giger, J., Davidhizar, R., Evers, S., & Ingram, C. (1994). Cultural factors influencing mental health. In Taylor, C. (Ed.), *Essentials of psychiatric nursing* (ed. 14) (pp. 215-238). St. Louis: Mosby.

Giger, J. & Davidhizar, R. (1995). *Transcultural nursing: assessment and intervention*. St. Louis: Mosby.

Giger, J., Davidhizar, R., Johnson, J., & Poole, V. (1997). The changing face of America. *Health Traveler, 4*(4), 11-17.

Gingerich, O. (1972). *The Amish of Canada*. Waterloo, Ont.: Conrad Press.

Gioscia, V. (1970). On social time. In Yaker, H., Osmond, H., & Cheek, F. (Eds.), *The future of time* (pp. 73- 141). New York: Doubleday.

Grpyma, S. (1993). Culture shock. *The Canadian Nurse, 89*, 33-37.

Guruge, S. & Donner, G. (1996). Transcultural nursing in Canada. *The Canadian Nurse, 92*, 34-39.

Hall, E., & William, F. (1960). Intercultural communication: a guide to men of action. *Human Organization, 19*, 7-9.

Hanson, A. (1988). Problems involved in delivering health care and social services to the inner city. In Young, (Ed.), *Health care issues in the Canadian north*. Edmonton: Boreal Institute for Northern Studies.

Hawley, A. (1986). *Human ecology*. New York: Ronald Press.

Hein, E.C. (1980). *Communication in nursing practice* (ed. 2), Boston: Little, Brown.

Hugey, R., & Buller, E. (1983). Drumming and dancing: a new rhythm in nursing care. *The Canadian Nurse, 79*(4), 28-31.

Hoppe, S., & Heller, P. (1974). Alienation, familism, and the utilization of health services by Mexican Americans. *Journal of Health and Social Behavior, 15*, 304.

Hymovich, D.P., & Chamberlin, R.W. (1980). *Child and family development*. New York: McGraw-Hill.

Iverson, P. (1992). *The Navajos*. New York: Chelsea House Publishers.

James, W. (1890). *Principles of psychology* (vol. 1). New York: Dover Publications.

Ketchum, J.D. (1951). Time, values, and social organization. *Canadian Journal of Psychology, 5*, 97-109.

Kluckhohn, F., & Strodtbeck, F. (1961). *Variations in value orientation*. Evanston, Ill.: Row, Peterson.

Kohn, M. (1977). *Class and conformity* (ed. 2). Chicago: Dorsey Press.

Landes, D. (1983). *Revolution in time*. Cambridge, Mass.: Belknap Press of Harvard University Press.

Lebhar, G. (1958). *The use of time* (ed. 3). New York: Chain Store.

Lefever, D., & Davidhizar, R. (1995). Eskimos. In Giger, J.N., & Davidhizar, R.E. (Eds.), *Transcultural nursing: assessment and intervention*. St. Louis: Mosby.

Levine, R., & Wolff, E. (1985, March). Social time: the heartbeat of culture. *Psychology Today*, 29-35.

MacStavic, R.E. (1978). Setting priorities in health planning: what does it mean? *Inquiry, 45*(1), 20-24.

Maguire, D.C. (1984). *Death by choice* (ed. 2). New York: Schocken Books.

Mbiti, S.S. (1990). *African religions and philosophies* (ed. 2). New York: Anchor Press.

McGrath, J., & Kelly, J. (1986). *Time and human interaction* (ed. 2). New York: Guilford Press.

McNiff, M. (1984). Getting organized—at last. *RN, 47*, 23-24.

McRae, L. (1994). Cultural sensitivity in rehabilitation related to native clients. *Canadian Journal of Rehabilitation, 7*(4), 251-256.

Meade, R. (1960). Time on their hands. *Personnel Journal, 39*, 130-132.

Morgenstern, I. (1960). *The dimensional structure of time*. New York: Philosophical Library.

Nash, M. (1967). *Machine age Maya*. Chicago: University of Chicago Press.

Nelkin, D. (1970). Unpredictability and life style in a migrant camp. *Social Problems, 17*, 472-487.

Nojima, Y., Oda, A., Nishii, H., Fukui, M., Seo, K., & Akiyoshi, H. (1987). Perception of time among Japanese inpatients. *Western Journal of Nursing Research, 9*(3), 288-300.

Nolt, S. (1992). *A history of the Amish*. Intercourse, Pa.: Herald Press.

Parkinson, C. (1970). *The law of delay.* London: John Murray.

Polick, F. (1973). *The image of the future* (vols. 1 & 2). New York: Oceana Publications.

Poussiant, A., & Atkinson, C. (1970). Black youth and motivation. *Black Scholar, 1,* 43-51.

Pyle, K. (1969). *The new generation of Meiji Japan.* Stanford, Calif.: Stanford University Press.

Randall-David, E. (1989). *Strategies for working with culturally diverse communities and clients* [Brochure]. Washington, D.C.: U.S. Department of Health and Human Services.

Ritzenthaler, R. (1953). The impact of small industry on an Indian community. *American Anthropologist, 55,* 143-148.

Ruiz, R. (1981). Cultural and historical perspectives in counseling Hispanics. In Sue, D. (Ed.), *Counseling the culturally different: theory and practice* (pp. 186-215). New York: Wiley.

Ruiz, R.A., & Padella, A.M. (1977). Counseling Latinos. *The Personnel and Guidance Journal, 55,* 401-408.

Salmond, S. (1986). Time management: the time is now. *Orthopedic Nursing* 5(3), 25-32.

Schilder, E. (1981). On the structure of time with implications for nursing. *Nursing Papers, 13*(3), 17-26.

Sheard, T. (1980). The structure of conflict in nurse-physician relations. *Supervisor Nurse, 11* (8), 14-16.

Sideleau, B. (1992). Space and time. In Haber, J., Leach-McMahon, A., Price-Hoskins, P., & Sideleau, B., (Eds.), *Comprehensive psychiatric nursing,* (ed. 4). St. Louis: Mosby.

Smith, J.A. (1976). The role of the Black clergy as allied health care professionals in working with Black patients. In Luckraft, J.D. (Ed.), *Black awareness: implications for Black care* (pp. 12- 15). New York: American Journal of Nursing Company.

Sorokin, P. (1964). *Sociocultural causality, space, time.* New York: Russell & Russell.

Spector, R. (1996). *Cultural diversity in health care* (ed. 4). Stanford, Conn.: Appleton & Lange.

Stauffer, R. (1995). Vietnamese Americans. In Giger, J., & Davidhizar, R. (Eds.), *Transcultural nursing: assessment and intervention.* St. Louis: Mosby.

Stoetzel, J. (1953). The contribution of public opinion research techniques to social anthropology. *International Social Science Bulletin, 5,* 494-503.

Strauss, G. (1963). Group dynamics and intergroup relations. In Lewis, A.O., Jr. (Ed.), *Of men and machines* (pp. 321-327). New York: E.P. Dutton.

Suto, M., & Frank, G. (1994). Future time perspective and daily occupations of persons with chronic schizophrenia in a board and care home. *American Journal of Occupational Therapy, 48*(1), 7-18.

Thompson, E. (1967). Time, work-discipline, and industrial capitalism. *Past and Present, 38,* 58-59.

Thompson, P., & McDonald, J. (1989). Multicultural health education: responding to the challenge. *Health Promoting, 28*(2), 8-11.

Toffler, A. (1970). *Future shock.* New York: Random House.

Tripp-Reimer, T., & Lively, S. (1993). Cultural considerations in therapy. In Beck, C.K., Rawlins, R.P., & Williams, S., (Eds.), *Mental health-psychiatric nursing* (ed. 3) (pp. 185-199). St. Louis: Mosby.

Veterans World Project. (1972). *Wasted men: the reality of the Vietnam veteran.* Edwardsville, Ill.: Southern Illinois University Foundation.

Weigert, A. (1981). *Sociology of everyday life.* New York: Longman.

Wenger, A. (1991). The culture care theory and the older order Amish. In Leininger, M., (Ed.), *Culture care diversity and universality: a theory of nursing.* New York: National League for Nursing.

Wessman, A., & Gorman, B. (1977). The emergence of human awareness and concepts of time. In Gorman, B.S., & Wessman, A.E. (Eds.), *Personal experience of time* (p. 3). New York: Plenum Press.

Weyer, E. (1961). *Primitive peoples today.* New York: Doubleday.

Wuest, J. (1992). Joining together: students and faculty learn about transcultural nursing. *Journal of Nursing Education, 31*(2), 90-92.

Yogman, M.W., Lester, B.M., & Hoffman, J. (1983). Behavioral rhythmicity and circadian rhythmicity during mother, father, stranger, infant social interaction. *Pediatric Research, 17*(11), 872-876.

Young, D., Ingram, C., & Swartz, L. (1990). *Cry of the eagle: encounters with a Cree healer.* Toronto: University of Toronto Press.

Young, L., & Hayne, A. (1988). *Nursing administration: from concepts to practice.* Philadelphia: W.B. Saunders.

Young, T. (1988). *Health care and cultural change: the Indian experience in the central subarctic.* Toronto: University of Toronto Press.

Zerubavel, E. (1979). *Patterns of time in hospital life.* Chicago: University of Chicago Press.

Ziac, D.C. (1984). Menstrual synchrony in university women. *American Journal of Physical Anthropology, 63*(2), 237.

CHAPTER 6

Environmental Control

BEHAVIORAL OBJECTIVES

After reading this chapter, the nurse will be able to:

1. Recognize relevant cultural factors that affect health-seeking behaviors related to environmental control.
2. Recognize relevant cultural factors that affect illness behaviors related to environmental control.
3. Identify factors affecting external locus of control for persons in selected cultural groups.
4. Recognize the relationship between external locus of control and fatalistic or health-seeking behaviors.
5. Recognize various types of cultural folk health practices and their influence on health-seeking behaviors.

Environmental control refers to the ability of an individual or persons from a particular cultural group to plan activities that control nature. Environmental control also refers to the individual's perception of ability to direct factors in the environment. This definition in itself implies that the concept of environment is broader than just the place where an individual resides or where treatment occurs. In the most practical sense, the term "environment" encompasses relevant systems and processes that affect individuals (Sideleau, 1992).

Systems are organized structures that may influence and be influenced by individuals. Processes may be viewed as organized, purposeful patterns of operations. Processes generally include the dynamics and interactions between families, groups, and the community at large. On the basis of these definitions, it is evident that the environment and humans have a reciprocal relationship in the sense that humans and the environment are constantly exchanging matter and energy. When this exchange has purpose and is goal directed, the interaction and exchange processes are considered functional and useful. However, when the exchange has no purpose and lacks goal direction, a dyssynchronous relationship occurs (Haber and Giuffra, 1992).

In the broadest sense, health may be viewed as a balance between the individual and the environment. Health practices such as eating nutritiously, subscribing to preventive health services available in the community, and installing hazard- and pollution-control devices are all believed to have a positive effect on the individual, who in turn can positively affect the environment (Giger and Davidhizar, 1995; Spector, 1996).

Complex systems of health beliefs and practices exist across and within cultural groups. In addition, variations, whether extreme or modest, to cultural beliefs and practices are found across ethnic and social class boundaries and even within family groups. Today the most widely accepted approach to health care is the biomedical model. This model emphasizes biological concerns, which are considered by those who support this model as more "real" and significant in contrast to psychological and sociological issues (Kleinman, Eisenberg, and Good, 1978).

Today in modern Western society, health care practitioners remain primarily interested in abnormalities in the structure and function of body systems and in the treatment of disease. According to Kleinman, Eisenberg, and Good (1978), the biomedical approach is culture specific, culture bound, and value laden. The biomedical model represents only one end of a continuum. At the opposite end of the continuum is the traditional model, which espouses popular beliefs and practices that diverge from medical science (Chrisman, 1977). Persons who subscribe to beliefs encompassed in the traditional model have varying health beliefs and practices, including folk beliefs and traditional beliefs, which are also shaped by culture (Spector, 1996).

DISTINCTION BETWEEN ILLNESS AND DISEASE

During the last decade, scientists and anthropologists began to make a distinction between the terms "illness" and "disease." The individual experiences that relate to illnesses do not necessarily correlate with the biomedical interpretation of disease. Illness can be defined as an individual's perception of being sick. On the other hand, disease is diagnosed when the condition is a deviation from clearly established norms based on Western biomedical science (Fabrega, 1971). Illness can and does occur in the absence of disease; approximately 50% of visits made by individuals to physicians are for complaints without a definite basis. According to Kleinman, Eisenberg, and Good (1978), illness is culturally shaped in the sense that it is individually perceived. In other words, how one experiences and copes with disease is based on the individual's explanation of sickness. Disease is described in detail in medical-surgical nursing textbooks. However, nurses need to remember to incorporate both personal and cultural reactions of the client to illness, disease, and discomfort to give culturally appropriate nursing care.

Just as culture influences health-related behavior, it also has a profound effect on expectations and perceptions of sickness that shape the labeling of sickness and on how, when, and to whom communication of health problems occurs (Campinha-Bacote, 1997). The astute nurse must keep in mind the fact that perceptions of health and illness are shaped by cultural factors. As a direct result of cultural shaping, individuals vary in health care behaviors, health status, and health-seeking attitudes (Grypma, 1993; Thompson, 1993; McRae, 1994; Guruge and Donner, 1996).

The term "health care behavior" is defined as the social and biological activities of an individual that are based on maintaining an acceptable health status or manipulating and altering an unacceptable condition (Bauwens and Anderson, 1988). The term "health status," on the other hand, is defined as the success with which an individual adapts to the internal and external environment (Bauwens and Anderson, 1988). Thus health care behavior influences health status, which in turn influences health care behavior. Because health care behavior and health care status are reciprocal in nature, they can both be affected by sociocultural forces such as economics, politics, environmental influences, and the health care delivery system itself (Elling, 1977).

CULTURAL HEALTH PRACTICES VERSUS MEDICAL HEALTH PRACTICES

Cultural health practices are categorized as efficacious, neutral, dysfunctional (Pillsbury, 1982), or uncertain.

Efficacious cultural health practices

According to Western medical standards, efficacious cultural health practices are those practices that are viewed as beneficial to health status, though they can differ vastly from modern scientific practices. Because efficacious health practices can facilitate effective nursing care, nurses need to actively encourage the use of these practices among and across cultural groups. Nurses must keep in mind that a treatment strategy that is consistent with the client's beliefs may have a better chance of being successful. For example, persons from cultural groups who subscribe to the theory of hot and cold, such as some Mexican Americans, may actually benefit from this particular belief. Individuals who subscribe to this theory may avoid hot foods in the presence of stomach ailments such as ulcers, a practice that is consistent with the bland diet used in a medical regimen for the treatment of ulcers. Thus scientific health care practices may be blended with efficacious cultural health practices (Giger and Davidhizar, 1995).

Neutral cultural health practices

Neutral cultural health practices have no effect on the health status of an individual. Although some health care practitioners may consider neutral health practices irrelevant, the nurse must remember that such practices may be extremely important because they may be linked to beliefs that are closely integrated with an individual's behavior (Pillsbury, 1982). Greene (1981) cited several examples of neutral practices, including the "ritual disposal of the placenta and cord," interpretation of signs in the cord, avoidance of sexual activity during various stages of pregnancy, certain hygiene practices, and avoidance of exposure to luminous rays of the moon during a lunar eclipse. Many Southeast Asian women believe that sitting in a door frame or on a step while they are pregnant will complicate labor and delivery. In waiting and examination rooms, these women will avoid areas near doors. These women may also think that overeating or inactivity during pregnancy will cause a difficult delivery. For many of these women, it is believed that sleeping late or during the day will have the same effect. Hill tribeswomen (Hmong and Mien) avoid contact with scissors and knives because they fear sharp instruments may cause cleft lip or abortion. There is a general belief among these women that reaching overhead for something or working too hard may cause miscarriage or birth defects (Lee, 1989; Mattson, 1995; Stauffer, 1995). Although these practices require no planned nursing interventions, the astute nurse must recognize their significance and respect the client's right to subscribe to and practice such beliefs.

Dysfunctional cultural health practices

Dysfunctional cultural health practices are harmful. An example of a dysfunctional health care practice found in the United States is the excessive use of such items as overrefined flour and sugar. The nurse must be aware of practices that are dysfunctional and should work to establish educational training programs that will help individuals identify dysfunctional health practices and develop beneficial practices.

A dysfunctional health care practice was noted among women of various racial, ethnic, and cultural groups in British Columbia (Hislop, Deschamps, Band, Smith, and Clarke, 1992). Findings from this study indicated that implementation of a population-based cervical cytology screening program in British Columbia that began in 1955 decreased the mortality from invasive squamous cervical cancer by over 70%. However, the mortality from cervical cancer, despite the implementation of this innovative program, remained high among the Canadian Native population (Inuit, Indians, the Metis). In fact, the mortality was four times higher among Canadian Native women, compared to their non-Native counterparts (Threlfall, 1986). Although approximately 85% of the women in the general population complied with screening recommendations, the compliance by Native women was approximately 30% less. Whether this underparticipation by Native woman resulted from beliefs and attitudes or lack of availability of resources was not determined.

Uncertain cultural health practices

In 1972 Williams and Jelliffe developed a cultural assessment system that included a category of cultural health practices with unknown effects. Classified as uncertain, these practices included such things as swaddling a newborn infant to maintain body temperature and using an abdominal binder for mother and infant to prevent umbilical hernias.

The nurse must remember that in most instances health practices do not fit perfectly into one category or another. According to Greene (1981), health practices are subjectively evaluated as more or less beneficial or harmful when they are compared with the alternative practices available to the user.

VALUES AND THEIR RELATIONSHIP TO HEALTH CARE PRACTICES

Values may be viewed as individualized sets of rules by which people live and are governed. They serve as the cornerstone for beliefs, attitudes, and behaviors. Cultural values are often acquired unconsciously as an individual assimilates the culture throughout the process of growth and maturation. It is important for the nurse to recognize that because cultural values are believed to exist almost solely on an unconscious level they are the most difficult to alter. Cultural values therefore have a pervasive and profound influence on the individual (Giger and Davidhizar, 1995; Giger, Davidhizar, Johnson, and Poole, 1997).

Value orientations

Kluckhohn and Strodtbeck (1961) defined value orientations as "complex but definitely patterned principles . . . which give order and direction to the ever-flowing stream of human acts and thoughts as they relate to the solution of common human problems." Kluckhohn and Strodtbeck also proposed that it is entirely possible for an individual to hold a value orientation different from that of the rest of the same cultural group. However, they concluded that, despite differences in value orientation within a cultural group, dominant value orientations can be identified for most persons of a particular cultural group.

Kluckhohn and Strodtbeck (1961) compared the way people in different cultural groups organize their thinking about such things as time, personal activity, interpersonal relationships, and the relationship to nature and the supernatural. They developed an orientation framework that includes temporal, activity, relational, people-to-nature, and innate human nature orientations.

Temporal orientation Temporal orientation refers to the method by which persons from particular cultural groups divide time. Time in Western cultures is generally divided into three frames of reference: past, present, and future. According to Kluckhohn and Strodtbeck (1961) and Haber et al. (1992), most cultures combine all three orientations, but one is more likely to dominate than another.

Activity orientation Activity orientation refers to whether a cultural group is perceived as a "doing"-oriented culture, which is oriented toward achievement, or as a "being"-oriented culture, which values "being" and views people as an important link be-

tween generations. In other words, the "doing"-oriented culture values accomplishments, whereas the "being"-oriented culture values inherent existence.

Relational orientation Relational orientation from a cultural perspective distinguishes among interpersonal patterns. More specifically, relational orientation refers to the way in which persons in a culture set goals for individual members. Relational orientations are found in three modes: lineal, individualistic, and collateral.

Lineal mode. When the lineal mode is dominant within a particular cultural group, the goals and welfare of the group are viewed as major concerns. Other major concerns are the continuity of the group and the orderly succession of the group over time. Cultures that are perceived as subscribing to the lineal mode view kinship bonds as the basis for maintaining lineage.

Individualistic mode. Cultures in which the dominant mode is individualistic value individual goals over group goals. Thus each individual is responsible for personal behaviors and ultimately is held accountable for personal accomplishments.

Collateral mode. When the collateral mode is dominant in a cultural group, the goals and welfare of lateral groups such as siblings or peers are of paramount importance. Examples are found in Russia and in Israel where the goals of individuals are subordinate to those that affect the entire lateral group.

People-to-nature orientation People-to-nature orientation implies that people either dominate nature, live in harmony with nature, or are subjugated to nature. The conceptual framework of people dominating nature is based on the view that humans dominate nature and further suggests that humankind can master or control natural events. When people live in harmony with nature, there is an integration among them, nature, and the universe. When the view that humans are subjugated to nature is held, a philosophy of fatalism is adopted; that is, fate is considered inevitable and individuals perceive themselves as having no control over nature or their future—they consider themselves powerless to guide personal destiny. An example is the belief held by some Appalachian people that "If I'm going to get cancer, I'm going to get it," so that taking preventive measures to avoid cancer would be of no benefit. This fatalistic attitude, however, is not completely consistent because most Appalachians will go to a physician or hospital if they believe they are extremely ill.

With the arrival of the White man, life for many Canadian Inuit in the North lost harmony with nature and turned to chaos. Without the stability of the known way of life, which included living off the land, many Canadian Inuit appeared to lose the balance with nature and fell pray to environmentally controlled government subsidies and the availability of alcohol. For example, in Inuvik in the Northwest Territories, a government-built town 124 miles north of the Arctic Circle, at least 80% of local crimes were reported as alcohol related. Van Itallie (1996) reported that Inuit "drink until the liquor is gone and then search for more." For some Canadian Inuit, there are other problem besides the high rate of alcoholism. For example, the suicide rate among the Inuit residing in the Northwest Territories is four times higher than the national average (van Itallie, 1996). It has been noted by some researchers that the Northwest Territories are hard regions to live in. In fact, just trying to survive in these regions is extremely difficult. It is perhaps the harshness of the terrain and its remoteness that contribute to the excessive drinking among the Inuit and causes some of these individuals to wander around outdoors and die from hypothermia. In addition, while intoxicated, some of these individuals fall through the ice (van Itallie, 1996).

Nurses who are located at the various "nursing stations" and hospitals throughout the Northwest Territories also experience feelings of isolation both professionally and socially and may suffer from fatigue, burnout, and alcohol abuse (Scott, 1991). Scott (1991) described an employee assistance program to assist nurses to cope with the desolation of the area in an effort to reduce burnout. Unfortunately, when Occupational Health was turned over to the Department of Health in the Northwest Territories, this federally mandated program ceased to exist. The loss of the federally funded Occupational Health program created a serious void in health care

access for all people residing in the Northwest Territories, but particularly for the Inuit. The Canadian government has attempted to correct the historic wrongs suffered by the Inuit by organizing these people to facilitate the election of legislators, providing land, and attempting to combat social ills. Nonetheless, many problems remain as the Inuit struggle to gain harmony with their environment (Red Horse, Johnson, and Weiner, 1989).

Health knowledge as well as health concerns are problems for many Native peoples in Canada in addition to those in the Far North. McKinnon, Gartrell, Kerksen, and Jarvis (1991) described the health knowledge of the Native youth in central Alberta. Although they noted that the Native youth reported knowledge about dental health, fire safety, and the effects of smoking, alcohol, and drugs, they were nevertheless less knowledgeable on first aid for burns, nutrition, communicable diseases, and personal health. There is a wealth of data available to indicate that Canadian Native youths have high rates of accidents and violence (Linwood, Kasian, and Irvine, 1990; Jarvis and Boldt, 1982), mental health problems (Armstrong, 1986; Jilek, 1982), and alcohol and substance abuse (Indian and Northern Affairs, 1980; Tousignant, 1985). McKinnon, Gartrell, Derksen, and Jarvis (1991) noted that the challenge remains as to how to convert these problems into better access and improved health care.

Innate human nature orientation The innate human nature orientation distinguishes an individual's human nature as being good, evil, or neutral. Some cultural groups view human beings as having a basic nature that is either changeable or unchangeable. For example, an individual may be viewed as evil and unchangeable, evil but changeable, or neutral (subject to both good and negative influences).

Locus-of-control construct as a health care value

The locus-of-control construct, which originated in social learning theory, is defined as follows:

When a reinforcement is perceived as following some action but not being entirely contingent upon (personal) action, in our culture it is typically perceived as a result of luck, chance, and fate, as being under the control of powerful others, or as unpredictable because of the great complexity of the forces surrounding [the individual]. When the event is interpreted in this way by an individual, we have labeled this belief in external control. If a person perceives that the event is contingent upon his own behavior or his own permanent characteristics, we have termed this a belief in internal control (Rotter, 1966).

The above definition presupposes that individuals who believe that a contingent relationship exists between actions and outcomes have internal feelings of control and thus act to influence future behaviors and situations. Individuals who believe that efforts and rewards are uncorrelated and who thus have external feelings of control view the future as the result of luck, chance, or fate and are less likely to take action to change the future. The locus-of-control construct can be applied to a variety of phenomena, including the weather, preventive health, curative health actions, and feelings of well-being. For example, individuals who believe that a contingent relationship exists between compliance to preventive and treatment regimens and health have an internal locus of control and are likely to respond positively to affect the future and thus promote good health. On the other hand, individuals who believe that compliance behaviors and health are unrelated have an external locus of control and have little motivation to develop behaviors that could affect the future and enhance good health. Rotter (1975) concluded that the locus of control does not in itself represent a behavior trait and can be modified by interaction with others.

The astute nurse should recognize that persons who subscribe to an external locus of control tend to be more fatalistic about nature, health, illness, death, and disease. For example, some Hispanics, Appalachians, and Puerto Ricans are reported to have an external locus of control. Some Canadian Indians, Chinese Canadians, and Japanese Canadians are said to be more or less in harmony with nature; therefore their cultural beliefs fall outside the locus-of-control construct. However, northern European Canadians and African Canadians are reported to fall within both the internal and the external locus-of-control

constructs (Kluckhohn and Strodtbeck, 1961). The nurse can help the client modify behaviors that fall within the realm of the external locus-of-control construct by showing the effects of certain behaviors on illnesses, health, and disease and thus promote the development of an internal locus of control.

FOLK MEDICINE

Folk medicine, or what is commonly referred to as "Third World beliefs and practices," is often called "strange or weird" by nurses and other health professionals who are unfamiliar with folk medicine beliefs (Snow, 1981; Giger, Davidhizar, and Turner, 1992; Giger and Davidhizar, 1995). In reality, whether something is considered "strange or weird" depends on familiarity with the beliefs. In most instances folk medicine practices will not be considered "strange or weird" once health care providers become familiar with them.

The astute nurse must distinguish between practices that are familiar and practices that are desirable because becoming familiar with something does not imply acceptance. In this situation tolerance becomes a two-way process: people who subscribe to folk medicine practices need not feel compelled to abandon these beliefs and practices when they become familiar with modern medicine, and health care practitioners should not feel compelled to abandon modern medical practices when they become familiar with folk medicine practices (Giger and Davidhizar, 1995).

An individual's world view largely determines beliefs about disease and the appropriate treatment interventions. For example, a belief in magic may lead to the assumption that a disease is a result of human behavior and that a cure can be achieved by magical techniques. A religious belief may lead to the assumption that the disease is a result of supernatural forces and that a cure can be achieved by appealing to supernatural forces. The scientific view may lead to the assumption that the disease is a result of the cause-and-effect relationship of natural phenomena and that a cure is achieved by scientific medicine (Henderson and Primeaux, 1981).

Data in a study of Anglo-Celtic, Chinese, and East Indian Canadians concerning long-term illness constructs indicated that although education is often cited as a predictor of biomedical beliefs concerning illness, a higher preference for biomedical treatment was predicted by education elsewhere (Rodin and Salovey, 1989). These results emphasize greater use of the popular nontraditional medicines by both East Indians and Chinese.

Folk medicine beliefs as a system

The folk medicine system classifies illnesses or diseases as natural or unnatural. This division of illnesses or diseases into natural and unnatural phenomena is common among Haitians, persons from Trinidad, Mexicans and Mexican Canadians, African Canadians, and some Southern White Americans (Snow, 1981).

Distinction between natural and unnatural events The simplest way to distinguish between natural and unnatural illnesses is to state that, according to this belief system, natural events have to do with the world as God made it and as God intended it to be. Thus natural laws allow a measure of predictability for daily life. Unnatural events, on the other hand, imply the exact opposite because they upset the harmony of nature. Unnatural events can therefore be viewed as events that interrupt the plan intended by God and at their very worst represent the forces of evil and the machinations of the devil. Unnatural events are frightening because they have no predictability. They are outside the world of nature, and so, when they do occur, they are beyond the control of ordinary mortals.

Germane to the tendency to view phenomena in terms of opposition, such as good versus evil and natural versus unnatural, is the belief held by some folk medicine systems that everything has an exact opposite. For example, some African Canadians who subscribe to a folk medicine system believe that for every birth there must be a death, for every marriage there must be a divorce, and for every person with good health there must be someone with bad health. This belief is so encompassing that such individuals believe that every illness has a cure, every poison has an antidote, every herb has a healing purpose, and so on (Snow, 1981). This belief contributes to the lack of acceptance by persons in some cultural groups to the chronicity of such diseases as AIDS, herpes, or syphilis.

Today, herbal medicine is enjoying a "rebirth" (French, 1996). Eisenberg, Kessler, Foster, Norlock, Calkins, and Delbanco (1993) noted that 34% of all United States citizens use herbal products in some way. In 1990 United States citizens spent $13.7 billion dollars on "unconventional" therapy, with 75% of this cost "out of pocket." Canadians are also participating in this rebirth with an increase use of herbal medicines (Abarts, 1995).

Distinction between natural and unnatural illnesses Illnesses are generally classified as natural or unnatural, which affects the type of cure or practitioner sought. All illnesses can be viewed as representing disharmony and conflict in some particular area of life and thus tend to fall into two general categories: (1) natural illnesses with environmental hazards and (2) unnatural illnesses with divine punishment.

Natural illness with environmental hazards. Natural illnesses in the folk medicine belief system are those that occur because of dangerous agents such as cold air or impurities in the air, food, and water. Natural illnesses are based on the fact that everything in nature is connected and that events can be both interpreted and directed by an understanding of these relationships. Sympathetic magic, the basis for popular folk medicine beliefs and practices, can be divided into two categories: contagious and imitative magic. At the root of contagious magic is the premise that the parts do represent the whole. Many witchcraft practices are based on contagious magic, including such practices as an evildoer obtaining a lock of the victim's hair or shavings from another victim's skin to do harm. Imitative magic, on the other hand, is based on the premise that like will follow like. For example, a knife under the bed will cut labor pains. To assist the client in preventing natural illnesses, the nurse must comprehend the direct connections between the body and natural phenomena such as the phases of the moon, the position of the planets, and the changing of the seasons. Because in this belief system good health is contingent on these phenomena, it is imperative that one be able to read these signs if the body is to remain in harmony with nature.

Unnatural illnesses with divine punishment. Unnatural illnesses are believed to occur because a person may become so grave a sinner that the Lord withdraws his favor. In fact, illnesses may be attributed to punishment for failure to abide by the proper behavior rules given to man by God (Gregory, 1988). The cause of unnatural illnesses, for those who subscribe to these beliefs, is based on the continual battle between the forces of good and evil as personified in God and the devil. Evil influences may be blamed for any unnatural illness, which may range from nightmares to tuberculosis or cancer (Boston, 1993). An example of a person subscribing to this belief would be a diabetic African-Canadian woman who consistently refuses to inject herself with insulin because she believes her illness is the direct result of punishment by the devil for her sinful youth. However, unnatural illnesses are also believed to occur as a result of witchcraft. Witchcraft is based on the belief that there are individuals who have the ability to mobilize unusual powers for good and evil.

Comparison of the folk medicine system and other medical systems To develop an understanding of folk medicine as a system, the system itself must be examined along with the ecological model, the Western medical system, alternative therapies, and religious systems. Every medical system is based on the philosophy of survival of the human organism (Giger and Davidhizar, 1995). According to the classic work of Thomas Weaver (1970), both folk practices and Western medical practices are social systems with interdependent parts or variables that include beliefs, attitudes, practices, and roles associated with the concepts of health and disease and with the patterns of diagnoses and treatment.

All medical systems have an adaptive nature. As such, the term "medical system" can be defined as the pattern of cultural tradition and social institutions that evolves from deliberate behavior to improve health status regardless of the outcome of a particular behavior (Dunn, 1975).

To achieve good health, a person must develop an idea of what constitutes disease, with its counterpart conditions of pain and suffering. Once a philosophy of health is adopted by that person, various health roles are delineated. These health roles require specific health care practitioners who are duly initiated into the rights of practice. Practitioner status may be granted by medical societies or, in the case of folk medicine practices, by supernatural forces. The body is an integral part of each person; therefore all medical systems use body parts or excreta for diagnostic purposes. In addition, folk medicine practices, in most cases, prescribe medicine to rub into the skin, to irrigate the body, or to anoint the sick.

Ecological model. The ecological model is closely related to the folk medicine system. Kay (1979) defined ecology as having three foci: (1) biological, or the branch of biology that deals with the relationship between organisms and the environment; (2) social, or the relationship between people and institutions, and the interdependence between the two; and (3) cultural, or the relationship between culture and the environment, which also includes culture and societies in the environment. Ecological dimensions of health care can assist the nurse in providing plausible explanations as to why certain persons contract specific diseases and why other persons do not. Over the past decade, health care practitioners have become increasingly concerned with the ecological dimensions of race and ethnic minority group health problems such as AIDS, sickle cell anemia, and other such diseases.

Western medical system. In contrast to the folk medicine system, which is an attempt to explain illness in terms of balances between an individual and the physical, social, and spiritual worlds, is the Western medical system of diagnoses and scientific explanations for illness. Western medical practices focus on preventive and curative medicine, whereas folk medicine practices focus on personal rather than scientific behavior. In the folk medicine system, it may make all the sense in the world to burn incense and to avoid certain individuals, cold air, and the "evil eye." According to Kay (1979), one person's religion is another person's magic, witchcraft, or superstition. However, it is very difficult for health care professionals to see these entities as directly relevant to medical practice or to recognize that for some cultural groups religion is the equivalent of a science.

Although many differences in focus can be seen when a comparison between Western and folk medicine health practice is made, some of these differences may not be that significant. For example, Western medical relationships are generally dyads, such as physician-client, physician-nurse, and nurse-client relationships, whereas folk medicine networks are generally multiperson health care networks that may depend on parents, other relatives, and nonrelatives as health caregivers. However, today multiperson health care networks are no longer dismissed by Western health care practitioners as being irrelevant and thus dysfunctional. In fact, multiperson networks are slowly being incorporated into the Western medical system of health care.

Ethnic diets are an important aspect of human ecology because health care providers are beginning to incorporate into practice the use of ethnic diets and to understand their significance. An individual, regardless of ethnic group, must consume enough food to meet nutritional requirements for energy, fat, protein, vitamins, and minerals to keep the body functioning. Rittenbaugh (1978) noted that very little is known regarding the range of human variability both among and within human populations, particularly regarding common parameters such as nutritional requirements, physiological response to malnutrition, and digestive capabilities. It is perhaps this lack of knowledge that has in the past resulted in Western-oriented health care providers prescribing diets unacceptable to persons from diverse and multicultural backgrounds. In fact, the constitution of some persons from diverse cultural backgrounds may be physically incompatible with certain Western foods. Therefore factors regarding ethnic diets and other such folk practices must be considered by the nurse when developing care plans for culturally specific nursing care.

Alternative therapies. In 1990, 34% of Americans, approximately 61 million people, used one or more nonmedical forms of therapy to treat illness. Most of these individuals used these alternative therapies without informing their health practitioner (Eisenberg, Kessler, Foster, Norlock, Calkins, and Delbanco, 1993). In contrast, Dr. William LaValley, founder of the Nova Scotia Medical Society's Complementary Medicine Section, estimates that 25% of the Canadian population seeks health care from alternative practitioners (University of Calgary Medicine Seminar, 1995). Other presenters at the University of Calgary Complementary Medicine Seminar (1995) reported that 18% of patients seen at the Calgary HIV/AIDS clinic and 27% of those seen at the University of Calgary gastroenterology clinic had tried alternative therapies. Some 44% of physicians from Alberta indicated that they made referrals to practitioners of alternative therapies, though only 10% considered themselves informed on the subject (Petersen, 1996).

Although Western medicine tends to focus on illness care, alternative therapy addresses the whole patient (Peterson, 1996). In alternative therapy, symptoms are seen as the tip of the iceberg and the body's means for communicating to the mind that something needs to be changed, removed, or added to one's life (Petersen, 1996). In alternative therapy, the mind and the body are seen as a whole. Acupuncture, holistic healing, therapeutic touch, aromatic therapy, meditation, guided imagery, and a variety of other techniques prevail as viable alternative therapies (Barnum, 1994). Practitioners of alternative therapies include homeopaths, naturopaths, massage therapists, and reflexologists (Cronsberry, 1996). According to Dossey (1993), scientists working in the new field of psychoneuroimmunology have demonstrated the existence of intimate links between parts of the brain concerned with thought and emotion and the neurological and immune system. Based on these discoveries, Dossey (1993) concluded that there is no doubt that thought can become biology (Dossey, 1993). In 1983 a group of nurses in Canada began efforts toward what is today the Canadian Holistic Nurses Association. This is a recognized interest group of the Canadian Nurses Association (Petersen, 1996). Although the scientific value of alternative or complementary therapies is yet to be proved, there is a psychological component that allows the client to have a sense of control. For this reason, nurses should be well informed about unconventional methods (Cronsberry, 1996).

Religious systems. Some religious groups have elaborate rules concerning health care behaviors, including such things as the giving and receiving of health care. Religious experiences are based on cultural beliefs and may include such things as blessings from spiritual leaders, apparitions of dead relatives, and even miracle cures. Healing power based on religion may also be found in animate as well as inanimate objects. Religion can and does dictate social, moral, and dietary practices that are designed to assist a person in maintaining a healthy balance and, in addition, plays a vital role in illness prevention. Examples of religious health care practices to prevent illness are the burning of candles, rituals of redemption, and prayer. Religious practices such as the "blessing of the throats" on St. Blaise Day are performed to prevent illnesses such as sore throats and choking. Baptism may be seen as a ritual of cleansing and dedication as well as a prevention against evil. In addition to being related to dedication to God's will and a preparation for death, anointing the sick is related by some religious and cultural groups to recovery and may be performed in the hope of a miracle. Circumcision is also a religious practice, in that it may be viewed as having redemptive values that may prevent illness and harm (Morgenstern, 1966; Spector, 1996).

It is important for the nurse to learn to distinguish between a shaman and a priest. A shaman derives power from the supernatural, whereas a priest learns a codified body of rituals from other priests and from biblical laws. In traditional folk medicine systems, some of the most significant religious rituals are those that mediate between events in the "here and now" and events in the hereafter, or "out there" in the "nether" world (Morley and Wallis, 1978).

Another example of a religious system is the Amish. For the Amish, religion and custom are inseparable and blend into a way of life (Randall-Davis, 1989). Religious considerations determine hours of work, occupation, means and destination of travel, and choice of friends and mates. The Amish value the importance of working with the el-

ements of nature rather than mastery over these elements. Closeness to soil, animals, plants, and weather is valued. Salvation is viewed as obedience to the community (Wenger, 1991). The Amish have the belief that the human body was created by God and should not be tampered with. Some Amish believe that although medication may help, it is God who heals (Randall-David, 1989).

Many Amish have been increasingly influenced by special health food interests—vitamins and food-supplement industries (Wenger, 1988). Folk medical practices and opposition to health care seems to be dominant in some family systems (Hostetler, 1980). Egeland (1967) hypothesized there is a relationship between the concept of family culture and health behavior. Clusters of family cultures serve as basic socializers of health (Egeland, 1967). *Friendshaft,* a concept that crosses church distinct lines, produces distinct patterns of behavior and personality in the Amish community related to choice of type of physician. It also influences choice of curative diet therapy, folk remedies, and family coding of preference of treatment in reference to presumed cause of symptoms (Brewer and Bonalumi, 1995; Wenger, 1995).

IMPLICATIONS FOR NURSING CARE

The nurse must keep in mind that regardless of whether a client believes in internal or external locus of control or whether the client uses a folk medicine system, religious system, or ecological system, there is still safety in harmony and balance, and there may be danger in anything that is done to the extreme. In other words, it is bad for the body if one eats too much, drinks too much, stays out too late, and so forth (Giger and Davidhizar, 1995). In a classic 1972 study in Harlem, it was reported that 90% of African-American adolescents surveyed believed that good health was largely a matter of looking after oneself. These adolescents concluded that the results of excess may not be immediately visible but sooner or later will affect the individual because the body has become weakened (Brunswick and Josephson, 1972).

Asians tend to believe that health depends on maintaining a balance within the body between opposing forces of *yin* and *yang*. It is believed that strong emotions and improper diet can disturb this balance (Randall-David, 1989; Gold, 1992; Stauffer, 1995). On the other hand, several studies have indicated that many Canadian First Nations women have a lack of concern for prenatal care and have substantially more reproductive health problems than their other Canadian counterparts (Baskett, 1977; Graham-Cummings, 1967; Sokoloski, 1995; Young, Horvath, and Moffatt, 1989). Many First Nations women have a higher incidence of adolescent pregnancy, complications of pregnancy, grand multiparity, and low and high birth weight babies and subsequently experience greater infant mortality after preterm births (Sokoloski, 1995). Godel, Pabst, Hodges, and Johnson (1992) investigated iron-deficiency anemia among women in the western Canadian Arctic and highly recommended iron supplement to increase prenatal ferritin levels.

There seemingly is a gender and age differential that is associated with strengths and weaknesses among individuals. Generally speaking, strength is correlated with a person's ability to withstand illness, whereas weakness is correlated with a person's heightened susceptibility. For example, strength has been related to the male species. In Canada, females may be regarded as weaker than their male counterparts, and this gender weakness is generally perceived as women being more prone to illness primarily because of functional blood loss and anatomical differences. Certain age groups have also been related to individual strength and weakness. Infants and unborn fetuses are considered the weakest of all and are perceived to be at the mercy of the mother's behavior, including prenatal behavior. During pregnancy, harmony and moderation are the keys to a healthy baby; thus the pregnancy period carries the greatest taboos among most cultural groups. For example, some Mexican Americans, Amish, Hutterites, and both White Canadians and African Canadians subscribe to the doctrine of maternal moderation in pregnancy (Bauer, 1969; Giger and Davidhizar, 1995). It is even believed that the mother's emotional state during pregnancy may affect the baby, particularly in the case of pity, fear, mockery, or hate. For example, some southern Afri-

can Americans believe that feelings of hate for a particular person may cause the baby to resemble that person or that a child could be subjected to seizures if the mother saw someone having a seizure and felt pity. Some African Canadians, persons from the southern United States, and Mexican Canadians also believe that when a pregnant woman makes fun of someone with a physical affliction the baby may be born with the same affliction, thus punishing the mother for lack of charity (Snow, 1981).

Because some cultural groups believe in a direct connection between the body and the forces of nature, it is important for the nurse to recognize the relevance of natural phenomena such as phases of the moon, positions of the planets, and seasons of the year.

In the rural South in the United States there is a dependence on natural signs to regulate behavior. Some of these people rely on the *Old Farmer's Almanac* to guide such events as planting crops, setting hens' eggs, destroying weeds, weaning babies, and fishing. The almanac is consulted for many health needs, such as the best time to extract teeth or to have teeth filled (according to the almanac, the best time to have teeth extracted is during the moon's increase, and the best time to have teeth filled is during the moon's decrease). The almanac may also be used to determine the optimal time to undergo surgical procedures. The nurse must remember that not only is the almanac used by rural southern people, but also in northern urban areas many African-American pharmacists give almanacs as gifts to their customers for the New Year. Interestingly, the first *Old Farmer's Almanac* is reported to have been written by a physician in 1897.

It is also important for the nurse to remember that many people from diverse cultural groups use the zodiacal signs to manipulate health regimens but do not mention this to health professionals for fear of being ridiculed. Use of zodiacal signs illustrates how external forces are brought to bear on the individual; these signs are the basis for a lively practice of self-medication, dietary regulation, and behavior modifications. The nurse should remember that some of these practices are harmful, some are neutral, and some are beneficial. For example, it would be extremely detrimental for a client in need of a lifesaving surgical procedure to wait for a full moon to have the procedure done. It is important for the nurse to devise training programs that will teach clients to modify behaviors and interpret zodiacal signs in a way that will maintain health and prevent illness and disease (Giger and Davidhizar, 1995).

The nurse should also appreciate that dreams may have a role in health. Many Haitians believe that dreams are important events that allow the individual to communicate with inhabitants of the supernatural world. When dead relatives appear in a dream, they bring messages from the other world, upon which the Haitian individual is likely to rely (Randall-David, 1989; Giger and Davidhizar, 1995).

In a study of the folk medicine system, it may become obvious that this system reflects a view of the world as a dangerous place, where the individual must be constantly on guard against nature, other individuals, and possible punishment from God. This world view teaches the individual that it is best to look out for oneself and that mistrust is wiser than trust. For example, Hispanics or Latinos may believe that illness has its roots in physical imbalances or supernatural forces that include God's will, magical powers, evil spirits, powerful human forces, or emotional upsets. For some Hispanics or Latinos, treatment comes primarily through a variety of healers, which include the *curandero* (using prayer and artifacts); *yerbero* (herbalist); *espiritista* (practitioner of *espiritismo,* a religious cult concerned with communication with spirits and the purification of the soul through moral behavior); *santero* (practitioner of *santería,* a religious cult concerned with teaching people how to control or placate the supernatural) (Randall-David, 1989; Richardson, 1982; Wanderer and Rivera, 1986; Ruiz, 1985; Weclew, 1975). It may be necessary to involve spiritual healers and priests in crisis intervention therapy to treat the client.

The presence of an alternative medical (folk medicine) system that is different from and possibly in direct conflict with the Western medical system can serve to complicate matters. It not only becomes a matter of offering health care in the place of no

health care, or offering superior health care in lieu of inferior health care, but the nurse must remember that persons from diverse cultural backgrounds have deeply ingrained beliefs about how to attain and maintain health. These beliefs, which may be linked to the natural and supernatural worlds, may adversely affect the physician-client and nurse-client relationships and thus influence the individual's decision to follow or not follow prescribed treatment regimens. For example, in certain cultures, the occurrence of cancer may be attributed to insufficient use of herbal medicine, an insult to an ancestor, or a perceived punishment. Thus standard Western medical approaches may not always appear relevant to certain clients in multicultural populations (Boston, 1993).

The nurse might correctly assume that when a low-income Black Canadian, Canadian from the southern United States, Puerto Rican, or Mexican Canadian arrives for professional health care, every home remedy known to the client has already been tried. It is important for the nurse to determine what the client has been doing to combat the illness. If the home remedy is harmless, it is best left in the treatment plan and the nurse's own suggestions added. However, harmful practices must be eliminated. One of the best ways for the nurse to eliminate harmful practices is to inquire whether the practice has worked. If the client assumes that it has not worked, the nurse can simply suggest that something else be tried. If the client perceives that a harmful practice is beneficial, the nurse must provide education that will illuminate the dangers of this harmful practice (Giger and Davidhizar, 1995).

Nurses have recently begun to explore the relationship of person and environment in nursing research. An exploratory study by Pyles (1989) related Etzioni's compliance theory to satisfaction by nursing employees in a school of nursing. Data from the study indicated that a normative power structure in the school and the resultant moral-involvement profile in the faculty were compatible for an organization such as a university, which displays cultural goals. In a clinical study, Gould (1989) studied 112 elderly residents in three metropolitan nursing homes. The data suggested that life satisfaction is an indicator of well-being, which is useful as a measure of quality of care because of its linkage to health. The data additionally indicated that bonding develops between institutionalized elderly persons and their caregivers, which precludes the drive for self-determination. Thus the data provided an explanation of why lower-income elderly persons demonstrated high levels of life satisfaction despite low levels of perceived influence over the institutional environment.

Case Study

Martha Ricardo is a 27-year-old Hispanic-Canadian woman who lives in northern Alberta in a small cabin in the hills that has no indoor plumbing. She lives with her husband and six small children. The public health nurse makes a home visit after three of the children have been diagnosed by the school nurse as having lice. While the nurse is explaining the use of Rid (lice treatment) to the mother, she observes that Mrs. Brown has a persistent cough that she states she has had for 2 years. The nurse notes that the cough is productive, that Mrs. Brown looks emaciated, and that her color is extremely ashen. She tires easily. Although health insurance is a benefit of her husband's job in a nearby mine, Mrs. Brown's children were born at home, and she has never had a complete physical examination. When asked why she has not gone to a nearby free health clinic, Mrs. Brown replies, "Sickness is God's will, and He will cure me if He wants to. Anyway, my family comes first, and I don't have the time. Besides, doctors can't be trusted. My Aunt Jane went to one once, and she died the next week."

STUDY QUESTIONS

1. Based on the fact that Mrs. Ricardo is Hispanic and taking into consideration the fact that every person is unique, decide whether Mrs. Ricardo is more likely to be "being" oriented or "doing" oriented in regard to activity orientation.
2. Decide what the relational orientation is for Mrs. Ricardo based on her reply to the public health nurse about why she has not sought treatment.
3. Based on Mrs. Ricardo's reply to the public health nurse and on the fact that she is Hispanic, what people-to-nature orientation is she likely to have?
4. Decide, on the basis of Mrs. Ricardo's comment and the fact that she is Hispanic, what view of human nature she is likely to hold.
5. List at least three reasons why Mrs. Ricardo might be apprehensive about seeking medical help.

References

Abarts, J. (1995). University of Calgary hosts complementary medicine society. *Holistic and Complementary Medical Society of Alberta Newsletter, 1*(1), 1.

Armstrong, M. (1986). *Exploring the circle: a journey into Native children's mental health.* Edmonton: Alberta Social Services and Community Health.

Barnum, B. (1994). *Nursing theory* (ed. 4). Philadelphia: J.B. Lippincott Co.

Baskett, T.F. (1977). Grand multiparity—a continuing threat: a 6-year review. *Canadian Medical Association Journal, 116*(9), 1001-1004.

Bauer, W.W. (1969). *Potions, remedies, and old wives' tales.* New York: Doubleday.

Bauwens, E., & Anderson, S. (1988). Social and cultural influences on health care. In Stanhope, M., & Lancaster, J. (Eds.), *Community health nursing: process and practice for promoting health* (ed. 2) (pp. 89-108). St. Louis: Mosby.

Boston, P. (1993). Culture and cancer: the relevance of cultural orientation within cancer education programmes. *European Journal of Cancer Care, 2,* 72-76.

Brewer, J., & Bonalumi, N. (1995). Cultural diversity in the emergency department. *The Journal of Emergency Nursing, 2*(6), 494-497.

Brunswick, A.F., & Josephson, E. (1972, October). Adolescent health in Harlem. *American Journal of Public Health, 72* (suppl.), 7-47.

Campinha-Bacote, J. (1997). Understanding the influence of culture. In Haber, J., Krainovich-Miller, B., McMahon, A., & Price-Hoskins, P. (Eds.), *Comprehensive psychiatric nursing* (ed. 5). St. Louis: Mosby.

Chrisman, N.J. (1977). The health seeking process. *Culture and Medicine in Psychiatry, 1,* 351-377.

Cook, P. (1994). Chronic illness beliefs and the role of social networks among Chinese, Indian, and Anglo-Celtic Canadians. *Journal of Cross-Cultural Psychology, 25*(4), 452-465.

Cronsberry, T. (1996). Alternative cancer therapies. *The Canadian Nurse, 92,* 35-40.

Dosey, L. (1993). *Healing words.* New York: Harper & Row.

Dunn, F.L. (1975). Transcultural Asian medicine and cosmopolitan medicine as adaptive systems. In Leslie, E. (Ed.), *Asian medical systems: a comparative study* (p. 135). Berkeley: University of California Press.

Egeland, J. (1967). Belief and behavior as related to illness: a community case study of the old order Amish. (Doctoral dissertation, Yale University). *Dissertation Abstracts International, X,* 1967.

Eisenberg, D.M., Kessler, R.C., Foster, C., Norlock, F.E., Calkins, D.R., & Delbanco, T.L. (1993). Unconventional medicine in the United States: prevalence, costs, and patterns of use. *New England Journal of Medicine, 328*(4), 246-252.

Elling, R.H. (1977). *Socio-cultural influences on health care.* New York: Springer Publishing.

Fabrega, H. (1971). Medical anthropology. In Siegel, B.J. (Ed.), *Biennial review of anthropology.* Stanford, Calif.: Stanford University Press.

French, M. (1996, July). The power of plants. *Advances for Nurse Practitioners,* 16-18.

Giger, J., Davidhizar, R., & Turner, G. (1992). Black American folk medicine. *The ABNF Journal,* 42-46.

Giger, J., & Davidhizar, R. (1995). *Transcultural nursing: assessment and intervention.* St. Louis: Mosby.

Giger, J., Davidhizar, R., Johnson, J., & Poole, V. (1997). The changing face of America. *Health Traveler, 4*(4), 11-17.

Godel, J., Pabst, H., Hodges, P., & Johnson, K. (1992). Iron status and pregnancy in a northern Canadian population: relationship to diet and iron supplementation. *Canadian Journal of Public Health, 83*(5), 339-343.

Gold, S. (1992). Mental health and illness in Vietnamese refugees. *Western Journal of Medicine, 157*(3), 290.

Gould, M. (1989, November 14). *The relationship of perceived social-environmental factors and functional health status to life satisfaction in the elderly.* Paper presented at the Sigma Theta Tau International Conference, Indianapolis, Ind.

Graham-Cumming, G. (1967). Prenatal care and infant mortality among Canadians Indians. *The Canadian Nurse, 63*(9), 29-31.

Greene, L. (1981). *Social and biological predictors of nutritional status, growth, and development.* New York: Academic Press.

Gregory, D. (1988). Nursing practice in native communities. In Baumgart, A., & Larson, J. (Eds.), *Canadian nursing faces the future.* Toronto: Mosby.

Grypma, S. (1993). Culture shock. *The Canadian Nurse, 89,* 33-37.

Guruge, S., & Donner, G. (1996, September). Transcultural nursing in Canada. *The Canadian Nurse, 92,* 34-39.

Haber, J., & Giuffra, M. (1992). Sociocultural issues. In Haber, J., Hoskins, P., Leach, A., & Sideleau, B. (Eds.), *Comprehensive psychiatric nursing* (ed. 4) (pp. 244-246). St. Louis: Mosby.

Henderson, G., & Primeaux, M. (1981). *Transcultural health care.* Reading, Mass.: Addison-Wesley.

Hislop, M., Deschamps, M., Band, P., Smith, J., & Clarke, H. (1992). Participation in British Columbia cervical cytology screening programme by Native women. *Revue Canadienne dé Sante Publique, 83*(5), 344-350.

Hostetler, J. (1980). *Amish society* (ed. 3). Baltimore: The Johns Hopkins University Press.

Indian and Northern Affairs. (1980). *Indian conditions: a survey.* Ottawa: Department of Indian Affairs and Northern Development (catalogue no. QS5141/000/EEA3).

Jarvis, G.K., & Boldt, M. (1982). Death styles among Canada's Indians. *Social Science and Medicine, 16,* 1345-1352.

Jilek, W. (1982). How young Indian people die. *Proceedings of the 1982 Canadian Psychiatric Association Meeting. Section on Native Mental Health.* Toronto: Canadian Psychiatric Association.

Kay, M. (1979). Clinical anthropology. In Bauwens, E.E.(Ed.), *The anthropology of health* (pp. 3-11). St. Louis: Mosby.

Kleinman, A., Eisenberg, L., & Good, B. (1978). Culture, illness and care. *Annals of Internal Medicine, 88,* 251-258.

Kluckhohn, K., & Strodtbeck, F. (1961). *Variations in value orientations.* New York: Row, Peterson.

Lew, L. (1989). *Southeast Asian Health Project: Application for mother, children and infants demonstration grant.* Unpublished manuscript (grant proposal), Ottawa.

Linwood, M.E., Kasian, G.F., & Irvine, J.D. (1990). Child and youth accidents in northern Native communities. *Canadian Journal of Public Health, 81,* 77-78.

Mattson, S. (1995). Culturally sensitive perinatal care for Southeast Asians. *Journal of Obstetric and Gynecological Nursing, 4*(4), 335-341.

McKinnon, A., Gartrell, J., Derksen, L., & Jarvis, G. (1991). Health knowledge of Native Indian youth in central Alberta. *Canadian Journal of Public Health, 82*(6), 429-433.

McRae, L. (1994). Cultural sensitivity in rehabilitation related to native clients. *Canadian Journal of Rehabilitation, 7*(4), 251-256.

Morgenstern, J. (1966). *Rites of birth, marriage, death, and kindred occasions among the Semites.* Chicago: Quadrangle.

Morley, P., & Wallis, R. (1978). *Culture and caring.* London: Peter Owen.

Petersen, B. (1996). The mind-body connection. *The Canadian Nurse, 92,* 29-31.

Pillsbury, B. (1982). Doing the month: confinement and convalescence of Chinese women after childbirth. In Kay, M. (Ed.), *Anthropology of human birth.* Philadelphia: F.A. Davis.

Pyles, C. (1989, November 13). *Power compatibility profile in a school of nursing.* Paper presented at the Sigma Theta Tau International Conference, Indianapolis, Ind.

Randall-David, E. (1989). *Strategies for working with culturally diverse communities and clients* [Brochure]. Washington, D.C.: U.S. Department of Health and Human Services.

Red Horse, J., Johnson, T., & Weiner, D. (1989). Commentary: Culture perspectives on research among American Indians. *American Indian Culture and Research Journal, 13*(3), 267-271.

Richardson, L. (1982). Caring through understanding: Part 2. Folk medicine in the Hispanic population. *Imprint, 29*(2), 21.

Rittenbaugh, C. (1978). Human foodways: a window on evolution. In Bauwens, E.E. (Ed.), *The anthropology of health.* St. Louis: Mosby.

Rotter, J.B. (1966). Generalized expectancies for internal versus external control of reinforcement. *Psychological Monographs, 80*(1), 1-28.

Rodin, J., & Salovey, P. (1989). Health psychology. *Annual Review of Psychology, 40,* 533-579.

Rotter, J.B. (1975). Some problems and misconceptions related to the construct of internal versus external control of reinforcement. *Journal of Consulting and Clinical Psychology, 43,* 56-67.

Ruiz, P. (1985). Cultural barriers to effective medical care among Hispanic-American patients. *Annual Review of Medicine, 36,* 63-71.

Scott, K. (1991). Northern nurses and burnout. *The Canadian Nurse, 87,* 18-21.

Sideleau, B. (1992). Space and time. In Haber, J., McMahon, A., Price-Hoskins, P., & Sideleau, B. (Eds.), *Comprehensive psychiatric nursing* (ed. 4). St. Louis: Mosby.

Snow, L.F. (1981). Folk medical beliefs and their implications for the care of patients: a review based on studies among black Americans. In Henderson, G., & Primeaux, M. (Eds.), *Transcultural health care.* Reading, Mass.: Addison-Wesley.

Sokoloski, E. (1995). Canadian first nations women's beliefs about pregnancy and prenatal care. *The Canadian Journal of Nursing Research, 27*(1), 89-100.

Spector, R. (1996). *Cultural diversity in health care* (ed. 4). Stamford, Conn.: Appleton & Lange.

Stauffer, R. (1995). Vietnamese Americans. In Giger, J., & Davidhizar, R. (Eds.), *Transcultural nursing: assessment and intervention.* St. Louis: Mosby.

Threlfall, W.J. (1986). Cancer patterns in British Columbia Native Indians. *Medical Journal, 28,* 508-510.

Thompson, K. (1993, September). Self-governed health. *The Canadian Nurse, 89,* 29-32.

Tousignant, M. (1985). *Youth health in Canada: trends, assessment, and psychosocial aspects.* Ottawa: Social Trends Analysis Directorate, Policy Coordination Analysis and Management Systems Branch. (catalogue no. A85-1).

University of Calgary—Complimentary Medicine Seminar. (1995). University of Calgary, Alberta.

van Itallie, N. (1996). *Fodor's Canada.* Toronto: Fodor's Travel Publications.

Wanderer, J., & Rivera, G. (1986). Black magic beliefs and white magic practice: the common structures of intimacy, tradition and power. *Social Science Journal, 23*(4), 419.

Weaver, T. (1970). Use of hypothetical situations in a study of Spanish-American illness referral systems. *Human Organisms, 29,* 141.

Weclew, R.V. (1975). The nature, prevalence, and level of awarenesss of *curanderismo* and some of its implications for community mental health. *Community Mental Health Journal, 11*(2), 145-154.

Wenger, A. (1988). *The phenomenon of care in a high context culture: the old order Amish.* (Doctoral dissertation, Wayne State University, Detroit, Michigan).

Wenger, A. (1991). The culture care theory and the older order Amish. In Leininger, M. (Ed.), *Cultural care diversity and universality: a theory of nursing.* New York: National League for Nursing.

Wenger, A. (1995). Cultural context, health, and health care decision making. *The Journal of Transcultural Nursing, 7*(1), 3-14.

Williams, C., & Jelliffe, D. (1972). *Mother and child health: delivering the services.* London: Oxford University Press.

Young, T., Horvath, J., & Moffatt, M. (1989). Obstetrical ultrasound in remote communities: an approach to health program evaluation. *Canadian Journal of Public Health, 80*(4), 276-281.

CHAPTER 7

Biological Variations

BEHAVIORAL OBJECTIVES

After reading this chapter, the nurse will be able to:

1. Articulate biological differences between individuals in various racial groups.
2. Relate the importance of knowledge of biological differences that may exist between individuals in various racial groups to the provision of health care by the nurse.
3. Describe nursing implications that may arise when providing care for individuals in different cultural and racial groups.
4. Describe nutritional preferences and deficiencies that may exist among persons in different cultural groups.
5. Explain how psychological characteristics may vary from one culture to another.
6. Explain how susceptibility to disease may differ between individuals in different racial groups.

It is a well-known fact that people differ culturally. Cultural differences are evident in communication, spatial relationships and needs, social organizations (family, kinships, and tribes), time orientation, and ability or desire to control the environment. Less recognized and understood are the biological differences that exist between people in various racial groups. It is becoming more evident to nurses that a body of scientific knowledge does exist about biological cultural differences. References to and information about biocultural differences are mushrooming in the literature and have resulted in a field of study known as biocultural ecology (Bennett, Osborne, and Miller, 1975), which has as its major focus the study of human adaptation and homeostasis. The purpose of biocultural ecology is to transcend the fragmentation inherent in the separation of culture, human biology, and ecology with environment. Biocultural ecology is the study of diverse human populations by means of this three-way interaction system and focuses on specific, localized individuals and populations within a given environment. Data relative to all the variables significant to people within a racial group are essential for complete understanding of the people. Not only are no two persons alike, but also no two cultural or racial groups are alike, and all phenomena relative to both individuals and cultural or racial groups must be understood.

Many biocultural studies can be noted in Canadian history. For example, in Newfoundland and Labrador, many families of fishermen lack fresh vegetables over the winter months and survived mainly on white bread. Consequently there was a higher incidence of beriberi because of the lack of thiamine in the diet. Legislation in the 1970s requiring the addition of vitamin A to certain foods has significantly improved the health status of Canadian people, and the incidence of beriberi has been dramatically reduced (Basch, 1990). In the 1960s, an epidemic of amebic dysentery occurred in a closely knit population of Native Americans in northern Saskatchewan causing more than 100 hospitalizations and 8 deaths. One third of the population was found to be carriers of the responsible pathogen related to poor nutrition and deficient sanitation (Basch, 1990). In Canada, the incidence of stomach cancer is double that in Japan, with almost twice as much of this type of cancer occurring in men as that in women. The etiology for this remains under investigation (Basch, 1990). In 1987 the Lubicon Lake band of Indians in northern Canada filed a complaint noting that state-sponsored oil and gas exploration threatened the Indians' means of subsistence and violated their right to life. In a precedent-setting action, the court supported the petitioners and the Indian's rights, and the terrain was protected (Brown, 1996).

Although the significance of biocultural ecology concepts has existed in other disciplines, such as sociology and medical anthropology, the nursing literature has only recently documented the importance of this field for nurses. A focus on transcultural issues that began in the mid-1960s with the impetus of nurses such as Madeleine Leininger (1970) has helped nurses to develop cultural insights and a deeper appreciation for human life and values from a cultural perspective. However, despite the introduction of transcultural nursing concepts, the nursing literature remains scanty on biological variations existing among people in various racial groups. The strongest argument for including concepts on biological variations in nursing education and subsequently nursing practice is that scientific facts about biological variations can aid the nurse in giving culturally appropriate health care. Nurses who care for people transculturally need to be cognizant of certain basic biological differences to give nonharmful and competent care.

The majority of nurses in Canada, similar to nurses in the United States, have been educated in a system of nursing practice based on biological parameters of the dominant White race. Because studies on biological baseline values in growth and development, nutrition, and other biological phenomena have been conducted using White subjects, standardized norms available to the nurse do not recognize biological variations existing among different racial groups. That people in various racial groups differ tremendously is evidenced externally and is related to biogenetic variations that have occurred internally. Therefore values uniracially normed are inappropriate when applied across racial groups. In Canada, White-standardized values for factors related to growth and development, nutrition, and susceptibility to disease are often applied to Blacks, Orientals, and First Nation people. Therefore significant deviations from the norm that may be labeled "nonnormal" might be more appropriately labeled "non-White" (Overfield, 1977). In fact, biological variations among racial groups are so diverse that multiple dimensions are encompassed. It must be remembered that data relative to all the variables significant to people within a racial group are essential for complete understanding of the people. Not only are no two persons, but also no two cultural or racial groups are alike, and all phenomena relative to both individuals and cultural or racial groups must be understood.

DIMENSIONS OF BIOLOGICAL VARIATIONS

A direct relationship exists between race and body structure, skin color, other visible physical characteristics, enzymatic and genetic variations, electrocardiographic patterns, susceptibility to disease, nutritional preferences and deficiencies, and psychological characteristics. Differences between people in various racial groups in each of these areas are discussed in the following sections.

Body Structure

One category of difference between racial groups is body structure, which includes both body size and shape. Newborn body proportions differ among racial groups. Although research on this topic remains scanty, it has been postulated that newborn body proportions appear to be genetically programed to conform to the pelvic shape of the mother (Overfield, 1977).

Body structure and bone density also differ among adults. For example, both the prevalence of osteoporosis and the incidence of vertebral fractures are reported to be substantially lower in African American women than in White American women (Cummings, Kelsey, Nevitt, and O'Dowd, 1985; Gilsanz, Roe, Mora, Costin, and Goodman, 1991; Melton and Riggs, 1987; Pollitzer and Anderson, 1990). This finding is generally attributed to racial differences in adult bone mass (Pollitzer and Anderson, 1990).

Among adults, bone density is greater in African Americans than in White Americans of either sex (Reid, Cullen, Schooler, Livingston, and Evans, 1990). However, differences in adult bone density are not necessarily confined to these two racial groups. In fact, the bone density of adult Polynesians is reported to be greater than that of age-matched Whites (Reid et al., 1990). In contrast, Asian Americans generally have lower values for bone density compared with other racial groups (Reid et al., 1990).

Biological markers that account for the variations in adult bone mass among racial groups are unknown. In addition, the time of life at which these differences are manifested is uncertain. According to Li, Specker, Ho, and Tsang (1989), prepubertal African-American children tend to have higher values for bone density than do their White counterparts. Some researchers (Garn, Nagy, and Sandusky, 1972; Li, Specker, Ho, and Tsang, 1989) have speculated that such findings indicate that racial differences in skeletal mass may develop early in childhood and persist throughout life.

In regard to body structure and size, the face is perhaps one of the most fascinating areas of the body because it has many parts that combine to make the whole. The face tends to be the one prominent area that can visibly categorize people by race. For example, eyelids vary from racial group to racial group. In some racial groups the eyelids droop over the cartilage plate above the eye, and in other racial groups the eyelids do not droop. The epicanthic fold, another variation of the eyelids, is found predominantly in persons with Oriental characteristics but may be present in other racial groups.

Ears are another fascinating part of the face because they have a variety of shapes. Earlobes can be free and floppy or attached close to the face as if the intent were to make sure the lobe stayed in place. Earlobes that are free and floppy are very handy for attaching earrings. When earlobes are attached, they are the least defined, and the wearing of objects such as earrings may be difficult.

Wiet, DeBlanc, Stewart, and Weider (1980), in a review of studies of the incidence of otitis media in Canadian Indian children, noted that chronic otitis media is estimated to be 15 times higher among Indians than among non-Indians. A screening in a northern Quebec community found 4% of Cree children and 23% of Inuit children had hearing loss (Julien, Baxter, Crago, Ilecki, and Thérien, 1979). Thérien (1988) conducted a study in Quebec and found 23% of Inuit to have unilateral hearing loss and 40% to have bilateral hearing loss. A genetic basis for dysfunction of the eustachian tube has been suggested as a cause of repeated episodes of otitis media in Native Canadian children (Gunby, 1979).

Noses come in all sizes and shapes; however, nose size and shape correlate directly with one's racial ancestry. It has been postulated that small noses were an evolutionary result of living in cold climates, such as the classic Oriental nose. On the other hand, noses with high bridges were a result of living in climates that were dry, such as the classic Iranian and American and Canadian Indian noses. People who lived in moist, hot climates developed broad, flat noses, such as those found on Africans, Black Canadians, and African Americans (Overfield, 1977, 1985).

Teeth offer another important variation in body size and shape. Tooth size, which is important because the teeth help shape the size of the lower face, varies among racial groups. For example, Australian aborigines have the largest teeth in the world, as well as four extra molars. Oriental, Black Canadian, and African Americans have very large teeth, whereas White Canadians and White Americans have very small teeth. People with very large teeth tend to have their jaws projecting beyond the upper part of the face. This projection tends to be a normal variation and not an orthodontic problem. There is also a tendency among some racial groups for fewer teeth. For example, some racial groups do not have a third molar or maxillary lateral incisors. Peg teeth are sometimes a step in the evolutionary process that facilitates the presence or absence of a particular type of tooth (Overfield, 1977).

As teeth vary among racial groups, so do tongues. The most common variances are scrotal tongues, which occur in 5% of the population in some racial groups; geographic tongues, which occur in 3% of the population in some racial groups; and fissured tongues, which occur in 5% to 40% of the population in some racial groups (Witcop et al., 1963).

The mandibular or palatine torus is also of concern to the nurse when inspecting the mouth. The torus is a bony protuberance, and the palatine torus occurs on the midline of the palate, whereas the mandibular torus occurs as a lump on the inner side of the mandible near the second molar. Tori are fairly common, with palatine tori occurring in up to 25% of the population in most racial groups studied. Mandibular tori occur in 7% of Whites, 2% of Blacks, and 40% of Orientals (Jarvis, 1972).

Another variation in body size and structure is attributable to muscle size and mass. In certain racial groups specific muscles are absent altogether. The peroneus tertius muscle, which is found in the foot, and the palmaris longus muscle, which is found in the wrist, are absent in individuals in some racial groups. However, muscle absence in general does not appear to be more prevalent in any particular racial group; nor does absence of a particular muscle correspond with absence of another muscle. Numerous studies have been conducted regarding inheritability of stature (Overfield, 1985). In general, the conclusions are that people by virtue of race vary in height. Individuals of higher socioeconomic status in all ethnic groups are taller (Overfield, 1985). In regard to physical growth and developmental rates, African Americans are generally advanced, whereas Orientals are generally retarded when these groups are compared with White norms.

A new phenomenon among Native Canadians appears to be excessively heavy birth weights among babies. Only 12.2% of Native infants were 4 kg or more in 1962, whereas 21.6% were considerably heavier in 1983 (Stewart, 1985). A study by Thomson (1990) suggested that heavy birth weight, by gestational age, occurred almost 50% more often in Na

tive Canadians than in non-Natives of British Columbia. It has been suggested that this may have resulted from forced adaptation through changing dietary habits. Today, Native peoples not only have a steady food supply but also have increased their sugar intake (Thomson, 1990).

Skin Color

When working with people from diverse cultural backgrounds, the nurse should have an understanding of how different races evolved in relation to the environment. Biological differences noted in skin color may be attributable to the biological adjustments a person's ancestors made in the environment in which they lived. For example, it has been scientifically postulated that the original skin color of humans on earth was black (Overfield, 1977). Further postulations suggest that white skin was the result of mutation and environmental pressures exerted on persons living in cold, cloudy northern Europe. The mutation is believed to have occurred because light skin was better able to synthesize vitamin D, particularly on cloudy days. It is believed that black skin became a neutral trait in climates where protection from the sun and heat of the tropics was not a factor (Overfield, 1977, 1985).

Skin color is probably the most significant biological variation in terms of nursing care. Nursing care delivery is based on accurate client assessment, and the darker the client's skin, the more difficult it becomes to assess changes in color. When caring for clients with highly pigmented skin, the nurse must first establish the baseline skin color, and daylight is the best light source for doing so. If possible, dark-skinned clients should always be given a bed by a window to provide access to sunlight. When daylight is not available to assess skin color, a lamp with at least a 60-watt bulb should be used. To establish the baseline skin color, the nurse must observe those skin surfaces that have the least amount of pigmentation, which include the volar surfaces of the forearms, the palms of the hands, the soles of the feet, the abdomen, and the buttocks. When observing these areas, the nurse should look for an underlying red tone, which is typical of all skin, regardless of how dark its color. Absence of this red tone in a cli ent may be indicative of pallor. Additional areas that are important to assess in dark-skinned clients include the mouth, the conjunctivae, and the nail beds. Generally speaking, the darkness of the oral mucosa correlates with the client's skin color. The darker the skin, the darker the mucosa; nevertheless, the mucosa is lighter than the skin.

The nurse must be aware that oral hyperpigmentation can occur on the tongue and the mucosa and is a condition that can alter the value of the oral mucosa as a site for observation. The occurrence of oral hyperpigmentation is directly related to the darkness of a person's skin. Oral hyperpigmentation appears in 50% to 90% of Blacks, compared with 10% to 50% of Whites. Another important consideration for the nurse is the appearance of a hard palate because it takes on a yellow discoloration, particularly in the presence of jaundice. The hard palate is frequently affected by hyperpigmentation in a manner similar to that of the oral mucosa and the tongue. The nurse should also assess the lips because they may be helpful in the assessment of skin color changes (such as jaundice or cyanosis). It is important for the nurse to remember, however, that the lips of some Black people have a natural bluish hue (Rouch, 1977). Thus it is important for the nurse to have established the baseline color of the lips if the colors are to be of value in detecting cyanosis (Branch and Paxton, 1976).

It is also important for the nurse to establish the normal color of both conjunctivae when working with persons from transcultural populations. The conjunctivae will reflect the color changes of cyanosis or pallor and are a good site for observing petechiae. Another excellent source for determining the presence of jaundice is the sclerae. The nurse should first establish a baseline color for the sclerae because the sclerae of dark-skinned persons often have a yellow coloration because of subconjunctival fatty deposits. A common finding of persons with highly pigmented skin is the presence of melanin deposits, or "freckles," on the sclerae.

The final area of assessment should be the nail beds, which are useful when there is an attempt to detect cyanosis or pallor. In dark-skinned persons it is difficult to assess the nail beds because they may be highly pigmented, thick, or lined or contain melanin deposits. Regardless of color, for baseline assessment it is important for the nurse to observe how quickly the color returns to the nail beds after pressure has been released from the free edge of the nail (Rouch, 1977). A slower return of color to the nail beds may be indicative of cyanosis or pallor. It is also difficult to detect rashes, inflammations, and ecchymosis in dark-skinned persons. It may be necessary to palpate rashes in dark-skinned persons because rashes may not be readily visible to the eye. When palpating the skin for rashes, the nurse should notice the induration and warmth of the area.

Other Visible Physical Characteristics

In addition to looking for changes in pallor and cyanosis, the nurse should notice other aberrations in the skin. For example, mongolian spots may be present on the skin of Blacks, Asians, Native Canadians, or Hispanic Canadian newborns. Mongolian spots are bluish discolorations that vary tremendously in size and color and are often mistaken for bruises. Another aberration that is more common in Blacks than in other racial groups is keloids. These ropelike scars represent an exaggeration of the wound-healing process and may occur as a result of any type of trauma, such as surgical incisons, ear piercing, or insertion of an intravenous catheter.

Enzymatic and Genetic Variations

The basic genetic makeup of a person is determined from the moment of conception. At the moment of conception, among other things, the upper limits of achievement are set; the "map," so to speak, is drawn. In other words, a person can be only what he or she is genetically determined to be. More specifically, growth and development cannot go beyond what the genes make possible. A person will not grow 1 inch taller than genetic structure allows regardless of the amount of exercise or vitamins consumed. By the same token, a person will be no more intelligent than genetic structure allows, despite the amount of tutoring or special schooling that the person receives (Burt, 1966; Lorton and Lorton, 1984).

In medical terms, a person's race represents his or her genetic makeup. Although race may be irrelevant in some situations, knowing the racial predisposition to a certain disease is often helpful in evaluating clients and diagnosing their illness as well as in assessing risks (Divan, 1989). The genetic and enzymatic predisposition to certain diseases is discussed in this chapter under the heading Susceptibility to Disease; lactose intolerance and glucose-6-phosphate dehydrogenase (G-6-PD) deficiency are discussed under the heading Nutritional Deficiencies.

The incidence of dizygote twinning is highest in Blacks, occurring in 4% of births. Dizygote twinning occurs in approximately 2% of births in Whites and in 0.5% of births in Asians (Bulmer, 1970; Giger, Davidhizar, and Wieczorek, 1993).

Some research interpretations (Jensen, 1969, 1974, 1977) have indicated that the small but persistent differences between the average intelligence quotients (IQs) of Black children and those of White children reflect a genetic difference. Jensen (1969) claimed to have controlled for variables, including income and education. He reported that he found a difference in IQ, which he believed to be indicative of a genetic difference. Others have refuted Jensen's claim (Kamlin, 1974). In 1977 Jensen conducted a study of children between 5 and 16 years of age in the rural South, in which analysis of the data suggested that the IQs of Black children, but not those of White children, drop substantially as they grow older. Jensen believed that this contrast between Blacks and Whites possibly meant that the decrement in IQ was genetically determined. This has not been supported by research by others.

Drug interactions and metabolism Reactions to drugs vary with race. Some evidence indicates that drugs are metabolized by different races in different ways and at different rates (Echizen, Horai, and Ishizaki, 1989). For example, Zhou, Koshakji, Silberstein, Wilkinson, and Wood (1989) demonstrated that Chinese subjects are more sensitive to the cardiovascular effects of propranolol than are White subjects. In the body there are three classes of reactions to foreign chemicals or drugs: hydrolysis, conjugation, and oxidation (Kalow, 1982, 1986, 1989). The following are examples of reactions to specific drugs.

Isoniazid is a drug commonly used to treat tuberculosis. People metabolize this drug in one of two ways: they will inactivate it either very slowly or very rapidly. Those persons who inactivate this drug very slowly are at risk for developing peripheral neuropathy during therapy (Vessell, 1972). Rapid inactivation of this drug occurs in 40% of Whites, 60% of Blacks, 60% to 90% of American and Canadian Indians and Inuits, and 85% to 90% of Orientals (Vessell, 1972). Pyridoxine is given with isoniazid, and the doses are spaced at larger intervals for slower reaction during treatment for tuberculosis. Primaquine is metabolized by oxidation and is used in the treatment of malaria. When this drug is given to individuals who lack the enzymes necessary for glucose metabolism of the red blood cells, hemolysis of the red blood cells occurs. Approximately 100 million people in the world are affected by this particular enzyme deficiency and thus are unable to ingest primaquine. Approximately 35% of Blacks have this particular enzyme deficiency.

Succinylcholine is a muscle relaxant used during surgery. It is inactivated by hydrolysis by the enzyme pseudocholinesterase. In most individuals it is rapidly inactivated, but some individuals have the atypical form of the enzyme and suffer prolonged muscle paralysis and an inability to breathe after administration of the drug. Blacks, Orientals, and Native Americans and Canadians are at risk for having pseudocholinesterase deficiency; Whites have a slightly higher risk than these groups. Some Jews and Inuits have a considerably greater risk: 1 out of 135 Inuit is unable to metabolize the drug succinylcholine normally (Kalow, 1982, 1986, 1989; Vessell, 1972).

Alcohol is metabolized differently depending on race. There are two enzymes involved in the metabolism of alcohol: alcohol dehydrogenase (ADH) and acetaldehyde dehydrogenase (ALDH). Alcohol metabolism is a two-step process: ADH converts alcohol to acetaldehyde, and ALDH converts acetaldehyde (a toxic substance) to acetic acid (a nontoxic substance). Both of these enzymes have more than one variant. Alcohol has a high-activity type of ADH, which converts alcohol to acetaldehyde rapidly, and a low-activity variant, which converts it slowly (Kalow, 1986; Kalow, 1972). ALDH has four variants (ALDH-1 through 4). Acetaldehyde dehydrogenase 1 (ALDH-1) is considered "normal"; other types are less efficient in their ability to metabolize acetaldehyde (Goedde, 1983, 1986).

In Whites, with "normal" levels of both ADH and ALDH-1, alcohol is metabolized fairly efficiently. In contrast, American Indians and Asians have an excessive level of high-activity ADH and a low level of ALDH-1. Consequently some studies have noted that alcohol is metabolized to acetaldehyde rapidly by persons in these groups. However, the metabolism to acetic acid is delayed. Because acetaldehyde is toxic and acetic acid is not, the net result is unpleasant effects such as facial flushing and palpitations (Keltner, 1994; Kudzma, 1992). Data from some studies indicate that American Indians and Orientals experience marked facial flushing and other vasomotor symptoms after ingesting alcohol, compared with their White and African-American counterparts, who experience less severe reactions (Fenna, Schaefer, Mix, and Gilbert, 1971). Facial flushing, after ingestion of alcohol, occurs in 45% to 85% of Asians versus 3% to 29% of Whites (Chan, 1986).

A study in Alberta compared White volunteers with Inuit and Indian hospital clients and found that, when clients were given alcohol intravenously, both Native groups had slower rates of disappearance of blood alcohol. This differential response persisted even after the investigators stratified for the history of usual alcohol consumptions. This study provides credence to the hypothesis that Native people take a longer time to "sober up" (Fenna et al., 1971; Young, 1994). However, this finding was not collaborated in a study of Ojibwa from northwestern Ontario and Whites. In this study, the Ojibwa had a faster metabolism than did Whites (Reed, Kalant, Gibbins, Kapur, and Rankin, 1976). Thus the genetic basis of alcohol abuse or alcoholism in Native Americans continues to be the subject of controversy among researchers (Young, 1994).

Caffeine, a component of many drugs as well as coffee, tea, and colas, appears to be metabolized and excreted faster by Whites than by Asians (Grant, Tang, Kalow, 1983). It is believed that the differences noted in caffeine metabolism are directly correlated with liver-enzyme differences (Kudzma, 1992).

Another category of drugs that is metabolized differently depending on race is antihypertensives. Several studies suggest that there are notable differences between Blacks and their White counterparts in the metabolism of antihypertensive drugs (Freis, 1986; Moser and Lunn, 1982; Zhou et al., 1989). Fries (1986) noted that Blacks tend to need higher doses of beta-adrenergic receptor blocking agents such as propranolol (Inderal). In contrast, Moser and Lunn (1982) found that angiotensin-converting enzyme inhibitors (captopril) tend to be less effective as a single therapy for Blacks compared with Whites with the same treatment regimen. Zhou et al. (1989) noted that even when body surface area and body weight were taken into account Chinese men tend to need only about half as much propranolol compared with White males.

Psychotropic drugs are also metabolized differently depending on race. When blood plasma levels of alprazolam (Xanax) were studied in 42 healthy men (14 American-born Asians, 14 foreign-born Asians, and 14 Whites), it was noted that the Asian clients needed smaller doses to achieve the same blood plasma levels as their White counterparts (Lin, Lau, Smith, Phillips, Antal, and Poland, 1988). Body heights and weights were not a factor in the study results. Nonetheless, in both Asian groups (American born and foreign born), the drug remained in the blood longer (Lin et al., 1988). It is important for the nurse to remember that certain psychotropic drugs can cause higher blood levels in certain individuals by virtue of race (such as Asians). It is essential to modify the dosage of these drugs based not only on body surface area and weight, but also on racial consideration.

Lawson (1986) noted that Third-World clients are routinely given smaller doses of neuroleptics because some racial groups metabolize drugs more slowly and therefore experience a greater drug effect. For neuroleptic medications, these same variations by race are found in the United States. In a prospective study of tardive dyskinesia, Glazer, Morgenstern, and Doucette (1993) found that among psychiatric outpatients treated with neuroleptic medications, race was a probable factor for this iatrogenic movement disorder. The data indicated that non-White clients, 97% of whom were African American, were about twice as likely to develop tardive dyskinesia as their White counterparts. To ensure the accuracy of the results, the researchers controlled for other demographic and clinical risk factors.

In a follow-up study, Glazer, Morgenstern, and Doucette (1994) found that, compared with Whites, non-Whites were more likely to be younger, less skilled, unmarried, and more likely to have a diagnosis of schizophrenia. Non-Whites were also more likely to receive higher doses of neuroleptics principally because they were frequently given more high-potency depot medications. Despite the control for known tardive dyskinesia factors, the estimated rate of tardive dyskinesia was nearly twice as high for non-Whites as that for Whites. According to Glazer, Morgenstern, and Doucette (1994), none of the other demographic, clinical, psychosocial, or general health variables measured in the study appeared to explain the association between race and the propensity for tardive dyskinesia. Despite these findings, the correlation between race as a biological marker for tardive dyskinesia remains unclear (Glazer, Morgenstern, and Doucette, 1994). Habits such as drinking and smoking are known to speed drug metabolism, and thus the fact that some White and Blacks drink significantly more alcohol than some Asians is an important consideration.

Lefley (1990) contends that Black clients are significantly misdiagnosed as psychotic. Because they are viewed as more violent, they receive more medication and spend more time in seclusion than Whites, Hispanics, or Asians (Lefley, 1990). The higher dose of medication prescribed for Blacks may result more from staff perception than a decision based on serum levels and careful observation (Keltner and Folks, 1992).

Some Native Canadian, Pakistani, and Sri Lankan Tamil women have reported a high degree of side effects from the use of contraceptives. Some researchers have suggested that although these women report numerous of problems they may not recognize depression, weight gain, amenorrhea, and dysmeno-rhea as side effects (Guruge and Donner, 1996). Consequently it is imperative that the nurse recognize the need for a thorough explanation of possible side effects and that appropriate action be taken. In many cultures, issues of sexuality, including birth control, are not openly discussed among immigrant women; therefore it is essential that the health care practitioner provide information about birth control (Guruge and Donner, 1996).

Tobacco use differs significantly across racial and ethnic groups. A causal relationship has been firmly established between tobacco use and a number of fatal diseases (Edwards and MacMillan, 1990). It is estimated that each year tobacco kills more than 30,000 Canadians 35 to 84 years of age (Health and Welfare Canada, 1987). In Canada, a 1987 survey of students in the Northwest Territories who smoked noted exceedingly high rates among Inuit and Indian youths. By age 19, 71% of Inuit and 63% of Indians, compared with only 43% of the nonindigenous population, were current smokers (Miller, 1990).

Gender is another cultural consideration that may have profound influence on the metabolism of drugs. Yonkers, Kando, Cole, and Blumenthal (1992) suggest that women have the potential for higher blood plasma levels of psychotropic drugs, especially when used with oral contraceptives. In addition, they note that women have greater efficacy of antipsychotic agents and a greater likelihood of adverse reactions such as hypothyroidism and, in older women, tardive dyskinesia. Although plausible explanations for these differences have been offered, women have traditionally been excluded from clinical trials measuring the efficacy and metabolism of certain drugs.

Electrocardiographic Patterns

A common finding in Blacks, particularly in Black men, is the occurrence of inverted T waves in the precordial leads of the electrocardiogram. This aberration is considered to be a normal variant in the Black population but could indicate a pathological condition if found in other racial groups, such as Whites.

Susceptibility to Disease

Another category of differences between racial groups is susceptibility to disease. The increased or decreased incidence of a particular disease may be genetically determined.

Tuberculosis In the United States, the number of reported cases of tuberculosis (TB) among certain racial groups has changed dramatically over the last several years. For example, in 1988, the incidence of tuberculosis was seven times higher among African Americans than among non-Hispanic Whites, nine times higher among Asian and Pacific Islanders, and four times higher among Native Americans and Hispanics (Centers for Disease Control, 1989a). Ethnic minorities now account for more than two thirds of all the reported cases of tuberculosis in the United States, partly as a result of the increased incidence of tuberculosis among ethnic minorities affected with the HIV (Centers for Disease Control, 1991). It is also interesting to note that, of the cases of tuberculosis reported for children, ethnic minorities account for nearly 83% of the number of cases (Healthy People 2000, 1990).

Historically, in Canadian schools of nursing at the close of the 1800s, the general assumption was that at least 1 student nurse from every class would die from tuberculosis (Zilm and Warbinek, 1994). By the turn of the century, tuberculosis was Canada's leading cause of death. The mortality in 1900 was established at about 200 per 100,000 (Wherrett, 1977). The rate of TB in Canada in 1994 was 7.1 cases per 100,000 people (Statistics Canada, 1996). However, in the Northwest Territories, the number of cases jumped from 35 in 1993 to 65 in 1994. In 1994, immigrants accounted for more than half of the Canadian TB cases. Aboriginal people, including Indians, Métis, and Inuit, account for nearly 20% of the cases. However, because of the many cases of TB that are related to HIV, the World Health Organization has declared this virulent strain of TB a global emergency and predicts it will kill 30 million people over the next 10 years (Editorial, 1996). Many persons with HIV infection have organisms that are resistant to most of the chemotherapeutic agents used to treat this type of tuberculosis. When a person has drug-resistant tuberculosis, he or she may pass the resistant organisms to others. In such cases, effective treatment of this type of tuberculosis becomes nearly impossible (Phipps, 1993).

It is important to remember that susceptibility to disease may also be environmental or a combination of both genetic and environmental factors. The evidence indicates that tuberculosis can occur in response to both socioenvironmental and psychological stress factors. In a classic study of clients in Seattle, Holmes et al. (1957) found that environmental factors appeared to be relevant in relation to the onset of tuberculosis. In this classic study, data in the life experiences of each client were plotted for a 12-year period preceding hospitalization. Analysis of the data revealed that in the majority of clients there was a gradual increase in experiences that were perceived by the individual as significant and stressful. The combination of stressful life experiences and personal perception resulted in a psychological crisis situation that was evidenced in the 2-year period preceding hospitalization. Further analysis of the data done by Holmes et al. suggested that clients who are poorly equipped to deal with social relationships, especially when a lot of tension is present, may be at risk for tuberculosis.

Blood groups, Rh factor, and disease Blood groups also differentiate people in certain racial groups. A prevalence for type O blood has been found among Canadian Indians and Native Americans, with some incidence of type A blood and virtually no incidence of type B blood. Almost equal incidences of types A, B, and O blood are found in Japanese and Chinese people, with the AB blood type found in only about 10% of the Japanese and Chinese population. Blacks and Whites have been found to have equal incidences of A, B, and O blood types. The predominant blood types of Blacks and Whites are A and O, with fewer incidences of AB and B types.

Statistically, persons with type O blood are at a greater risk for duodenal ulcers, whereas persons with type A blood are more likely to develop cancer of the stomach. In addition, there is some evidence that women with type O blood have a diminished chance of getting thromboembolic disease, particularly when taking birth control pills, than women with other ABO blood types (Jick, Slone, Westerholm, et al., 1969).

The Rh-negative factor in blood is most common in Whites, much rarer in other racial groups, and apparently absent in Inuits (Lewis, 1942). Because there are at least 27 different antigens in the Rh system, this system is complex and difficult to understand. Of clinical significance is the D antigen because it is more immunogenic than any other Rh antigen and is usually the antigen involved in hemolytic disease of the newborn. When antigen D is present, the term "Rh-positive" is used. Approximately 85% of persons in the world have Rh-positive blood. The term "Rh-negative" is used when antigen D is absent. Persons with the Rh-negative factor who are exposed to Rh-positive blood form Rh antibodies. After continued exposure to Rh-positive blood, the Rh antibody will bind to corresponding antigens on the surface of red blood cells, which contain the Rh antigen. Ordinarily Rh antibodies do not fix complement. As a result, there is no immediate hemolysis, as occurs with ABO incompatibility. Rather, Rh-antigen red blood cells are broken down rapidly by macrophages in the spleen, resulting in a conversion of hemoglobin to bilirubin, which causes jaundice. Thus the multigravida woman with the Rh-negative factor who has an Rh-positive mate and has either delivered or aborted an Rh-positive infant will be more likely to have babies who are susceptible to jaundice. This condition can be prevented in subsequent pregnancies if the Rh-negative woman is given RhoGAM immediately after aborting or delivering an Rh-positive infant.

Diabetes Other conditions that appear to have biocultural or racial prevalence include diabetes mellitus, hypertension, sickle cell anemia, and systemic lupus erythematosus (SLE). Reportedly there is a high incidence of diabetes mellitus in certain American Indian tribes, including the Seminole, Pima, Papago, Sioux, and Northern Utes (Jacobson, 1994).

It is important to note that the prevalence of diabetes varies according to race and gender. The prevalence of diabetes increases with age and at all ages is highest among African-American women. In 1988, in the United States, the prevalence rate of diabetes for Black women (50.9 per 1000) was twice as high compared with their White counterparts (23.4 per 1000) (Horton, 1992).

There are three types of diabetes: insulin-dependent diabetes mellitus (IDDM), non-insulin dependent diabetes mellitus (NIDDM), and gestational diabetes mellitus (GDM). IDDM has a peak incidence between 10 and 14 years of age, apparently affects boys at a somewhat higher frequency than girls, has a higher incidence in Whites, and accounts for 10% to 20% of cases (Krolewski and Warram, 1994). NIDDM dramatically increases with age, has a higher frequency in women, has a higher incidence in non-White persons (particularly Hispanics and Native Americans), and accounts for 80% to 90% of cases (Carter Center of Emory University, 1985). GDM has been reported in 20% of all pregnant women and increases with maternal age but is not affected by race or culture (Rifkin, 1984).

In the United States, diabetes mellitus is a major health problem affecting some 3% of the total population (American Diabetic Association, 1991). However, in Canada, diabetes mellitus occurs to a lesser degree. Diabetes accounts for 1.3% of the deaths among United States males 25 to 44 years of age and 1.9% of the deaths among females in the same age group. In contrast, in Canada, in this same age group (25 to 44), diabetes mellitus accounts for only 0.7% of deaths for males and 1.3% for females. In the United States, diabetes accounts for 2.1% of the deaths among males 45 to 64 years of age and 3.3% of the females in the same age group. Again in stark contrast, in Canada, diabetes mellitus accounts for only 0.8% of the deaths for males and 1.9% of the deaths for females. Interestingly enough, in the age category 65 years and over, diabetes mellitus accounts for 1.9% of the deaths for males and 2.6% of the deaths for females in both the United States and Canada (International Health Statistics, 1993).

Daniel and Gamber (1995) noted that the high prevalence of NIDDM in Canada's Native communities corresponds with high diabetes prevalence in other populations of indigenous people who have undergone changes associated with acculturation.

Because indigenous people of the Americas, South Pacific, New Zealand, and Australia have similar histories, it is postulated that the similarities in the incidence of diabetes may be expected (Zimmet, Dowse, Finch, Serjeantson, and King, 1990; Prior and Tasman-Jones, 1981; West, 1974). Daniel and Gamble (1995) also note that behavioral risk factors can be particularly amenable to public health and actions that will reduce risk or onset by early detection and treatment. Among some researchers, there is general agreement that NIDDM has a genetic basis or component (Knowler, Williams, Pettitt, and Steinberg, (1988). This predisposition to diabetes may to some extent explain the disproportionately high incidence of diabetes found among American Indians, an incidence that has dramatically increased over the last several decades (Knowler, Pettitt, Saad, and Bennett, 1990). Similar increases in the frequency of diabetes over time also appear to have occurred in other populations characterized by major socioeconomic changes and increasingly obesity (Zimmet et al., 1990). Data over time indicate that the majority of Native Canadians have developed their disease relatively recently, indicating an increase in the incidence of diabetes in Canada's Native communities (Young, McIntyre, Dooley, and Rodriguez, 1985; Montour, Macaulay, and Adelson, 1989).

Data from the 1978 Canada Health Survey indicated that the prevalence of self-reported diabetes in the Canadian population was about 1.7%. According to the 1985 General Social Survey, the prevalence of diabetes among Canadians has significantly increased to about 2.4%. The age-adjusted prevalences for the Native population in most regions was two to three times the overall general population rate, except in British Columbia, Yukon, and the Northwest Territories (Young, 1988, 1989). Within geographical areas, which reflect aboriginal lifestyles, the lowest rate is in the Arctic area (represented exclusively by the Inuit) and the highest rate is in the Northeast regional area (the St. Lawrence-Great Lakes basin). However, among the Algonquians, who belong to the three geographical areas (subarctic, plains, and the Northeast), no significant difference was found in the prevalences, an indication that geographical

area may not be of primary importance (Young, 1988, 1989). Hagey (1984) described how the Ojibwa story of Nanabush, a legendary teacher, serves as an exemplary model for explaining cultural balance. This story was used to explain the origin and nature of diabetes and to identify appropriate coping strategies while preserving the right of each individual to choose a unique path (Health and Welfare Canada, 1991). MacDonald, Shah, and Campbell (1990) used Hagey's recommendations to develop a cross-cultural program to improve self-care among several tribes in southern Alberta.

Hypertension The incidence of hypertension has been reported to be significantly higher in Blacks than in White Americans. The onset by age is earlier in African Americans, and hypertension is more severe and associated with a higher mortality in African Americans than in White Americans. Studies that demonstrated obvious differences in blood pressure between African Americans and their White counterparts date back to 1932 (Adams, 1932). Since that time other studies have also clearly indicated that there is a remarkable difference in blood pressure levels between African Americans and individuals of other races (Lerner and Kannel, 1986; Stokes, Kannel, Wolf, Cupples, and D'Agostino, 1987).

For a number of years, it has been postulated that 35% of Blacks more than 40 years of age are hypertensive (Tipton, 1974). In a study with a random sample of adults 18 to 79 years of age, 9% of non-Blacks and 22% of Blacks were found to be hypertensive according to standards set by the World Health Organization, wherein hypertension is indicated when a diastolic blood pressure of 95 mm Hg or greater is evidenced (Boyle, 1970). In another study done by the Chicago Health Association, the analysis of the data confirmed previous findings of a higher prevalence for hypertension among Blacks in all age groups than for Whites. Further analysis of the data suggested an equal prevalence of hypertension among both sexes in the Black race and an increased incidence with advancing age (Merck, Sharp, and Dohme, 1974). However, contrasting opinions indicate that hypertension occurs slightly more often in men than in women (Joint National Committee, 1993).

Data from the 30-year follow-up study to the classic Framingham study conducted in the United States indicate that hypertension is an independent risk factor for coronary heart disease for both men and women between 35 and 64 years of age (Stokes, Kannel, Wolf, Cupples, and D'Agostino, 1987).

Other data indicate that the prevalence of hypertension is highest among Black-American, non-Hispanic women (National Center for Health Statistics, 1991). In the Maryland Statewide Household Survey of 6425 adults 18 years of age and older, 28.2% of the Black population showed a prevalence of mild to moderate hypertension (a systolic blood pressure greater than 160 mm Hg and a diastolic blood pressure greater than 95 mm Hg) compared with 20.1% of their White counterparts (Saunders, 1985; State of Maryland Demonstration, 1977-1983).

Since the traditional terms "mild hypertension" and "moderate hypertension" failed to convey the major effect of high blood pressure as a risk factor for cardiovascular disease (CVD) in the United States, the Joint National Committee on Detection, Evaluation, and Treatment of High Blood Pressure (1993) has attempted to clarify terminology. According to the committee report, 50 million Americans have elevated blood pressure, which by current definition implies a systolic blood pressure 140 mm Hg or greater or a diastolic blood pressure 90 mm Hg or greater, or both (Joint National Committee, 1993). The committee concluded that the prevalence of hypertension increases with age, is greater in African Americans than in Whites, is greater in both races in less educated individuals than in more educated individuals, and is especially prevalent and devastating in lower socioeconomic groups (Joint National Committee, 1993). In addition, the data indicate that in young adulthood and early middle age, high blood pressure prevalence is greater in men than in women. However, after middle age the reverse is true (Joint National Committee, 1993)

The prevalence for hypertension is also greater by geographical region. For example, both Blacks and Whites residing in the southeastern United States have a greater propensity for hypertension and a greater stroke death rate as a direct result of the condition than Blacks and Whites residing in other areas of the country (Roccella and Lenfant, 1993). The new classifications for hypertension as proposed by the Joint Committee on Detection, Evaluation, and Treatment of Hypertension (1993) are as follows:

Category	Systolic (mm Hg)	Diastolic (mm Hg)
Normal	<130	<85
High normal	130-139	85-89

Hypertension (based on the average of two or more readings)

Stage 1 (Mild)	140-159	90-99
Stage 2 (Moderate)	160-179	100-109
Stage 3 (Severe)	180-209	110-119
Stage 4 (Very severe)	>210	>120

As indicated previously, a diagnosis of hypertension is confirmed when there is a consistent systolic blood pressure level of 140 torrs or above and a consistent diastolic blood pressure level of 90 torrs or above (based on the average of two or more readings). Reportedly, as a result of this definition, hypertension is of concern for approximately 50 to 60 million Americans (Joint National Committee, 1993; Walsh, 1993). It is essential to remember that hypertension should never be diagnosed on the basis of a single measurement except when the systolic blood pressure is 210 mm Hg or greater or the diastolic blood pressure is 120 mm Hg, with average levels of diastolic blood pressure of 90 mm Hg or greater and systolic blood pressure levels of 140 mm Hg or greater (Joint National Committee, 1993).

Many individuals who are hypertensive remain symptom free for a long time; thus researchers at the National Heart, Lung, and Blood Institute have estimated that more than 50% of persons with hypertension do not know that they are hypertensive. Hypertension continues to be the major cause of heart failure, kidney failure, aneurysm formation, and congestive heart failure. Primary hypertension is evidenced in 90% of reported cases, whereas only about 10% of reported cases are classified as secondary.

The diagnosis for primary hypertension may be supported when the following risk factors are present:

1. Positive family history
2. Increased sensitivity to the renin-angiotensin system
3. Obesity
4. Hypercholesterolemia
5. Hyperglycemia
6. Smoking
7. Abnormal sodium and water retention

The diagnosis for secondary hypertension is made when the following causes are present (Walsh, 1993):

1. Coarctation of the aorta
2. Pheochromocytoma (a catecholamine-secreting tumor)
3. Cushing's disease
4. Chronic glomerulonephritis
5. Toxemia from pregnancy
6. Thyrotoxicosis
7. Effects of certain drugs such as contraceptives
8. Collagen disease

Primary hypertension affects more Black Americans than White Americans. Researchers at the National Health Examination Survey indicated that in persons 24 to 34 years old, 3.6% of non-Black men and 12.5% of Black men have primary hypertension, as well as 2.3% of non-Black women and 8.6% of Black women. According to this study, these figures appear to rise steadily with age and are at all age levels conspicuously higher in Blacks. Thus the overall ratio of African Americans to non-Blacks for incidence of primary hypertension is estimated to be 2:1. In addition, primary hypertension is believed to be more severe for Blacks regardless of age level. The death rate for primary hypertension at all age levels up to 85 years of age is higher in Blacks than in non-Blacks. It was reported that men between 24 and 44 years of age have a mortality from primary hypertension of 14.8% for Blacks and 1% for non-Blacks. In this same age group female mortality from primary hypertension was reported to be 12.3% for Blacks and 0.8% for non-Blacks (Merck, Sharp, and Dohme, 1974). These data indicate that Blacks succumb to primary hypertension almost 15 times more often than non-Blacks. Furthermore, the death

rate for hypertension is probably an underestimation. The nurse must be aware of significant risk factors for hypertension to assist in early detection and continued maintenance and treatment, which can aid in reducing the mortality.

There are data available to indicate that Black Americans have a higher propensity for hypertension (Centers for Disease Control, 1992b; Joint National Committee, 1993; Lerner and Kannel, 1986; National Center for Health Statistics, 1991; Stokes, Kannel, Wolf, Cupples, and D'Agostino, 1987). It remains controversial as to whether there are genetic markers such as skin color that can be related to hypertension prevalence among Black Americans and other persons with dark skin color (Braithwaite and Taylor, 1992; Centers for Disease Control, 1993). However, in a classic study of African Americans residing in Charleston, South Carolina, it was noted that these subjects showed significant association between blood pressure and skin darkness among both men and women (Boyle, 1970). The effect for this study was independent of age but was minimized by consideration of socioeconomic status.

A later but totally different study was done with Black Americans as the population from the same geographical location. Contrary to the earlier study, the data indicated that skin color was not significantly associated with a 15-year incidence of hypertension noted in African-American women over 35 years of age in this geographical location (Keil, 1981). In this study, skin color was measured by a photoelectric reflection meter on the medial aspect of the upper arm. In addition, the effect for the study was independent of socioeconomic status. Both these studies differ remarkably from a study reported by Braithwaite and Taylor (1992) that was conducted in Detroit on Black men. According to Braithwaite and Taylor (1992), the data from this study indicate that there is a significant relationship between high blood pressure and skin color as measured by subjective coding of skin color of the forehead, between the eyes.

In a recent study, Klag, Whelton, Coresh, Grim, and Kuller (1992) found that there was an association between skin color and higher systolic and diastolic blood pressures in darker-skinned persons. In the study, 457 African Americans were surveyed in three United States cities with use of a reflectometer to measure the intensity of skin color and the correlation with blood pressure. The findings from the study indicate that both systolic and diastolic blood pressures were higher in darker persons and increased by 2 mm Hg for every 1-standard-deviation increase in skin darkness. However, the data indicated that the association was dependent on socioeconomic status, whether measured by education or on another index consisting of education, occupation, and ethnicity. Significant findings were present only in persons on the lower level of either index (Klag et al., 1992). Using multiple linear regression, the researchers found that both systolic and diastolic blood pressures remained significantly associated with darker skin in the lower socioeconomic status, independent of age-body mass index, and concentration of blood glucose. The researchers concluded that the findings may be attributed to two factors:

1. The inability of such groups to deal with psychosocial stress associated with darker skin, or
2. The findings may be consistent with an interaction between the environmental factors associated with low socioeconomic status and a susceptible gene that has a higher prevalence in persons with darker skin (Klag et al., 1992).

Regardless of the race of the client, to obtain blood pressure measurements with values that are representative of the client's usual levels, it is important that the individual be seated with the arm bared, supported, and at heart level. The client should not have smoked or ingested caffeine within 30 minutes before the measurement is taken (Joint National Committee, 1993). If the measurement must be repeated, it should not be taken for at least 5 minutes after the first reading. To ensure an accurate measurement, the appropriate cuff size must be used. In addition, it is also essential that the bladder of the cuff should nearly (or at least 80%) or completely encircle the arm (Joint National Committee, 1993).

Sickle cell anemia The most common genetic disorder in the United States is sickle cell anemia, which occurs predominantly in Black Americans. It has been projected that 50,000 Black Americans have sickle cell anemia (Wyngaarden and Smith, 1996). Sickle cell anemia or the asymptomatic trait also occurs in people from Asia Minor, India, the Mediterranean, and the Caribbean area but to a lesser extent than has been reported in Black Americans. Sickle cell anemia is characterized by chronic hemolytic anemia and is a homozygous recessive disorder. In sickle cell anemia the basic disorder lies within the globin moiety of the hemoglobin (Hb), where a single amino acid (valine) is substituted for another (glutamic acid) in the sixth position of the beta chain. It is believed that this single amino acid substitution profoundly alters the properties of the Hb molecule; Hb S is formed instead of normal Hb A as a result of the intermolecular rearrangement. The normal oxygen-carrying capacity of the blood is found in Hb A. As a result of deoxygenation, however, there is a change in solubility of the protein, which causes the Hb molecules to lump together, causing the cell membrane to contract, with the resultant sickle cell shape.

The affected cells have a shortened life span of 7 to 20 days, which is profoundly different from the life span of normal cells, which is 105 to 120 days. Hb SA is the heterozygous state and is often an asymptomatic condition referred to as sickle cell trait.

Sickle cell anemia is believed to have occurred for many years in Africa along the Nile River valley as an adaptive disease. In Africa this disorder was believed to produce resistance from malaria transmission by the *Anopheles* mosquito (Williams, 1975). In Africa, sickle cell anemia or the asymptomatic trait affects approximately 10% of the Black population, and the death rate before 21 years of age has been 100% in those affected with the disease. Before full recognition of the clinical significance of sickle cell anemia in the United States, the death rate was almost of the same magnitude as that in Africa. Today in the United States, as a result of improved and comprehensive care and early recognition of the crisis of the disease, persons with sickle cell anemia may live through their third and fourth decades of life.

A differential diagnosis for sickle cell anemia should be made for all Black persons who (1) have chronic anemia of undetermined origin, (2) demonstrate an increased susceptibility to infections, or (3) have unexplained attacks of joint, bone, or abdominal pain. Making the diagnosis of sickle cell anemia is done in the laboratory through a technique called "hemoglobin electrophoresis." Hemoglobin electrophoresis provides a definitive diagnosis. In addition to hemoglobin electrophoresis, a complete history including a physical examination and laboratory data base should be done. The laboratory data base should include a complete blood cell count (CBC) with a differential and reticulocyte count, electrolytes, blood urea nitrogen (BUN), glucose, direct bilirubin, and urinalysis (Satcher and Pope, 1974). In addition, radiographs of the chest, abdomen, and bones are indicated if there is evidence of pain or fever. However, a bone scan is preferable.

For persons with sickle cell anemia the indications for prompt admission to a hospital include the following (Leffall, 1974):

1. Vaso-occlusive pain crisis that does not respond to analgesics within 4 hours of administration.
2. Aplastic crisis.
3. Splenic sequestration, a life-threatening condition that requires immediate admission to the intensive care unit for continuous observation and therapy.
4. Hyperhemolytic crisis, which can occur if the hemoglobin and hematocrit levels continue to drop.
5. Infections indicated by a temperature greater than 101° F or a white blood cell count greater than 15,000/mm. (However, viral, ear, nose, and throat infections may not indicate admission for pediatric clients.)
6. Thromboembolic phenomena in the lungs, cerebrum, and long bones.
7. Pregnancy, which indicates an increased risk.

A common problem associated with sickle cell anemia is drug use and abuse. At the Martin Luther King, Jr., Hospital, a team of health professionals working through the National Sickle Cell Center was involved in the care of clients with sickle cell anemia.

Their work revealed three kinds of problems (Satcher et al., 1973):

1. Clients with sickle cell anemia were typically stereotyped as drug abusers by many health professionals.
2. The delay in seeking medical care during a sickle cell crisis was attributable to the client's desire to tolerate pain and avoid drug dependence.
3. Drug abuse in clients with sickle cell anemia was found in those clients with severe and disabling conditions. These clients required drugs so frequently that they often became mentally and physically dependent.

The nurse must be able to identify early signs of sickle cell crisis and teach the client to recognize these symptoms when they occur. The nurse should impress on the client the significance of early recognition and treatment of crisis symptoms. Ongoing surveillance of signs and symptoms of sickle cell crisis can promote appropriate treatment and perhaps early death (Platt et al., 1994).

Systemic lupus erythematosus Systemic lupus erythematosus (SLE) is a chronic disease of unknown cause that affects organs and systems individually or in a variety of combinations. The disease affects women eight to ten times more often than it does men. The age distribution for the disease spans from 2 to 97 years. SLE was named after the classic butterfly rash, which is erosive and thus "likened to the damage caused by a hungry wolf" (Schumacher, 1993). This disease was once believed to be relatively rare and always fatal. However, with the advent of better techniques for recognition, the disease has come to be thought of as fairly common, and its course can be controlled by corticosteroids. Even today, however, some clients do die as a result of lesions that affect major organs or as a result of secondary infections. Although the etiology for the disease is still unknown, three major causative factors are being investigated. The first factor is an aberration of the immune system that causes immune complexes containing antibodies to be deposited in tissue, which in turn causes tissue damage. The second factor is a viral infection that is caused by or results from some immunological abnormality. The third factor is the combination of the above factors to produce the disease. In addition, some drugs are known to induce lupuslike syndromes, including procainamide (Pronestyl), isonicotinic acid hydrazide (INH, isoniazid), and penicillin (Schumacher, 1993).

As previously indicated, SLE was believed to be a very rare disease. However, because of sophisticated detection procedures, researchers now postulate that this is not so—its incidence has been estimated to be 2.6 per 100,000 population. Although it occurs more frequently in Blacks than in non-Blacks, it is reported to be extremely rare among the Asian population.

The nurse who understands that signs and symptoms of arthritis may be indicative of SLE, especially when combined with weakness, fatigue, and weight loss, can assist in early detection. In addition, the nurse should look for symptoms of sensitivity to sunlight, including development of a rash or symptoms of fever or arthritis as a result of exposure to sunlight. The butterfly lesions of SLE generally appear over the cheeks and bridge of the nose. These lesions are often bright red and may extend beyond the hairline, thus causing alopecia (loss of hair), particularly above the ears. Lesions may also be noted on the neck and may spread slowly to the mucous membranes and other tissues of the body. These lesions generally do not ulcerate; however, they do cause degeneration and atrophy of tissues. Other clinical findings may also be present, depending on the organs involved, including glomerulonephritis, pleuritis, pericarditis, peritonitis, neuritis, and anemia. The most severe manifestations of SLE are renal and neurological in nature.

Laboratory tests used to diagnose SLE may need to be specific to the organs involved, such as proteinuria, abnormal cerebrospinal fluid, or radiographic evidence of pleural reactions. Before the advent of the LE-cell preparation, or what is commonly referred to as the "LE-cell test," the diagnosis was made by the presentation of the butterfly rash and systemic complications, and the prognosis for the client was generally fatal. However, as a result of the LE-cell test and other sensitive tests, including the antinuclear antibody (ANA) or the antinuclear factor (ANF) test, clients with more varied symptoms have been confirmed earlier. Thus through early detection appropriate treatment has been initiated. Client teaching by the nurse should include instructions on the need for appropriate exercise, appropriate balance of rest and activity, and the necessity of avoiding direct exposure to sunlight. As indicated earlier, SLE is a disease with prevalence among some racial groups, and the nurse who recognizes the biocultural significance of the disease is more apt to give culturally appropriate nursing care.

AIDS AIDS data are available from all industrialized and developed countries through various disease-surveillance programs. As of mid-1993, cumulative rates of the incidence of AIDS were substantially higher in the United States (1267.8 per million) compared to Canada (309.5 per million). Although Canada's rate is only one fourth that of the United States, it is dramatically higher than that of Japan, which is 4.4 per million. AIDS cases in the United States through mid-1993 were 315,390 compared with 8232 in Canada (Health and Welfare Canada, 1993). In Canada, AIDS-related deaths are at a significantly lower level than in the United States. In 1989, although AIDS-related deaths were the second leading cause of deaths for males 25 years to 44 years of age and older (14.7), in Canada AIDS-related deaths accounted for only 8.3% of the deaths in this same population. In the United States, for women in this same age group, AIDS or AIDS-related deaths were the sixth leading cause of deaths (5.6%). In stark contrast, in Canada, AIDS or AIDS-related deaths accounted for only 0.8% of all deaths in women. Likewise, in the United States, for men 45 to 64 years of age, AIDS or AIDS-related deaths were the ninth leading cause of death (1.8%) for men but caused only 0.8% of the deaths for women (U.S. Congress, Office of Technology and Assessment, 1993).

In Canada there has generally been more state support for community responses than in the United States (Altman, 1994). In addition, federal and provincial governments are major players in the AIDS field in terms of providing direct health and social services and in supporting community-based organizations (Rayside and Linquist, 1992). In addition there are local incentives and provincial incentives across Canada for AIDS community action, treatment, care, and support (Cain, 1995).

Health and Welfare Canada (1991) reported that a national strategy on aboriginal AIDS education and prevention was almost complete. A study reported in *AIDS in Canada* (1990) noted that as of January 29, 1990, of the number of reported cases of AIDS, 3469 were Indians with half of the reported cases in Quebec, 5 in Ontario, 3 in British Columbia, 1 in Alberta, and 2 from the reminder of the country. In Canada, homosexual or bisexual activity is reported to be the paramount risk factor with 79.6% of all AIDS cases being directly related to such activity. In Canadian Indians, homosexual or bisexual activity is reported to be the paramount risk factor in only 68.2% of the cases. With regard to overall knowledge of AIDS, Native youth were found to be slightly less knowledgeable than non-Native young people in Canada but more Native youth than non-Native youth felt they needed more information about AIDS (Radford, 1989).

Nutritional Preferences and Deficiencies

Another category of differences among cultural groups is nutritional preferences and deficiencies. Although Canadian food at one time was strongly influenced by the British "bland is beautiful" tradition, today, Canada's wide ethnic diversity of immigrants has resulted in Canadian cuisine that ranks among the best in the world for its quality and variety (Fodor's staff, 1988; Bailey and Bailey, 1995; Lightbody and Smallman, 1994). Canadians pay less for their food than any other country in the world except the United States. They also eat out at least one third of the time, and such a pattern contributes to the wide range of dining-out experiences available. Canadian chefs consistently win top awards at international competitions.

Nutritional preferences Nutritional preferences include habits and patterns. When it comes to food choices, people are creatures of habit (Zifferblatt, Wilbur, and Pinsky, 1980). The term "habit" connotes inflexibility, though people do change their habits for many reasons. The term "food patterns" is more descriptive of food choices. Many factors are associated with the formation of food patterns and preferences. Food patterns are developed during childhood as a result of family lifestyle and ethnic or cultural, social, religious, geographical, economic, and psychological components. All these variables influence an individual's attitudes, feelings, and beliefs about certain foods. Adults in a particular culture set the tone for cultural food patterns, which establish the foundation for a child's lifelong eating customs regarding the timing of meals, the number of meals per day, foods acceptable for specific meals, methods of preparation, dislikes and likes, and table manners. Over time, children develop a sense of stability and security in regard to certain food patterns and attitudes (Schwerin, Stanton, and Smith, 1982; Katz, Hediger, Valleroy, 1974; Pangborn, 1975; Riggs, 1980; Saldana and Brown, 1984). Food also has symbolic meaning, in some cultures, that has nothing to do with nutritional value. In these cultures eating becomes associated with sentiments and assumptions about oneself and the world (Chang, 1974; Farb and Armelagos, 1980). Food becomes symbolic to people not only because of religious connotations, but also because it can be used as a reward. For example, a mother who gives a child candy or ice cream as a reward for good behavior may be reinforcing that food as a good food. On the other hand, a mother who serves a particular food (such as broccoli or cabbage) and says she is doing so because of bad behavior may be reinforcing that food as a bad food or as punishment.

When people relocate, they carry established food habits to the new location, but these habits are retained only if the foods are available in the new location and are affordable. Although Greek, Italian, East Indian, Chinese, and other ethnic specialty restaurants can be found in most Canadian cities, many Canadians today are eating foods produced only in Canada and choose foods found in the region or province where they reside (Lightbody and Smallman, 1994). Thus, although individuals follow the food traditions related to their culture of origin, adaptations of favorite recipes are frequently made to suit the local ingredients available. Canadians also enjoy locally produced chocolate bars, Caramilk and

Crispy Crunch, and a truly Canadian candy, the butter tart.

On the other hand, many Canadian Natives have changed their traditional food habits and patterns related to eating foods available in nature and choose instead to purchase commercially available food products because this food has become accessible in stores. For many Canadian Natives, commercially available food has resulted in a deterioration of healthy food habits. The traditional Native foods are based on wild game such as deer (venison) and pheasant and buffalo (bison) meat, which is lean and has more protein and less cholesterol than beef. Greens, edible only in the springtime, can be picked in the woodlands of the Maritime Provinces. Wild rice, with its black husks and almost nutty flavor, often accompanies the traditional Native meal.

British Columbia. Foods commonly available in British Columbia include fish and shellfish of many kinds. Salmon, crab, shrimp, black cod, and halibut are among the best. Lamb, from the marshes of Saltspring Island, is served with mint sauce, not mint jelly. Cheddar cheese is produced in Armstrong, whereas the Okanagan River valley has a wealth of produce including cherries, peaches, pears, apples, and vegetables.

The Prairies. World-famous grain-fed beef is produced in the Alberta foothills, which yields juicy thick steaks and chuckwagon stew. Honey is found in the Peace country. Bison are naturally available in this area. In Saskatchewan, a variety of grains, especially wheat, is produced, and whitefish, trout, and pickerel are found in the streams. Gamebirds such as partridge and prairie chicken are used in preparing tasty dishes. Saskatoon is known for pie with thick cream made from a berry that gave its name to the city. In Manitoba smoked Winnipeg goldeye, wild rice, and whitefish are available. Honey comes from the Dauphin area.

Ontario. This region is famous for freshwater fish including whitefish, lake trout, pike, and smelt from its many lakes. Fruits and vegetables are grown in the Niagara Peninsula. Macintosh applies are plentiful in their place of origin in eastern Ontario. Ontario is also known for cheddar cheese and corn,

which is served roasted or steamed, dripping in melted butter.

Quebec. Most of Canada's few semioriginal repasts come from the French of Quebec. Quebec is famous for maple sugar, which is served on hotcakes or ice cream, made into candy, as part of sugar pie, or made into taffy. Brome Lake duckling, oka (a cheese made from Trappist monks), and Ermite cheese are specialties of this region. Pork is essential to the rural French-Canadian meal and may be served spiced as *cretons* or in *tourtière* (a minced pork pie). French-Canadian pea soup is flavored with ham hock or salt pork. French fries (chips) in Quebec, where they are known simply as *frites,* or *patates,* can be bought at small roadside chip wagons (Lightbody and Smallman, 1994).

Maritimes. In New Brunswick, steamed fiddleheads (a large fern) with melted butter, salmon, oysters, lobster, and clam are readily available. Dulse (a dried seaweed snack), blueberries, strawberries, and rhubarb are commonly enjoyed. In Prince Edward Island, soused mackerel, Malpeque Bay oysters, and some of the finest potatoes in the world are available (Foder's staff, 1988). In Nova Scotia there are famous Digby scallops, tuna, and swordfish. Apples are famous in the Anapolis Valley. Mahone Bay is famous for steamed brown bread, Lueneburg sausage, and blueberry grunt. In Newfoundland specialty fish dishes are baked cod cheeks or cod tongue, or seal-flipper pie. Baked-apple berry pie is a dish rich in vitamin C.

The Arctic. In the Arctic char-broiled caribou steak is a unique delicacy with flavor. Wild berries include blueberries and soapberries.

Beers, Wines, and Whiskey Canadians have always made good beer (Bailey and Bailey, 1995). The range traditionally offered from Labatt and Molson has been extended by the products of microbreweries, which are developing all over Canada.

Wine making in Canada dates back to the 1600s when early Jesuit missionaries made their own sacramental wines. Today, wine is produced in seven provinces, but the two main centers are the Niagara Peninsula of Ontario and the Okanagan river valley of British Columbia. The wines produced in Canada have tended to be cheap and to have a poor reputation (Lightbody and Smallman, 1994). More recently, Canadian wineries are taking great care to produce higher-quality wine, with the best known wine coming from the Niagara district. Canada also has a wide range of imported wines. Alberta, with no domestic wine industry and therefore no tariff protection, has the lowest prices in the country on imported wines. Quebec shows a definite preference for imported French wines. Many wines unavailable in North America can be found in Quebec restaurants and liquor stores.

Canada produces its own gins, vodkas, rums, liqueurs, brandies, and coolers. Canadian rye whiskey is the best known with a legendary reputation. Canadian whiskey has been distilled since the mid 1800s and has been popular in the United States as well as Canada. Tax contributes to the high price of some spirits.

Nutritional deficiencies Racially related nutritional deficiencies include lactose intolerance and glucose-6-phosphate dehydrogenase (G-6-PD) deficiency. Lactose intolerance, or intolerance to milk, is a relatively common condition that is considered normal in many ethnic groups. It is found in over 66% of Mexican Americans and Orientals (Bayless, 1975; Burns and Neubort, 1984; Kisch, 1953). It has been reported to be found in approximately 100% of American and Canadian Indians and as many as 90% of Blacks, Mediterraneans, Asians, and Jews (Gerchufsky, 1966). Although lactose intolerance is very common among these racial groups, it is reported to be much less common among Whites of northern European descent, with only 5% to 15% of this population having the disorder. Yet the statistical significance reported among Whites of northern European descent indicates that this condition is more than a rare phenomenon.

The cause of lactose intolerance is an insufficient amount of lactase, the enzyme responsible for converting the nonabsorbable milk sugar lactose into the absorbable sugars glucose and galactose. With lactase deficiency, any undigested lactose will remain in the small intestine, where, because of its osmotic capacity, it draws water. When the lactose reaches the colon, it begins to combine acetic acid and hydrogen gas, which results in the symptoms of lactose intol-

erance: cramping, flatulence, abdominal bloating, and diarrhea. These symptoms are dose related, meaning that they occur only if the person ingests more food containing lactose than the person's supply of available lactase can metabolize. Foods containing large amounts of lactose include milk, yogurt, and milk chocolate. Of these food items, nonfat dry milk contains the most lactose. Foods containing moderate amounts of lactose include cream, cottage cheese, and most cheeses. Even unlikely foods such as dried soup, cookies made from prepared mixes, cold cuts, and bread and butter contain small amounts of lactose (When Patients, 1976).

The nurse must be cognizant of foods that can cause lactose-intolerance symptoms, particularly when working with persons who are extremely lactose intolerant. For the majority of clients, treatment of this condition is usually a matter of restricting lactose-containing foods rather than eliminating them altogether. An adult who is advised to restrict milk and milk products but otherwise eats a well-balanced diet should not need any nutritional supplements. However, for pregnant or lactating women, nutritional supplements (such as calcium tablets) may be necessary. Lactose intolerance does not generally develop until after childhood; children who are lactose deficient should be encouraged to eat aged cheeses because the aging process changes lactase to lactic acid. In addition, some physicians may recommend a soybean-based milk substitute as well as vitamins and calcium supplements. Even for the adult lactose-deficient client, the astute nurse can suggest alternatives to milk products, such as cheese aged over 60 days. The nurse should be aware that telling the client to drink milk may not necessarily be good advice for many adults in the world and should give special consideration to the pregnant or lactating woman because most racial groups, except for Whites, cannot tolerate milk in adulthood (Bayless, 1975).

G-6-PD deficiency is another enzyme deficiency disorder that is more prevalent in certain racial or ethnic groups. Although it is more prevalent in certain groups, these groups may have different forms of the deficiency. Williams (1975) reported that the type A variety, which moves rapidly on starch-gel electrophoresis, is found in 35% of Blacks who have the deficiency. The slower-moving type B variety is found in 65% of Blacks who have the deficiency and in nearly all non-Blacks who have the deficiency. However, all forms affect males more than females because the genetic inheritance is carried on the X chromosome. The Canton/Chinese disorder of G-6-PD has been found among the Chinese and the people of Southeast Asia. The incidence of the Canton or Chinese form ranges from 2% to 5% (Williams, 1975). Still another form of G-6-PD deficiency is the Mediterranean variety, which is the most clinically severe type. This form of G-6-PD deficiency affects up to 50% of male Greeks, Sardinians, and Sephardic Jews.

G-6-PD is an enzyme constituent of the red blood cells and is involved in the hexose monophosphate pathway, which accounts for 10% of glucose metabolism of the red blood cells. Under normal circumstances the proportion of glucose metabolized through this pathway may increase greatly if the cells are subjected to oxidants causing metabolic stress. The result is the formation of increased methemoglobin and degradation of hemoglobin. In addition, certain medications tend to overwhelm the protective mechanism, especially when older red blood cells are involved, because of a decline in G-6-PD activity with the aging of these cells. Red blood cells with a genetically determined deficiency of G-6-PD are unable to withstand lesser oxidative stresses, and as a result, a hemolytic process ensues and precipitates a significant anemia.

In the presence of certain conditions, G-6-PD-deficient red blood cells hemolyze, resulting in hemolytic anemia. Conditions that precipitate hemolytic anemia in susceptible persons include the administration of certain drugs such as quinine, aspirin, phenacetin, chloramphenicol, probenecid, sulfonamides, and thiazide diuretics. The presence of infection and the ingestion of fava beans (also called broad beans, or horse beans) are also linked to the precipitous onset of hemolytic anemia. The fava bean is a dietary staple in some of the Mediterranean countries such as Greece and those of North Africa. Favism, a condition induced by ingesting the fava bean, is one of the most severe forms of G-6-PD

hemolysis. G-6-PD deficiency has also been related to an adaptive process that prevents malaria. The discerning nurse should assist the client in identifying substances that are likely to precipitate hemolytic episodes. In addition, the client should be taught to exercise caution to prevent serious infections. G-6-PD deficiency is a condition that remains asymptomatic until an exposure occurs. The nurse must understand that hemolytic episodes are the result of culturally related nutritional habits and geographical and environmental location.

Psychological Characteristics

Gaitz and Scott (1974) have indicated that although cultural factors may influence mental health scores in research studies, such scores are not indicative of whether one cultural group has more or fewer incidences of mental illness than another. There are many different definitions of mental health, one of which postulates that a person is mentally healthy when there is a balance in the person's internal life and adaptation to reality. Thus it can be determined that normal behavior is relative to a specific culture and that different psychological characteristics are promoted by each culture. Other variables that influence mental health include family relationships, childrearing practices, language, attitudes toward illness, and social and economic status.

Some cultural groups have a low socioeconomic status, which consequently affects mental health. For example, some Native Canadians have a low socioeconomic status in terms of substandard housing, education, physical health, political influence, communication, and social exclusion. The concept of social exclusion must be considered as a contributing factor in the failure of any particular cultural group to assimilate the culture of the wider society. Broad exposure to other lifestyles, cultures, environments, and ideas facilitates an understanding and flexibility on the part of an individual when dealing with other people or when solving problems. Feelings of insecurity may also be related to cultural background. For example, psychological adjustment may be difficult for a Native Canadian who has lived on a reservation and goes to a college where there are few other Native Canadians. The difficulty in adjustment may be attributable to the fact that this person has lived in an isolated environment in which there is a failure to become assimilated into the mainstream of society. Therefore health care providers must consider both ethnicity and economic factors when assessing mental health status.

Given the proliferation of new and growing ethnocultural communities in Canada, professionals who serve the mental health needs of Canadians must become increasingly prepared to modify program and treatment strategies to accommodate families from multicultural and diverse backgrounds (Short and Johnston, 1994). Sue has noted that, in general, mental health services are underutilized by ethnocultural group members (Sue, 1977). Researchers have cited several reasons for this phenomenon including, for example, language barriers (Beiser and Wood, 1986), fear of stigmatization (Sue and Morishima, 1982; Sue, Sue, and Sue, 1983), and a lack of culture-compatible programing (Flaskerud, 1986). Furthermore, among those ethnocultural group members who do seek treatment, there in a disproportionately high rate of attrition relative to "mainstream" program recipients (Sue, 1977; Sue and Morishima, 1982). Researchers have found that utilization is increased when services are made more culturally appropriate (Allodi and Fantini, 1985; Flaskerud, 1986). Powell (1988) noted that "goodness of fit" is important to create services that meet the special needs of Canadian families from ethnocultural communities. Teram and White (1993) noted that it is important to address bureaucratic disentitlement of clients from cultural minority groups. Additionally they also note that it is important to monitor newcomer-serving agencies to negotiate and monitor that adequate efforts are made to address the needs of culturally diverse communities.

There has been no consistent attack on problems of mental illness around the world. Although no continent or island area has been immune from mental illness, the study of mental illness in relation to culture has been restricted and often localized. There may have been a hesitancy to study cultures and mental illness because of possible implications of racism (Griffith and Griffith, 1986). Some authorities state that psychiatry has also not seriously

discussed the possibility that racism may be a manifestation of an individual psychological disorder (Poussaint, 1995). In any case, research on mental illness on a broad world perspective has been seriously lacking.

Although research, for the most part, is lacking, some interesting cultural data and implications are available in the studies that have been reported. Not only do mental illnesses seem to vary among cultures, but treatment does also. In Japan, psychiatric institutions are small; in the United States and Canada they are growing smaller. Societies also have differing demands on individuals emerging from the treatment milieu. Not only do hospitals and treatment milieus differ around the world, but also the paths into illness show a different pattern in each culture. Variations in class identity or in the pace of acculturation of class segments may produce differences in deviant types. Similarly, personalities seem to vary among persons from different geographical regions. There is some evidence that the cultural backgrounds and forms of illness vary apart from the question of how these illnesses are treated. For example, stresses placed on a traditional Chinese family are different from those placed on Hindus and Malays (Opler, 1959).

Lawson (1986) reported findings indicating that racial and ethnic differences exist in the clinical presentations of psychiatric disorders. Significant racial differences have been noted among proposed biological markers for various psychiatric disorders, such as serum creatinine phosphokinase, platelet serotonin, and HLA-A2 determinations. Racial and ethnic differences in response to psychotropic medication, such as higher blood levels of the drugs found among Asians, affect dosage requirements and potential side effects. All these developments underline the importance of considering ethnic and racial factors in caring for psychiatric clients.

The statistics on schizophrenia in Canada suggest that it is similar to that throughout the world with approximately 1 in 100 persons having schizophrenia (Morris, Clarke, and Bingham, 1989). Thus approximately 288,206 persons are afflicted (World Almanac, 1997). According to the 1994-1995 National Population Health Survey, close to 6% of Canadians

18 years of age and over had experienced a major depressive episode in the previous 12 months. Univariate analysis indicated that prevalence of depression was higher among women than among men but tended to decline at older ages in both sexes. For both sexes, chronic strain, recent negative events, lack of closeness, and low self-esteem increased the odds of depression. A substantial number of persons reported using drugs (Beaudet, 1996).

There are no empirical data available to indicate that Native people in Canada are more prone biologically to schizophrenia (Health and Welfare Canada, 1991). However, the working group suggested that among Canadian Natives, a high rate of depression seems to exist and it may be correlated with other symptomatic behaviors such as sexual abuse, suicide, and alcoholism. Suicide rates are higher among Natives than among Canadians in general (Health and Welfare Canada, 1991). Seasonal affective disorder (SAD) is a type of depression related to biological rhythms that is mediated by the hormone melatonin produced in the pineal gland (Lahaie, 1990). Typically SAD occurs at a rate in the southern regions of the United States of 6 per 100,000 but is disproportionately higher in the northern regions of Canada where it occurs at 100 per 100,000 (Wurtman and Wurtman, 1989). Thus, when these figures are applied to 28 million Canadians, the cases of SAD would number approximately 28,000. However, it is reasonable to assume that SAD is underdiagnosed. Phototherapy, which allows the biological clock to be reset, is an important intervention in the North where the summer is characterized by long days and the winter by long nights (Lahaie, 1990).

It is evident from the increasing quantities of literature on culture and mental health that there is a growing awareness among health professionals that care for clients with mental problems must be culturally appropriate and that cultural factors do affect mental health. Although rice and tea may not be the most potent tools of modern psychiatry, they may play an important role in making psychiatric care acceptable to the acutely disturbed Asian or South Pacific psychiatric client (Lu, 1987). It is important

for the nurse to study what is available about the population groups being served and to consider the important differences that may be required in the care provided. Not only must nurses appreciate that caring for clients from different cultural groups may require different care methods, but they must also assist other mental health workers in being sensitive to differing care needs.

Domestic Violence

Abuse in the family or living situation may be targeted at persons at any age, such as at elders, spouses, and, most frequently, helpless infants and children (Carlson, 1995; Fishman, 1995; Anonymous, 1995, Nov. 22; Chittister, 1995; WIN News, 1995; Heneson, 1992; Johnson and Sigler, 1995). Abuse to a spouse may be called by an assortment of terms: "battering," "spousal abuse," or "domestic abuse." Physical abuse to the family may range from a pinch or a slap to the extreme act of violence, murder (Gelles and Straus, 1988). Regardless of whether the abuse is targeted at a child, teenager, or spouse, abuse in the family is often sexual (Federation, 1986; Ward, 1991; Klingbeil, 1991).

Pilowsky (1993) notes that one of the most serious issues affecting Canadian immigrant is violence. Violence is understood differently in different cultures, and for many immigrant women, wife abuse is "normalized" in their own culture. Without a linguistically "friendly" support system, the social isolation of immigrant women may be keenly felt. Pilowsky (1993) sited that for Latin-American immigrant women denial and socialization into acceptance of abuse in the family were factors that additionally contributed to women in the study group to remain in abusive situations. Breton & Burston (1992) noted that homeless women in Canada are especially vulnerable to violence. Residents in one Toronto hostel for homeless women all reported having experienced some type of violence—child abuse, incest, rape, or assault (Breton and Burston, 1992). In a follow-up study involving 10 Toronto hostels and two drop-in centers three fourths of the 84 women in the study reported being physically or sexually assaulted (Breton and Burston, 1992). This study corroborated the growing documentation of the high incidence of violence against women in general (Appleby, 1991). The findings are congruent with research on the incidence of date and acquaintance rapes as well as with statistics from a study by the Canadian Advisory Council on the Status of Women that found that women are seven times more likely to be assaulted by someone they know intimately than by a stranger (Breton and Burston, 1992).

Family violence in aboriginal communities appears to be linked to acculturation, which has resulted in altered lifestyles and altered family relationships. It is also connected with alcohol abuse (Health and Welfare Canada, 1991). In some communities, denial of the problem of family violence leads to difficulties in trying to overcome it. Frequently aboriginal women are hesitant to report abuse because the consequences might be dissolution of the family, children separated from the parents, and loss of status as a member of the community for the women involved (Health and Welfare Canada, 1991). In addition to the fear of family breakup, factors such as shame, fear, lack of awareness of available services, threats, and loss of privacy may contribute to the low level of reporting of family violence (Breaking free: a proposal for change to aboriginal family violence, 1989). The Ontario Native Women's Association assessed abuse of aboriginal women in Ontario in 1987 and 1988. Of the 104 responses, only one indicated that family violence did not occur, 15% said they did not know, and 84% indicated that family violence occurred in their communities. A total of 80% indicated that they had personally experienced family violence (Breaking free: a proposal for change to aboriginal family violence, 1989). In a study of Canadian primary care physicians in 10 provinces all reported that cultural barriers were a concern with respect to wife abuse (Ferris, 1994). The physicians indicated that cultural norms made it difficult for the physician to deal with abuse since "natives are more secretive that whites," "there are different laws in those communities based on tradition," and "it's only alcohol." Other physicians noted that "band councils seem to condone wife abuse and resist physicians who oppose it" and "most Indian women are very scared and will put up with abuse."

Butler, Atkinson, Magnatta, and Hood (1995) noted a significant problem in the disposition of child maltreatment cases in Toronto. Although there was significant agreement among child welfare, mental health, and judicial systems regarding recommendations or dispositions for child custody in serious cases of child maltreatment, significant disagreements existed in parental access rights. Court decisions sometimes increased the distance from the family and its natural ecology and were thus increasingly ill informed.

Case Study

Sarah Jennings is a 21-year-old Canadian Black married woman and the mother of a 12-month-old daughter. She is originally from the United States. Mrs. Jennings was diagnosed at age 11 as having sickle cell anemia. For the last 3 years, she has remained largely asymptomatic. She was admitted to the hospital in sickle cell crisis. Her admitting complaints include severe joint pains in both the upper and the lower extremities, a temperature of 101.8° F, and shortness of breath. On physical examination, the nurse notes that Mrs. Jennings has coarse rales in the base of both lungs and that her lips are cyanotic and dry. Her nail beds are also cyanotic, and when they are blanched, capillary refill is slow. Initial laboratory examination reveals a hemoglobin of 8 g/dL. While the nursing history was being taken, it was revealed that Mrs. Jennings has also had problems drinking milk and eating certain dairy products for most of her adult life.

STUDY QUESTIONS

1. List at least two contributing factors for Mrs. Jennings' sickle cell anemia that relate to biological variations by race and ethnic heritage.
2. List at least one other racial group with a predisposition for sickle cell crisis.
3. List the basic etiology of sickle cell anemia.
4. List at least two other conditions that Mrs. Jennings could be at risk for developing because of her race and ethnic heritage.
5. Describe at least two differences noted when the skin color of dark-skinned individuals is being assessed.

References

Adams, J.M. (1932). Some racial differences in blood pressures and morbidity in groups of white and colored workmen. *American Journal of Medical Science, 184,* 342-350.

AIDS in Canada. Cross tabulations on selected variables by race/ethnic origin for reported AIDS cases. (1990). Ottawa: Bureau of Epidemiology and Surveillance, Federal Centre for AIDS.

Allodi, F., & Fantini, N. (1985). The Italians in Toronto: a data system for psychiatric services to an immigrant community. *Annals of Psychotherapy and Psychopathology, 2,* 49-58.

Altman, D. (1994). *Power and community: organizational and cultural responses to AIDS.* London: Taylor & Francis.

American Diabetic Association. (1991). *Vital statistics.* Alexandria, Va.: the Association.

Anonymous. (1995, November 22). Social discrimination against women is on the rise. *Current Digest of the Post-Soviet Press, 47*(43), 18-19.

Appleby, T. (1991, July 13). Who gets killed in Canada? *The Globe and Mail,* pp. D1, D4.

Bailey, E., & Bailey, R. (1995). *Discover Canada.* Princeton, N.J.: Berlitz Publishing Co.

Basch, P. (1990). *Textbook of international health.* Oxford: Oxford University Press.

Bayless, T. (1975). Lactose and milk intolerance: clinical implications. *New England Journal of Medicine, 292*(5), 1156-1159.

Beaudet, M. (1996). Depression. *Healthreports.* Ottawa: Health Statistics Division: Statistics Canada.

Beiser, M., & Wood, M. (1986). *Canadian task force on mental health issues affecting immigrants and refugees: review of the literature on migrant mental health.* Ottawa: Health and Welfare Canada.

Bennett, K.A., Osborne, R.H., & Miller, R.J. (1975). *Biocultural ecology: annual review of anthropology.* Palo Alto, Calif.: Annual Reviews.

Boyle, E. (1970). Biological patterns in hypertension by race, sex, body weight, and skin color. *Journal of the American Medical Association, 213,* 1637-1643.

Braithwaite, R.L., & Taylor, S.E. (1992). *Health issues in the Black community.* San Francisco: Josey-Bass.

Branch, M., & Paxton, P. (1976). *Providing safe nursing care for ethnic people of color.* East Norwalk, Conn: Appleton-Century-Crofts.

Breaking free: a proposal for change to aboriginal family violence. (1989, December). Ottawa: Ontario Native Women's Association.

Breton, M., & Burston, T. (1992). Physical and sexual violence in the lives of homeless women. *Canadian Journal of Community Mental Health, 11*(1), 29-44.

Brown, L. (1996). *The state of the world.* New York: W.W. Norton.

Bulmer, M. (1970). *The biology of twinning in man.* New York: Oxford University Press.

Burns, E., & Neubort, S. (1984). Sodium content of koshered meat [letter]. *Journal of the American Medical Association, 252*(21), 2960.

Burt, C.L. (1966). The genetic determination of difference in intelligence: a study of monozygote twins reared together and apart. *British Journal of Psychology, 57,* 137-153.

Butler, S., Atkinson, L., Magnatta, M., & Hood, E. (1995). Child maltreatment: the collaboration of child welfare, mental health, and judicial systems. *Child Abuse and Neglect, 19*(3), 355-362.

Cain, R. (1995). Community-based AIDS organizations and the state: dilemmas of dependence. *AIDS and Public Policy Journal, 10*(2), 83-94.

Carlson, M. (1995, October 16). Preventable murders. *Time,* 65.

Carter Center of Emory University. (1985). Closing the gap: the problem of diabetes mellitus in the United States. *Diabetes Care, 8,* 391-401.

Centers for Disease Control. (1989a). A strategic plan for the elimination of tuberculosis in the United States. *Morbidity and Mortality Weekly Report 38*(suppl. 3), 1-27.

Centers for Disease Control. (1992b). Recommendations of the Advisory Council for the reduction of hypertension among minority populations. *Morbidity and Mortality Weekly Report, 40,* 1-7.

Chan, A.W. (1986). Racial differences in alcohol sensitivity. *Alcohol and Alcoholism, 21*(1), 93-104.

Chang, B. (1974). Some dietary beliefs in Chinese folk culture. *Journal of the American Diet Association, 65*(4), 436.

Chittister, J. (1995, September 8). Commentary. *National Catholic Reporter, 31*(39), 13.

Cummings, S., Kelsey, J., Nevitt, N., & O'Dowd, K. (1985). Epidemiology of osteoporosis and osteoporotic fractures. *Epidemiology Review, 7,* 178-208.

Daniel, M., & Gamble, D. (1995). Diabetes and Canada's aboriginal peoples: the need for primary prevention. *International Journal of Nursing Studies, 32*(2), 243-259.

Department of Health and Human Services. (1990). *Healthy people 2000: National health promotion and disease prevention objectives,* (DHHS Publication No. PHS 91-50212). Washington, D.C.: U.S. Government Printing Office.

Divan, D. (1989). Letter to the editor. *New England Journal of Medicine, 321*(4), 259.

Echizen, H., Horai, Y., & Ishizaki, T. (1989). Letter to the editor. *New England Journal of Medicine, 321*(4), 258.

Editorial (1996). Modest increase in Canadian rate in midst of global emergency. *The Canadian Nurse, 92,* 18.

Edwards, N.C., & MacMillan, K. (1990). Tobacco use and ethnicity: the existing data gap. *Canadian Journal of Public Health, 81*(1), 31-34.

Farb, P., & Armelagos, G.J. (1980). *Consuming passions: the anthropology of eating.* Boston: Houghton Mifflin.

Federation, S. (1986). Treatment modalities for the younger child. *Sexual Abuse, 24*(7), 21-24.

Fenna, D., Schaefer, O., Mix, L., & Gilbert, J. (1971). Ethanol metabolism in various racial groups. *Canadian Medical Association Journal, 105,* 472-475.

Ferris, L. (1994). Detection and treatment of wife abuse in aboriginal communities by primary care physicians: preliminary findings. *Journal of Women's Health, 3*(4), 265-271.

Fishman, R. (1995, July 15). Concern grows over domestic abuse in Israel. *Lancet, 346*(8968), 174.

Flaskerud, J.H. (1986). The effects of culture-compatible intervention on the utilization of mental health services by minority clients. *Community Mental Health Journal, 22*(2), 126-141.

Fodor's staff. (1988). *Fodor's Canada.* New York: Fodor's Travel Publications (David McKay Co., Inc.).

Freis, E. (1986). Antihypertensive agents. In Kalow, W., Goedde, H.W., & Agarwal, D. (Eds.), *Ethnic differences in reactions to drugs and xenobiotics.* New York: Liss.

Gaitz, C.M., & Scott, J. (1974). Mental health of Mexican-Americans: do ethnic factors make a difference? *Geriatrics, 29*(11), 103-110.

Garn, S., Nagy, A., & Sandusky, S. (1972). Differential sex dimorphism in bone diameters of subjects of European and African ancestry. *American Journal of Anthropology, 37,* 127-130.

Gelles, R.J., & Straus, M.A. (1988). *Intimate violence: the causes and consequences of abuse in the American family.* New York: Simon & Schuster.

Gerchufsky, M. (1996, July). Milk: does it really do a body good? *Advance for Nurse Practitioners,* 39-41.

Giger, J., Davidhizar, R., & Wieczorek, S. (1993). Culture and ethnicity. In Bobak, I., & Jensen, M. (Eds.), *Maternity and gynecologic care* (ed. 5) (pp. 43-67). St. Louis: Mosby.

Gilsanz, V., Roe, T., Mora, S., Costin, G., & Goodman, W. (1991). Changes in vertebral bone density in Black girls and White girls during childhood and puberty. *New England Journal of Medicine, 325*(23), 1597-1600.

Glazer, W.M., Morgenstern, H., & Doucette, M.T. (1993). Predicting the long-term risk of tardive dyskinesia in outpatients maintained on neuroheptic medications. *Journal of Clinical Psychiatry, 54*(4), 133-139.

Glazer, W., Morgenstern, H., & Doucette, M.T. (1994). Race and tardive dyskinesia among outpatients at a CMHC. *Hospital and Community Psychiatry, 45*(1), 38-45.

Goedde, H.W. (1983). Population genetic studies on aldehyde dehydrogenase isoenzyme deficiency and alcohol sensitivity. *American Journal of Human Genetics, 35,* 769.

Goedde, H.W. (1986). Ethnic differences in reactions to drugs and other xenobiotics: outlook of a geneticist. In Kalow, W, Goedde, H.W., & Agarwal, D. (Eds.), *Ethnic differences in reactions to drugs and xenobiotics* (pp. 9-20). New York: Liss.

Grant, D., Tang B.K., & Kalow, W. (1983). Variability in caffeine metabolism. *Clinical Pharmacology Therapy, 33*(5), 591-602.

Griffith, E.E., & Griffith, E.J. (1986). Racism, psychological injury, and compensatory damages. *Hospital and Community Psychiatry, 37*(1), 71-75.

Gunby, P. (1979). The changing picture of otitis media in childhood. *Journal of American Medical Association, 245,* 707-709.

Guruge, S., & Donner, G. (1996, September). Transcultural nursing in Canada. *The Canadian Nurse, 92,* 34-39.

Hagey, R. (1984). The phenomenon, the explanations and the responses: metaphors surrounding diabetes in urban Canadian Indians. *Social Science and Medicine, 18,* 265-272.

Health and Welfare Canada. (1987). *Mutual aid as a mechanism for health promotion and disease prevention.* Ottawa: Minister of Supply and Services.

Health and Welfare Canada. (1991). *Health status of Canadian Indians and Inuit 1990.* Ottawa: Health and Welfare Canada.

Health and Welfare Canada. (1993, July). *AIDS in Canada surveillance update.* Ottawa: Health and Welfare Canada.

Heneson, L. (1992). The secretary's initiative on child abuse and neglect. *Children Today, 21*(2), 4-5.

Holmes, T.H., et al. (1957). Psychosocial and psychophysiological studies of tuberculosis. *Psychosomatic Medicine, 19,* 134-143.

International Health Statistics. (1993). Office of Technology Assessment, United States Congress.

Horton, J. (Ed.) (1992). *The women's health data book: a profile of women's health in the United States* (pp. 60-62). Washington, D.C.: The Jacob's Institute of Women's Health.

Jacobson, S.F. (1994). Native American health. *Annual Review of Nursing Research, 12,* 193-213.

Jarvis, A. (1972). Minor orofacial abnormalities in an Eskimo population. *Oral Surgery, 33,* 417-427.

Jensen, A.R. (1969). How much can we boost IQ and scholastic achievement? *Harvard Education Review, 29,* 1.

Jensen, A.R. (1974). Cumulative deficits: a testable hypothesis? *Developmental Psychology, 10,* 996.

Jensen, A.R. (1977). Cumulative deficit in IQ of Blacks in the rural South. *Developmental Psychology, 13,* 184.

Jick, H., Slone, D., Westerholm, B., et al. (1969). Venous thromboembolic disease and ABO blood type. *Lancet, 1,* 539-542.

Johnson, I., & Sigler, R. (1995). Community attitudes: a study of definitions and punishment of spouse abusers and child abusers. *Journal of Criminal Justice, 23*(5), 477-487.

Joint National Committee. (1993). *The fifth report of the Joint National Committee on Detection, Evaluation and Treatment of High Blood Pressure.* Washington, D.C.: National Institutes of Health, National Heart, Lung, and Blood Institute.

Julien, G., Baxter, J., Crago, M., Ilecki, H., & Thérien, F. (1987). Chronic otitis media and hearing deficit among native children of Kuujjuaraapik (northern Quebec): a pilot project. *Canadian Journal of Public Health, 78,* 57-60.

Kalow, W. (1972). Pharmacogenetics of drugs used in anesthesia. *Human Genetics, 60,* 415-427.

Kalow, W. (1982). The metabolism of xenobiotics in different populations. *Canadian Journal of Physiological Pharmacology, 60,* 1-19.

Kalow, W. (1986). Outlook of a pharmacologist. In Kalow, W., Goedde, H., & Agarwal, D. (Eds.), *Ethnic differences in reactions to drugs and xenobiotics.* New York: Liss.

Kalow, W. (1989). Race and therapeutic drug response. *New England Journal of Medicine, 320*(9), 588-589.

Kamlin, L.J. (1974). *The science and politics of IQ.* New York: John Wiley & Sons.

Katz, S.H., Hediger, M.L., & Valleroy, L.A. (1974). Traditional maize processing techniques in the New World. *Science, 184,* 765.

Keil, J. (1981). Skin color and education effects on blood pressure. *American Journal of Public Health, 71,* 532-534.

Keltner, N. (1994, October), Birmingham, Alabama, Personal communication to J.N. Giger.

Keltner, N., & Folks, G. (1992). Psychopharmacology update: culture as a variable in drug therapy. *Perspectives in Psychiatric Nursing, 28*(1), 33-35.

Kisch, B. (1953). Salt poor diet and Jewish dietary laws. *Journal of the American Medical Association, 153*(16), 1472.

Klag, M.J., Whelton, P.K., Coresh, J., Grim, C.E., & Kuller, L.H. (1991). The association of skin color with blood pressure in U.S. Blacks with low socioeconomic status. *Journal of the American Medical Association, 265*(5), 599-602.

Klingbeil, K. (1991). Keynote address at a conference on battering of women. Seattle, Wash.

Knowler, W.C., Williams, R.C., Pettitt, D.J., & Steinberg, A.G. (1988). Gm 3,5,13,14 and type 2 diabetes mellitus: an association in American Indians with genetic admixture. *American Journal Human Genetics, 43,* 520-526.

Knowler, W.C., Pettitt, D.J., Saad, M.F., & Bennett, P.H. (1990). Diabetes mellitus in the Pima Indians: incidence, risk factors and pathogenesis. *Diabetes/Metabolism Reviews, 6,* 1-27.

Krolewski, A., & Warram, G. (1994). Epidemiology of diabetes mellitus. In Krall, L.P., & Beaser, R.S. (Eds.), *Joslin's diabetes mellitus* (ed. 12). Philadelphia: Lea & Febiger.

Kudzma, E.C. (1992). Drug response: all bodies are not created equal. *American Journal of Nursing, 92*(12), 48-50.

Lahaie, U. (1990, January, March). Seasonal affective disorder. *Canadian Psychiatric Nursing, 86,* 9-11.

Lawson, W. (1986). Racial and ethnic factors in psychiatric research. *Hospital and Community Psychiatry, 37*(1), 50-54.

Leffall, L.D. (1974). Cancer mortality among Blacks. *CA: A Cancer Journal for Clinicians, 24,* 42-46.

Lefley, H. (1990). Culture and chronic mental illness. *Hospital and Community Psychiatry, 41,* 277.

Leininger, M. (1970). *Nursing and anthropology: two worlds to blend.* New York: John Wiley & Sons.

Lerner, D., & Kannel, W. (1986). Patterns of coronary heart disease morbidity and mortality in the sexes: a 26-year follow-up of the Framingham population. *American Heart Journal, 11,* 383-390.

Lewis, J.H. (1942). *The biology of the Negro.* (Chicago University Monographs in Medicine). Chicago: University of Chicago Press.

Li, J., Specker, B., Ho, B., & Tsang, R. (1989). Bone mineral content in Black and White children 1 to 6 years of age: early appearance of race and sex differences. *American Journal of Disorders in Children, 143,* 1346-1349.

Lightbody, M., & Smallman, T. (1994). *Canada: a travel survival kit.* Australia: Lonely Planet Publications.

Lin, K.M., Lau, J., Smith, R., Phillips, P., Antal, E., & Poland, R.E. (1988). Comparison of alprazolam plasma levels in normal Asian and Caucasian male volunteers. *Psychopharmacology, 96*(3), 365-369.

Lorton, J., & Lorton, E. (1984). *Human development through the life span.* Belmont, Calif.: Brooks/Cole.

Lu, F. (1987). Culturally relevant inpatient care for minority and ethnic patients. *Hospital and Community Psychiatry, 38*(11), 1126-1127.

MacDonald, F., Shah, W.M., & Campbell, N.M. (1990). Developing the strength to fight diabetes: assessing the education needs of Native Indians with diabetes mellitus. *Beta Release, 14*(1), 13-16.

Melton, L., & Riggs, B. (1987). Epidemiology of age-related fractures. In Avioli, L. (Ed.), *The osteoporotic syndrome: detection, prevention, and treatment* (ed. 2) (pp. 1-30). Orlando, Fla.: Grune & Stratton.

Merck, Sharp, & Dohme. (1974). *Hypertension handbook for clinicians.* Westpoint, Pa.

Miller, W. (1990). Smoking prevalence in the Canadian arctic. *Medical Research, 49*(suppl 2), 23-28.

Montour, L.T., Macaulay, A.C., & Adelson, N. (1989). Diabetes mellitus in Mohawks of Kahnawake, PQ: a clinical and epidemiologic description. *Canadian Medical Association Journal, 141,* 549-552.

Morris, R., Clarke, M., Bingham, B. (1989). Schizophrenia and the family. *Canadian Journal of Psychiatric Nursing, 20,* 17-19.

Moser, M., & Lunn, J. (1982). Responses to catopril and hydrochlorothiazide in Black patients with hypertension. *Clinical Pharmacology Therapy, 32,* 307-312.

National Center for Health Statistics. (1991). *Health, United States, 1990* (DHHS Publication No. PHS 91-1232). Hyattsville, Md.: Public Health Service.

Opler, M. (Ed.). (1959). *Culture and health.* New York: Macmillan.

Overfield, T. (1977). Biological variations. *Nursing Clinics of North America, 12*(1), 19-27.

Overfield, T. (1985). *Biologic variations in health and illness: race, age and sex differences.* Reading, Mass.: Addison-Wesley.

Pangborn, R.M. (1975). Cross-cultural aspects of flavor preferences. *Food Technology, 29*(6), 34.

Phipps, W. (1993). The patient with pulmonary problems. In Long, B.C., Phipps, W.J., & Cassmeyer, V. (Eds.), *Medical surgical nursing: concepts and clinical practice.* St. Louis: Mosby.

Pilowsky, J. (1993). The courage to leave: an exploration of Spanish-speaking women victims of spousal abuse. *Canadian Journal of Community Mental Health, 12*(2), 15-27.

Platt, O., Brambilla, D., Rosse, W., Milner, P., Castor, O., Steinberg, M., & Klug, P. (1994, June 9). Mortality in sickle cell disease: life expectancy and risk factors for early death. *New England Journal of Medicine, 330* (23), 1639-1644.

Pollitzer, W., & Anderson, J. (1990). Ethnic and genetic differences in bone mass: a review with a hereditary vs environmental perspective. *American Journal of Clinical Nutrition, 52,* 181.

Poussaint, A.F. (1995). Interracial relations. In Freedman, A.M., Kaplan, H.I., & Sadock, B.J. (Eds.), *Comprehensive textbook of psychiatry* (ed. 2, vol. 2). Baltimore: Willians & Wilkins.

Powell, D. (1988). Emerging directions in parent-child early intervention. In Powell, D. (Ed.), *Parent education as early childhood intervention: emerging directions in theory, research and practice: vol. 3. advances in applied development* (pp. 1-21). Norwood, N.J.: Ablex Publishing.

Prior, D., & Tasman-Jones, C. (1981). New Zealand Maori and Pacific Polynesians. In Trowell, H.C. &. Burkitt, D.P (Eds.), *Western diseases: their emergence and prevention* (pp. 227-267). London: Edward Arnold.

Radford, J. (1989). *Street youth and AIDS.* Social Program Evaluation Group, Queen's University at Kingston, Kingston, Ontario.

Rayside, D., & Lindquist, E. (1992). Canada: community activism, federalism, and the new politics of disease. In Kirp, D. & Bayer, R. (Eds.), *Aids in industrialized democracies: passions, politics, and policies* (pp. 49-98). Montreal, P.Q., and Kingston, Ont.: McGill-Queen's University Press.

Reed, T., Kalant, H., Gibbins, R., Kapur, B., & Rankin, J. (1976). Alcohol and acetaldehyde metabolism in Caucasians, Chinese and Amerinds. *Canadian Medical Association Journal, 115,* 851-855.

Reid, I.R., Cullen, S., Schooler, B.A., Livingston, N.E., & Evans, M.C. (1990). Calcitropic hormone levels in Polynesians: evidence against their role in interracial differences in bone mass. *Journal of Endocrinology Metabolism, 70,* 1452-1466.

Rifkin, H. (Ed.). (1984). *The physician's guide to type II diabetes (NIDDM): diagnosis and treatment.* New York: The American Diabetes Association.

Riggs, S. (1980). Tastes of America: regionality. *Institutions, 87*(12), 76.

Roccella, E., & Lenfant, C. (1989). Regional and racial differences among stroke victims in the United States. *Clinical Cardiology, 12*(IV), 1213-1220.

Rouch, L. (1977). Color changes in dark skin. *Nursing '77, 7*(1), 48-51.

Saldana, G., & Brown, H.E. (1984). Nutritional composition of corn and flour tortillas. *Journal of Food Science, 49*(4), 202.

Satcher, D., & Pope, L. (1974). *Emergency evaluation and management of persons with sickle cell disease.* Bethesda, Md.: National Institutes of Health.

Satcher, D., et al. (1973). *Sickle cell counseling: a committee's study and recommendations.* New York: National Foundation—March of Dimes.

Saunders, E. (1985). Special techniques for management of hypertension in Blacks. In Hall, W.D., Saunders, E., & Shulman, N.B. (Eds.), *Hypertension in Blacks: epidemiology, pathophysiology, and treatment* (pp. 209-236). St. Louis: Mosby.

Schumacher, H. (1993). *Primer on the rheumatic diseases* (ed. 10). Atlanta: Arthritis Foundation.

Schwerin, H.S., Stanton, J.L., & Smith, J.L. (1982). Food, eating habits, and health: a further examination of the relationships between food eating patterns and nutritional health. *American Clinical Nutrition, 35*(suppl. 5), 1319.

Short, K., & Johnston, C. (1994). Ethnocultural parent education in Canada: current status and directions. *Canadian Journal of Community Mental Health, 13*(1), 43-54.

State of Maryland Demonstration of Statewide Coordination for the Control of High Blood Pressure. (1977-1983, October). NHLBL Contract No. 1-HV-2986.

Statistics Canada. (1996). *Report of the royal commission on Aboriginal peoples.* Ottawa: Minister of Indian Affairs and Northern Development.

Stewart, P. (1985). National database on breastfeeding among Indian and Inuit women: survey of infant feeding practices from birth to six months, Canada, 1983. Health and Welfare Canada, Medical Services Branch, Ottawa, 1995.

Stokes, J., Kannel, W., Wolf, P., Cupples, L., & D'Agostino, R. (1987). The relative importance of selected risk factors for various manifestations of cardiovascular disease among men and women from 35 to 64 years old: 30 years of follow-up in the Framingham study. *Circulation, 75*(6), 65-73.

Sue, D., Sue, D.W., & Sue, D.M. (1983). Psychological development of Chinese-American children. In Powell, G.J. (Ed.), *The psychosocial development of minority group children* (pp. 159-166). New York: Brunner/Mazel.

Sue, S. (1977). Community mental health services to minority groups. *American Psychologist, 32,* 616-624.

Sue, S., & Morishima, J.K. (1982). *The mental health of Asian Americans.* San Francisco: Jossey-Bass.

Teram, E., & White, H. (1993). Strategies to address the bureaucratic disentitlements of clients from culturally minority groups. *Canadian Journal of Community Mental Health, 12*(2), 59-70.

Thérien, F. (1988). Otitis and hearing loss among northern Quebec Inuit. *Arctic Medical Research, 47,* (suppl. 1), 657-658.

Thomson, M. (1990, November-December). Heavy birthweight in Native Indians of British Columbia. *Canadian Journal of Public Health, 81,* 443-446.

Tipton, D. (1974, May). Physiological assessment of Black people. In *Care of Black patients* (X428.1). A group of papers presented at a conference on care of the Black patient, sponsored by Continuing Education in Nursing, University of California, San Francisco.

U.S. Congress, Office of Technology Assessment. (1993). *International health statistics: what the numbers mean for the United States—background paper.* Washington, D.C.: U.S. Government Printing Office.

Vessell, E. (1972). Therapy-pharmacogenetics. *New England Journal of Medicine, 287*(18), 904-909.

Walsh, E. (1993). The patient with peripheral vascular problems. In Long, B.C., Phipps, W.J., & Cassmeyer V. (Eds.), *Medical surgical nursing: concepts and clinical practice* (pp. 705-742). St. Louis: Mosby.

Ward, W. (1991). When teens are sexually abused. *Oakleaves, 16*(3), 1-2.

West, K.M. (1974). Diabetes in American Indians and other populations of the New World. *Diabetes, 23,* 841-855.

When patients can't drink milk. (1976, August). *Nursing Update,* pp. 10-12.

Wherrett, G.J. (1977). *The miracle of empty beds: a history of tuberculosis in Canada.* Toronto: University of Toronto Press.

Wiet, R.J., DeBlanc, G.B., Stewart, J., & Weider, D.J. (1980). Natural history of otitis media in the American native. *Annals of Otology, Rhinology and Laryngology, 89* (Suppl. 68), 14-19.

Williams, R.A. (Ed.). (1975). *Textbook of Black-related disease.* New York: McGraw-Hill.

WIN News. (1995). *Sexual violence grounds for political asylum, 21*(3), 44.

Witcop, E., et al. (1963). Oral and genetic studies of Chileans, 1960: 1. Oral anomalies. *American Journal of Physical Anthropology, 21,* 15-24.

World Almanac. (1997). Mahwah, N.J.: World Almanac Books.

Wurtman, R.J., & Wurtman, J.J. (1989). Carbohydrates and depression. *Scientific American, 260*(1), 68-75.

Wyngaarden, J.B., & Smith, L.H. (Eds.). (1996). *Cecil textbook of medicine* (ed. 20). Philadelphia: W.B. Saunders.

Yonkers, K.A., Kando, J.C., Cole, J.O., & Blumenthal, S. (1992). Gender differences in pharmacokinetics and pharmacodynamics of psychotropic medication. *American Journal of Psychiatry* 149(5), 587-595.

Young, T. K., McIntyre, L. L., Dooley, J., & Rodriguez, J. (1985). Epidemiologic features of diabetes mellitus among Indians in northwestern Ontario and northeastern Manitoba. *Canadian Medical Association Journal, 132,* 793-797.

Young, T.K. (1988). *Diabetes among the Canadian native population: a national survey.* Interim report, March.

Young, T.K. (1989). *National diabetes survey—Preliminary results.* Unpublished report, Medical Services Branch, January.

Young, T. (1994). *The health of Native Americans.* New York: Oxford University Press.

Zhou, H.H., Koshakji, R.P., Silberstein, D.J., Wilkinson, G.R., & Wood, A.J.J. (1989). Racial differences in drug response: altered sensitivity to and clearance of propranolol in men of Chinese descent as compared with American Whites. *New England Journal of Medicine, 320,* 565-570.

Zifferblatt, S.M., Wilbur, C.S., & Pinsky, J.L. (1980). Understanding food habits. *Journal of American Diet Association, 76*(1), 9.

Zilm, G., & Warbinek, E. (1994). *Legacy: history of nursing education at the University of British Columbia 1919-1994.* Vancouver: UBC Press/UBC School of Nursing, p. 42.

Zimmet, P., Dowse, G., Finch, C., Serjeantson, S., & King, H. (1990). The epidemiology and natural history of NIDDM: lessons from the South Pacific. *Diabetes Metabolism Review 6,* 91-124.

Application of Assessment and Intervention Techniques to Specific Cultural Groups

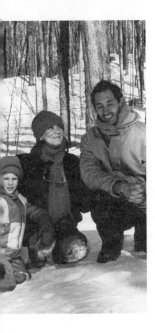

CHAPTER 8
French Canadians of Quebec Origin

Mary Reidy and Marie-Elizabeth Taggart

BEHAVIORAL OBJECTIVES

After reading this chapter, the nurse will be able to:

1. Understand the communication patterns and the dialectical variations of the French-Canadian people of Quebec.
2. Describe the spatial needs, distance, and intimacy behaviors of the French-Canadian people of Quebec.
3. Describe the time orientation and effects on treatment regimes of the French-Canadian people of Quebec.
4. Describe the social organization of family systems among the French-Canadian people of Quebec.
5. Identify the illness, wellness, and health-seeking behaviors of the French Canadians of Quebec.
6. Identify folk beliefs, folk practices, and folk healers unique to the health value systems of the French Canadians of Quebec.
7. Identify susceptibility of the French-Canadian people of Quebec to specific disease or illness conditions.

OVERVIEW OF QUEBECKERS

Conflict concerning French Canadians is an integral part of Canadian history. The history of the White man began in Canada in 1497, when John Cabot, an Italian in the service of Henry VII of England, reached Newfoundland. However, Canada was taken

This chapter was prepared with the financial support of ESSPOIR-FRSQ and with the collaboration of research assistant Louise Mercier, master's student at the Faculty of Nursing, University of Montreal, and Stéphanie Simard, library assistant, master's student in Library Science, University of Montreal.

for France in 1534 by Jacques Cartier. The actual settlement of New France, as it was then called, began in 1604 in Nova Scotia. In 1608 Quebec was founded. By the seventeenth century French explorers had penetrated beyond the Great Lakes to the western prairies. However, conflict for possession by England and France continued. The conflict climaxed in the Seven Years' War (1756-1763), which ended in a conquest by England. Nevertheless, at that time the population of Canada was almost entirely French. In the next few decades, thousands of British colonists emigrated to Canada (Johnson,

1997). Over the years, the rivalry between the French and the British in Canada has been ongoing.

Despite the vastness of Canada, some two thirds of the population is concentrated in the southeastern part of the country (southern areas of Ontario and Quebec provinces), especially in the highly industrialized areas of Toronto, Hamilton, London, Windsor, and Montreal. Other densely populated areas include the Edmonton-Calgary axis in the plains of the eastern slope of the Rocky Mountains, the Pacific harbor of Vancouver, the region around Ottawa and the St. Lawrence lowlands with the historic city of Quebec (Johnson, 1997). Today some 24.4% of the Canadian population are French speaking (Bailey and Bailey, 1995). However, because these individuals are spread throughout Canada and have a profoundly different history, French Canadians across Canada differ significantly. This chapter focuses on the French Canadians whose origin is the province of Quebec. Although Canadians pride themselves on tolerance toward diverse ethnic cultures in the country, the uniqueness of native and ethnocultural groups requires that health care knowledge of specific groups be utilized to provide culturally appropriate care (Ntetu and Fortin, 1996).

QUEBEC PROVINCE

Quebec (English /kwuh-bek'/, French /kay-bek'/, from Micmac *kepek* 'narrows') is a province of Canada that reaches almost to the Arctic Circle. Geographically Quebec borders on Labrador, Newfoundland, and New Brunswick in the east; the American states of New York and Vermont in the south and southeast; and Ontario province and Hudson Bay in the west. The border with Labrador remains a matter of dispute. Quebec encompasses the Canadian land mass north of the Ottawa and the St. Lawrence Rivers. To the south of the St. Lawrence it takes in the lowlands as far as the United States border, as well as the Gasppé Peninsula projecting into the Gulf of St. Lawrence. In the west, an artificial line divides Quebec from Ontario (Bailey and Bailey, 1995).

Quebec is a vast province about one sixth of the whole of Canada. Quebec is so vast that it could accommodate the United Kingdom five times over, but it has a population of only 7.4 million (Statistics

Canada, 1996) with most of the people living in the two largest cities, its capital, the city of Quebec (645,500), and Montreal (3,127,242) (Statistics Canada, 1991 Census; Metropolitan areas). The lifeline of this province is the St. Lawrence River, which is almost 750 miles long. The St. Lawrence River along the St. Lawrence Seaway has been the direct link between the Atlantic Ocean and the Great Lakes since 1959.

Quebec is the largest of the 10 Canadian provinces. Because of its geographical location, Quebec is divided into three climate zones: humid continental in the central southern areas (warm summers, cold winters), subarctic farther to the north, and arctic in the far northern regions (long, intensely cold winters, short cool summers). The greater part of Quebec's territory is covered by forests; only 2.5% is agricultural or urban.

The people and the culture of French Quebec

Quebec traces its cultural origins to approximately 500 Catholic colonists who came from Normandy and west central France to the land called "New France" in 1604 (Laberge, 1992; Johnson, 1997). These colonists along with other immigrants to follow formed the cornerstone of a distinct sociocultural entity. A cholera epidemic and a poor potato crop in Ireland that caused a widespread famine prompted a later wave of immigrants. The trip to Quebec took many lives, resulting in many Irish children arriving as orphans. Although they were adopted by French-speaking families, they often kept their own names, which explains family names such as McNeill and Ryan among the current French-speaking population of Quebec. Their assimilation was such that the culture acquired a high degree of homogeneity while becoming rapidly differentiated from the French culture from which it was derived (Rioux, 1974).

Today the descendants of these French colonists call themselves "Québecois" or, in popular speech, *nous autres,* which one might translate as 'our people.' The term "French Canadians" has been largely replaced by *Québecois de souche* designating 'old-stock Quebeckers', or the Quebec people of French origin. Other colonists from France who emigrated to the United States became known as Franco-Americans and settled mainly in the Lake Champlain valley and in the states of New York, Vermont, Connecticut, and Massachusetts. In Canada other, though distinctively different, French-speaking communities developed in New Brunswick, Ontario, and Manitoba. In the United States, the Cajuns of Louisiana are descended from the Acadians who underwent forced immigration from the Maritime Provinces of Canada. Historical and geographical factors caused each of these groups to evolve into very different cultural communities.

Many factors have contributed to the distinct character of the French-speaking people of Quebec. After the Treaty of Paris in 1763, which recognized English authority over former French possession, the urban centers of Montreal and Quebec City became predominantly English speaking. However, until the midnineteenth century, agriculture, law, and medicine proved to be, almost exclusively, the professions of the French in Quebec. This historical and political evolution reinforced the isolation and homogeneity of the French-speaking community (Rioux, 1974).

From its beginning, Quebec society has been characterized by a fierce nationalism intent on preserving the French language and culture. This process has led to the creation of various movements in favor of a political independence for Quebec, separate from Canadian provinces. These political tendencies are responsible for certain tensions in relations between Quebec's citizens and those in the rest of Canada. A charged emotional climate exists between those for and those against separatism.

Tensions exist between provincial and federal governments, between separatists and nonseparatists, between old immigrants and new, and between White Quebeckers and the Native peoples, who were the first inhabitants of this land. The recent massive arrival of immigrants has added a further dimension to the political and human problems of Quebec. This has caused a population increase despite a declining birth rate (Labrie, 1990; Tétu de Labsade, 1990). During the eighteenth and nineteenth centuries, immigration came primarily from English-speaking countries (Scotland, Ireland, and

so on) and to a certain extent from Eastern Europe (Poland, Czechoslovakia, and so on). More recently, Quebec has received French North Africans, Chileans, Vietnamese, Cambodians, Italians, Greeks, and Haitians.

The issue of separatist sentiments in French-speaking Quebec flared most recently in the Quebec referendum on succession of French-speaking Quebec in October 1995. Although the referendum yielded a narrow rejection, the separatists vowed to try again (Johnson, 1997).

POLITICAL DEVELOPMENT

After the English conquest, the political system of Canada took on the form of a parliamentary democracy. In 1867, the British North America Act established Canada as a federal state, with strong central powers, uniting several dependent provinces. This system is, in fact, a constitutional monarchy: the queen of England remains the queen of Canada and holds the title of head of state. Each province has its own government and parliament. In Quebec, the parliament is known as the National Assembly (Assemblée nationale). The federal government shares legal, fiscal, and social powers with the provinces. Criminal and international law are under federal jurisdiction in conformity with the British Common law tradition, whereas the provinces retain the power to enact civil legislation affecting private property, family affairs, social welfare, and health. The Quebec civil code is unique to Canada because it was inspired by French legal tradition.

Health care

Before 1970, Canadian and Quebec health services were privately organized and funded. In 1969, Quebec put into place a medical insurance program guaranteeing free and universal access (Anctil and Bluteau, 1986). This program was followed in 1970 by the development of a network of social services for those in need of social or financial assistance.

Education

During the nineteenth and most of the twentieth centuries, free schooling to the eighth grade was provided. For Canadian students, high schools and colleges were private, maintained for the most part by religious orders who charged tuition. In 1943, attendance became compulsory in the Canadian school system (Gagnon, 1992). School systems were still organized according to religion. The Catholic School Commission and the Protestant School Board operated schools for French-speaking and English-speaking children in their denomination.

In 1960 and 1961, a series of laws was enacted that provided free universal education through the eleventh grade and compulsory education to 15 years of age (Audet and Gauthier, 1967). This parent report led to a reorganization of the educational system with free schooling up to the university level. A system of postsecondary junior colleges was established, replacing the last year of high school and first year of university. Universities provide 3-year undergraduate programs as well as graduate and professional education.

In June 1993, the Supreme Court of Canada upheld the constitutionality of a 1988 law that reorganized school boards along linguistic lines rather than religion. Reorganization of these new school boards is presently underway (Authier, 1993). Today, private schools, at all levels, coexist with the public system.

"Quiet revolution"

In the years after World War II, Quebec underwent a rapid transition from a rural to an urban technological society. This pattern of change did not correspond to the classical steps of the industrial revolution seen in the urban centers of England and Europe. Until the 1960s, Quebeckers were very traditionally oriented. The so-called "Quiet Revolution" resulted in social, political, and behavioral transformations as profound and permanent as those produced by armed and violent revolution. The state progressively replaced the church in most of its functions. The school, health care, and social welfare systems were now controlled by the Quebec government. A widespread movement against the clergy resulted in a newfound sexual liberty. The divorce rate increased dramatically. Individuals became more interested in business. Women acquired a place in the work force (Bouchard, 1992, Lanthier and Rousseau, 1992). The social classes in Quebec evolved to the current four classes: nonspecialized

workers, cyclically employed workers, and welfare recipients make up the lower or disadvantaged class; specialized workers, small businessowners, and merchants are included in the middle class; executives, industrialists, professionals, and technocrats form the upper middle class; and intellectuals and artists are the intelligentsia (Lacroix and Simard, 1984).

Economy

Starting in the 1950s the control of political institutions and business enterprises shifted into the hands of French-speaking Quebeckers. Closely related to change in world economy during the 1980s, Quebec experienced a slowing of economic growth, a decrease in industrial jobs, and the deterioration of the economic climate (Langlois, 1992). Under these conditions, more families needed two sources of income to maintain living standards. Women with higher education began to pursue demanding careers, and underprivileged women worked longer hours for less pay. By 1990, the decline in the birth rate, the increase in the number of women in the work force, and the increase in the number of elderly persons produced a profound change in the Quebec economy.

COMMUNICATION
Language and culture

The French-Canadian people of Quebec are a linguistic minority in North America and as such fear the eventual loss of their cultural identity. Despite their ongoing efforts to preserve the distinct nature of the French-speaking culture, they are bombarded by pervasive American political and cultural influences exerted through various media, including film, radio, television, magazines, and recordings (Lamonde, 1991).

A Charte des Droits et des Lois was established to protect Quebec's language, culture, and identity (Bills 178, 101, 86, and so forth). These laws established French as Quebec's official language and enabled the French-speaking people to live and prosper. In addition, the laws promote the use of French among newly arrived immigrants and within commercial enterprises and public institutions. Several organizations have been created to monitor and encourage the use of French. The Commission for the Protection of the French Language handles complaints concerning the unavailability of health or social services by French-speaking professionals. Another task of this commission is to handle violations of the French sign law. Another organization, the Office de la Langue Française, administers French competency tests to individuals entering health and other professions, and maintains the quality of the French language.

French

French is the everyday language of most of the people of Quebec and the foundation of their cultural identity. However, maintaining purity of one language is difficult in this era of mass communication when opinions, attitudes, values, and world views are constantly formed, reformed, and influenced by the flood of images, advertisements, and slogans of the mass media (Labrie, 1990). The language brought from the old country was shaped and refined for two centuries from an amalgam of accents and expressions of various regions of France with the assimilation of American Indian words designating places, lakes, flora, and fauna. In speaking this language, the *r*'s can be rolled, and the long vowels, *t*'s, and *d*'s slide into certain vowels with a postconsonantal *s* sound (Tétu de Labsade, 1990).

Normative values of certain prosodic parameters of French-speaking persons have been evaluated to provide acoustic data to assist French-speaking subjects with communication disorders (Le-Dorze, Lever, Ryall, and Brasard, 1995).

With the migration of rural populations to the cities and the common use of English in the workplace a popular level of language often referred to as *joual* [literally 'stock of an anchor'] was created. This type of speech, reserved for oral communication, incorporates English words into a syntax and grammatical system that is essentially French (Hamelin, 1973). The resulting speech patterns are, at times, quite remote from the standard French used by intellectuals, writers, and those in the media. *Joual* belongs, for the most part, to the poorly educated and economically underprivileged class (Tétu de Lab-

sade, 1990.) Some 83% of the population of Quebec are French-speaking descendants of the French (Bailey and Bailey, 1995). English is the language of 12% of the people. Although the English-speaking population has decreased and appears to be decreasing, 30% of the urban population is bilingual, speaking both French and English. Another 35 languages are spoken in the province, including Italian, Greek, Chinese, Native Indian, Inuit, Slavic, Spanish, Chinese, Vietnamese, Persian, and Tamil (Statistics Canada, 1989). These immigrants usually learn French as a second language and frequently learn English as a third language.

COMMUNICATION BEHAVIOR

As the French language evolved in Quebec, so did the behavioral patterns of its speakers. For example, in Quebec there is a tendency to use the familiar pronoun *tu* very soon after a first meeting or being introduced to someone, a habit frowned on in France (Tétu de Labsade, 1990). Native French Quebeckers are warm-hearted people who express their thoughts and opinions openly. They are quite expressive and use their hands for emphasis when speaking. However, they do not use so many nonverbal movements as the Italians, Spaniards, or the continental French. They enjoy social gatherings and celebrating important dates. They have a quick sense of humor and are very resourceful.

With the older and more rural French Quebec population, conversation tends to center on subjects having to do with farm work and day-to-day life. Within the home, discussions take place between women in the kitchen about subjects of mutual concern such as children. Men appear to talk less; however, when they do converse, they prefer speaking to other men in the barn, the garage, the club, or the tavern. Little use is made of the living room of the home except on very special occasions.

Young people of both sexes discuss politics, art, or world events. When they are married and have young children, they tend to associate with others in similar life situations. Family and friends enjoy meals together, but the women soon leave for the kitchen and the men retire to the balcony or another room to watch sports on television.

Women tend to be well aware of feminist concerns and are increasingly vocal concerning issues of status, needed services, and treatment by various government agencies. French Quebec women demand respect and heatedly discuss the right to "freedom of choice" versus the "right to life."

The problem of illiteracy can be found in Quebec among those who have dropped out of school as well as in the immigrants from certain Third-World countries. The problem of illiteracy has become more apparent now that the computer has become a part of daily life. Consequently government efforts to retrain unemployed workers and to help the young workers enter the work force through job development and placement programs are under way.

Implications for nursing care

In Canada as elsewhere the nurse must respect the client's choice of language. This respect is necessary not just to ensure clear communication and out of concern for the individual, but also to meet the requirements of Quebec law. The nurse should be familiar with the popular expressions used to designate parts of the body (such as *passage* equals 'vagina') or certain infections (such as *chaude pisse* equals 'gonorrhea'). A Quebecker will say that if the individual is able to resist illness, this individual is as "strong as an ox" or "able as a bear." However, if illness occurs, an expression such as "weak constitution" is used. If someone faints, they "fall into the apples" or "into the plums" and someone who is unconscious is said to "hit the canvas" or "hit the floor" (Dulong and Bergeron, 1980). When interacting with the older generation, the nurse should avoid using the familiar *tu* form because this is considered to show lack of respect.

The ethnic mosaic that exists in Quebec requires that the nurse be sensitive to the style, mode, and context of the communication patterns of different ethnic groups. For example, although the native Quebecker will not hesitate to ask for a pain medication, the Asian client, who does not manifest pain in the same way, may continue to suffer silently, waiting for someone to bring relief instead of requesting it. Because certain immigrant groups have high rates of illiteracy or are not comfortable with

written information, communication should be tailored to the client's ability to understand.

SPACE
Interpersonal space

In public, Quebeckers tend to avoid physical contact and to maintain a certain physical space. At work they may be in closer contact, but individuals generally attempt to maintain a distance of 18 to 30 inches between themselves and others (Hall, 1966). Among friends and close relations, greater intimacy is permitted: men may pat each other on the back or shake hands when they meet; women of the same family may embrace but seldom walk arm in arm down the street. Normally, physical contact in public is limited to young lovers, between adults and young children, or between adults at emotional or difficult moments when they require support. However, when family members are in public, the norms of interpersonal space are present. Although the kitchen used to be the key area for social interaction, today, social interaction, beyond the immediate family, tends to occur in sidewalk cafes, restaurants, shopping centers, bars, and taverns.

Physical space

Families generally live in apartments, condominiums, single-family dwellings in the suburbs, or single-family dwellings in rural areas. Housing is plentiful in Quebec, and, except in the poorest parts of the inner cities, overcrowding is not a problem. However, some older, poorer, chronically mentally ill or alcoholic persons of French-Canadian descent live in poorly maintained rooming houses. In 1986, 83.8% of French Canadians living in Quebec lived as part of a family, with an average of 3.1 persons, of whom 1.2 were under 25 years of age. The majority of those living alone are women (Shirley and Duchesne, 1989).

In 1901, the rural population of Quebec formed 60% of the total population. However, by 1961 this number had decreased to 25% and continues to decrease. Today the urban population of Quebec totals some 7,366,883 people (Johnson, 1997). Nearly half of the population lives in 0.7% of Quebec. Thus the population is concentrated mainly in Montreal and

Quebec City and in the regions of Sherbrooke, Trois-Rivières, and the St. Lawrence River valley (Thibault, 1989).

Implications for nursing care

French Canadians generally maintain their distance when speaking with other individuals. The nurse should avoid overly familiar attitudes and respect the privacy needs of the client. Some French Canadians tend to be rather modest, particularly when receiving intimate care. It is important for the nurse to remember to draw the bed curtains or use the drawsheet to cover certain parts of the body to maintain the client's sense of dignity.

SOCIAL ORGANIZATION
Family and church

In early colonial days in French Quebec, families were large and stable, and family members felt a sense of belonging. They attached great importance to the traditional values of "the Holy Mother, the Church" and accepted its dominance in health care, education, and population management (Fahmy-Eid and Dumont, 1983). During the period preceding the world wars, rural Quebeckers practiced what was known as the "Revenge of the Cradle." In other words, families had many children to provide additional help with farm work and out of respect for the teachings of the church.

With the advent of the Quiet Revolution of the 1960s, the state assumed responsibility for the Quebec family (health and social resources and services) (Fahmy-Eid and Dumont, 1983). From 1971 to 1976, changes in social and political attitudes, coupled with the introduction of the contraceptive pill, destroyed one of the fundamental values of Quebec society: the role of the family as a generous lifegiver. In the 1970s young Quebec women learned to control their fertility through contraceptives. They no longer accepted the birth of eight or more children. Most wanted only one or two, as they strove for a higher standard of living and a greater degree of personal liberty (Henripin, Huot, Lapierre-Adamcyk, and Marcil-Gratton, 1981). Consequently, during the past 30 years, the family has undergone radical and disruptive changes

(Rapport de la Commission d'Enquête sur les Services de santé et les Services sociaux, 1988).

Evolution of the family

In the past, family roles were well defined. The father was head of the family and responsible for its material well-being. The mother had specific household duties and was caregiver and religious educator. In addition to these duties, rural mothers also had specific farm duties. These roles remained relatively unchanged until women, in great numbers, began to join the work force and to become the heads of single-parent families. Amidst social change, the mother has remained the principal health caregiver in the Quebec family (Thibaudeau and Reidy, 1985). From colonial times through the 1950s, the mother would depend on her eldest daughter, usually unmarried, who shared and later, if necessary, would assume this caregiver role. In her role as natural caregiver, the mother took responsibility for the maintenance of the health of all family members. She instilled and supervised the practice of healthy habits within the family.

With the transition to the new generation of families of the seventies, eighties, and nineties, men and women began to reevaluate their familial roles. However, the new model of family functioning has not evolved smoothly. Often the mother has maintained a double burden, still encumbered with her former tasks while assuming the obligations that come with outside employment. Meanwhile, the two-parent family remains the ideal in Quebec, and the fathers of young children today are beginning to play a larger role in the care of their children and in maintaining their home environment. The increase in the number of single-parent families has brought about the formation of new family units composed of the woman and her children, the man and his children, and ultimately their children.

Statistics confirm the seriousness of the breakup of the nuclear family. In 1985, Quebec had the lowest birth rate in Canada and one of the lowest in the world (Dandurand, 1990; Rapport de la Commission, 1988). Unmarried couples living together represent 10.8% of families (Shirley and Duchesne, 1989). Approximately 40% of Quebeckers over 18 years of age live with a child or adolescent under 18 years of age, many of whom are single parents, making a ratio of approximately one single-parent family per eight families (Rapport de la Commission, 1988). Nearly 80% of single-parent families are headed by women, with over half of them living in poverty (Lazure, 1990).

New models of interdependence

Quebec society has evolved in such a way as to seriously undermine the traditional network of support built around family and relatives, the neighborhood, and various religious institutions (Rapport de la Commission, 1988). However, the changes that have occurred over the last few years have stimulated the creation of new models of interdependence, founded on changing cultural options, emerging lifestyles, or shared problems. This regrouping of individuals and communities into new networks of mutual help or self-help is particularly significant. Community and volunteer organizations have assumed many social functions within Quebec society; they have become essential in providing support to individuals and services to the citizens. These models of informal social support and care are often inspired by needs no longer met by traditional means or by emerging social and health needs (such as those for persons with AIDS).

Aging of the population

Profound demographic changes of the last 20 years leave Quebec with a higher percentage of older citizens and fewer children. The number of persons over 65 years of age is increasing rapidly and now totals more than 650,000 (Rapport de la Commission, 1988). This general aging of the population entails an increase in the number of elderly women in relation to men of the same age and an increase in the number of the "old" old (Rapport de la Commission, 1988). These persons often experience chronic illness and serious financial difficulties.

Youth

Unemployment is one of the most pressing concerns of Quebec's youth. Although the general unemployment rate in Quebec is currently at 12.8%, it is 18.3% for persons 18 to 24 years of age. This untapped work force, in great part untrained for Quebec's increasing technological demands, presents a considerable drain on the province's resources.

Religion

With the British military conquest, the Catholic church became a social and political force defending faith, language, and culture. Until the Quiet Revolution of the sixties, the church was actively involved in financial, educational, and health affairs. In the sixties, however, the Quiet Revolution brought about greater separation of Church and State. At this time, attendance at church declined greatly, and religious affiliations became more diversified (Orr, 1992). By 1981, 132,000 Quebeckers stated they "had no religious preference." Despite the decline in religious influence and practice in Quebec, many individuals continue to conform to a model whereby one not only calls oneself "Catholic" and marks certain important events in life by a church ceremony (baptism, marriage, funeral, and so on), but also continues to support both a school system organized on religious grounds and, in general, Catholic religious instruction in the schools (Laperrière, 1992).

The population of Quebec supports a wide variety of religions, including Catholicism, Protestantism, Judaism, Buddhism, Islam, Sikhism, Hinduism, and Seventh-Day Adventism.

Implications for nursing care

Despite Quebec's complex social problems, the social canvas of the province appears to be held together through the influence of the older generation, sense of family, and sharing and mutual aid between generations.

In working with single-parent families headed by women with limited financial means, the nurse may work with families whose members suffer from a variety of health problems and behavioral or learning difficulties. Problems unique to children often require prolonged interaction with the health and social welfare system and the intervention of several specialists. As the feelings of powerlessness increase among the single mothers of Quebec, their self-confidence is increasingly undermined. The nurse must help the mother understand her situation, participate in the care process, and deal with the health system. With an increase in feelings of confidence as a parent and of self-esteem as an individual, the single mother may be able to function in her role as principal health agent in the family.

Because of economic conditions and widespread poverty, malnutrition and hunger have resurfaced among children. Children may fall asleep at their desks from hunger and from tiredness because of watching television into the early hours of the morning. These children have increased likelihood of suffering from repeated respiratory infections and increased absenteeism.

It is necessary both to develop or reinforce family support networks both for exchange of services and to stimulate a sense of empowerment (that is, to help maintain neighborhoods free from drugs and prostitution). Within the family itself, efforts must be made to improve functioning in health matters, whether improving competencies, direct support, information, and advice or arranging access to resource people. The nurse may also be asked to become an advocate for these families so that they may obtain the social and health services to which they are entitled (Thibaudeau and Reidy, 1985; Thibaudeau, Reidy, d'Amours, and Frappier, 1984).

An aging population and a diminishing national health budget require that more community services be available to enable elderly people to remain in their own homes. "Day" hospitals and centers, staffed by multidisciplinary teams, that offer various social and health services are increasing in numbers. Cossette, Levesque, and Laurin (1995) note that both gender and kinship should be considered with respect to support when assisting French-speaking primary caregivers who provide care for aging and disabled relatives in the home. However, to attain the ultimate goal of health and autonomy of the aged, additional innovative nursing approaches must be created.

The extreme diversification of ethnic and cultural groups concentrated in Quebec's cities constitutes a challenge for the practice of nursing. The nurse must determine cultural attitudes of the client toward health, human reproduction, illness, and health care to be assured of the client's participation in the care. The client and the family caregiver must be included in planning, carrying out, and evaluating health interventions. Adaptation of a health care approach to cultural realities must involve consideration of a variety of factors, including behavioral patterns (verbal and nonverbal), use of health services, types and availability of family and group support networks, cultural attitudes toward health, illness and health services, degrees of assimilation into society, and sociodemographic characteristics (Schoolcraft, 1984).

TIME
Past and present

The people of Quebec tend to attach primary importance to day-to-day affairs and to living in the present (Paquet, 1989). Decisions are often made on a short-term basis; pleasure and sorrow are generally accepted as they occur; life goes on from one day to the next. However, climatic and historic conditions have prompted planning to survive long and cold winters and a context of stability that provides structure for these values and attitudes.

Although time is determined by the flow of the successive seasons for rural populations, urban life is characterized by variations in the relationship of time devoted to work, to family, and to leisure (Pronovost, 1989). For older Quebeckers, time is intimately associated with religion. They envision the future with the hope of life after death. Anniversaries of the death of family members are often celebrated by commemorative masses. However, younger urban Quebec people tend not to follow these traditions because they tend to reject traditional institutions.

Time, for women in modern Quebec society, has taken on a new meaning. Working women assume a variety of roles (wife, mother, professional person). Many children wear a house key around their necks and spend the time between 4 and 6 o'clock alone at home. In such households, mothers are often exhausted when they get home from work and can provide little parental nurturance.

Implications for nursing care

The nurse must consider the present time orientation, often demonstrated by the importance attributed to short-term goals, in interacting with families and individuals and in the approach and content of health education and information. A verbal "contract" between health professional and client often proves advantageous in increasing client self-care and in promoting compliance with prescribed medical regimens. The school nurse must support parents' and teachers' efforts in establishing study periods or activities during the after-school hours for children whose time is unsupervised.

ENVIRONMENTAL CONTROL
Attitudes toward health

The practice of medicine has always held a place of prestige and political power in Quebec. The Quiet Revolution, however, saw changes in nursing care and nursing services. The religious orders, responsible for hospitals and the care of the sick since colonization, began to withdraw their services. Their withdrawal left a vacuum within hospitals that professional nurses often have not seemed to recognize or fill. Consequently, medical dominance within the health system further increased.

The older generation has complete confidence in their doctors for the preservation of life and the restoration of health. With the advent of consumerism, the people of Quebec began to participate more directly in health care decision making. The ideology of the powerful medical establishment is now being questioned by both ordinary citizens and government health administrators (Vail, 1995). The latter have increased responsibilities for health services, particularly with the control of health costs and with encouraging the medical profession to practice a greater degree of efficiency and economy.

In Quebec, having adequate financial resources or at least a regular job is often seen as more important than health itself. In intellectual circles, health is perceived as being in complete possession of one's physical and mental capacities and as a way of improving one's status, professional or otherwise. A global notion of health is found more frequently among the well-to-do, but even here the concept remains abstract (Paquet, 1989).

For financially secure families, health is seen as an ideal state in which illness is absent. These individuals view illness as a slow and insidious degradation of health that occurs over time. In the lower classes, health is defined as the ability to work, to be self-sufficient, and to satisfy primary needs. The disadvantaged often attach less value to a general state of good health than the well-to-do because they tend to seek the satisfaction of immediate needs rather than engage in the pursuit of long-term goals (Paquet, 1989). Illness is seen as accidental, causing a momentary rupture in one's normal state of health, or as a chance stroke of bad luck. The popular French phrase "to catch an illness" supports this perception (Rapport de la Commission, 1988). Religion has greatly encouraged the perception of illness as a necessary evil, brought on by sins committed by the individual, and therefore as a form of divine punishment.

In the last 10 years, various "alternative medicine" approaches have appeared on the Quebec health scene. For some people, alternative forms of medicine have apparently answered a need for therapies that allow for greater control of the bodily functions (Laforest, 1985). Such practices have gained ground in Quebec: 14% of individuals over 18 years of age use alternative treatments (Rapport de la Commission, 1988). However, this relatively low proportion, in relation to international rates, is a partial result of their recent introduction and because they are generally administered in Quebec by nonmedical therapists (Rapport de la Commission, 1988; Renaud, Jutras, and Bouchard, 1987). The usual pattern of behavior is consultation with practitioners of alternative medicine only when ordinary medicine has failed to bring about a cure or to avoid chemically derived treatments. Also consulted are certain individuals with the reputation of having the "gift" of healing or stopping the flow of blood by the laying on of hands (Renaud, Jutras, and Bouchard, 1987). These folk healers and bonesetters are still quite popular in rural areas. They have learned through knowledge passed from generation to generation and are often expert in the massage of strained muscles and ligaments or in the setting of certain bones (Desautels, 1984).

The people of Quebec seek long and prosperous lives, and death is perceived as the ultimate failure.

They usually withdraw from the reality of death and avoid speaking of it. With earlier generations, death was formalized and dealt with by adherence to the symbols and ceremonies of the church and by a strong belief in an afterlife. Today, death is more often treated as taboo because it cannot be mastered or controlled by technology. The inherent repulsiveness of the final agony of death and all the emotions it provokes are concealed from public view because death usually occurs in an institution. Although many hospitals have palliative care units, the practice of caring for the chronically ill at home is increasing.

Physical environment

Problems of pollution and waste management constitute a serious challenge to the environment in terms of costs, contamination, and health. A water-purification program, under way in Quebec since 1981, involves water-processing plants and greater control of industrial waste. Effective pollution control has been estimated between 3.2 and 5 billion dollars per year, or 600 dollars per person per year (Thibault, 1989).

A new partnership is evolving in Quebec between the environment and the people. Not only has the government enacted laws specifying serious penalties in case of infringement, but also public awareness programs concerning recycling, composting, using natural products, cleaning up lakes and rivers, disposing of dangerous household wastes, and so on have been created. Cities, towns, and villages have organized projects for beautifying their settings. In sum, Quebeckers are taking concrete steps to protect their environment and reduce the effects of toxic elements and other pollution on health.

Illness-wellness behavior

Since 1969, when free access to health care was instituted in Quebec, user satisfaction has been at a high level (80%), and heavy use has been made of the health care network (Renaud, Jutras, and Bouchard, 1987). Clients belonging to the middle or upper classes usually consult private doctors, outpatient clinics in hospitals, or community centers. Underprivileged people of Quebec often wait until a physical or psychological crisis occurs before consulting a doctor. When these individuals do seek treatment, it is often at a hospital emergency department. These visits for nonemergency situations often cause crowded conditions in units that should theoretically be reserved for accidents, heart attacks, or other actual emergencies. Distrust of the system plays a particular role in reluctance and hesitancy seen in clients who delay seeking treatment. Many of these individuals will consult family members or close friends as to whether they should see a doctor. In disadvantaged environments, state services are often viewed with distrust as a menace to privacy.

Women in Quebec make greater use of preventive services than men. Women's groups have been formed both for and against abortion and home birth. Women seek favorable work conditions, day-care facilities, and support for health promotion and illness prevention programs. They also tend to pay more attention to symptoms than do men. In addition, women tend to seek treatment in health centers, where they submit to more radical treatments than men in terms of medication, hospitalization, and surgery (Conseil du Statut de la Femme, 1981). Upper-class women engage more often in health-promotion activities such as aerobics, aesthetic treatments, and cosmetic surgery than lower-class women (Chanlat, 1985).

According to Taggart (1983), French Canadians are weak in compliance with medical treatment at all social levels. Some French Canadians will stop medication use and medical consultation as soon as they feel better. When they are admitted to hospitals, French Canadians are generally cooperative clients.

Exercise

The importance of exercise in relation to health and general well-being has been widely recognized (Rapport de la Commission, 1988). The physical condition of the people of Quebec is estimated to be equal or slightly inferior to that of other North American populations (Roy, 1985). Between 40% and 50% are estimated to be quite active, whereas 15% to 20% may be classified as sedentary. Nevertheless, no more than one third of the population engage in a physical exercise to a degree that is potentially beneficial to health. Therefore the Quebec government has inaugurated programs designed to increase public awareness of the importance of exercise on one's overall health.

Married individuals exercise less than unmarried persons, men more than women, and well-educated individuals more than less-educated (Paquet, 1989; Roy, 1985). Sports and health clubs that provide aerobic dance classes and fitness exercises are the privilege of prosperous Quebeckers. In Quebec, ice hockey has the widest appeal for both spectators and participants (Paradis, 1992).

Implications for nursing care

In the larger cities, nurses are likely to encounter clients who are suffering from the harmful effects of polluted air and water or soil contamination. Air pollution is responsible for such problems as asthma, bronchitis, and allergies affecting the skin, eyes, and respiratory systems and is seasonal as well as situational. For example, parents should avoid exposing infants to automobile fumes during the rush hour and should minimize use of possible allergy-producing substances found in rugs and humidifiers in homes in which there are young children, older people, or individuals with symptoms of acquired immunodeficiency. The problem of eliminating symptoms caused by stagnant air and old materials in large buildings or factories also falls within the domain of the nurse concerned with the work environment and the reduction of worker absenteeism.

Hunting and fishing are popular activities in Quebec. However, both of these activities can be detrimental to an individual's health because of the pollution present in freshwater and soil. Therefore, pregnant women should be advised against consuming freshwater fish or game during pregnancy. Even when women are not pregnant, the federal government recommends that fish from contaminated lakes be consumed no more than once a week, to prevent accumulation of PCB (polychlorinated biphenyl) in body tissues. The nurse's role includes participation in awareness campaigns, in short-term and long-term preventive measures, and in research to determine possible interrelation between such aspects as pollution, health, lifestyle, and heredity.

The low level of physical activity observed in members of Quebec's less educated classes should stimulate the community health nurse to participate in educational campaigns in various community sectors. Because women are usually the principal health agents in the family, nursing interventions should be directed toward encouraging their collaboration in fostering healthy living habits.

The nurse should participate in setting up and maintaining programs designed to reduce malnutrition in schools serving underprivileged children. School nurses are in a good position to assess needs and seek ways to foster healthy living habits among children and to act as liaison between parents and teachers.

BIOLOGICAL VARIATIONS
Genetic factors

The various social, economic, and cultural practices of a given population influence the eventual formation of a genetic "pool" that determines the biological characteristics of a community (Bouchard and DeBraekeleer, 1991a). Quebeckers of French origin have a specific genotype inherited from the original group of 5000 colonists. Such phenomena as migrations, successive waves of immigration, family inbreeding, and concentration of certain groups in specific areas have directly contributed to reducing or increasing the frequency of certain genes in the Quebec population. For example, the genetic abnormalities found in the populations of the Saguenay and Charlevoix regions of Quebec represent an important public health problem in these areas. The most striking example is that of muscular dystrophy, a disorder of genetic origin characterized by a progressive increase of muscular debility (Bouchard, 1991). Its worldwide frequency is approximately 1 in 25,000 persons. In the Saguenay region, the frequency is estimated to be 1 in 514 (DeBraekeleer, 1991). Familial hypercholesterolemia has a worldwide frequency of 1 in 500 in the general population; in eastern Quebec its frequency is estimated to be l in 150 (DeBraekeleer, 1991). Familial hypercholesterolemia has probably been the most carefully studied of dominant chromosome abnormalities. The principal complication of this disease is coronary thrombosis in the young adult, which is often fatal (Bouchard and DeBraekeleer, 1991b). Cystic fibrosis is the most common fatal hereditary illness among White French Canadians. Its frequency of 1 in 895 births in the Saguenay region is higher than in most populations. Tay-Sachs disease also seems to occur frequently in Quebec. No treatment has been discovered for this condition, which occurs in infants from 2 to 6 months of age (DeBraekeleer, 1991).

Life expectancy

During the past 30 years, the life expectancy of Quebeckers has increased: women now live, on average, to 80.2 years of age and men to 72.8 years of age (Côté, 1992). However, after 70 years of age a rapid deterioration of quality of life occurs, accompanied by various chronic illnesses associated with aging. It is also important to understand that wide differences in mortalities exist between the sexes, socioprofessional categories, and urban and rural areas of Quebec (Rapport de la Commission, 1988).

The most important cause of death in Quebeckers is heart disease, with cardiac malfunction responsible for 40% of all deaths. Recognized risk factors for heart disease include smoking, hypertension, and hypercholesterolemia. It is estimated that 70% of the population between 18 and 74 years of age have at least one of these risk factors. Poor eating habits and lack of physical exercise compound risk of heart failure (Rapport de la Commission, 1988). A new cause of death appeared in the eighties, and the possibility exists that, by the next century, AIDS may replace heart failure as the primary form of high mortality in Quebec. At present, the second leading cause of death is cancer, accounting for approximately 30% of all deaths. The most typical forms are lung cancer in men and breast cancer in women, the latter occurring especially after 25 years of age (Côté, 1992).

Although Quebec has a very low rate of perinatal and infant mortality (6.9 and 6.3 out of 1000 births respectively), premature birth (weight less than 2500 g) remains a serious health problem, with rates of 5.7 per 1000 in 1980 and 6.6 per 1000 in 1990. Rates for low birth weight are 6.5 per 1000 in 1980 and 5.9 per 1000 in 1990. The unsatisfactory health status of these infants may be the result of lack of resources among very young mothers, unsatisfactory nutrition caused by poverty, and lack of or poorly applied contraceptive practices, particularly among adoles-

cent girls in disadvantaged environments (Côté, 1992).

Premature death among French Canadians has two primary causes: highway accidents and suicide. Trauma and accidents account for 60% of these deaths and are the major causes of death for persons 30 years of age or younger. Each year, there are 60,000 highway accident victims, and 1200 of these victims die from injuries received (Côté, 1992; Rapport de la Commission, 1988). Each year, more than 1000 suicides occur in Quebec. Most suicide attempts and suicidal tendencies occur in persons 15 to 24 years of age. Quebec's suicide rate exceeds that of the United States, Japan, and Sweden (Rapport de la Commission, 1988). Family breakup (divorce, reconstitution of family units, lack of attachment), upheaval of traditional values, social isolation, and the current depressed economic climate contribute to the high suicide rate among these young people.

Susceptibility to disease

Osteoarthritic disorders Because of Quebec's harsh climate and its very low temperatures and high humidity in winter, approximately 19% of the population suffers from some form of osteoarthritic condition, which hampers them in their occupational or personal activities (Pampalon, Gauthier, Raymond, and Beaudry, 1990).

Allergies An estimated 13.3% of the population suffers from one or more allergies. This occurrence is primarily an urban phenomenon caused by smog, pollen, and lack of air circulation in buildings. Women and children are the principal groups affected (Pampalon, Gauthier, Raymond, and Beaudry, 1990).

Sexually and intravenously transmitted diseases Diseases transmitted sexually and through the bloodstream constitute a serious public health problem in Quebec. It is estimated that 12,500 persons annually contract genital herpes (Stében, 1985). Every year in Canada 125,000 cases of *Chlamydia* infection and 50,000 cases of gonorrhea occur (Soumis, 1987). Both are widespread in adolescent girls and adult women. In Quebec, half the cases of these diseases occur in persons 15 to 24 years of age (Côté, 1992; Rapport de la Commission, 1988). The repercussions of these sexually transmitted diseases are particularly critical in relation to feminine reproduction, causing pelvic inflammation, which in turn results in salpingitis, producing infertility (Bryant, 1990; Lavoie-Roux, 1989).

Among Canadian provinces, Quebec currently has the second highest number of cases of AIDS: 2192 cases reported up to 1993. Bisexual and homosexual men 25 to 39 years of age and intravenous drug users account for 89% of all AIDS cases (Côté, 1992). Women infected with HIV and their children infected by vertical transmission constitute a growing group in Quebec. They are concentrated in the Montreal area, and the women contract the disease either from infected male sexual partners or through intravenous drug use.

In Quebec, a person's knowledge about AIDS increases with the degree of education and socioeconomic status. However, the level of knowledge is inferior to that of persons in other Canadian provinces. Women are more knowledgeable than men on this subject (Ornstein, 1989). Unfortunately a commonly held view of AIDS is that it is a problem that concerns only homosexuals and intravenous drug users. The population of Quebec demonstrates a generally negative attitude toward the adoption of preventive behavior patterns such as the use of condoms. In Montreal, 51.6% of adults having occasional partners and 75% having a regular partner report that they never use a condom (Dupras, 1989).

Lévy-Marchal et al. (1995) studied diabetes in relation to evaluated bovine serum albumin (BSA) antibody levels. They concluded that elevated IgC anti-BSA levels are associated with the low incidence of insulin-dependent diabetes mellitus (IDDM) in the French population studied. Thus their results support an immunological role of BSA in diabetic autoimmunity.

Nutritional preferences

For some French Canadians, food constitutes a whole system of meanings. There is a "language of food," which includes how society views eating and how it designates foods into categories of normal and healthy. In addition, there is the personal adaptation that an individual or group makes concerning eating habits. Although socioeconomic and cultural factors influence the way these two concepts function, both must be considered when attempts are made to improve living habits.

From early colonial times, because of the harsh climate, the diet of French Canadians has been rich in starchy foods and fat. The people of Quebec have consistently continued to devote a considerable portion of their family budget to food. Fish has been a favorite food because it is much less costly than red meat. In the sixties and seventies the practice of eating in restaurants became more frequent, and "fast foods" became popular because of their low price and convenience. Unfortunately these foods are rich in fatty substances and salt and poor in fibers and vitamins.

A portion of the population of Quebec is reported to have improved their eating habits over the last 10 years (Rapport de la Commission, 1988). In a study conducted by Renaud, Jutras, and Bouchard (1987), a majority of respondents claimed to have made a particular effort to balance their diets. Although they consume foods with less fat, they still consume too much sugar and too few milk products, fruits, and vegetables. Since the economic recession, there have been experiments such as the "community kitchen," where women buy healthful foods in large quantity. Because of the high cost of living and rampant unemployment, students and people out of work are often undernourished. To combat the problem of undernourishment in schools and in disadvantaged neighborhoods, cafeterias are subsidized by the government, and free milk is regularly distributed.

In Quebec, men are more likely than women to be prone to poor eating habits (Renaud, Jutras, and Bouchard, 1987; Rapport de la Commission, 1988). Women of all ages attempt to control their weight. The perceived social requirement of staying slim, coupled with the burdens of motherhood and outside employment, causes many women to be undernourished and to fall victim to "miracle diets." Given the importance of the relationship between nutrition, the health of newborns and adolescents, and osteoporosis in older women, much remains to be accomplished in the area of proper diets for women. In Quebec, women have a predominant role in the choice and preparation of food. Consequently the way women nourish themselves and their families is of vital importance to the health of the community.

Psychological characteristics

Alcoholism and drug abuse Alcoholism and the abuse of psychotropic and illegal drugs are serious problems in Quebec. More than 6% of Quebeckers over 15 years of age have dependency problems with alcohol, with the highest proportion of drinkers being males 20 to 24 years of age (Côté, 1992; Moisan, 1991). Women have a tendency to abuse antidepressants and sleeping pills. Older people tend to abuse psychotropic drugs, which are often routinely prescribed.

Users of illegal drugs, such as cocaine, crack, and hallucinogenics, are becoming younger and younger. The current drug use curve is different from that of the seventies, when addiction tended to be progressive, beginning with "soft" drugs such as marijuana and ending with "hard" drugs such as heroin. Today's drug users often go right to hard substances and intravenous drugs as they make contact with the world of illegal drugs. However, the use of heroin in Quebec is restrained by its limited availability, even in urban centers.

Smoking is another behavior with an unfavorable effect on health. Although there has been a recent decrease in the number of smokers, approximately 35% of men and 31% of women still smoke. Each year, tobacco use is responsible for 8000 deaths occurring as a result of cardiovascular and respiratory diseases and lung cancer (Lavoie-Roux, 1989; Rapport de la Commission, 1988).

Mental health One member of the Quebec population in five will suffer a mental health problem at some point during his or her life. Women suffer more psychological distress than men and consult health professionals three times more frequently (Gouvernement du Quebec, 1989; Perreault, Légaré, and Boyer, 1988-1989).

Chronic mental illness, deinstitutionalizing, and drug and alcohol abuse problems have combined with the depressed economy to produce a new subpopulation: the homeless. It has been estimated in Montreal that during a 1-year period between 10,000 and 15,000 people have no fixed address and roam the streets. These individuals include adult men and women, young people who have run away from home, and families with young children. Many of these individuals are former psychiatric patients who are no longer taking their medications (Côté, 1992; Lavoie-Roux, 1989).

Implications for nursing care

Regardless of the biological variations, the nurse needs to consider the relationship between social integration, social support, and health. Mortality and morbidity rates, in different cultural communities, are partially determined by the degree of an individual's integration into a society and the social support supplied by the community. Social support has a preventive value if it is associated with networks that are stable, homogeneous, and dense and that provide for a variety of links between individuals (Bozzini and Tessier, 1985).

Given the ethnic variety in Quebec society, the nurse should include the following three differentiating factors in health care assessment. First, note should be made of the meaning of health and illness in terms of the underlying significance of these concepts in the cultural group. Second, consideration must be given to the social class of the individual requiring care. Descriptions of symptoms, compliance with treatment, and reaction to pain will differ according to social level and ethnic origin. Third, the client's gender must be considered because gender influences how individuals view their bodies and the adoption of dependent or independent behavior patterns with regard to health (Dorvil, 1985). These three factors have a dominant influence on one's representation of illness. French-Canadian people tend to adopt terms of reference of one of the various subcultural groups (French-speaking, English-speaking, and so on) as the "dominant," or reference, group in the creation of these representations. These terms influence the way the clients explain their illness and participate in care and the degree to which they comply when following the advice of health professionals.

Bellevance and Perreault (1995) interviewed eight French-Canadian gay men living with AIDS in Quebec and noted that Herzlich's framework of health and illness as socially constructed concepts can be used to assist individuals with AIDS to make behavioral changes that will generate health throughout the course of the illness.

Perinatal, physical, and mental health services for women exposed to venereal disease should be promoted in parallel with preventive and health programs. These programs should be designed to educate the public considering the dangers of sexually transmitted diseases, especially AIDS, and the part played by illegal drugs in the transmission process. Nurses are also subject to the influence of these fears and prejudices. However, nurses need to maintain open, nonjudgmental attitudes in their interactions with clients suffering from AIDS (Taggart, Reidy, and Grenier, 1992).

The particular mortality and morbidity curves occurring in the Quebec population, combined with severe budget limitations placed on health services, call for the creation of new approaches in the care of those affected by illness. Target populations include those who suffer from chronic illnesses or are infected by viruses (as in AIDS) or other agents (as in tuberculosis). The evolution of these latter illnesses follows a pattern in which brief hospitalizations occur periodically, followed by long periods of time when the client must learn to function at home within the limits imposed by the condition. As the periods of allowed hospitalization become shorter, nurses must develop home care approaches facilitating the participation of the client's family caregiver. The participation of client and caregiver enables individuals to make those decisions that will maintain quality of life at an acceptable level.

With the aging of the population and the subsequent increase in the incidence of chronic illnesses has come an intensification in the use of various drugs and medicines in the community. It is the nurse's responsibility to help clients maintain their medical regimen and to inform them about the dangers of uncontrolled and irrational use of prescription or nonprescription drugs, of accidental or intentional intoxication, of teratogenic and iatrogenic effects, and of physical and psychological dependency. It is also important for the Canadian nurse to be active in administrative boards that play a strategic role in making decisions about health and social service establishments. The public-centered approach is at the heart of health and social service reform in Quebec. Nursing input is being welcomed as new public policy is being designed (Trudel, 1995). Additionally, Dumas, Plouffe, Boutin, and Desaulniers (1995) describe the important role the nurse can serve in providing interdisciplinary care.

SUMMARY

The people of Quebec have a long, colorful past. It is essential for the nurse to remember that the people of Quebec represent a multicultural, heterogeneous, pluralistic society. Thus the illness or wellness behaviors of these people are difficult to characterize as unique to a specific cultural group. To understand the cultural significance of behaviors noted among Quebec people, it is essential that the nurse develop an understanding of the different cultural, ethnic, and racial groups that blend to make Quebec society.

Case Study

Marguerite Tremblay (born McNeill) married in 1929 at 16 years of age. Her husband, Théophile Tremblay, worked at a farm in the Laurentians. They were for the most part self-sufficient, with cows, a few sheep, and a market garden. They traded for certain goods and had a small cash crop. life was hard, with a day that began before dawn and continued until bedtime.

In 1960, at the death of Théophile, the eldest son, Étienne, took over running the family farm, where he had continued to live with his wife, Estelle, and their children. Several years later, the land was expropriated to make room for a highway. The family, now composed of Mrs. Tremblay, Rose (her unmarried daughter), and Étienne and his children, moved to a small farm property in Ste-Rose. Mrs. Tremblay, with the help of Rose, raised Étienne's children, after their mother died in childbirth.

Mrs. Tremblay, a good Catholic and farm wife, had 15 children between 1930 and 1956, eight of whom survived to maturity (see Fig. 8-1). Two of these children were born dead, two died after premature births, one died of meningitis, one died of polio, and one did not survive a hard winter. One son died in an automobile accident, when he was drinking, at 18 years of age.

The life situation of the surviving family members demonstrates how the family structure and religious practices have changed within the life span of one family.

Rose

age 63; unmarried; lives with mother; suffers from obesity, diabetes, and osteoporosis; attends church and receives the sacraments regularly.

Étienne

age 62; widower; farmer and truck driver; father of seven children, five of whom survived to maturity, all of whom have left home; suffers from severe arthritis.

Philippe

age 59; notary; father of six children, five of whom lived to maturity; smoker; suffers from hypertension and hypercholesterolemia; wife has recovered from breast cancer.

Line

age 56; married a farmer; worked as a volunteer for the parish church; mother of four children, all of whom survived to maturity.

Victor

age 55; missionary in Africa; smoker; suffers from certain chronic parasitical infections.

Marie-Madeleine

age 45; was a nun in a nursing order; after leaving the convent, has worked with adolescents with drug problems; does not practice her religion.

Catherine

age 43; former teacher; divorced from a doctor; mother of two children; suffers from chronic anxiety and mild abuse of tranquilizers; has become a Christian Scientist.

Denise

age 34; former commercial artist; unmarried; mother of one child whose father, an actor, died of AIDS; mother and child HIV positive; activist in AIDS self-help group; very interested in spiritual renewal but refuses her mother's pleas to return to the church.

Mrs. Tremblay has remained active and involved in the life of her children and grandchildren. At 80 years of age, she suffered a cerebrovascular accident that left her with left-sided hemiplegia. She has made only moderate recovery. She requires help with transfer but can stand with a walker. She requires help with many activities of daily living and spends much of her time in a wheelchair. She speaks slowly but is lucid, if somewhat anxious.

She has been admitted to a long-term care unit because of her physical limitations and her immediate family's inability to care for her at home. She alternates between understanding the need for long-term care and the fear that her family no longer needs her. Her family, particularly her eldest son and daughter, with whom she lived, feel guilty and fear that they are not doing their "duty," despite their own health problems and physical limitations.

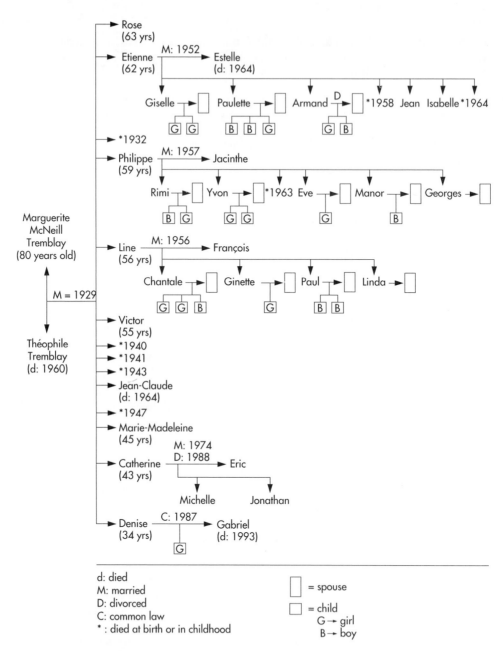

Figure 8-1 The Tremblay family tree. (From Giger, J.N.: [1995] *Transcultural nursing* [ed.2]. St. Louis: Mosby.)

CARE PLAN

 Nursing Diagnosis   Anxiety, related to situational crises (Adapted from Sparks and Taylor, 1993, p. 41).

Client Outcomes

1. Client will identify the factors in the situation that provoke anxiety (such as strange room, room shared with other resident).
2. Client will identify those activities, feasible in the new situation, that have helped her relax in the past.
3. Client will begin to accept the limits imposed by stroke and to control the anxiety provoked by life in a long-term care setting.

Nursing Interventions

1. Take the time, daily, to talk personally with client in an informal setting such as the lounge or kitchen.
2. When talking about client's stroke, as much as possible, use the language and words she uses. Verify client's comprehension of new or technical language.
3. Use the techniques of reminiscence therapy to remind client of past strategies for dealing with anxiety.
4. Identify those strategies appropriate to new environment that have previously helped control anxiety.

 Nursing Diagnosis   Powerlessness, related to the health care environment (Adapted from Sparks and Taylor, 1993, p. 221).

Client Outcomes

1. Client will understand and express her feelings of powerlessness.
2. Client will understand that her powerlessness is not universal.
3. Client will identify factors she can learn to control in the current situation.
4. Client will succeed in learning to control these factors.
5. Client will learn to use her interpersonal skills to exercise some control over her social environment.

Nursing Interventions

1. Help client arrange her room and equipment such as telephone, radio, call-bell so that she is comfortable in using them.
2. Arrange with client's family to have a telephone with memory for frequently called numbers and remote control for television (both with "user friendly" boards).
3. Develop with client daily routine that incorporates, as much as possible, strategies that give client control in current situation.
4. Develop with the client a prosthetic and secure environment where she compensates for her physical limits and maintains some control on her physical environment.
5. Encourage client to participate in social and recreational activities such as group singing and bingo.
6. Encourage client's interest and sense of responsibility in building the morale of other residents whom she seems to like.

 Nursing Diagnosis   Role performance, altered, related to ineffective coping (Adapted from Sparks and Taylor, 1993, p. 515).

Client Outcomes

1. Client will maintain and strengthen those aspects of her former social and familial roles that are possible within the current situation.
2. Client will identify, with the participation of her family, modified social roles within the family.
3. Client will identify a role, within the long-term unit, that she considers as her limit but makes use of her abilities and the prosthetic environment.

Nursing Interventions

1. Encourage the client to express her feelings and wishes concerning the roles she would like to play and the activities she would like to do.
2. Help client's daughter to aid the client to explore the sustainable aspects of her former roles and to develop new roles within the family.
3. Help the client to understand and play her role in maintaining effective interrelationships between the generations of her family.
4. Develop a "caring" relationship with the client and explore with her the relationships she can develop and the roles she can play in interacting with other staff members, volunteers, and other residents.

Nursing Diagnosis Self-esteem, situational low, related to hospitalization and forced dependence on health care team (Adapted from Sparks and Taylor, 1993, p. 515).

Client Outcomes	*Nursing Interventions*

Client Outcomes

1. Client will express opinions and her preferences to both staff and family.
2. Client will participate in the various aspects of her care process (such as decision making, physical care, assessment).
3. Client will experience and express, through her body language, an increase in self-esteem.

Nursing Interventions

1. Address the client by her name, Madame Tremblay, never "Mama" or other diminutives.
2. Respect the client's privacy and her physical space and go slowly in manifesting a physical display of affection. Permit client to set the parameters of her social space.
3. Listen to the client, encourage her to use "I" in her conversation, respect her opinion, encourage her to make decisions, and respect these decisions.
4. Encourage the family to help client maintain her personal appearance by providing clothes that fit and are attractive, personal grooming equipment, and the like. Compliment her on any improvements in appearance.
5. Work with occupational and physiotherapy personnel to develop appropriate but practical and worthwhile projects (such as weaving, food preparation).

 Nursing Diagnosis Sensory or perceptual alteration (kinesthetic), related to sensory reception, transmission, or integration (Adapted from Sparks and Taylor, 1993, p. 256).

Client Outcomes

1. Client will understand the relationship between her neurological pathological condition ("stroke") and the sensory and perceptual changes she has experienced.
2. Client will begin to compensate for inability to identify position of body parts by developing other senses (sight, sensations of unaffected members, and so on).
3. Client will learn to master prosthetic aids to compensate for diminished motor coordination.
4. Client will understand the importance of practicing preventive and safety measures (such as skin care and proper shoes).

Nursing Interventions

1. Validate with the client that she understands the effect of the "stroke" on her ability to function and that she realizes that certain false perceptions can occur because of this condition.
2. Work with the client so that she learns to use her "good" hand routinely and to use visual inspection to verify the position and location of her affected limbs.
3. Develop with the client compensatory routines such as turning her head to improve her visual field or repositioning items in her physical environment.
4. Show the client how to inspect her skin for pressure points and help her develop a routine for turning and relieving these pressure points.

 Nursing Diagnosis Coping, ineffective family, related to caring for dependent, aging family member (Adapted from Sparks and Taylor, 1993, p. 496).

Client Outcomes

1. Family will improve communications leading to clarification of needs and expectations and to evolution of the roles of family members.
2. Family will maintain and strengthen those aspects of existing family roles appropriate to the current situation.
3. Family will develop appropriate involvement of all family members in the client's current situation (such as involvement that encourages both affiliation and autonomy).
4. Family will mutually accept new roles of the client and the principal caregiver in the family.
5. Family will experience reduction in destructive feelings, such as guilt, on the part of family members.

Nursing Interventions

1. Clarify with the daughter the mutual affiliative role of mother and daughter.
2. Clarify with the daughter, in terms of her limits and abilities, her new role as principal health care giver in the family, emphasizing the essential nature of this new role.
3. Clarify with family members (especially the eldest son) the importance of visits, family celebrations, development of relationships with grandchildren, and keeping client informed of family events.
4. Include the daughter in the planning of the client's care.
5. Encourage family members to develop joint family projects such as a family photo album.

References

Anctil, H., & Bluteau, M.A. (1986). *La santé et l'assistance publique au Québec, 1886-1986* [Quebec health and social welfare, 1886-1986]. Québec: Ministère de la Santé et des Services sociaux, Direction des communications.

Audet, L.P., & Gauthier, A. (1967). *Le système scolaire du Québec: organisation et fonctionnement* [Quebec educational system: structure and function]. Montréal: Librairie Beauchemin Limitée.

Authier, P. (1993). New rules allow bilingual signs for all stores. *The Montreal Gazette, A3,* (June 15).

Bailey, E., & Bailey, R. (1995). *Discover Canada.* Oxford, England: Berlitz Publishing Company, Ltd.

Bellavance, M., & Perreault, M. (1995). AIDS, health and illness and socially constructed concepts in gay Quebecois men living with AIDS. *Canadian Journal of Nursing Research, 27*(1), 57-75.

Bouchard, G. (1992). Sur les perspectives de la culture québécoise comme francophonie nord-américaine [On the perspectives of Quebec culture as a French-speaking community in North America]. In Lanthier, P., & Rousseau, G. (Eds.), *La culture inventée, stratégies culturelles aux XIXe et XXe siècles.* [Cultural tendencies and cultural strategies of the nineteenth and twentieth centuries] (pp. 319-328). Québec: Institut Québécois de Recherche sur la Culture.

Bouchard, G. (1991). Pour une approche historique et sociale du génome québécois [Historical and social approach to the Quebec genome]. In Bouchard, G., & DeBraekeleer, M. (Eds.), *Histoire d'un génome: population et génétique dans l'Est du Québec* [History of a genome: population and genetics in eastern Quebec] (pp. 3-18). Québec: Les Presses de l'Université de Québec.

Bouchard, G., & DeBraekeleer, M. (Eds.). (1991a). *Histoire d'un génome: population et génétique dans l'Est du Québec* [History of a genome: population and genetics in Eastern Quebec]. Québec: Les Presses de l'Université du Québec.

Bouchard, G., & DeBraekeleer, M. (1991b). Mouvements migratoires, effets fondateurs et homogénéisation génétique [Migratory shifts, founder effects, and genetic homogenization]. In Bouchard, G., & DeBraekeleer, M. (Eds.), *Histoire d'un génome: population et génétique dans l'Est du Québec* [History of a genome: population and genetics in eastern Quebec] (pp. 281-321). Québec: Les Presses de l'Université de Québec.

Bozzini, L., & Tessier, R. (1985). Support social et santé. [Social support and health]. In Dufresne, J., Dumont, F., & Martin, Y. (Eds.), *Traité d'anthropologie médicale.* [Medical anthropology treatise] (pp. 905-939). Québec: Les Presses de l'Université du Québec.

Bryant, H. (1990). *L'infertilité à l'heure de la procréatique . . . et la prévention?* [Infertility in the age of artificial reproduction . . . and prevention?]. Ottawa: Conseil consultatif canadien sur la situation de la femme.

Chanlat, J.F. (1985). Types de sociétés, types de morbidités: la socio-génèse des maladies [Types of societies, types of morbidities: socio-genesis of illness]. In Dufresne, J., Dumont, F., & Martin, Y. (Eds.), *Traité d'anthropologie médicale* [Medical anthropology treatise] (pp. 293-304). Québec: Les Presses de l'Université du Québec.

Conseil du Statut de la Femme. (1981). *Pour les Québécoises: egalité et indépendance* [For the women of Quebec: equality and independence]. Québec: Éditeur officiel.

Cossette, S., Lévesque, L., & Laurin, L. (1995). Informal and formal support for caregivers of a demented relative: do gender and kinship make a difference? *Research in Nursing and Health, 18*(5): 437-451.

Côté, M.Y. (1992). *La politique de la santé et du bien-être* [Health and welfare policy]. Québec: le Ministère.

Dandurand, R.B. (1990). Peut-on encore définir la famille? [Can we still define the family?]. In Dumont, F. (Ed.), *La société québécoise après 30 ans de changements* [Quebec society after 30 years of change] (pp. 49-66). Québec: Institut Québécois de Recherche sur la Culture.

DeBraekeleer, M. (1991). Les gènes délétères [Deleterious genes]. In Bouchard, G., & DeBraekeleer, M. (Eds.), *Histoire d'un Génome: Population et génétique dans l'Est du Québec* [History of a genome: population and genetics in eastern Quebec] (pp. 343-363). Québec: Presses de l'Université de Québec.

Desautels, Y. (1984). *Les coutumes de nos ancêtres* [Customs of our ancestors]. Montréal: Édition Paulines.

Dorvil, H. (1985). Types de sociétés et représentations. [Types of societies and representations]. In Dufresne, J., Dumont, F., & Martin, Y. (Eds.), *Traité d'anthropologie médicale* [Medical anthropology treatise]. Québec: Les Presses de l'Université du Québec.

Dulong, G., & Bergeron, G. (1980). Le parler populaire du Québec et de ses régions voisines [Popular language of Quebec and its neighboring regions]. *La documentaion québécoise, 8*, 3124-3655.

Dumas, L., Plouffe, M., Boutin, D., & Desaulniers, M. (1995). University and community service center (CLSC) and collaboration. *The Canadian Nurse, 91*(8), 45-49.

Dupras, A. (1989). *La sexualité des montréalais et le sida* [Sexuality of Montrealers and AIDS]. Longueuil: Éditions IRIS.

Fahmy-Eid, N., & Dumont, M. (1983). *Maîtresses de maison, maîtresses d'écoles: femmes, familles et éducation dans l'histoire du Québec* [Housewifes, school mistresses: women, families, and education in Quebec history]. Montréal: Boréal Express.

Gagnon, S. (1992). L'École élémentaire québécoise au XIXe siècle [Quebec elementary school in the nineteenth century]. In Lanthier, P., & Rousseau, G. (Eds.), *La culture inventée, stratégies culturelles aux XIXe et XXe siècles* [Cultural tendencies and cultural strategies of the nineteenth and twentieth centuries] (pp. 135-153). Québec: Institut Québécois de Recherche sur la Culture.

Gouvernement du Québec. (1989). *Politique de santé mentale* [Mental health policy]. Québec: le Ministère.

Hall, E.T. (1966). *The hidden dimension.* New York: Doubleday & Co., Inc.

Henripin, J., Huot, P.M., Lapierre-Adamcyk, E., & Marcil-Gratton, N. (1981). *Les enfants qu'on n'a plus au Québec* [Children that we no longer have in Quebec]. Montréal: Les Presses de l'Université de Montréal.

Johnson, O. (Ed.). (1997). *Information please almanac.* Boston & New York: Houghton Mifflin Company.

Laberge, H. (1992). Culture nationale et cultures ethniques: l'interculturalisme à la québécoise [National and ethnic cultures: interculturalism in Quebec]. *Action Nationale, 82*(7), 897-906.

Labrie, N. (1990). La question linguistique et les communautés culturelles au Québec [Quebec linguistic issue and cultural communities]. In Guilbert, L. (Ed.), *Identité ethnique et interculturalité: état de la recherche en ethnologie et en socio-linguistique.* [Ethnic identity and interculture: state of research in ethnology and in sociolinguistics] (pp. 33-46). Sainte-Foy: CELAT (Centre d'Études sur la Langue, les Arts, et les Traditions populaires des Francophones en Amérique du Nord), Université de laval.

Lacroix, B., & Simard, J. (1984). Religion populaire, religion de clercs [Popular religion and clergymen]. Collection: *Culture populaire,* No. 2. Québec: Institut Québécois de Recherche sur la Culture.

Laforest, L. (1985). Pratiques médicales et évolution sociale [Medical practices and social evolution]. In Dufresne, J., Dumont, F., & Martin, Y. (Eds.), *Traité d'anthropologie médicale* [Medical anthropology treatise] (pp. 267-280). Québec: Les Presses de l'Université du Québec.

Lamonde, Y. (1991). *Territoires de la culture québécoise* [Quebec cultural territories]. Québec: Les Presses de l'Université de laval.

Langlois, S. (1992). Niveaux de vie et consommation de 1960 à 1990 [Standards of living and consumption from 1960 to 1990]. In Lanthier, P., & Rousseau, G. (Eds.), *La culture inventée, stratégies culturelles aux XIXe et XXe siècles* [Cultural tendencies and cultural strategies of the nineteenth and twentieth centuries] (pp. 303-316). Québec: Institut Québécois de Recherche sur la Culture.

Lanthier, P., & Rousseau, G. (Eds.). (1992). *La culture inventée, stratégies culturelles aux XIXe et XXe siècles* [Cultural tendencies and cultural strategies of the nineteenth and twentieth centuries). Québec: Institut Québécois de Recherche sur la Culture.

Laperrière, G. (1992). La place du catholicisme [The place of Catholicism]. Dossier: Catholicisme et société distincte [Catholicism and distinct society]. *Présence, 2*(5), 21-23.

Lavoie-Roux, T. (1989). *Pour améliorer la santé et le bien-être au Québec: orientations* [Improving health and well-being in Quebec: orientations]. Québec: le Ministère.

Lazure, J. (1990). Mouvance des générations. Condition féminine et masculine [Generational sphere of influence. Female and male status]. In Dumont, F. (Ed.), *La société québécoise après 30 ans de changements* [Quebec Society after 30 years of change] (pp. 27-40). Québec: Institut Québécois de Recherche sur la Culture.

Le-Dorze, G., Lever, N., Ryalls, J., & Brassard, C. (1995). Normative values of certain prosodic parameters obtained with French-speaking persons without a communication disorder. *Folia Phoniatrica et logopaedica, 47*(1), 39-47.

Lévy-Marchal, C., Karjalainen, J., Dubois, F., Karges, W., Czernichow, P., & Dosch, H. (1995). Antibodies against bovine albumin and other diabetes markers in French children. *Diabetes Care, 18*(8), 1089-1094.

Moisan, C. (1991). *Portrait de la consommation d'alcool et de drogues au Québec: principales données de l'enquête nationale sur l'alcool et les autres drogues* [Portrait of alcohol and drug consumption in Quebec: principal data of the national survey on alcohol and other drugs]. Collection: Données statistiques et Indicateurs. Québec: Ministère de la Santé et des Services sociaux.

Ntetu, A., & Fortin, J. (1996). Reconsidering nursing interventions among Native people. *The Canadian Nurse, 92*(3), 42-46.

Ornstein, M. (1989). *AIDS in Canada: knowledge, behavior and attitudes of adults.* Ontario: Institute for Social Research, York University.

Orr, R. (1992). Notre héritage catholique. [Our Catholic heritage]. Translated by Serge Gagnon. Dossier: Catholicisme et société distincte [Catholicism and distinct society]. *Présence, 1*(5), 11-13.

Pampalon, R., Gauthier, D., Raymond, G., & Beaudry, D. (1990). *La santé à la carte: une exploration géographique de l'Enquête Santé Québec* [Health map: a geographic exploration of the Quebec Health Survey]. Québec: Ministère de la Santé et des Services sociaux.

Paquet, G. (1989). *Santé et inégalité sociales: un problème de distance culturelle* [Health and social inequality: Cultural gap]. Québec: Institut Québécois de Recherche sur la Culture.

Paradis, J.M. (1992). La pratique du sport en Mauricie: du fair play britannique à la compétition nord-américaine. [Sport practices in Mauricie: British fair play in North American Competition]. In Lanthier, P., & Rousseau, G. (Eds.), *La culture inventée, stratégies culturelles aux XIXe et XXe siècles* [Cultural tendencies and cultural strategies of the nineteenth and twentieth centuries] (pp. 87-97). Québec: Institut Québécois de Recherche sur la Culture.

Perreault, C., Légaré, G., & Boyer, R. (1988-1989). La santté mentale des Québécois [Mental health of Quebeckers]. *Santé et Société, 2*(1), 50-53.

Pronovost, G. (1989). Les transformations des rapports entre le temps de travail et le temps libre [Transformation in work time and leisure time]. In Pronovost, G., & Mercure, D.(Eds.), *Temps et sociétés* [Time and societies] (pp. 37-61). Québec: Institut Québécois de Recherche sur la Culture.

Rapport de la Commission d'Enquête sur les Services de santté et les Services sociaux. (1988). *Commission d'Enquête sur les Services de santé et les Services sociaux* [Inquiry commission on Health and Social Services]. Québec: Les Publications du Québec.

Renaud, M., Jutras, S., & Bouchard, P. (1987). *Les solutions qu'apportent les québécois à leurs problèmes sociaux et sanitaires* [Solutions brought forth by Quebeckers concerning social and health problems]. In *Commission d'Enquête sur les Services de santé et les Services sociaux.* [Inquiry Commission on Health and Social Services]. Québec: Les Publications du Québec.

Rioux, M. (1974). *Les québécois* [The Quebeckers]. Paris: Seuil.

Roy, L. (1985). *Le point sur les habitudes de vies: l'activité physique* [Focusing on health patterns: physical activity]. Québec: Gouvernement du Québec.

Schoolcraft, V. (1984). *Nursing in the community.* Toronto: Wiley & Sons.

Shirley, J., & Duchesne, L. (1989). Population et ménage [Population and household]. In Asselin, R. (Ed.), *Le Québec statistique 1989* [1989 Quebec's statistic] (ed. 59) (pp. 293-323). Québec: Les Publications du Québec.

Soumis, L. (1987, August). La guerre aux MTS et au sida [The war on STD and AIDS]. Commercial: radio-Canada refuse diffuser les messages au Québec. *Le Devoir, 1*(25).

Sparks, S.M., & Taylor, C.M. (1993). *Nursing diagnosis reference manual: an indispensable guide to better patient care* (ed. 2). Pennsylvania: Springhouse Corporation.

Statistics Canada. (1991). *Statistics Canada, 1991 census: metropolitan areas.* Ottawa: Ministre des Approvisionnements et Services, Canada.

Statistiques Canada. (1989). *Annuaire du Canada 1990* [1990 Canadian annual]. Ottawa: Ministre des Approvisionnements et Services Canada.

Statistiques Canada. (1996). *Annuaire du Canada 1996* [1996 Canadian annual]. Ottawa: Ministre des Approvisionnements et Services Canada.

Steben, M. (1985). Les maladies transmises sexuellement: l'épidémie catastrophique [Sexual transmitted diseases: a catastrophic epidemic]. In Dupras, A., & Lévy, J.J. (Eds.), *La sexualité au Québec: perspectives contemporaines* [Sexuality in Quebec: contemporary perspectives]. Longueuil: Éditions IRIS.

Taggart, M.E. (1983). *Acquisition de connaissances et de comportements chez les primipares à la suite de deux types de programmes èducatifs postnatals* [Acquisition of knowledge and behaviors in primiparas after two types of postnatal educational programs]. Montréal: Universitté de Montréal. Doctoral thesis in education (not published).

Taggart, M.E., Reidy, M., & Grenier, D. (1992). Attitudes d'infirmières francophones face au sida [French-speaking nurses' attitudes towards AIDS]. *Infirmière canadienne/Canadian Nurse, 88*(1), 48-52.

Tétu de Labsade, F. (1990). *Le Québec: un pays, une culture* [Quebec: a country, a culture]. Montréal: Boréal Express.

Thibaudeau, M.F., & Reidy, M. (1985). A nursing care model for the disadvantaged family. In Stewart, M. (Ed.), *Community health nursing in Canada* (pp. 269-286). Toronto: Gage Publishing Co.

Thibaudeau, M.F., Reidy, M., d'Amours, F., & Frappier, G. (1984). *La santé de la famille défavorisée: évaluation de l'application d'un modèle de soins infirmiers auprès de familles défavorisées qui utilisent les services du CLSC* [Health of the disadvantaged family: assessment of the application of a nursing care model in disadvantaged families using community health clinics]. Montréal: Faculté des Sciences infirmières, Université de Montréal.

Thibault, M.T. (1989). Environnement [Environment]. In Asselin, R. (Ed.), *Le Québec statistique 1989* [1989 Quebec statistics] (ed. 59) (pp. 261-291). Québec: Les Publications du Québec.

Trudel, A. (1995). Nurses as members of administrative boards. *The Canadian Nurse, 91*(5), 37-40.

Vail, S. (1995). Rationing health care. *Canadian Nurse, 90*(60), 59-60.

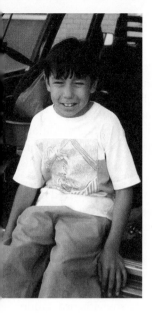

CHAPTER 9
The Cree Living in Urban Settings

Olive Yonge and Mardi Bernard

BEHAVIORAL OBJECTIVES

After reading this chapter, the nurse will be able to:

1. Describe the communication patterns of Cree Indians living in inner-city settings in Canada.
2. Describe the adjustment the Cree have had to make in going from a nomadic lifestyle to the restricted life on the reserves.
3. Describe the social organization of the Cree into clans and how this had changed as the Cree are moving to the inner city.
4. Explain the effect of the present-time orientation of many Cree in relation to preventive health care.
5. Relate the traditional orientation of the Cree to control by the Great Spirit as well as the need to stay in harmony with the environment.
6. Describe biological variations that have been identified among the Cree.

HISTORIC ORIGIN OF THE CREE

The Cree are a subarctic group whose name is derived from the name of specific Indian bands in the region between Lake Superior and Hudson Bay, known to the early French explorers, as "Kristino" (of uncertain original meaning). The name was later shortened to "Cree" and was associated with Indians who spoke the language described by the Europeans as Cree (Levinson, 1991). Each Cree band has a regional designation by which it is known including names such as "Rainy River" or "Rocky Bay" (Levinson, 1991). The first reference to the Cree in the literature is in a Jesuit account describing an interaction in 1640 with the Kiristinon, who lived on the shores of the North Sea (James Bay) (Thwaites,

1901). Little is known about the distribution of the Cree-speaking natives at the time the Europeans arrived in Canada. However, the literature indicates that they seem to have occupied lands surrounding James Bay, the western shores of Hudson Bay, and north to the Churchill River (McMillan, 1988). They also occupied lands extending as far as Lake Winnipeg to the west and Lake Nipigon to the south. Seventeenth-century accounts indicate that they frequently visited the northern shores of Lake Superior, and on several occasions they were reported to be fishing at Sault Saint Marie as guests of the Ojibwa (McMillan, 1988).

In response to the opportunity to trade firearms for fur with the Europeans on Hudson Bay, some of the Cree living in the east expanded far to the west, eventually occupying southern portions of the western Subarctic as far as the Peace River of Alberta. Some moved out into the plains, allying with the Assiniboine against their enemies and adapting their culture to become Plains warriors and bison hunters. By the early nineteenth century, the Cree occupied the largest geographic extent of any Canadian native group, reaching from Labrador to the Rockies (Wright, 1971; Tanner, 1979; Rogers, 1973; Rogers, 1963; Feit, 1986; Preston, 1975; Dewdney, 1978). However, although the fur trade caused a relocation for some Cree, La Vérendrye traveling in Manitoba in 1730 reported that some bands of Cree were already established in the plains, prairies, and mountains, and existed before the movement west by Cree armed with European weapons obtained in trade on Hudson Bay (McMillan, 1988). However, the Cree were seriously affected by a smallpox epidemic in 1781, and later they would also be affected by other European-introduced diseases to which they had no immunity (Levinson, 1991).

Historically, the primary source of food staples for many Crees living in the subarctic region of Canada was caribou, moose, bear, beaver, and fish. Although berries were available in the summer, plant foods played a less valued role in their diet. In contrast to subarctic Crees, Crees who lived in the plains consumed bison as their primary sustenance. Bison was not only an important food staple, but it also provided hides for shelter and clothing. In addition, various implements were fashioned from the bones and horns of bison, and dried dung served as fuel on the treeless plains. In addition to bison, antelope, mule deer, elk, prairie chicken, and a variety of edible plants including wild turnips and berries helped vary the diet (McMillan, 1988).

The arrival of the horse, acquired from Spanish settlements in the Southwest, was a feature of southern plains life as early as 1640. Within a generation, the Plains Indians had become master horsemen, which enabled raiding for the accumulation of wealth because transportation of possessions was now possible, and it also increased interactions with others (Dempsey, 1986; Corrigan, 1970; Wissler, 1914; Vickers, 1986). Many Plains tribes preferred

bows and arrows over the traders' guns, which were not only difficult to load on the scared animals but contributed significantly to further frightening these animals because of their noise (Dyck, 1977).

The Plains Crees had many unique traditions such as painting. In fact, many everyday items were embellished with painting. Tipi covers and shields commonly bore depictions of bison or other images arising from visions. The Plains Cree preferred floral motifs over geometric designs and used floral patterns in beadwork (Fisher, 1986; Mandelbaum, 1979).

The Plains Cree had a single society to which men gained entry by a valorous deed. The societies kept order in the camp and on the hunt and guarded against enemy attack. Rituals strengthened group solidarity and fostered a pride in military prowess.

Religion permeated everyday life for the Plains Cree (Ahenakew, 1973). Some Cree believed that the universe was filled with supernatural beings with power to harm or to help. Manifestations of spiritual power could be seen in nature or could come in a vision. Sacred objects, which often represented a gift from a supernatural encounter, were carefully wrapped in a medicine bundle. Contents could include skins from various animals, eagle feathers, braided sweetgrass used for incense, fossils, or supernaturally charged stones. Sacred pipestems were of particular importance because smoking was a method of communicating with the supernatural. The most important religious festival of the Plains tribes was the "thirsting dance." This festival was held during the summer when large encampments assembled. Although all Plains groups shared the basic ritual, procedures varied by tribe. Among the Plains Cree, a man might pledge to hold a "thirsting dance" if he returned safely from a war expedition. The ceremony included construction of a lodge. While the sponsor fasted, warriors cut down a tree to serve as the sacred central pole. A "thunderbird nest" was constructed at the top, and cloth and offerings were hung from it. Dancing then occurred around the central pole. This was the time when young men, also in fulfillment of vows, had the muscles of their chests pierced and wooden skewers pushed through. Ropes tied to the skewer were attached to the central pole, and the young men danced while leaning back on the ropes until they tore free. Scars acquired in the dance were bore proudly throughout life. The days of the dance strengthened people in their shared faith, and the gathering of bands allowed such social activities as visiting friends, courting, gambling, and horse racing (McMillan, 1988; Sharrock, 1974; Mandelbaum, 1979).

In Plains mythology, a common theme was the trickster or transformer. The Plains Cree brought Wisakedjak (properly *Wisahkechahk*) from their original subarctic homeland telling of his actions that put the world into its present order (McMillan, 1988).

When a person died, the body was usually placed in a tree or scaffold. The death was frequently believed to be the result of witchcraft and was sometimes followed by the survivors performing an act of revenge on those considered accountable. However, men of distinction were left in their lodges with their valued possessions. Horses were sometimes shot so that they could accompany the man to the spirit world. A gun was fired in the tent to drive away evil spirits (Levinson, 1991). Sometimes men would immediately leave on a war party attempting to ease grief by striking the enemy. A grieving mother or wife might gash her legs or chop off a finger joint.

Although many Cree pushed across the northern plains and to the Rockies in search of furs for the Europeans, many Plains Cree established themselves as middlemen between the posts on Hudson Bay and the western tribes. Huge profits could be made from taking furs to the posts and bringing back European goods to trade with more distant groups. Later when the companies established posts across the plains, these Cree became major suppliers of pemmican and bison hides. This close association with the fur trade led to the rise of the Métis (always pronounced /may-tee'/), persons whose fathers were fur traders and their mothers were Cree or Ojibwa. Thus many Métis are biologically related to the Cree.

The Algonquian Cree became more closely allied with the Siouan Assiniboine, and intermarriage with this Indian group began to occur. Many Cree became bilingual, and the intermingled traditions became a "fused ethnicity" in which they were neither Cree nor Assiniboine, but a new hybrid identity. Mid-nineteenth century accounts describe large camps of Assiniboine, Cree, Ojibwa, and Métis. However, as more and more Europeans came, cultural change began to occur. The disappearance of the bison removed the potential for self-sufficiency. Some bands began to scorn fish and the diet they had been used to over the years in preference for European food.

With the loss of the bison, the traditional garb of bison hide and canvas for tipis was also gone. Unfortunately, with their economy destroyed, the Cree were essentially in no position to resist government offers of assistance in exchange for signing treaties. The Indian Act of 1876 is the treaty most often referred to in the literature (McMillan, 1988). This treaty outlined the definition of "Indian," the recognition, protection, management, and sale of reserves, the payment of money to support and benefit the Indians, the election of councils and chiefs, Indian privileges, the provision of receiving evidence of "non-Christian Indians" in criminal prosecutions, the control of intoxicants, and provisions of enfranchisement. This treaty is commonly thought of as an act legalizing the Canadian federal government's actions and position toward the Indians and representative of the ultimate goal of assimilating the Native people in Canada. By 1877 the Canadian tribes had ceded by treaty all claims to their lands. The treaties allocated reserves and provided small payments of money and farm equipment. As the Canadian government organized the Native peoples into reserves, the Plains Cree lacked a tribal organization to tie them together into bands. As a result, they were scattered into small reserves that were concentrated in Alberta and Saskatchewan and frequently shared with the Assiniboine or Ojibwa (Vickers, 1986; Tarasoff, 1980; Skinner, 1914). Although the Canadian government attempted to end aboriginal title to Indian lands in return for reserves and small annuities, a small number of remote and isolated Bush Cree bands were overlooked. They neither entered into treaty relations nor surrendered their lands or sovereignty.

In only a few decades the Cree, a proud and self-sufficient nomadic people, were reduced to destitute and dependent groups confined to small areas of land without any adequate means of support. Rather than becoming self-sufficient farmers, starvation set in and many died from meager rations, tuberculosis, influenza, whooping cough, and other diseases. Children were taken away and placed in residential schools. Missionaries and government agents made major efforts to Christianize and acculturate the Cree. By the end of the 1800s, tipis, horses, and bison had essentially been replaced by cabins, cattle, and gardens. Agricultural efforts began to have some success. However, reserves generally continued to lack any real economic base and were generally not considered a desirable place to live. Interestingly the discovery of oil on reserve land has been a source of great tension between the bands and the Canadian government (Levinson, 1991). However, on one Indian reserve of the Cree people just southeast of Hobbema, Alberta, is the Samson Cree nation, and the profits from oil have been used to make this reserve the most prosperous in Canada (Nemeth and Hiller, 1996). The royalties have allowed for a medical clinic, a band-owned pharmacy, a gas station and grocery store, a federally chartered trust company, a recreation center, an educational trust for the young people, and 10,000 acres of land are being developed into farms. Although the reserve still has a high unemployment rate, they have been able to distribute some funds among the members and to diversify their economy (Nemeth and Hiller, 1996). Unfortunately Native interests have not been so well addressed on reserves without this advantage, and this story is the exception to a general climate of fiscal restraint in relation to the reserves (Nemeth and Hiller, 1996).

According to Statistics Canada Indian register data (1997) there are 348,732 persons in Indian bands living both on and off reserves in Canada that are identified as Cree. Some 191,161 Cree individuals are on reserves, whereas 157,571 live off reserves. A total of 15,784 Cree live in Quebec, 138,379 in Ontario, 50,320 in Manitoba, 94,947 in Saskatchewan, and 49,302 in Alberta. The number of status Indians (persons registered as Indians and able to prove descendance from an Indian band) who live off the reserves is steadily increasing. In 1971, 27% of the status Indians lived off the reserve. By 1986 this number had increased to 40% (Hanvey, Avard, Graham, Underwood, Campbell, and Kelly, 1994). However, data available on the Cree vary depending on source. Accurate data on the aboriginal groups are difficult to obtain, and statistics often underrepresent the actual numbers because not all Indians are recognized as Indians and not all choose to be or are registered as Indians (Young, 1994). Persons with Indian ancestry but who cannot prove that they are descendants from a band are called "nonstatus Indians" and are therefore not registered (Aboriginal Health Unit, Alberta Health, 1995).

THE MOVE TO URBAN SETTINGS

Not only has there been a tendency for the Cree to leave reserves, but also the desire to escape reserve community problems of poverty, crime, unemployment, and poor services and the hope of economic opportunity and a new life have drawn the Indian population to large urban settings such as Regina, Winnipeg, and Edmonton (McMillan, 1988; Krotz, 1980; La Prairie, 1995). Migration to urban centers has steadily increased over the past 50 years. Unfortunately the expectation of better opportunity and education has not usually proved to be reality. Many Cree living in urban settings have instead encountered a poor quality of life, feelings of isolation, lack of a support system, inability to practice and live within their traditions, difficulty accessing health care services, and poor employment opportunities (Aboriginal Health Unit, Alberta Health, 1995). The Cree as well as other Indians leaving the reserves have also experienced racism, discrimination, crowding, and inadequate living conditions in urban settings (Royal Commission on Aboriginal Peoples, 1996; Frideres, 1992). Significant health concerns, including alcohol, drug, prescription drug abuse, fetal alcohol syndrome, injury, violence, teen pregnancy, AIDS, tuberculosis, and diabetes have also been documented (Aboriginal Health Unit, Alberta Health, 1995).

The city of Edmonton in Alberta is one example of an urban setting with a population of Cree. According to the 1991 census, 63%, or 6403, of the Native population was Cree (Royal Commission on Aboriginal Peoples, 1996). However, these statistics are likely very conservative because only Native persons living within the boundaries of the inner city were counted in the census and low-cost housing and poor living conditions present where Native persons also live are found adjacent to the boundaries of the city.

Although data pertaining specifically to the number of Edmonton Natives living in the inner city are not available, data for Winnipeg Natives are available. In the 1991 census, 42% of Winnipeg's Native population lived in the inner city rather than in rural outlying areas (Gaede, 1993). It can be hypothesized that there is a similar situation in Edmonton because the two cities have similar situations with Native residents. The urban inner city Natives (UICN) are considerably younger than the general population. In a comparison of Native and non-Native urban populations, based on data from the 1991 census, 36.6% of the UICN population are between 0 and 14 years, whereas only 19.7% of the urban non-Native population are in this age category (Royal Commission on Aboriginal Peoples, 1996). The level of education is also much lower for UICN. Data from the 1991 census indicate that 49.7% of UICN over the age of 15 have less than a high school certificate, whereas only 35.6% of the non-Native population have less than a high school certificate. In addition, only 3.8% of UICN have a university degree, whereas 13.0% of the non-Native population have a degree (Royal Commission on Aboriginal Peoples, 1996). Although compared to that of non-Native urban residents, the UICN level of education is low, in relation to Native persons living on reserves there is not much difference (Frideres, 1988). Because their level of education is lower, UICN in Edmonton also have a lower mean salary. The average total income for UICN living in urban areas is $16,560 compared to an average income of $24,876 for non-Native urban residents (Royal Commission on Aboriginal Peoples, 1996). The life expectancy of UICN is also much lower than that for the general Canadian population as a whole. In the 1991 census, the life expectancy of Native persons in general was 67.9 for males and 75.0 for females. For the total population it was 74.6 for males and 80.9 for females. The life expectancy for registered North American Indians living in urban, nonreserve areas was 72.5 for males and 79.0 for females (Royal Commission on Aboriginal Peoples, 1996). Although the urban statistics on life expectancy for North Americans Indians living in urban settings are higher than that for the total Indian population, they are still lower than the average life expectancy in Canada.

Acculturation is an important phenomenon for the Cree person who is attempting to make the rural urban shift. McClure, Boulanger, Kaufert, and Forsyth (1992) describe acculturation as the ways in which indigenous cultures adapt to accommodate to or are ultimately assimilated by a dominant culture. The difficulties Cree and other Native persons have with acculturation stem from different values (Mason, 1967). Urban cultures have a high priority on competitiveness, material success, and commitment to one's employment, whereas the Native culture values sharing of property, hospitality, and flexible use of time (Drew, 1988). Drew postulates that alcohol abuse, the cheapest form of recreation in the UICN, is a product of difficulties with acculturation. The stress of urban life such as being on time, noise, increased potential for children to get into trouble, and lack of familiarity with all the systems ranging from transportation to education to cramped housing hinder acculturation. Another stressor affecting acculturation is the blending of different cultures because half of all Native people marry non-Natives (Drost, Crowley, and Schwindt, 1995). The practice of traditional religion or speaking one's own language must be negotiated in a culturally mixed household.

COMMUNICATION

The Cree language is the northern variant of Central Algonquian, extending from the Montagnais-Naskapi of the Labrador Peninsula to the Rocky Mountains (Levinson, 1991; Helm, 1981; Smith, 1987). Although a single language was spoken throughout this vast area by the Cree, differences in dialect means that over the years only neighboring groups could easily converse. In fact, nine major

Cree dialects have been identified and related to a geographic region of Canada (McMillan, 1988). For example, Plains Cree was spoken on the plains and the western woodlands, whereas Woods Cree is spoken in the woodlands of central Saskatchewan and Manitoba (McMillan, 1988). In a study of indigenous languages of Canada, only three (Cree, Ojibwa, and Inuktitut) were considered to have excellent chances for survival. All others were considered endangered and listed as verging on extinction. Federal educational policy, which once used the schools as instruments of assimilation, punishing children for speaking their own languages, now strongly supports preservation of indigenous languages throughout the schools. Native communities across Canada are experimenting with language and cultural programs, and a substantial percentage of children now receive some form of native language instruction (Campbell and Mithun, 1979; Foster, 1985). The *Profile of Canada's Aboriginal Population* (Statistics Canada, 1991) identified that 73,375 persons claimed aboriginal origins and that Cree was their mother tongue. On the other hand, 50,850 persons identified aboriginal origins and identified Cree as their home language. An additional 92,180 claimed to have knowledge of the Cree language (Statistics Canada, 1995).

Today, most Cree coming to urban settings are bilingual and speak English. Only recent arrivals from remote rural areas or elders may be unfamiliar with English. However, Crees who do not speak English will not necessarily be able to communicate with each other if they come from a different dialectal area.

The Cree generally have nonverbal communication patterns found among other Canadian Indian groups. Long gaps in conversation are easily tolerated, and Cree are frequently comfortable with silence (Brant, 1990; McClure et al., 1992). The gaps are used for assimilation and reflection. The Cree are likely to be nonassertive and slow to anger. Face-to-face conflict is almost always avoided (Levinson, 1991). A consequence of this is that they may not challenge racist remarks but rather choose to let them pass. Personal autonomy is respected. This is reflected in the common nonverbal communication

pattern of leaning back and avoiding eye contact. Eye contact may be interpreted as an effort to control another and can be interpreted by the Cree as interference and an invasion of privacy (Farkas, 1987).

Implications for nursing care

Accurate assessment of the client is the first priority in establishing a plan of care. The culturally sensitive nurse should be aware that guidelines for assessment that are appropriate for non-Native clients may not be suitable for Cree clients. A study by Burke, Sayers, Baumgart, and Wray (1985) suggested that the commonly used Denver Developmental Screening Test appeared to have major pitfalls in cross-cultural use when used on Cree children.

When possible a nurse caring for a non-English speaking Cree client should be Cree and be able to communicate to the client in Cree (Lloyd, 1994). Fortunately, some nursing schools in Canada are making a serious effort to attract Cree students who will then be able to return to their local communities to practice (Lloyd, 1994). An organization for aboriginal nurses had developed in Canada and is growing as the population of Native nurses increases (Aboriginal Nurses Association of Canada, 1995). When this is not possible, a Cree interpreter should be used. However, the Cree language does not have words for some concepts that are used in nursing, and so it is important that the interpreter have some understanding of medical terminology and that the nurse provide simple and understandable explanations. Nurses should support the development of paraprofessional Native persons to provide clinical, educational, and social support in health care settings (Anishinawbe Health Toronto, 1990).

It is important for the nurse interacting with Cree clients in an urban setting to appreciate the nonverbal communication patterns that are part of their cultural heritage. Therefore, when interacting on a one-to-one basis, direct eye contact should be avoided, particularly if working with an elder. Respect can be communicated by looking at their heart or brain. The culturally sensitive nurse should be aware that the Cree traditionally do not like to talk a great deal, seldom disclose personal information, do not seek or ask advice, and do not complain.

Frequently the Cree use a story as a form of communication and may indirectly answer questions or communicate through this medium. The nurse should be alert to the significance a story may have in relation to the client's condition. Hagey (1984) describes how she used the story of Nanabush and the Pole Stranger to educate Natives about diabetes. She advocates carefully choosing the right story for the right culture. Since Native women in particular prefer one-on-one sessions rather than groups, teaching by means of a story may not be automatically used by nurses because in the non-Native culture, stories are associated with groups. Nevertheless, it is important for the nurse to capitalize on the use of the oral tradition in teaching Cree clients (Krotz, 1980). Cree are also used to learning by observation rather than by long discussions, and so whenever possible the nurse should demonstrate and use motions to communicate, particularly when a language barrier is present (Lloyd, 1994).

The Cree are often reluctant to volunteer detailed descriptions of their problems (Mobbs, 1986), and the consequence of lack of disclosure is living with undetected chronic illness (Hanson, 1988). The nurse needs to be patient and knowledgeable and listen actively to what is being communicated through a story (Aboriginal Health Unit, Alberta Health, 1995). Problems frequently arise when non-Native nurses give advice and find that the Cree clients do not comply. The noncompliance may be attributable to the manner of communication, particularly if the nurse speaks rapidly and conveys the attitude of being in a hurry.

It is important for the nurse to be attentive to techniques that build trust with a Cree client. Because of the difficulties in trusting the government, many Cree may mistrust the service systems claiming to help them. Because of the dark Canadian history of traumatic attempts to acculturate generations of Cree children, including both the churches' rigorous residential schools in the midtwentieth century and the current child welfare system, many parents are fearful when an unknown "suit" knocks at their door. For many, "social worker" has become a name to be feared, whereas a "nurse" will ease many of the built-up fears and will open doors. The nurse can sometimes use trust that has been established to facilitate needed compromise with the five major governmental services dealing with the Cree family: health, education, child welfare, social services, and justice (Aboriginal Health Unit, Alberta Health, 1995).

SPACE

Over the centuries Crees have been accustomed to a nomadic lifestyle that allowed bands freedom to roam across the Canadian prairies or woodland country following sources of food in their autumn-winter-spring hunting ranges (Levinson, 1991). Living spaces usually were small, with their basic shelter being a conical lodge, made of moose or caribou hides. It usually contained the extended family, including several hunters. Animal hides were later replaced by canvas coverings, often made into ridge-pole tents. At the end of the nineteenth century log cabin settlements developed, reflecting a higher degree of sedentariness. In recent times, federal and provincial governments have provided relatively modern houses, band offices, schools, and health facilities. However, even today, many Crees are confined to cramped living conditions on reserves or in crowded and poor housing conditions in urban locations (Gaede, 1993). Today freedom to roam at will is restricted, which sometimes results in a feeling of confinement (Aboriginal Health Unit, Alberta Health, 1995).

Implications for nursing

McClure et al. (1992) noted that space affects the comfort level in communication and that interviews should be done in a private space. Katz (1981) noted that 50-minute sessions in the office setting were not effective. Katz (1981) noted more success when he saw clients in the community in their own space.

The nurse who is doing discharge planning and planning for care for an illness in the home should be aware that the setting in which the client lives may be small and modifications in the plan may need to be made based on space available.

SOCIAL ORGANIZATION

Crees have typically been organized into bands. The basic unit was a small hunting group or local band made up of one or more extended families and numbering about 25 persons (Levinson, 1991). Unity was based on father-son relationships and co-operation among brothers. Marriages were arranged by parents between opposite-sex cross cousins. Marriage with parallel cousins, first or classificatory, was prohibited because they were considered siblings. Arranged marriages ensured that the son-in-law would be a good hunter and provider. Bilateral cross-cousin marriage tended to establish or maintain cooperative relationships between hunting groups. Some marriages were arranged with distant groups and marriage to a fur trader was considered especially desirable. Divorce in the past was highly informal, but marriages are now performed in Roman Catholic or Anglican churches or by civil authorities and are subject to religious restraints and civil law.

Children were raised permissively, and control and discipline were instilled gradually. Mothers trained their daughters, and boys were gradually taught hunting and trapping skills by their fathers. These traditional practices have disappeared, and children now receive education through attending schools on the reserves. Some children go on to the university or other postsecondary institutions. Traditional values of the Cree culture including love, courage, respect, silence, generosity, chastity, and honesty are present today in family life and are evident in childrearing (Pompana and Grumbly, 1994). Children are allowed a great deal of freedom short of injuring themselves. In part this is based on the value of noninterference. In a safe environment this approach to parenting results in generally well-behaved and respectful children; in the inner city this permissiveness results in wary behaviors.

Elders are respected in the Cree culture because of their vast experience and knowledge. Among the Cree, it is considered inappropriate to conceal signs of aging. Many of the elderly Cree actively assist with childrearing, particularly if a family has a single parent or is trying to manage issues of abuse. The Cree value the extended family. Aunts are often considered to be mothers, and uncles are called "fathers." Cousins are called "brothers" and "sisters." Even if there is no relationship to other members of the group, they will be called "relatives." Their orientation is to inclusivity of kinship (Cardinal and Steinhauer, 1994). For those moving from traditional Cree communities to urban settings, the disconnection from the guidance of elders is a problem. There is often no easy way to find the services of an elder in a big city. Many newly arrived Crees express confusion as they seek credible elder services. In Edmonton, organizations such as the Meskahnow Aboriginal Society are attempting to fill this void. The program is designed to meet the needs of Cree and other Native children by providing an "at-home atmosphere" to families. Spirituality rather than religion is the core of meaning for Crees and other Canadian Native peoples. Key elements in promoting spirituality are wholeness, energy, noninterference and maintaining balance and harmony (Pompana and Grumbly, 1994). The most common symbol of spirituality is the *circle,* which depicts harmony of mind, body, and spirit. Everything in the world is intertwined, connected, and continuous (Pompana and Grumbly, 1994). The circle has four directions or aspects: physical, spiritual, mental, and emotional. All directions have to be present to have health. The sacred circle also represents the four elements of nature—fire, earth, air, and water—all being necessary for life. The circle also teaches that the four races—red, yellow, black, and white—are part of the universal family (Aboriginal Health Unit, Alberta Health, 1995). The Native peoples believe that sacred traditional ceremonies can facilitate new understanding about life, death, and the afterlife and are important not only for maintenance of tradition, but also for the vitality of spiritual life (Cardinal, Steinhauer, and Harrison, 1994). The ceremonies "protect the future of the grandchildren and offer healing, guidance, love, sharing, and trust among all the people of the world. They reflect Native ethics such as love, respect, silence, generosity, and honesty. They symbolize the universe, nature, purity, and harmony. The ceremonies present a balance of past, present and future. Native spirituality and Native healing involve the elders, the community, the family and the individual. It is a way of life" (Cardinal, Steinhauer, and Harrison, 1994).

Traditionally Crees survived by sharing resources, exchange of services, working collectively, and using consensual decision making. They focused on the meaning of their work and recognized that they co-existed with a Higher Spirit (Drost, Crowley, and Schwind, 1995). This social organization cannot and does not flourish in an urban setting and has contributed to the difficulty Cree have had adjusting to urban life.

Implications for nursing care

Nurses can have a vital role in addressing the rural urban migration through involvement with health care delivery systems at the planning level. Because the factors for leaving the rural areas and difficulties experienced in the urban settings are well documented, proactive planning guided through a prevention philosophy would help ensure valid interventions. One feasible service delivery model is the establishment of a migration center for Natives. A successful migration center was established in Thompson, Manitoba, Canada. The center formally is in liaison with selected rural Native communities. A worker from the center visits each rural community at least three times per year. Information about employment, housing, costs, health, and education are given. If a Native chooses to migrate to an urban center, job interviews and housing are arranged before his or her arrival. Families are asked to stay in the rural area until the person seeking employment is established. This decreases the stress of relocation. After the person arrives in the urban center, he or she is mentored and partnered, and nothing is left to chance (Sealey and Lussier, 1994). Nurses could take active roles in planning and coordination like-minded immigration centers.

The sense of isolation and loneliness of Native persons can also be decreased by outreach work in the school systems. Nurses working in the schools can provide services and programming for at-risk Native students, their families, and the community. By working with Native children in urban settings nurses can gain entry into their homes and assist them in negotiating the legal, health, and social ser-

vice systems. Home visits can be used to establish trust, engage in health teaching, and provide basic counseling. In the school setting, supportive educational groups can be provided for children. In some school systems, Native-awareness days have been organized to promote self-esteem for Native children as well as cultural awareness and education for non-Native children in the school. In schools with such programs truancy and absences have decreased for both Native and non-Native children.

Many of the Native families moving into Edmonton have few relatives or friends in the city. Relatives who do live there are often not within their neighborhood, making a lack of support and isolation a significant issue. Nurses working in the schools have been able to promote a sense of belonging and connectedness with these families. Programming includes intense rapport building, anticipatory problem solving and counseling, advocacy, and liaison with the multiple service systems the Native persons are involved with. A high level of holistic assessment and cultural sensitivity is essential for this role to be effective (Bernard, 1997).

It is important for the nurse to appreciate the traditional view of spirituality that many Cree adhere to. For many Cree spirituality and the sacred circle, which involves harmony of mind, body, and spirit, is essential to health and in seeking health care. The nurse should appreciate that for many Cree the sacred circle does not limit healing to Native healers. All healers, Native and non-Native, may use the circle. The sacred circle allows for a variety of cultural differences in healing techniques.

TIME

Traditionally the Cree have had a present time orientation. McClure et al. (1992) note that, for the Cree, "Time is always with us." Brandt (1990) describes their time concept as "intuitive, personal, and flexible" (p. 536), noting that originally they were regulated by the seasons and that they understood the importance of the "right time." Doing something at the right time ensures consideration of multiple environmental stimuli, and the outcome is success. The Cree have traditionally worked to satisfy their present needs. Because time is present, many Cree have no difficulty taking time to reach consensus when making a decision or taking time in the form of silence to answer a question. Their perception of time also underlies their value of giving. Because some Cree are present-time oriented, they will share and give away their possessions, knowledge, and experiences freely. This time orientation also gives rise to a valuable virtue for many Cree of patience. In addition, for some Cree, waiting is considered a sign of respect. Things are done as they are needed. For many Cree coming to an urban setting, the need to add a future orientation, which will enable them to meet future-oriented time frames and to plan for the future, is a difficult and significant adjustment.

Implications for nursing care

It is often quite difficult for individuals who hold a Western orientation to time to work only in the present. Mobbs (1986) found that having a present-time orientation led to errors in establishing a medical history. Mobbs (1986) gave the example whereby trying to establish the timing, frequency, and periodicity of a common pain symptom is not only unreliable but also frustrating.

A system of appointments between UICN and nurses usually results in "no shows." Gaede (1993) recommended the use of walk-in street clinics, evening availability, and hiring more Native state members. Services to Natives need to be accessible, affordable, and flexible. In this sense, services cannot be limited to rigid time schedules or structured health care professional availability.

The issue of time may present challenges for UICN children especially in the area of punctuality and school attendance. In Edmonton, nurses working in the schools are creating and delivering programs to assist Native students and their families to make efforts to attend school daily on time. The nurses are working within the educational system to impart a greater understanding of the cultural influence of the time dimension (Bernard, 1997). Cree clients have reported dissatisfaction with the amount of time doctors and nurses are willing to spend with them. It has been suggested that this re-

lates to noncompliance in suggested preventive health care measures (Morse, Young, and Swartz, 1991). For example, chemoprophylaxis for tuberculosis has only a 5% compliance rate among the Cree in Saskatchewan (Wobeser, To, and Hoeppner, 1989). Thus it is important for caregivers to be aware that although a high level of verbalization may not be considered important to the Cree client, the Cree client may feel strongly about the importance of time for a positive nurse-client relationship.

ENVIRONMENTAL CONTROL

Traditionally the Cree and other Native peoples linked illness to spiritual beliefs and the context of their environment (Frideres, 1992). Illness was a result of breaking a taboo. The Cree, like some other Native peoples, identified three kinds of illnesses: visible injuries such as lacerations, those caused by an invisible external event like cancer, and others that did not fit the former two categories like mental illness. The ill person would be treated first with medicines, and if this did not work, shamanistic methods of prayers and chants were used. These methods not only were used for healing, but were also a form of social control. Many of these beliefs and practices continue in the present.

In the Cree culture, shamans, or healers, are selected by the Elders, may inherit the position, or may assume the position after having a "called experience" (Pompana and Grumbly, 1994). These medicine people are believed to have specialized knowledge that help them understand the spirit world and Mother Earth. They are accountable for their knowledge and are obligated to engage in spiritual maintenance and pass on their knowledge through oral traditions from generation to generation. Part of their knowledge is the use of herbs to promote healing and the use of rituals (Morse, Young, and Swartz, 1991). Cree healing rituals are not solely dependent on the therapist, but also include the active participation by the patient, the healer's spirit helpers, and the Great Spirit. The spiritual nature of Cree healing requires purification of the immediate surroundings, the participants, the healer, the healer's medicine bundle, and his pipe. This purification process opens the doors to the spiritual world, which is the source of the healer's power and represents a supplication for spiritual forces to enter the room. In addition to opening the door to the spiritual world, purification encourages an attitude of receptivity in the participants. At the same time, it places the healer in a position of control and establishes his credentials. Purification also symbolizes the healer's sharing of spiritual power, which allows the patient to participate in the healing process. The healer's interaction with the Great Spirit continues throughout the healing rituals; all movements are clockwise, and all actions are geared to maintaining a balance with nature. When possible, healing rituals are conducted outside where spiritual forces are believed to be stronger (Morse, Young, and Swartz, 1991). It is important in Cree culture that the patient desire and request healing before treatment occurs. The patient symbolizes this by bringing a gift of tobacco and a square meter of cotton cloth to the healer (Morse, Young, and Swartz, 1991). The traditional Cree healer completes the healing ceremony by emphasizing that it is the Great Spirit that heals, not the healer. The healer also provides instructions on how patients are to care for themselves at home, such as preparation of herbal decoction (Morse, Young, and Swartz, 1991).

Generally the Cree do not act individualistically when ill. Their health status is determined by what the group believes to be norms for illness or sickness. Given their state of constant unremitting poverty, many Cree may focus instead on their basic needs to survive and ignore illness unless incapacitated (Frideres, 1992).

Implications for nursing care

It is important for the nurse to recognize that Cree clients may have negative attitudes toward health care providers because of past encounters, clashing value systems, perception of facilities, and being stereotyped as "irresponsible, dirty, and incapable of carrying out orders or taking responsibility for themselves" (Frideres, 1992). Education and value clarification sessions may help health care providers

determine if negative attitudes and stereotypes are present because they will interfere with care.

Perhaps the most important concept in improving health care is the feeling of self-governance and personal autonomy for the Cree. As primary caregivers in remote Cree and other Indian communities, nurses are often witness to the inequities between the health care available to Indians and that of other Canadians (Thompson, 1993). Currently, Health and Welfare Canada, under the guidance of the Department of Indian Affairs, provides health care to Indians through the Medical Services branch. To some Crees and other Indians, health care policy is imposed by an alien society not tailored to their community. It is critical that the nurse serve as a client advocate promoting health programs that are defined and directed at the communities themselves. It is only with the feeling of self-governance that good health practices can be developed (Thompson, 1993).

In a recent project by the Canadian Nurses Association (CNA), concerns about the health care system's inadequacy to meet the needs of aboriginal Canadians, particularly in urban areas, were addressed (Shestowsky, 1995). Data collected in this project were suggestive that if health services are to respond to the real needs of urban-dwelling aboriginal Canadians major changes are required. An integrated, community-based continuum of care is needed to provide coordinated access to a range of types and levels of services, such as health promotion, disease and disability prevention, restoration, rehabilitation, and support. The researchers concluded that it is essential that the aboriginals have an enhanced role in defining health care services that are culturally sensitive (Shestowsky, 1995). However, it is also important that the culturally competent nurse be aware that not all Crees subscribe to traditional views of the Great Spirit or the sacred circle or to the usefulness of traditional healers. It is important for the nurse to obtain the belief system of the Cree client. When traditional beliefs are important to the client, whenever possible these should be incorporated into the plan of care. In a hospital setting the nurse should respect the client's right to have a shaman or healer present and assist in providing opportunity including time and location for healing rituals to occur. Nurses should function in the role of client advocates when necessary mediating conflicts between traditional healers and Western medicine and promoting the benefits of traditional healing methodologies for the Cree and other Native peoples (McClure et al., 1992).

BIOLOGICAL VARIATIONS

Infant morbidity and mortality are high among the Cree and other Canadian Native people. Bottle feeding continues to be the most common method of feeding infants despite the fact that public health campaigns encourage breast feeding (Neander and Morse, 1989). Neander and Morse noted that the medicament of childbirth and the occurrence of childbirth in the hospital has resulted in loss of support for pregnant and postpartum mothers who feel insecure and afraid at this time and are consequently less likely to breast feed. Solid foods are introduced relatively early. Traditional mothers premasticated the infants' food rather than using commercial baby food or a blender. In the study of Cree infant-feeding practices it was noted that mothers believed that it was important to keep the breasts warm when lactating, and they were reluctant to feed the infant colostrum immediately after delivery (Neander and Morse, 1989). It is also suggested that the increase in bottle feeding has contributed to the increase in the total fertility rate, which Romaniuk (1981) noted in the James Bay Cree from 1927 to 1972. The increase from about 40 of 1000 in the preWorld War II years to just under 50 of 1000 in the early 1960s was related to a shortening of birth intervals (Romaniuk, 1981).

Skin color and other visible characteristics

The Cree are generally dark skinned and dark haired. In the early days tattooing was commonly practiced by the Plains Cree. Men had their upper bodies tattooed, whereas women limited tattoos to lines on their chins. The hair of both men and women was generally long, greased, and arranged in a variety of styles. Today, most Cree in the inner city do not have select dress or skin alterations that would make them different from other individuals (McMillan, 1988).

Genetic variations

The Cree, Indiana's Amish, and Oklahoma's Cherokee Indians have recently been discovered to have a genetic predisposition for lower rates of Alzheimer's disease. It is thought that the Cree have a lower incidence of apolipoprotein E4, the gene associated with the development of Alzheimer's disease. A University of Texas Southwestern neurologist reported to the Associated Press that an unknown protective gene appears to be at work and may assist in developing drugs effective against the disease (Neergaard, 1997).

Susceptibility to disease

The Cree and Ojibwa Indians in Canada have the highest-known incidence of type II diabetes of any group in the world. Researchers have found that 40% of the 728 Indian people studied among the 1500 residents of the Sandy Lake reserve, 450 km northeast of Winnipeg, are affected by the non-insulin dependent form of diabetes, with children as young as 10 years of age showing symptoms. Dr. Bernard Zinman, a diabetes expert from Toronto's Mount Sinai Hospital, told *Maclean's* that the Cree have a superior ability to store nutrients in their bodies to survive periods of famine. However, now that feature, combined with a lack of exercise and a reliance on fast-food products, is making the Cree more susceptible to obesity and at risk for diabetes.

During the twentieth century, the mortality from tuberculosis has declined substantially among the Cree and other Indians. The decline, in fact, preceded the availability of effective antituberculosis therapy in the 1950s (Young, 1994). However, despite the improvement, the disparity between Natives and non-Natives remains great with Natives having an incidence as much as 10 times higher than non-Natives in Canada (Young, 1994). A regional study of the Cree and Ojibwa in northwestern Ontario support the national trend toward leveling off (Young and Casson, 1988).

In the 1980s, the Cree in the James Bay area of northern Quebec suffered from severe epidemics of

Escherichia coli and rotavirus gastroenteritis. A population-based stool survey found 21 different serotypes of enteropathic *E. coli* in 7% of those sampled (Brassard et al., 1985).

Nutritional and lifestyle preferences

Traditionally the Cree lived off the land primarily subsisting off big game animals and supplemented by fish and fowl. Today, although a few raise some food from farming, most dietary needs are met through the local store where fast-food products are commonly purchased (Levinson, 1991). It is becoming recognized that dietary change is a major factor in the changing pattern of disease experienced by Native Americans (Young, 1994).

Psychological characteristics

Findings from one study indicate that there was a high incidence of abuse among Cree and other Indian children who were placed in some 80 residential schools across Canada between 1880 and continuing into the 1970s (Crary, 1996). During this time, pressure from Indian leaders forced the schools to close. Canadian investigators are amassing evidence of widespread physical and sexual abuse inflicted on the children decades ago in these government-funded, church-run boarding schools. Victims across Canada are reporting rapes, beatings, suicides, suspicious deaths, and humiliating punishments, even the use of a homemade, low-voltage electric chair (Crary, 1996). In many cases, children were forced to attend residential schools, separated from their families 10 months of the year while Catholic and Protestant instructors tried to steer them away from their native spiritual beliefs (Crary, 1996). Students were punished for speaking their native languages and were force-fed white culture. Constable Jerry Peters, who oversees the 3-year-old task force from the Vancouver police headquarters told the Associated Press News Service that "we've been talking about thousands of people who attended these schools and hundreds, perhaps thousands of people who were abused" (Crary, 1996). The probe covers 10 schools run by the Catholic church, two by the Anglican church, and two by the United Church. St. Anne's operated from 1904 to 1973 in an isolated Cree community on the west coast of James Bay 600 miles north of Toronto and was the unhappy home for many Cree in that area during that time (Moon, 1996). Because Canada has no statute of limitations for serious crimes, including sexual assault, some cases are presently active (Crary, 1996).

Interestingly enough, in northern Ontario, in the adult Cree population only 20% of these individuals are classified as "ever-drinkers" compared with 80% of "ever-drinker" in the general Canadian population. Although the prevalence of drinking declined with age, it was significantly higher among highly educated individuals (Young, 1982). Nevertheless, although some data are suggestive that Crees are less likely to be ever-drinkers, Beauvais et al. (1989) reported that, for some 5 or 6 Native tribes studied between 1975 and 1987, alcohol use was prevalent among 81% of the youth. Burd and Moffatt (1994) noted that fetal alcohol syndrome (FAS) occurred at higher rates in Black, Alaskan Native, aboriginal peoples of Canada, and American Indian populations. Findings from this study indicate that because theirs is a contingent relationship between FAS and childhood morbidity and mortality in these high-risk groups, health care professionals should be particularly cognizant of this unique susceptibility among this vulnerable population.

Implications for nursing care

The susceptibility to type II diabetes that is so noteworthy among the Cree has serious implications for nursing education. It is essential that the nurse use culturally appropriate ways to assist the Cree client to understand the serious complications that can arise from this illness including loss of eyesight, amputation of limbs, and kidney and heart problems. Becoming more physically active and eating less fatty foods are two actions that can be taken to help prevent this illness and to assist in limiting complications. Because of the difficulties Cree clients have with being told directly what they should do, it is important that health care implications be given using communication styles that will be received and will increase compliance (Editorial, 1997).

The abuse suffered by some Cree children in residential schools has serious implications for relationships with White health care providers with whom they relate because this trauma can cause mistrust and fear. Because many of the children who survived the horrors of school and have bitter memories of the abuse and punishment are still alive, many Cree still suffer from psychological trauma as a result of the abuse (Moon, 1996). Some Cree have received counseling since they left the school for the trauma they still experience because of the sexual abuse witnessed (Moon, 1996). It is important for nurses to be aware that a significant shortage of culturally appropriate psychological services for the Cree and other Native peoples has been identified by various studies (Armstrong, 1990).

SUMMARY

Discussion is ongoing in Canada about whether Quebec should separate and declare its own sovereignty. Some Cree are part of this dispute and are part of a huge backlog of Native land claims now under consideration requesting that land taken away be returned to them so that the rights of all people in Canada will be protected (Goar, 1996; Editorial, 1996). Whether Cree are isolated on reserves or struggling to adjust to life in the inner cities of Canada, unresolved issues of acculturation remain for the Cree in the multicultural country in which they live. Tom Jackson, Cree star of the CBC hit television series "North of 60," is one testimonial that the Cree can succeed. He is also helping draw national attention to the plight of the problem of the poor in the inner cities in Canada. In 1995 Jackson began taking a benefit concert tour on the road directed at nine cities from Vancouver to Halifax to raise money for food banks and homeless shelters (Jenish, 1995). As a Cree who has made it, he provides a role model of what one Cree can do to help a Canadian problem.

Case Study

Developed by Ruth Scherer, MSN, RN, Assistant professor of Nursing, Bethel College, Mishawaka, Indiana.

Bobby, a 9-year-old male of Cree descent, attends a public school in a urban area of poverty. He is referred to the school mental health nurse because of his poor school attendance and poor interpersonal skills in school. He is small for his age, weighing 60 pounds and standing 3 feet 10 inches. His face has many malformed features congruent with fetal alcohol syndrome, such as bilateral ptosis, short upturned nose, and flattened facial appearance. His IQ is 81, with math as a relative strength, but he is two grade levels behind in reading. The family has been referred to the new fetal alcohol syndrome clinic at a city hospital, but his mother has not followed through to attend.

During a home visit the nurse found Bobby's mother to be initially mistrustful until she was assured that the nurse was not from child welfare services and was not going to take away her kids. The home, in the center of a large low-cost housing complex, is just three blocks away from school. The home is untidy but clean with sparse furnishings that include two mattresses on the living room floor. The front yard is littered with empty beer cans.

Bobby's mother speaks in a low tone and avoids eye contact. She states that Bobby shows many negative behaviors at home and that, as a single mother, she is having difficulty. She confides that Bobby was caught stealing, but "it's because of the gang. . . . They tell him to do it and he just does." She describes her own harsh experiences with a residential school and adds that she doesn't really want Bobby to attend a White man's school.

Bobby's mother is in her fifth month of pregnancy but has not begun prenatal care. She is continuing to drink but only on weekends and drinks lots of coffee afterwards. She states that she is trying hard to gain only 10 pounds with this pregnancy "because I don't want to be fat."

CARE PLAN

 Nursing Diagnosis   Altered health maintenance related to insufficient knowledge of effects of alcohol consumption as evidenced by continued use of alcohol while pregnant and stating that she drinks but only on weekends and drinks lots of coffee afterwards.

Client Outcomes	*Nursing Interventions*
1. Client will stop drinking alcohol during this pregnancy.	1. Use storytelling technique of explaining effects of alcohol on mother's body. 2. Include myths about coffee decreasing effects of alcohol in the story. 3. Explain about the consumption of alcohol causing fetal alcohol syndrome even when drinking on the weekend (binge drinking). 4. Provide culturally appropriate alcohol counseling and rehabilitation. 5. Refer to public health nurse for Milk For Two program.

 Nursing Diagnosis   Body image disturbance related to pregnancy as evidenced by statement that she is trying hard to gain only 10 pounds because she didn't want to be fat.

Client Outcomes	*Nursing Interventions*
1. Client will eat healthful foods during pregnancy. 2. Client will gain about 20 to 25 pounds during this pregnancy.	1. Use storytelling technique to explain normal pregnancy, proper nutrition, and effects of good nutrition on delivery of a healthy normal-weight baby. 2. Encourage prenatal care. Initiate home visit by public health nurse. 3. Encourage client to share concerns about getting fat. 4. Encourage her to share expectations for self and significant others during and after pregnancy. 5. Assist her in identifying sources of love and affection.

 Nursing Diagnosis   Altered growth and development (of Bobby) as related to fetal alcohol syndrome as evidenced by IQ of 81 and functioning two grade levels behind in reading while math is a relative strength.

Client Outcomes	*Nursing Interventions*
1. Bobby will remain in educational program that fosters his intellectual and social development.	1. Assist school in building a cultural component into Bobby's education. 2. Refer mother to community Native agencies for support. 3. Involve school Native liaison services. 4. Use storytelling with Bobby and his mother to portray the value of school. 5. Explore school community activities that interest Bobby. 6. Encourage Bobby and his mother to become like other Natives in the school so that it is no longer viewed as the White man's school.

Nursing Diagnosis   Altered parent-child attachment possibly related to fetal alcohol syndrome and lack of supportive spouse.

Client Outcomes

1. Mother will demonstrate attachment behaviors towards Bobby.

Nursing Interventions

1. Encourage mother to discuss expectations that she had during pregnancy with Bobby.
2. Use storytelling techniques to encourage prenatal care and breast feeding.
3. Assist mother in identifying who can be with her when she comes home from the hospital with the baby and who can watch Bobby while she is in the hospital.
4. Provide support and positive reinforcement when the mother demonstrates attachment behaviors.

STUDY QUESTIONS

1. List several factors that may contribute to alcoholism among the Canadian Crees.
2. Describe at least two communication barriers encountered by the nurse from the dominant Canadian society when providing care to the Canadian Cree.
3. Describe at least one health care practice that Bobby's mother may adhere to that may be perceived as negative.
4. Describe the structure of the traditional Canadian Cree family.
5. Describe at least one health care practice Bobby's mother may adhere to that may be considered efficacious.

References

Aboriginal Health Unit, Alberta Health. (1995). *Strengthening the circle: what aboriginal Albertans say about their health.* Alberta: Aboriginal Health Unit. Aboriginal Nurses Association of Canada.

Ahenakew, E. (1973). *Voices of the Plains Cree.* Toronto: McClelland & Stewart.

Anishinawbe Health Toronto. (1990). *Anishinawbe Health Toronto—budget proposal 1990-1991.* Toronto, Ont.: Anishnawbe Health Toronto.

Armstrong, H.A. (1990). The development and evolution of mental health services in the Sioux Lookout Zone over a 19-year period. In *Circumpolar health 90: Proceedings of the 8th international conference on circumpolar health.* Canadian Society for Circumpolar Health.

Beauvais, F., Oetting, E., Wolf, W., & Edwards, R. (1989). American Indian youth and drugs 1976-87: a continuing problem. *American Journal of Public Health, 79,* 634-636.

Bernard, M. (1997). Personal conversation with school nurses in Edmonton.

Brant, C.C. (1990). Native ethics and rules of behaviour. *Canadian Journal of Psychiatry, 35,* 534-539.

Brassard, P., Hoey, J., Ismail, J., & Gosselin, F. (1985). The prevalence of intestinal parasites and enteropathogenic bacteria in James Bay Cree Indians—Quebec. *Canadian Journal of Public Health, 76,* 322-325.

Burd, L., & Moffatt, M.E.K. (1994). Epidemiology of fetal alcohol syndrome in American Indians, Alaska Natives, and Canadian aboriginal peoples: a review of the literature. *Public Health Reports, 109*(5), 688-693.

Burke, S.O., Sayers, L.A., Baumgart, A.J., & Wray, J.G. (1985). Pitfalls in cross-cultural use of the Denver developmental screening test: Cree Indian children. *Canadian Journal of Public Health, 76,* 303-307.

Campbell, L., & Mithun, M. (Eds.). (1979). *The languages of Native America: historical and comparative assessment.* Austin, Texas: University of Texas Press.

Cardinal, N., & Steinhauer, H. (1994). An experience with the elders. In Smyth, D. (Ed.), *The Intercultural Health Association of Alberta sixth annual seminar on: Culture, health, and healing* (pp. 57-59). Edmonton, Alberta: Intercultural Health Association of Alberta.

Corrigan, S.W. (1970). The Plains Indian powwow: cultural integration in Manitoba and Saskatchewan. *Anthropologica, 12,* 253-277.

Crary, D. (1996, November 24). *Canada probes Indian abuse.* The Associated Press News Service.

Dempsey, H.A. (1986). *Indian tribes of Alberta* (ed. 2). Calgary: Glenbow Museum.

Dewdney, S. (1978). Birth of a Cree-Ojibway style of contemporary art. In Getty, I.A.L, & Smith, D.B. (Eds.), *One century later,* pp. 117-125. Vancouver: University of British Columbia Press.

Drew, L. (1988). Acculturation stress and alcohol usage among Canadian Indians in Toronto. *Canadian Journal of Public Health, 79,* 115-118.

Drost, H., Crowley, B.L., & Schwindt, R. (1995). *Market solutions for Native poverty: social policy for the third solution.* Toronto: C.D. Howe Institute.

Dyck, I.G. (1977). *The Harder site: a middle period bison hunter's campsite in the northern great plains.* Ottawa: National Museum of Man Mercury Series, Archaeological Survey of Canada Paper No. 67.

Editorial. (1996, February 24). A first nation message for Canadians. *Economist,* 44.

Editorial. (1997). A survival gene. *Maclean's, 110*(9), 58.

Farkas, C. (1987). Ethnospecific communication in diabetes education. In Canadian Diabetes Association (Ed.), *Diabetes in the Canadian Native population.* Biocultural perspectives (pp. 123-132). Winnipeg, Manitoba: Diabetes Association.

Feit, H.A. (1986). Hunting and the quest for power: the James Bay Cree. In Morrison, R.B., & Wilson, C.R. (Eds.), *Native peoples: the Canadian experience,* (pp. 171-207). Toronto: McClelland and Stewart.

Fisher, A.D. (1986). Great Plains ethnology. In Morrison, R.B., & Wilson, C.R. (Eds.), *Native peoples: the Canadian experience,* pp. 358-375. Toronto: McClelland & Stewart.

Foster, M.K. (1985). Native people, languages. In *The Canadian encyclopedia,* pp. 1217-1219. Edmonton: Hurtig.

Frideres, J.S. (1992). Racism and health: case of the Native people. In Boland, B., & Dickinson, H. (Eds.), *Health, illness, and health care in Canada* (pp. 202-220). Toronto: Harcourt.

Frideres, J.S. (1988). *Native peoples in Canada: contemporary conflicts.* Scarborough, Ont.: Prentice-Hall Canada, Inc.

Gaede, L. (1993). *Agency perspectives of native health in Edmonton's inner city.* Unpublished manuscript.

Goar, C. (1996, September 26). U.S. panel examines breakup of Canada but few legislators on hand to listen. *Toronto Star,* p. A21.

Hagey, R. (1984). The phenomenon, the explanations and the responses: metaphors surrounding diabetes in urban Canadian Indians. *Social Science and Medicine, 18*(3), 265-272.

Hanson, A. (1988). Problems in delivering health care and social services to the inner city. In Young, D.E. (Ed.), *Health care issues in the Canadian north* (pp. 25-28). Edmonton, Alberta: Boreal Institute for Northern Studies.

Hanvey, L., Avard, D., Graham, I., Underwood, K., Campbell, J., & Kelly, C. (1994). *The health of Canada's children: A CICH profile.* Ottawa, Ont.: Canadian Institute of Child Health.

Helm, J. (Ed.). (1981). *Handbook of North American Indians* (vol. 6). Washington, D.C.: Smithsonian Institution.

Jenish, D. (1995). A guardian angel for the derelicts. *Maclean's, 108*(49), 12.

Katz, P. (1981). Psychotherapy with Native adolescents. *Canadian Journal of Psychiatry, 26,* 455-459.

Krotz, L. (1980). *Urban Indians: the strangers in Canada's cities.* Edmonton, Alberta: Hurtig Publishers Ltd.

La Prairie, C. (1995). *Seen but not heard: native people in the inner city.* Ottawa, Ont.: Minister of Public Works and Government Services Canada.

Levinson, D. (Ed.). (1991). *Encyclopedia of world cultures,* volume 1, *North America.* Boston: G.K. Hall & Co.

Lloyd, N. (1994). Cowboy and Snowboy. *The Canadian Nurse, 90,* 59-60.

Mandelbaum, D.G. (1979). *The Plains Cree: an ethnographic, historical, and comparative study.* Canadian Plains Research Center, University of Regina.

Mason, L. (1967). The swampy Cree: a study in acculturation. Ottawa: National Museum of Canada.

McClure, L., Boulanger, M., Kaufert, J., & Forsyth, S. (1992). *First nations urban health bibliography: a review of the literature and exploration of strategies.* Winnipeg, Manitoba: Northern Health Research Unit.

McMillan, A.D. (1988). *Native peoples and cultures of Canada.* Vancouver/Toronto: Douglas & McIntyre.

Mobbs, R. (1986). But I do care! Communication difficulties affecting the quality of care delivered to Aborigines. *The Medical Journal of Australia, 144*(13), S3-S5.

Moon, P. (1996, October 25). Native victims of Canadian assimilation school abuse want judgment. *Toronto Globe and Mail.*

Morse, J.M., Young, D.E., & Swartz, L. (1991). Cree Indian healing practices and Western health care: a comparative analysis. *Social Sciences Medicine, 32*(12), 1361-1366.

Neander, W.L., & Morse, J.M. (1989). Tradition and change in the northern Alberta woodlands Cree: implications for infant feeding practices. *Canadian Journal of Public Health, 80,* 190-194.

Neergaard, L. (1997, January 8). Alzheimer's clues probed. The Associated Press News Service.

Nemeth, M., & Hiller, S. (1996). Paying the price. *Maclean's, 109*(49), 16.

Pompana, C., & Grumbly, J. (1994). *Inipi kagipi:* a native healing model. In Smyth, D. (Ed.), *The Intercultural Health Association of Alberta sixth annual seminar on: Culture, health, and healing* (pp. 57-59). Edmonton, Alberta: Intercultural Health Association of Alberta.

Preston, R.J. (1975). *Cree narrative: expressing the personal meaning of events.* Ottawa: National Museum of Man Mercury Series, Canadian Ethnology Service Paper No. 30.

Rogers, E.S. (1963). Changing settlement patterns of the Cree-Ojibwa of northern Ontario. *Southwestern Journal of Anthropology, 19,* 64-88.

Rogers, E.S. (1973). *The quest for food and furs: the Mistassini Cree, 1953-1954.* Ottawa: National Museum of Man, Publications in Ethnology No. 5.

Romaniuk, A. (1981). Modernization and fertility: the case of the James Bay Indians. *Canadian Review of Social Anthropology, 11,* 344-359.

Royal Commission on Aboriginal Peoples (1996). *Report of the Royal Commission on Aboriginal peoples.* Ottawa: Minister of Supply and Services Canada.

Sealey, D., Bruce, & Lussier, A.S. (1994). *The Métis: Canada's forgotten people.* Winnipeg, Manitoba: Pemmican Publications Inc.

Sharrock, S.R. (1974). Crees, Cree-Assiniboines: interethnic social organization on the far northern plains. *Ethnohistory, 21*(2), 95-122.

Shestowsky, B. (1995). Health-related concerns of Canadian Aboriginal people residing in urban areas. *International Nursing Review, 42*(1), 23-26.

Skinner, A. (1914). Political organization, cults, and ceremonies of the Plains-Ojibway and Plains-Cree Indians. *Anthropological papers of the American Museum of Natural History,* vol. 11, pt. 6, pp. 474-542.

Smith, J.G.E. (1987). Western Woods Cree: anthropological myth and historical reality. *American Ethnologist, 14,* 434-448.

Statistics Canada. (1995). *Profile of Canada's aboriginal population.* Ottawa: Industry, Science and Technology, 1991 Census of Canada. Catalogue number 94-325.

Statistics Canada. (1997). *Indian register population data.*

Tanner, A. (1979). *Bringing home animals: religious ideology and mode of production of the Mistassini Cree hunters.* St. John's, Newfoundland: Institute of Social and Economic Research, Memorial University of Newfoundland.

Tarasoff, K.J. (1980). *Persistent ceremonialism: the Plains Cree and Saulteaux.* Ottawa: National Museum of Man Mercury Series, Canadian Ethnology Service Paper No. 69.

Thompson, K. (1993, September). Self-governed health. *The Canadian Nurse, 89,* 29-32.

Thwaites, R.G. (Ed.). (1901). *The Jesuit relations and allied documents,* (vol. 18). Cleveland: Barrows Brothers.

Vickers, J.R. (1986). *Alberta plains prehistory: a review. Occasional Paper No. 27.* Edmonton: Archaeological Survey of Alberta.

Wissler, C. (1914). The influence of the horse in the development of Plains culture. *American Anthropologist, 16,* 1-25.

Wobeser, W., To, T., & Hoeppner, V.H. (1989). The outcome of chemoprophylaxis on tuberculosis prevention in the Canadian Plains Indian. *Clinical and Investigative Medicine, 12,* 149.

Wright, J.V. (1971). Cree culture history in the southern Indian Lake region. *Contributions to anthropology VII: archaeology and physical anthropology, 1-31.* Ottawa: National Museum of Man, Bulletin 232.

Young, T. (1982). Self perceived and clinically assessed health status of Indians in northwestern Ontario: analysis of a health survey. *Canadian Journal of Public Health, 73,* 272-277.

Young, T. (1994). *The health of Native Americans.* New York: Oxford University Press.

Young, T., & Casson, I. (1988). The decline and persistence of tuberculosis in a Canadian Indian population: implications for control. *Canadian Journal of Public Health, 79,* 302-306.

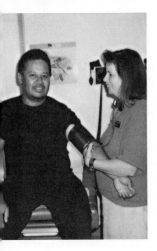

CHAPTER 10
The Canadian Ojibwa

JoLynn J. Reimer and Coleen Redskye

BEHAVIORAL OBJECTIVES

After reading this chapter, the nurse will be able to do the following:

1. Describe the influence of acculturation on the Canadian Ojibwa.
2. Develop a sensitivity and a understanding for the communication styles within and across the Canadian Ojibwa culture to avoid stereotyping and to provide culturally appropriate care.
3. Describe the time orientation of some Ojibwa people and its influence on wellness and illness behavior.
4. Discuss the spatial needs and implications for culturally appropriate care for the Canadian Ojibwa client.
5. Discuss the influence of family and social organization on behavior.
6. Explain the health care beliefs, folk beliefs, and folk practices of Canadian Ojibwa and the influence on health-seeking behavior.
7. Recognize physical, biological, and psychological variances that exist within and across the Canadian Ojibwa culture to provide culturally appropriate care.

HISTORIC OVERVIEW OF THE OJIBWA

The name "Ojibwa" originally came from one small group of native Indians north of modern Sault Sainte Marie. The term was later extended to other groups sharing the same culture and language in the Upper Great Lakes area including the Ojibwa, Ochipwe, and Chippewa (McMillan, 1988). According to legend, the Ojibwa called themselves *Anishinaabe,* which meant 'first man', or 'original man' (Kubiak, 1970; Johnston, 1976). The concept of "Anishinaabe nation" has emerged to link the widespread speakers of the Ojibwa language (Stan, 1989).

In the past, the English preferred to use the name Chippewa, or Chippeway, and it is these forms of the name that appeared on the treaties with the British government and later with the United States government. Today, many Ojibwa demonstrate interest in their native cultural identity by preferring to be called *Anishinaabe* (Galens, Sheets, and Young, 1995). However, the term "First Nations people," which is widely used by other aboriginal groups native to Canada, is also used by the Ojibwa (Royal Commission on Aboriginal People, 1995).

The origin of the term "Ojibwa" is also reported by legend. Some say it is related to the word 'puckered' that refers to the distinctive type of moccasin that had high cuffs and a puckered seam of the Ojibwa. Others say it was adopted because of the Anishinaabe practice of roasting their enemies until the corpses were puckered (Vecoli, 1995). Still others say the French used the word *o-jib-i-weg,* or 'pictograph' because the Anishinaabe employed a written language based on pictures or symbols (Galens, Sheets, and Young, 1995).

After the arrival of the Europeans in the 1660s, the Ojibwa underwent a major geographical expansion. After getting deeply involved with the fur trade and the Hudson Bay Company, the Ojibwa became heavily dependent on the European trade goods (Howard, 1965; McKay and Silman, 1995). When the Huron were defeated by the Iroquois in 1649-1650, in their contest for control of the western fur trade, the Ojibwa came under strong pressure from the Iroquois, which contributed to relocation. From their early historic homeland along the northern shores of Lake Huron and Lake Superior, with its center on the major fishery at the rapids of Sault Sainte Marie, some Ojibwa moved to the southeast into the formerly Iroquoian lands of southern Ontario. Others moved south into Wisconsin and Minnesota, often forcefully displacing others including the Dakota with firearms obtained from the French (McMillan, 1988; Ritzenthaler, 1978; Rogers, 1978). The lucrative fur trade lured many far to the north and west, into the Canadian Shield country of northern Ontario and Manitoba, in search of new trapping grounds (Rogers and Taylor, 1981). Some even spread out onto the plains, becoming the Plains Ojibwa of southern Manitoba and Saskatchewan.

Although some common traditions remained, the relocation to other geographical areas resulted in major cultural differences that evidently emerged among the Ojibwa people. This diversity was manifested by new traditions such as the use of different names by various subgroups. In fact, as many as 70 different names have been used to describe the people collectively known as "Ojibwa" (Hilger, 1992; McMillan, 1988; O'Leary and Levinson, 1991). Some of these names are still in use. For example, the term "Saulteaux" came from the French *Saulteurs,* or 'people of the rapids', referring to their origins at Sault Sainte Marie. Although the term "Saulteaux" is sometimes used as a near-synonym for Ojibwa, it is more commonly applied to western groups, such as those around Lake Winnipeg in Manitoba and Lake of the Woods in Ontario. Today, the American

Ojibwa, along with those of southern Ontario, are generally known as the "Chippewa" (McMillan, 1988).

The Ottawa (or *Odawa,* with stress on the second syllable) occupied much of the north shore of Georgian Bay and Manitoulin Island as well as the Bruce Peninsula, where they bordered on the Huron and Petun. Their lifestyle and language were virtually indistinguishable from the neighboring Ojibwa and the Potawatomi of lower Lake Michigan. In fact, these three groups formed a confederacy known as the "three fires" (Kubiak, 1970; Galens, Sheets, and Young, 1995). Several modern reserve communities in Ontario trace their ancestry to all three of these groups.

Much of the indigenous culture and religion of the Ojibwa remained intact until the early 1800s. At this time the fur trade began to decline, and more and more Ojibwa required assistance to meet their needs. However, the fur trade had changed an essential traditional pattern of life of the Ojibwa and that was that "you only take what you need" (McKay and Silman, 1995). The Ojibwa had become oriented to taking all the furs that could be found in order to trade for desirable commodities at the trading post thus violating a traditional value of the people. It was also at this time that the Canadian government began to restrict where the Ojibwa could live, violating another fundamental tradition of their lifestyle, that of following the source of food. Reserves were created, and children were placed in residential schools. For many Ojibwa, the changes in the traditional pattern of life brought social and cultural upheaval.

With the arrival of the Europeans there was also exposure to illnesses that had previously been unknown or rare in Canada. Infectious diseases were passed from the newcomers to the Native people with devastating results. As the larger sociodemographic fabric of the country changed during the postcontact period, the capacity for diseases to afflict the Native communities was enhanced. The growth of cities and communities, which increased population density, also supported acute community infections in endemic form. Poor living conditions on reserves ensured that chronic infections, like tuberculosis, took firm root in the communities, and thousands of the Native people died (Waldrum, Hering, and Young, 1995; Royal Commission on Aboriginal People, 1995). However, over the past 50 years, improved lifestyle has dramatically reduced the morbidity and morality associated with infectious disease and starvation, and a shift has occurred so that present health concerns include chronic diseases such as obesity, diabetes, and cardiovascular disease. However, among the Native population, including the Objiwa, the incidence of infectious diseases is still higher than the national average, as with respiratory and gastrointestinal infections, especially in children.

The Ojibwa are one of the largest American Indian groups north of Mexico. In the midseventeenth century, the Ojibwa numbered at least 35,000. Today, the Ojibwa located in Ontario, Manitoba, and Saskatchewan in Canada and Michigan, Wisconsin, Minnesota, North Dakota, Montana, and Oklahoma in the United States number about 160,000 (O'Leary and Levinson, 1991). Of the number of more than 76,000 registered Canadian Ojibwa, some 36,000 live on reserves (Statistics Canada, l995). This number is an underestimate of the Ojibwa because some choose not to be registered (Young, 1994).

To provide culturally competent care to this unique group of Native Canadians, it is important that the nurse understand their unique history. It is also important to assess each client for specific areas that typically vary across cultural groups.

COMMUNICATION

Algonquian is by far the largest and most widespread language family in Canada. It contains such well-known languages as Cree, spoken from northern Quebec to the Rockies, and Ojibwa, spoken from southern Ontario to Saskatchewan (McMillan, 1988). Spoken Ojibwa, or *Ojibwemowin,* has regional dialectal differences (Galens, Sheets, and Young, 1995). Because it is a spoken rather than a written language, the spelling of Ojibwa words varies. Common Ojibwa expressions include: *Boozhoo* (/bō-zhō/, from French *Bonjour* 'Good day'), 'Hello'; 'Greetings'; *Miigwech* (/mée-gwaych/), 'Thank you'; *Aniin ezhi-ayaayan?* (/uh-néen ay-zhée uh-yáw-

yun/), 'How are you?'; *Nimino-ayaa* (/nuh-mínno uh-yáw/), 'I am fine'; *Mino-ayaag!* (/mínno uh-yáwg/), 'All of you be well!' Young (1994) notes that, of the hundreds of Native American languages in Canada, only three languages still have large enough numbers of speakers not to be threatened with extinction—Inuit language, Cree, and Ojibwa. Today, over 29,000 Canadians report knowledge of the Ojibwa language, and over 12,000 report Ojibwa as their home language (Statistics Canada, 1995).

As the geographic movement of the Ojibwa was restricted by the Canadian government and children were placed into English-speaking schools, Ojibwa children became bilingual. Consequently, as the children became adults, use of the Ojibwa language decreased, and so by the mid-1940s only the elderly were bilingual. However, although for a time Ojibwa was spoken only by elders, there is currently a resurgence of interest in and promotion of the language (Galens, Sheets, and Young, 1995). Instruction is available in some public as well as tribally directed educational settings. Classes and workshops offered at community colleges and state universities are sometimes broadcast to more distant locations. Language texts as well as instructional material in workbooks, bilingual texts, audiotapes, and multimedia formats have also been developed. Tribal newspapers carry regular Ojibwa-language columns (Tanner, 1992). Today, many young Ojibwa adults are bilingual. However, bilingual speech is often limited to Ojibwa or English.

The communication patterns of the Ojibwa include complex nonverbal behaviors (McRae, 1994). For many Ojibwa eye contact is considered disrespectful because it is believed that to look into someone's eyes is to look into that person's soul (Henderson and Primeaux, 1981). Eye contact is considered acceptable when greeting an individual and occasionally throughout an interview, but maintenance of eye contact is not considered acceptable. In many tribes, nonverbal communication is a highly practiced art (Orque, Bloch, and Monrroy, 1983). For example, an Indian child is taught to organize thought processes before verbalizing them. Some Ojibwa assess body language for congruency with verbal messages to evaluate the truthfulness of what is said (Hagey and Buller, 1983).

Silence is a culturally related behavior for the Ojibwa. The lack of response to a question does not mean a refusal to respond. It is socially acceptable for an Ojibwa not to answer a question immediately but in a few days or even weeks, or not to respond at all to certain types of probing questions (Hagey and Buller, 1983).

The value of respect for all people is an important tradition of the Ojibwa. For example, if a person has a disability of some type, he or she is valued because of other sensitivities. Children are taught that people who are different physically, mentally, or emotionally must be respected because they have something to give that the community needs to learn. Traditionally respect was also demonstrated in ways such as learning multiple languages in order to honor guests. Even today old trappers or grandmothers talk of the time when they would go to their isolated winter traplines and encounter another group of people. They would show respect for one another by learning one another's language and caring for each other. Depending on whose camp it was, they would welcome the stranger. Welcoming strangers into one's midst and honoring them is a strong community motif (McKay and Silman, 1995).

Implications for nursing care

It is important for the nurse to appreciate the importance of verbal speech etiquette when relating to the Ojibwa people (Hagey and Buller, 1983). Direct, factual, and personal questioning, which is often the typical approach of a health care professional doing an assessment, can be interpreted by the Ojibwa as a form of violation of dignity. Such questions may be met with complete silence or meaningless answers. It is also expedient for the nurse to question the validity and completeness of information that is obtained by direct questioning because the use of hurried questions violates a deeply embedded cultural principle of noninterference (Hanson, 1988). An example of a factual question that is taboo and would likely be met by silence, anger, or avoidance, would be, "What kind of exercise do you get?" A better way to obtain information is the indirect approach such

as, "Sometimes Natives who live in the city don't get the exercise they need." This information gives the hearer the opportunity to interpret the statement as a question about activity level and to make the choice of responding (Hagey and Buller, 1983). It is important for the nurse to develop a level of comfort with silence because some Ojibwa find health care professionals too talkative, tending to fill every gap in the conversation with words.

To establish credibility with an Ojibwa client the nurse must be prepared to compromise, to trust, and to be open to the belief system of the client (McRae, 1994). Nurses who are competent with cultural assessment and negotiation will be most successful in relating to the Ojibwa client (Tripp-Reimer and Afifi, 1989). The culturally competent nurse must also be acutely aware of the value the Ojibwa place on showing respect. When respect is not felt, communication will be ineffective (McKay and Silman, 1995).

Since Ojibwa tend to enjoy humor in interpersonal interactions, the nurse may want to incorporate cartoons in client education. Humor is also a way to relieve tension when interacting with the Ojibwa (Hagey and Buller, 1983). However, caution should be used in using cartoons in teaching because some Ojibwa may regard this as a suggestion of lower intelligence and therefore an indication of the nurse's lack of respect.

The nurse should consider that questions need to be varied depending on the level of acculturation. For example, if an outhouse is used, the client complaining of gastrointestinal symptoms may have a difficult time answering a question such as, "Did you notice blood in your stool?"

SPACE

Traditional life for the Ojibwa was altered dramatically through contact with the Europeans in Canada. The Canadian Ojibwa had historically spent much of their year moving in dispersed groups in search of subsistence. During the summer they congregated at fishing sites in proximity to trading posts, where they procured their supplies for the coming year (O'Leary and Levinson, 1991). When the Canadian government established reserves for the Indians, seasonal travel was restricted and relocation policies dispersed tribe members. Around the beginning of the twentieth century Indian residential schools, or industrial schools as they were called on the prairies, began to be a central focus of the church missions. Children were taken away from their families and placed into boarding schools (McKay and Silman 1995). To this day, the Ojibwa tend to feel restricted in meeting their spatial needs, and many retain the feeling that their land and consequently part of their cultural heritage was unfairly taken away (Fennell, 1995). Some blame the social problems experienced today on the residential school system saying that children lost their sense of identity and family and even experienced physical and sexual abuse during separation from their families.

Traditionally the Ojibwa lived in wigwams that could be taken down and moved from one place to the next. However, by the late 1880s, few wigwams could be found and most Ojibwa lived in one-room log cabins, frame cabins, or tar-paper shacks. Today, although most Ojibwa live in prefabricated homes, living spaces may be cramped, and the high incidence of poverty and unemployment cause living conditions that are less than optimal. Although the actual living space of the traditional living quarters was small, the Ojibwa enjoyed a nomadic style with miles of open space for their living domain. Today, many Ojibwa find the space designated to them on the reserve too confining and feel that the treaties made for the land do not provide the space to which they are entitled (Royal Commission of Aboriginal Peoples, 1995). Living conditions vary greatly between different reserves. Some communities still have no running water or very basic water systems, whereas others have had modern conveniences for many years.

Implications for nursing care

It is important for the nurse caring for the Ojibwa client and family to appreciate the importance of the wide open spaces and the value of being able to commune with nature. Although Ojibwa clients may be accustomed to living close to others, for many the urge for the wide open spaces still remains. It is important for the nurse to contribute to efforts made to improve quality of life in the patient's living space and to facilitate efforts made to move the Ojibwa patient toward employment and an adequate income. The nurse should be aware that if the home environment does not provide running water this can create great hardships in keeping children clean. The nurse needs to assess the client's living conditions in order to develop appropriate plans; that is, will a mother be able to wash all bedclothes as a treatment for head lice or are other methods appropriate or more current?

SOCIAL ORGANIZATION

Traditionally the basic social unit for the Ojibwa was the extended family. However, relatives in the extended family were referred to with kinship terminology, thus drawing the relationship even closer. Parallel cousins were merged terminologically with siblings. Parallel aunts and uncles were merged terminologically by sex with mother and father. However, closeness to the extended family has given way to the nuclear family as Ojibwa youth have begun to leave the reserves and to become acculturated in large White cities.

Traditionally, children were raised in a permissive fashion and rarely reprimanded or punished physically. The most important phase of a boy's life occurred at puberty when he sought a guardian spirit through a vision quest involving several days of isolation, fasting, and prayer. Some young men were believed to receive spiritual powers through their vision quest, and it was these persons who in later life became shamans. Girls were also isolated at the time of first menstruation but did not undergo a vision quest. Some Plains Ojibwa girls were visited by a spirit and in this way were believed to have been given curing powers (Densmore, 1979). Today some Ojibwa are still attributed with having healing powers, and shamans can still be found practicing in some areas.

Traditionally, for the Ojibwa, division of labor between the genders involved shared responsibility for numerous economic activities such as fishing and trapping, and sometimes they cooperated in the same tasks such as canoe construction. Men's labor focused on hunting, trapping, and trading, and women's labor was concerned more with processing hides, making clothes, preparing foods, caring for children, and collecting plant foods and firewood (O'Leary and Levinson, 1991).

Historically the Ojibwa people were linked by autonomous politically independent bands that shared common traditions, their own chief, and a hunting territory. Bands dispersed into family hunting units much of the year, assembling in greater numbers in the spring and summer. Band organization was loose and flexible, and social relations, apart from divisions along the lines of age and sex, were egalitarian. Bands of the Ojibwa in Canada numbered from 50 to 75 members. Chiefs frequently held their position by virtue of prowess in hunting, warfare, or shamanism (McMillan, 1988). Ojibwa society was further divided into clans, each identified by a clan symbol, or totem. Warren (1984) listed 21 totems, of which the most important were the crane, catfish, bear, marten, wolf, and loon. The living totem animals were not worshipped, nor did clan members refrain from killing them for food, though a certain respect had to be shown. Clan membership was patrilineal; that is, children inherited their totem animal from their fathers. Persons sharing the same totem were considered to be close kin, and intermarriage was forbidden (McMillan, 1988).

On cold and dark winter evenings, as the Ojibwa people sat around the fires in their wigwams, a favorite pastime was listening to stories told by elders. Ojibwa mythology served both to instruct and to entertain. The rich oral traditions were filled with supernatural humans and animals, one of the most prominent being the culture hero Nanabush (or Nanabozho). It was Nanabush who put the earth and animals into their present form, many prominent features of the landscape were attributed to his actions, and he served an ambiguous role as both benefactor to humans and a self-indulgent and occasionally obscene trickster (McMillan, 1988). A most terrifying legendary figure was Windigo (Ojibwa *Wīntīko*, Cree *Wīhtikōw*), a supernatural giant with an insatiable hunger for human flesh (Densmore, 1979). Any unexplained disappearance would be taken to mean that the person had fallen pray to Windigo. This monster was particularly

feared because ordinary humans could be transformed into one by conditions of near starvation, which were not uncommon during the later months of winter. Anyone suspected of becoming a Windigo could immediately be put to death (McMillan 1988).

The Fox word for 'owl' is a *wi:teko:wa*, meaning an 'animate being that is called by higher [or demonic] powers' because "persons about to die hear the owl call their name . . . [which acts] as an agent of those powers" (Hewson, 1992). Many other powerful supernatural beings inhabited the Ojibwa world as well as lesser spirits who were also attributed with powers to help or hinder humans. The Jesuit Father Allouez, who traveled among the people in the mid-1660s, described religious beliefs of many spirits who could be either hurtful or helpful (Thwaites, 1896-1901).

Today, bands are sometimes larger than the size reported for earlier bands (Stan, 1989). Some modern bands include 300 to 400 people (Stan, 1989), whereas others may be as large as 1000 people. A single band may include persons living on a reservation as well as persons who do not.

Ojibwa religion was very much an individual affair and centered on the belief in power received from spirits during dreams and visions. For this reason, dreams and visions were accorded great significance, and much effort was given to their interpretation. Missionization by the Church of England, the Roman Catholic church, and later the Methodist church began during the nineteenth century, but conversion and Christian influence were limited before the twentieth century. In the midtwentieth century, the religious orientation of many Ojibwa was a mixture of Christian and traditional native elements (Rogers and Taylor, 1981; McKay and Silman, 1995).

Traditionally, special rituals surrounded death. If a person died inside a wigwam, the body was removed through a hole made in the west-facing side of the dwelling. The body was wrapped in birch bark and buried with items of special significance. During the next 4 days the individual's spirit or ghost was said to be walking westward to a place where the soul would swell after death. Food and beverage were left at the grave site for the spirit's consumption during the walk. Grave sites were marked by the erection of gabled wood houses over the length of the grave. A wooden marker was painted with the pictograph illustrating the individual's achievements and clan affiliation; the totem animal was painted upside down, denoting death. Families mourned for periods of up to 1 year, with some family members expressing grief by blackening their faces, chests, and hands with charcoal and maintaining an unkempt appearance. A feast of the dead service, scheduled each fall, was sponsored by families who had lost members over the previous year. Food continued to be left at the grave site at regular intervals over a period of many years (Galens, Sheets, and Young, 1995). For some Ojibwa these traditions are still maintained with a ceremonial "giveaway" taking place at strategic times after the death, such as 1 year. Such practices vary depending on the community and the religious beliefs of the family. In any case, whether maintained or not, the burial grounds of the ancestors have a special significance and are the basis of current legal action (Bolstering a Case, 1997).

Traditionally the Ojibwa were more concerned with comforts of their dress and less worried about their appearance than some Indian tribes. Deerskins, dressed with the hair still on, composed their shirt or coat, which was usually encircled around the waist with a belt or sash and hung halfway down the thigh. Moccasins were worn, and leggings were sewn fastened to a belt. A collar or scarflike garment circled the neck, and the skin of a deer's head was formed into an unusual type of hoodlike cap. They also wore turbans made of fur and in later years of woven sash. A robe was made of several deerskins sewn together. More attention made paid to women's hair, which was worn long, oiled with bear's grease, and braided (Kubiak, 1970). Today most Ojibwa have adopted modern clothing, and traditional dress is worn only for ceremonial occasions (Buffalohead, 1986).

Implications for nursing care

A central Ojibwa value is that everything belongs to everyone in the extended family. Traditionally, personal property had a very limited place in tribal community (McKay and Silman, 1995). Women were generally the keepers of the gifts of the community, balancing the economy so that food was distributed throughout the whole community. Today it is important for the nurse working with Ojibwa people to appreciate the strong ethic of sharing and of hospitality. When clients are following special diets, it is important that this concept be taken into consideration so that the nurse can help the client plan to meet dietary needs.

The nurse should appreciate the importance of family for Ojibwa clients. Family members will generally want to be involved in decisions regarding health care and will want to remain close to the hospitalized client.

TIME

Many Ojibwa people have a past and present time orientation (Brant, 1983; England, 1986). Orientation to the past is actualized by respect for tradition, the elders, and adherence to time-honored respect for harmony with nature. Orientation for the present is demonstrated by a present-time orientation. What is happening in the present is to be enjoyed and should receive undivided attention. The Ojibwa have generally been taught not to be concerned with the future. However, as the Ojibwa people adopt values of the society around them, more are becoming future oriented. Increasing numbers are leaving the reserve and migrating to predominantly White cities, going to school to learn a trade, and becoming part of a society oriented around future goals (Burke, Kisilevsky, and Maloney, 1989).

Implications for nursing care

It is generally held that there are differences in time orientation between Canadian Indians and their predominantly White health care providers (Burke, Kisilevsky, and Maloney, 1989). However, it has also been noted that time differences vary with Indians who are in urban versus rural settings and in situations where individuals are sick and need treatment as opposed to social settings (Burke, Kisilevsky, and Maloney, 1989).

There are general cultural considerations related to time of which the nurse working with the Ojibwa people should be cognizant. For example, it is important for the nurse working with the Ojibwa people to appreciate that Ojibwa speech etiquette involves taking time to get familiar with the health care professional before discussing health care problems (Hagey and Buller, 1983). Proceeding quickly in a health assessment to a discussion of the problem violates the appreciation for the present and the need to first establish a relationship. The Ojibwa client will be quick to notice if the health care professional is hurried or impatient and does not take the necessary time for relationship building. A smile will generally be accepted as reassuring on greeting a client but must be accompanied by an unhurried approach that establishes rapport. Relationship building and establishing rapport are very important and frequently take a long time when relating to an Ojibwa client. First Nations people have many reasons not to trust non-Natives.

The culturally sensitive nurse also needs to appreciate that individuals with a present-time orientation may not be compliant with keeping medical or clinic appointments though this may make a difference if the appointment is for a preventive purpose or to treat a health situation that exists (Burke, Kisilevsky, and Maloney, 1989). When a health situation exists, it is essential for the nurse to emphasize the importance of careful management. The nurse should work with the client to develop a nursing care plan that is relevant to the client's life situation and their understanding of their health problem. Additionally the nurse should help the client to plan how care activities can be incorporated into the client's daily activities so that health care needs can be met (McRae, 1994).

ENVIRONMENTAL CONTROL

Before the arrival of the Europeans the Ojibwa lived in close harmony with their environment. Rather than controlling the environment the Ojibwa emphasized living in harmony and respecting the environment. The environment was not abused, and only what was needed was taken. However, the environment also was respected for providing essentials needed for life.

Unfortunately harmony with the environment was disrupted by the Europeans, and there were significant differences in values about the land. The British attempted to make treaties with the Ojibwa. Unfortunately for the Indians and the British, treaties served two entirely different purposes. The British expected the Ojibwa to acknowledge the authority of the monarch and to cede large tracts of land to British control. To the Ojibwa the notion of giving up land was a concept foreign to their culture. The treaties that were signed in good faith were soon seen as domination. Many Ojibwa believed that policies were made to suppress the Native people, remove them from their homelands, undermine their culture, and stifle their identity (Royal Commission on Aboriginal People, 1995). Although Colonial and Canadian governments established "reserves" of land for the Native people, they were usually regarded as having inadequate size and resources (Royal Commission on Aboriginal People, 1995).

Policies on domination and assimilation have created poverty, ill health, and social disorganization among the Ojibwa people. In 1969 the federal government's white paper on Indian policy that offered "equality" was unanimously rejected by the First Nations people. Rather than assimilation being seen as positive, the First Nations people identified that assimilation was causing social dysfunction and family breakdown, suicide and attempted suicide among youth, substance abuse, and trouble with the law (Royal Commission of Aboriginal People, 1995). After a dozen years of intense political struggle by the Native people in Canada, including appeals to the queen and the British Parliament, a historic breakthrough occurred in the Constitution Act, 1982, in which existing aboriginal and treaty rights were recognized. This set the stage for profound changes in the relationship among the peoples of Canada.

However peaceful coexistence and agreement that Indian claims are being honored does not exist (Indians of North America, 1995). The Ojibwa (Chippewa) in Ontario are in the spotlight regarding this debate. An article entitled "Bolstering a Case" in the March 24, 1997, edition of *Maclean's* described a $36 million lawsuit against the federal government by the Kettle and Stony Point First Nation. The Indian Claims Commission, a federal advisory body, issued a nonbinding recommendation that Ottawa should compensate the Ojibwa in Ontario's Ipperwash area on Lake Huron for being cheated out of 33 hectares of land. Another recent conflict on an Ontario reserve involved the shooting of a native Ojibwa man over a conflict over sacred burial ground (Fennell, 1995). Yet another conflict involved the Ojibwa community at Kettle and Stony Point. Reserve land was taken to make an armed forces base in 1942 with the provision that the land would be returned after the war. Up to now, the land has not been officially returned (Steele, 1995). Thus the cultural value of ownership of land and the relationship to the environment is still keenly felt by the Ojibwa, and the battle over environmental control continues continues even to this day.

The Native people have traditionally believed that health is a spiritual experience. "The intimacy of religion and medicine is seen in the Native American theory of disease and illness causation, treatment, and prevention" (Henderson and Primeaux, 1981). Disease and illness are caused by soul loss, spiritual intrusion, taboo violation, object intrusion, sorcery or witchcraft, natural phenomena, or lack of harmony (Atcheson, 1987). Disease could also be retribution for improper conduct toward the supernatural or some social trangression (O'Leary and Levinson, 1991). The Weendigo [Windigo] myth as described by Darnell (1981) is the symbolization of the Ojibwa belief in the spirit of excess. Weendigo is the opposite of Nanabush. If an individual is overpowered by Weendigo, a lack of balance is created. It is believed by some Ojibwa that alcoholism is caused by Weendigo. There is also a widespread belief among the Ojibwa that diabetes is the result of excesses of one's ancestors (Hagey and Buller, 1983).

Folk medicine for the Ojibwa has generally involved a holistic approach, including the physical, spiritual, and psychological (Atcheson, 1987). Curing was traditionally performed by members of the *midéwiwin*, or Medicine Lodge Society, into which both men and women were inducted after instruction by *midé* priests, payment of fees, and formal initiation. Shamans, with their powers derived from dreams and visions, were and in some cases are the present curers of sickness. Others knowledgeable in the use of medicinal plants are attributed with healing skills (O'Leary and Levinson, 1991). Traditional herbal cures include sumac fruit made into a decoction with crushed roots to stop bleeding, blackberry roots boiled and drunk to stop diarrhea or prevent spontaneous abortion, wild onions cooked and sweetened with maple sugar to treat children's colds, yarrow roots mashed into creams for treating blemishes, strawberry roots boiled and eaten to treat stomachaches, and plantain leaves chopped and used as a poultice for bruises, rheumatism, and snake bites (Galen, Sheets, and Young, 1995). Today the Ojibwa tend to use a blend of traditional and modern treatment methods to improve health.

Among the most serious health problems affecting Native Canadians are injuries from accidents and violence. In the younger age groups, injuries are by far the most important cause of illnesses and death, and overall they may account for as many as 24% to 40% of all deaths (Young, 1994). Motor vehicle accidents (MVA) are the single most important cause of injury deaths, associated for just under 30% of all injury mortality among Native Canadians. MVAs have been observed to occur more frequently in areas of low per capita income and in rural areas (Baker, Whitfield, and O'Neill, 1987). In many remote Native communities where roads and motor vehicles are few, the risk of death from motor vehicles is comparable to or even lower than that of the national population. On the other hand, the risk of death from other transport accidents (such as railway and boats), where these are the chief means of transportation, is extremely high (Young, 1994). In recent years injuries associated with off-the-road recreational vehicles have become increasingly of public health concern (Postl, Moffatt, and Sarsfield, 1987). Fires and burns accounted for twice the number of deaths in Native Americans in Canada as in the United States during the period 1979 to 1988 (8% versus 4%) (Young et al., 1991).

Implications for nursing care

Today, the health of the Native Americans is generally at a lower level than that of the rest of the Canadian population. Health education including information about nutrition, exercise, oral hygiene, and other aspects of self-care are essential if health is to be increased among the Ojibwa people. Information about immunizations, basic hygiene principles, and the importance of rest are important concepts that need to be communicated for the overall health of the Ojibwa to be improved. However, it is important for the culturally sensitive nurse to appreciate that health education can be accomplished only by first establishing the need to know and by working with the key people in the community in developing a plan for what needs to be taught. The successful plan for education must be related to perceived need (Hagey and Buller, 1983; Lechky, 1991). It is important to work with the community elders and leaders to determine health education needs. It is also crucial to understand how they want information presented to the community, that is, in regard to sensitive issues such as sexuality, acquisition of HIV, or suicide. Information regarding nutrition must be appropriate to the circumstances of the client; that is, those in isolated communities may have limited access to fresh fruit or vegetables or the cost may be prohibitive and thus irrelevant. Knowledge of the traditional eating patterns is important to incorporate the use of these foods, such as some wild meat and fish. Respect for the nurse doing the teaching is also a critical aspect for success in the teaching-learning environment. Whether the client is familiar with the nurse, it is wise to offer directions to the Ojibwa client as suggestions or advice rather than firm directives because the Ojibwa client may be sensitive to a non-Native using an authoritarian approach.

Providing prenatal care is also an important area needing culturally competent intervention. Research indicates that Native Canadian women do not regularly attend prenatal care (Sokoloski, 1995). Generally Ojibwa women conceptualize pregnancy in a spiritual context and believe that it is a healthy, natural process requiring no intervention. Unfortunately this belief occurs despite the fact that the Ojibwa tend to be a high-risk group (Sokoloski, 1995). Since Ojibwa women believe that they are responsible for taking care of themselves during pregnancy, cultural

practices that are regarded as promoting a healthy pregnancy are espoused. Sokoloski (1995) noted that Native women believed that their expectations of freely offered explanations and a friendly nonauthoritarian approach were often not realized when health care was sought. Additionally they noted that their beliefs about health care were often in conflict with beliefs of the health-care providers. To reduce barriers in providing prenatal care holistic culturally appropriate care needs to be provided. On the other hand, it has been noted that Ojibwa women are compliant with suggestions about prenatal care when such suggestions are given in a low-key approach and when the reasons behind the recommendations are explained (Sokoloski, 1995).

The nurse working with the Ojibwa people should not automatically expect that instructions given will be followed and must not be frustrated when noncompliance becomes evident. To increase effectiveness of patient teaching and discharge planning, it is necessary for the nurse to be aware of the range of values and beliefs of the client related to health and the meaning of illness as well. To do this it becomes necessary to assess the degree to which individual clients are influenced by their cultural background. The importance of traditional healing practices and the possibility of blending them with Western biomedicine for a more holistic approach to health care for the individual client needs to be considered. It is important to be sensitive when the belief system of the Ojibwa client is being assessed. Some are comfortable with traditional healers and prefer to use only Indian medicine, whereas others complement Western medicine with it. Others have strong Christian beliefs and would be offended at the suggestion of using traditional techniques. Some are comfortable talking about the spirit world with the nurse, whereas others prefer to avoid such topics with non-Natives. In any case, it is important that client teaching make sense within a cultural as well as a social context.

Ferris (1994) notes that the cultural upheaval that has occurred among the aboriginal communities in Canada has contributed to increased family violence. This was specifically identified in one study in Ontario that included Ojibwa clients (Ferris and Tudiver, 1992). Health care professionals need to work with communities for community-based action against wife abuse. Health professionals must work closely with women to help them disclose abuse because community values regarding family preservation can be very strong. Advocating safe community options for women and children is important as well as working on prevention issues.

BIOLOGICAL VARIATIONS
Body size and structure
Similar to other Native Indians, the Ojibwa people are generally robust and tall in stature, their complexions are dark, their features are broad, and their hair is straight and jet black (Kubiak, 1970). Fat distribution appears to be a significant factor for Ojibwa. Among the Cree-Ojibwa, overall, 38% of men had a waist-to-hip ratio greater than 0.99, compared to only 11% among women. Central obesity was much less evident among women (Young and Sevenhuysen, 1989).

Enzymatic and genetic variations
Physiological responses to alcohol ingestion, such as facial flushing, and unpleasant symptoms, such as headaches and tachycardia, also have been found to vary between ethnic groups. In a comparative study of Whites, Chinese, and Ojibwa Indians, Reed et al. (1976) noted that, in tandem with the fastest decline in blood ethanol concentration among the three groups, the Indians also showed the highest levels of acetaldehyde at various times after the ingestion of ethanol.

Susceptibility to disease
Tuberculosis Although the incidence of tuberculosis (TB) has been believed to be present among Native Americans since prehistoric times, there is little doubt that after the influx of European settlers to Canada the effect of the disease became devastating (Rieder, 1989; Young, 1994). It has been speculated that the high incidence of TB was the result of enforced changes in ecological factors such as poor nutrition rather than exposure to a new, introduced infectious disease (Clark et al., 1987). During the twentieth century, the mortality from TB has declined substantially. However, despite improvements, the disparity in incidence between Natives and non-Natives remains great, with Native peoples having an incidence as much as 10 times higher than non-Native peoples in Canada (Young, 1994). The rates were lowest in eastern Canada and higher in the prairie provinces and northern territories (Enarson and Grzybowski, 1986). Region studies, such as those among the Cree-Ojibwa in northwestern Ontario (Young and Casson, 1988), supported the national trend toward a leveling off in the decline.

Hypertension The prevalence of hypertension has been determined in small population studies of Native American groups in Canada (Casper, Rith-Najarian, et al., 1996). A survey among the Ojibwa and Cree in the 1980s showed a higher mean diastolic blood pressure in all age-sex groups compared with that of Canadians nationally, whereas for systolic blood pressure, the Indians' level was lower above 45 years of age (Young, 1991).

Diabetes Diabetes has been studied extensively among the American Indians. Diabetes among North American Indians is overwhelmingly of the non-insulin dependent type (NIDDM) (Young, 1993; Young and Harris, 1994). There is wide geographical variation in prevalence. Although the factors that contribute to differences are not well understood, they probably reflect the differential effects of genetic susceptibility, overall level of "acculturation," and the contributions of specific risk factors such as physical activity, diet, and obesity (Young, 1994). Young, Szathmary, Evers, and Wheatley (1990) noted that there were significantly elevated levels of diabetes among Algonquian-speaking Indians, whether in the Subarctic, Plains, or Northeast (Woodland) cultures. However, Harris et al. (1997) found prevalence rates of NIDDM in a remote Algonquian-speaking reserve of 1600 Ojibwa-Cree persons of Sandy Lake, Ontario, to be the highest reported in the world. Native females on this reserve appeared to be at a much higher risk of becoming obese and developing impaired glucose tolerance and NIDDM and at a younger age than Native males. Measures of obesity and fasting insulin levels were significantly associated with NIDDM in the 18 to 49 year age group (Harris et al., 1997). In other studies, the risk of diabetes in Canadian Indians has been reported to be greater by a factor of two for men and greater by a factor of four for women than the risk for Canadian men and women in general (Mao et al., 1986). It appears that the lifestyle changes occurring on some reserves in which there is high unemployment, lack of exercise, and consumption of a diet high in fat, which have replaced the nomadic hunter-gatherer existence, are significantly contributing to diabetes (Harris et al., 1997).

Some evidence supports the ideology that diabetes is a health problem of relatively recent origin with the Ojibwa. Among the Cree-Ojibwa about half of all existing and still-living cases have been diagnosed in the last 5 years of a 25-year period (Young et al., 1985). Among the Cree-Ojibwa, several factors have been found to be associated with diabetic status or high plasma glucose levels (as measured by fasting plasma glucose and glycosylated hemoglobin) on multivariate analysis. Although age, triglycerides, and body-mass index were predictive of diabetic status, fasting plasma glucose, and glycosylated hemoglobin levels, it was education and waist-to-hip ratio that were associated with elevated glycosylated hemoglobin levels only (Young et al., 1990). Among Cree-Ojibwa diabetics, the duration of illness and coexisting hypertension were associated with the prevalence of complications, whereas the initial glucose level and weight status were not (Young et al., 1985).

Nutritional preferences and deficiencies

Traditionally, Ojibwa cuisine was closely influenced by the seasons. For example, because the Ojibwa who lived in southern Canada used maple sugar as a seasoning, during the late spring they lived near maple trees. Camps were moved in the summer to be close to gardens and wild berry patches. The Ojibwa cultivated gardens of corn, pumpkins, beans, and squash for trading. Dried berries, vegetables,

and seeds were stored in underground pits. They drank decoctions boiled from plants and herbs and sweetened with maple sugar. The Ojibwa fished throughout the year, using hooks, nets, spears, and traps. On the prairies and northern tundra there were vast migrating herds of bison and caribou. Fish and meat were dried and smoked so that they could be stored. In the late summer the Ojibwa moved again to be near wild rice fields. The rice harvest was a time of community celebration with the medicine man blessing the first rice harvested. Rice was often boiled and sweetened with maple sugar or flavored with venison or duck broth. Up to one third of the annual harvest was stored, usually in birch-bark baskets (Galens, Sheets, and Young, 1995).

Today, many of these old traditional nutritional patterns are gone. In fact, an improper diet has been identified as a major problem among the Native Americans because northern stores tend to stock processed foods high in fat content and low in nutritional value. The fruits and vegetables that are available are often prohibitively expensive and of poor quality (Lechky, 1991). Even when adequate food is available, the Ojibwa often lack knowledge of proper nutrition, and thus dietary intake is not well balanced.

Psychological characteristics

High rates of suicide and homicide are universal across all tribes and regions of Native Canadians. There are tribal differences demonstrated in a study between 1973 and 1982 where the mean annual rate of suicide for the Northern Ojibwa was 5, Chipewyan 13, Cree 22, Saulteaux 48, and Sioux 80 per 100,000 respectively. This correlated with their degree of isolation. The more isolated the tribe, the lower was the rate (Garro, 1988). An excess was observed in all ages for homicide, whereas for suicide the Native peoples had a lower risk beyond 45 years of age. Since the 1960s the tend appeared to be one of increasingly earlier onset. This trend, however, began to be reversed in the 1980s for both suicide and homicide (Ross and Davis, 1986).

Alcohol consumption and chemical dependency is discouraged among the Ojibwa. Traditionally alcohol and drugs were banned from powwow sites, and some powwows were organized to celebrate sobriety (Galens, Sheets, and Young, 1995). In fact, although alcohol use is high among some Native populations in Canada, alcohol use has been found to be lower than with non-Natives in some groups including the Ojibwa. For example, only about 20% of adult Ojibwa in northwestern Ontario, compared to 80% in the general population, were ever drinkers. The prevalence declined with age but was highest among those with the most education (Young, 1982). In a survey of residents over 5 years of age in an Ojibwa community in eastern Manitoba, it was found that adults and school pupils who participated in hobbies were less likely to use alcohol. Young people who reported good family relationships were also less likely to use alcohol and marijuana (Longclaws et al., 1980).

Implications for nursing care

The benefits of early diagnosis and prompt initiation of therapy for tuberculosis are well documented in the health care literature (Anonymous, 1994). Thus it is important for the nurse working with Native Canadians to assist these communities to participate in surveillance programs as well as to teach individuals of the early signs and symptoms so that they can be reported for evaluation.

In one study of an Ojibwa community in southern Manitoba it was determined that cultural beliefs can be at odds with the prevalent biomedical view on the chronicity of the illness and the importance of "compliance" with treatment. Hypertension was conceived by the Ojibwa in this study as episodic in nature, accompanied by perceptible symptoms, and treatment was therefore needed only when symptoms were present (Garro, 1988). It is therefore important for the nurse who is attempting a culturally appropriate intervention to provide education about the cause of hypertension and the need for ongoing monitoring.

Because of the prevalence of diabetes among the Ojibwa, it is important for the nurse working with the Ojibwa to be involved in client education and to try to help the client to understand the importance of diet and exercise in relation to control of symp-

toms. However, as was demonstrated by a native diabetes project for Ojibwa people living in Toronto it is very important for the nurses to keep in mind that for the culturally unique Ojibwa people true self-care can result only when a client's dignity and sovereignty have not been violated and a feeling of personal control is present (Hagey and Buller, 1983). Some nurses have found it useful to take the Nanabush approach when presenting information on food, medicine, and exercise to the Ojibwa. The Nanabush principle of balance can assist the client to see the appropriateness of diet, exercise, and insulin in keeping in balance (Hagey and Buller, 1983). Because of cultural values, client adherence to a diet that involves monitoring of nutritional intake on an individual basis rather than eating the same foods as other family members presents a significant challenge to the nurse. Although the major focus of strategies should be primary prevention of diabetes, improved glycemic control and regular surveillance for the complications of diabetes are needed for those affected by this disorder (Harris et al., 1997).

SUMMARY

Today there are many barriers to good health care for the Canadian Ojibwa people. Some prefer the traditional folk medicine utilized in the past. Even if there is interest in modern health care, some lack familiarity with health care services and how to get access to them. When provided with health care information, they may be hesitant in being compliant with the recommended treatment. Differences in communication patterns with care providers may result in an Ojibwa client not providing needed information and being seen by health care providers as uncooperative. When a chronic illness is present, medical records and information on a client's medical history are often not available. Presenting competent health care to the Ojibwa people requires sensitivity and appreciation for their unique cultural traditions and values. It is only when genuine respect and concern is communicated and felt that members of the health care team will be able to make a significant difference in the quality of care provided.

Case Study

Developed by Ruth Shearer, MSN, RN, Assistant Professor, Bethel College, Mishawaka, Indiana

John Yellowfish, a 43-year-old obese Ojibwa man, came into the reserve clinic accompanied by his wife. Although he would offer few complaints, his wife stated that he was complaining of dry mouth, tingling feet, and difficulty with vision. She said that she has been giving him tea made from herbs for the past several weeks but it appeared to have no effect. She was concerned that it was diabetes because some of their friends had recently been told that they had this problem. Her husband's father had used alcohol excessively, and she suggested that this probably was caused by the supernatural spirit Weendigo, who punished children and grandchildren for excesses of their ancestors with diabetes. When the nurse said, "Sometimes men don't get much exercise here on the reserve," the wife said, "Yes, he just watches TV most of the time since he lost his job."

CARE PLAN

 Nursing Diagnosis   Spiritual distress related to current symptoms as evidenced by wife stating that the spirit Weendigo punishes children for excesses of ancestors (use of alcohol) with diabetes. The Native people traditionally believe that health is a spiritual experience.

Client Outcomes	*Nursing Interventions*
1. Client will express spiritual satisfaction.	1. Display respect by using indirect rather than direct approach. Rephrase wife's comment about Weendigo punishing the offspring for ancestors' use of alcohol in excess.
	2. Allow silence.
	3. Make indirect comment about job loss contributing to social isolation.
	4. Explain the balance of correct diet, exercise, and medication as being like Nanabush, a principle of balance.
	5. Explain that the healthful diet for the client can be eaten by all family members.
	6. Encourage client and family to seek counsel of native healer who incorporates modern medicine with traditional healing techniques.

 Nursing Diagnosis   Altered peripheral tissue perfusion related to insufficient circulation secondary to diabetes mellitus or immobility.

Client Outcomes	*Nursing Interventions*
1. Client will define vascular problem in his own words.	1. Establish rapport with client by showing respect. Do not use direct eye contact except when greeting him and occasionally throughout the interview.
	2. Do not ask direct, factual, personal questions because this can be interpreted as a form of violation of dignity.
	3. Make indirect statements that client can choose to respond to, such as, some Native men have noticed strange sensations in their feet and hands, increased thirst, blurred vision, nausea, stomach problems, or vomiting.

2. Client will allow assessment to determine underlying cause of tingling feet.

4. Accept client's silence when asked a question. It is socially acceptable for him not to answer immediately. He may answer it at the next clinic visit or not at all.
5. Explain actions before, during, and after each part of the assessment.
6. Assess skin temperature and color and look for ulcerations. Assess peripheral pulses bilaterally (radial, posterior tibial, dorsalis pedis). Assess for edema, capillary refill (normal less than 3 seconds).
7. Assess blood glucose level (normal 70 to 110 mg/dL).
8. Assess temperature, pulse, respirations, blood pressure for baseline value.
9. Refer client to physician if any assessment data are abnormal or indicative of untreated diabetes mellitus.

3. Client will state when to contact physician.

10. Inform client about importance of seeking medical care immediately. Dangers of nontreatment include loss of eyesight, loss of function in feet and legs, possible amputation, loss of consciousness, and even death.
11. Give specific details regarding time and location of appointment.
12. Smile and be unhurried with care and instructions.
13. It is best to put in terms of present time; therefore set appointment immediately after nursing assessment rather than in the future.

STUDY QUESTION

1. Describe the communication barriers that may be encountered by the nurse from a different culture when interacting with the Ojibwa client.
2. Identify spiritual themes relevant to the rendering of culturally competent care to this client.
3. Describe at least three diseases or conditions that have a high prevalence among the Ojibwa.

4. Describe the spatial needs of the Ojibwa client and relevance to culturally competent care.
5. Identify the role assignments that are typically found in the Ojibwa family.

References

Anonymous. (1994). Essentials of tuberculosis control for the practicing physician. *Canadian Medical Association Journal, 150*(10), 1561-1571.

Atcheson, J.A.R. (1987). Traditional health beliefs and compliance in Native Indian tuberculosis patients. Unpublished master's thesis, McMaster University, Hamilton, Ont.

Baker, S.P., Whitfield, R.A., & O'Neill, B. (1987). Geographic variations in mortality from motor vehicle crashes. *New England Journal of Medicine, 316,* 1384-1387.

Bolstering a case. *Maclend's, 110*(12), 23. Editorial.

Brant, C. (1983). *Native ethics and rules of behaviour.* London, Ont.: University of Western Ontario.

Buffalohead, P. (1986). Farmers, warriors, traders: a fresh look at Ojibway women. In Nichols, R.L. (Ed.), *The American Indian* (ed. 3). New York: Alfred A. Knopf.

Burke, S.O., Kisilevsky, B.S., & Maloney, R. (1989). Time orientations of Indian mothers and white nurses. *The Canadian Journal of Nursing Research, 21*(4), 5-20.

Casper, M., Rith-Najarian, S., et al. (1996). Blood pressure, diabetes, and body mass index among Chippewa and Menominee Indians. *Public Health Reports, 3,* 37.

Clark, G.A., Kelley, M.A., Grange, J.M., & Hill, M.C. (1987). The evolution of mycobacterial disease in human populations. *Current Anthropology, 28,* 45-62.

Darnell, R. (1981). Taciturnity in Native American etiquette: the Cree example. *Culture, 1,* 55-60.

Densmore, F. (1979). *Chippewa customs.* St. Paul: Minnesota Historical Society.

Enarson, D.A., & Grzybowski, S. (1986). Incidence of active tuberculosis in the native population of Canada. *Canadian Medical Association Journal, 134,* 1149-1152.

England, J. (1986, December). Cross-cultural health care. *Canada's Mental Health,* 13-15.

Fennell, T. (1995). Deadly confrontation on an Ontario reserve. *Maclean's, 108*(38), 22.

Ferris, L.E., & Tudiver F. (1992). Family physician's approach to wife abuse: a study of Ontario Canada practices. *Family Medicine, 24,* 276.

Ferris, L.E. (1994). Detection and treatment of wife abuse in aboriginal communities by primary care physicians: Preliminary findings. *Journal of Women's Health, 3*(4), 265-271.

Galens, J., Sheets, A., & Young, R.V. (Eds.). (1995). *Gale encyclopedia of multicultural America* (vol. 2). Detroit, Mich.: Gale Research Inc.

Garro, L.C. (1988). Explaining high blood pressure: variation in knowledge about illness. *American Ethnologist, 15,* 98-119.

Hagey, R., & Buller, E. (1983). Drumming and dancing: a new rhythm in nursing care. *The Canadian Nurse, 79*(4), 28-31.

Hanson, A. (1988). Problems involved in delivering health care and social services to the inner city. In Young, D.E. (Ed.), *Health care issues in the Canadian north.* Edmonton, Alb.: Boreal Institute for Northern Studies.

Harris, S.B., Gittelsohn, J., Hanley, A., Barnie, A., Wolever, T.M.S., Gao, J., Logan, A., & Zinman, B. (1997). The prevalence of NIDDM and associated risk factors in Native Canadians. *Diabetes Care, 20*(1), 185-187.

Henderson, G., & Primeaux, M. (1981). *Transcultural health care.* Don Mills, Ont.: Addison-Wesley Publishing Co.

Hewson, J. (1992). Owls and Windigos. *International Journal of American Linguistics, 58*(2), 234-235.

Hilger, M. (1992). *Chippewa child life and its cultural background.* St. Paul: Minnesota Historical Society Press.

Howard, J.H. (1965). *The Plains Ojibwa or Bunji: hunters and warriors of the northern prairie, with special reference to the Turtle Mountain Band.* Vermillion, S.D.: University of South Dakota.

Johnston, B. (1976). *Ojibway heritage.* Toronto: McClelland & Stewart.

Kubiak, W.J. (1970). *Great Lakes Indians.* Grand Rapids, Mich.: Baker Book House.

Lechky, O. (1991). Transfer of health care to Natives holds much promise, lecturers say. *Canadian Medical Association Journal, 144*(2), 195-197.

Longclaws, L., Barnes, G.E., Grieve, L., & Dumoff, R. (1980). Alcohol and drug use among the Brokenhead Ojibwa. *Journal of Studies on Alcohol, 41,* 21-36.

Mao, Y., Morrison, H., Semenciw, R., & Wigle, D. (1986). Mortality on Canadian Indian reserves, 1977-1982. *Canadian Journal of Public Health, 77,* 263-268.

McKay, S., & Silman, J. (1995). *The first nations.* Geneva: World Council of Churches Publications.

McMillan, A.D. (1988). *Native peoples and cultures of Canada.* Vancouver/Toronto: Douglas & McIntyre.

McRae, L.A. (1994). Cultural sensitivity in rehabilitation related to native clients. *Canadian Journal of Rehabilitation, 7*(4), 251-256.

O'Leary, T.J., & Levinson, D. (Vol. Eds.). (1991). *Encyclopedia of world cultures,* Volume I: *North America.* Boston: G.K. Hall & Company.

Orque, M.S., Bloch, B., & Monrroy, L.S.A. (1983). *Ethnic nursing care: a multicultural approach.* Toronto: Mosby, Inc.

Postl, B., Moffatt, M., & Sarsfield, P. (1987). Epidemiology and intervention for Native Canadians. *Canadian Journal of Public Health, 78,* 219.

Reed, T.E., Kalant, H., Gibbins, R.J., Kapur, B.M., & Rankin, J.G. (1976). Alcohol and acetaldehyde metabolism in Caucasians, Chinese and Amerinds. *Canadian Medical Association Journal, 115,* 851-855.

Rieder, H.L. (1989). Tuberculosis among American Indians of the contiguous United States. *Public Health Report, 104,* 653-657.

Ritzenthaler, R.E. (1978). Southwestern Chippewa. In Trigger, B.G. (Ed.), *Handbook of North American Indians* (Vol. 15). Washington, D.C.: Smithsonian Institution.

Rogers, E.S. (1978). Southeastern Ojibwa. In Trigger, B.G. (Ed.), *Handbook of North American Indians* (Vol. 15). Washington, D.C.: Smithsonian Institution.

Rogers, E.S., & Taylor, J.G. (1981). Northern Ojibwa. In Helm, J. (Ed.), *Handbook of North American Indians* (Vol. 6). Washington, D.C.: Smithsonian Institution.

Ross, C.A., & Davis, B. (1986). Suicide and parasuicide in a northern Canadian Native community. *Canadian Journal of Psychiatry, 31,* 331-334.

Royal Commission on Aboriginal People. (1995, June 15). Looking forward, looking back. *CMA webspinners http://www.ma.ca/canmed/policy/female.htm.*

Sokoloski, E.H. (1995). Canadian First Nation's women's beliefs about pregnancy and prenatal care. *Canadian Journal of Nursing Research, 27*(1), 89-100.

Stan, S. (1989). *The Ojibwe.* Vero Beach, Fla.: Rourke.

Statistics Canada. (1995). *Profile of Canada's aboriginal population.* Ottawa: Industry, Science and Technology, 1991 Census of Canada. Catalogue number 94-325.

Steele, S. (1995). Last stand at CFB Ipperwash. *Maclean's, 108*(33), 15.

Tanner, H.H. (1992). *The Ojibway.* New York: Chelsea House.

Thwaites, J.R. (1896-1901). *The Jesuit relations and allied documents* (73 vols.). Cleveland: Borrows Brothers.

Tripp-Reimer, T., & Afifi, L.A. (1989). Cross-cultural perspectives on patient teaching. *Nursing Clinics of North America, 24*(3), 613-619.

Vecoli, R.J. (Contributing Ed.). (1995). *Gale encyclopedia of multicultural America* (vol. 2). Detroit, Mich.: Gale Research Inc.

Waldrum, J., Hering, A., & Young, K. (1995). *Aboriginal health in Canada.* Toronto: University of Toronto Press.

Warren, W. (1984). *History of the Ojibway people.* St. Paul: Minnesota Historical Society Press.

Young, K. (1994). *The health of Native Americans.* New York: Oxford University Press.

Young, T.K. (1982). Self-perceived and clinically assessed health status of Indians in northwestern Ontario: analysis of a health survey. *Canadian Journal of Public Health, 73,* 272- 277.

Young, T.K. (1991). Prevalence and correlates of hypertension in a subarctic Indian population. *Preventive Medicine. 20,* 474-485.

Young, T.K. (1993). Diabetes mellitus among Native Americans in Canada and the United States: an epidemiological review. *American Journal of Human Biology, 5,* 399-413.

Young, T.K., Bruce, L., Elias, J., O Neil, J.D., & Yassi, A. (1991). *The health effects of housing and community infrastructure on Canadian Indian reserves.* Ottawa: Department of Indian Affairs and Northern Development.

Young, T.K., & Casson, I. (1988). The decline and persistence of tuberculosis in a Canadian Indian population: implications for control. *Canadian Journal of Public Health, 79,* 302-306.

Young, T.K., & Harris, S.B. (1994). Risk of clinical diabetes in a northern Native Canadian. *Arctic Medical Research, 53*(2), 64-70.

Young, T.K., McIntyre, L.L., Dooley, J., & Rodrìguez, J. (1985). Epidemiologic features of diabetes mellitus among Indians in northwestern Ontario and northeastern Manitoba. *Canadian Medical Association Journal, 132,* 793-797.

Young, T.K., & Sevenhuysen, G. (1989). Obesity in northern Canadian Indians: patterns, determinants, and consequences. *American Journal of Clinical Nutrition, 49,* 786-793.

Young, T.K., Szathmary, E.J.E., Evers, S., & Wheatley, B. (1990). Geographical distribution of diabetes among the Native population of Canada: a national survey. *Social Science and Medicine, 31*(2), 129-139.

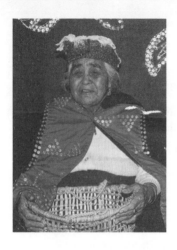

CHAPTER 11

Kwa-kwa'ka-wakw First Nation

Evelyn Voyageur

BEHAVIORAL OBJECTIVES

After reading this chapter the nurse will be able to:

1. Understand important historical events that have had an effect on health, social, political, economic, and spiritual systems of the Kwa-kwa'ka-wakw through an overview of precontact history to the present day profound effect of colonization.
2. Understand the barriers (racism, stereotyping, and so on) faced by Kwa-kwa'ka-wakw people to the achievement of self-sustaining healthy communities.
3. Explore factors that hinder and enhance communications between Kwa-kwa'ka-wakw people and nurses.
4. Appreciate the cultural values, beliefs, practices, and rituals of Kwa-kwa'ka-wakw people that have contributed to their survival as distinct societies.
5. Examine important health and socioeconomic issues and concerns that require intervention, such as poor housing, unemployment, family violence, and addictions.

OVERVIEW OF THE KWA-KWA'KA-WAKW FIRST NATION

The Kwa-kwa'ka-wakw people are found on the northwest coast of British Columbia, the north end of Vancouver Island, on the mainland of British Columbia, and on smaller islands adjacent to the mainland. These First Nation people have their own tribal names but are called the "Kwa-kwa'ka-wakw" (pronounced more accurately as /kwa-kwa'-kay-wakw/) because they speak *Kwa'kwa-la* (the apostrophe represents a glottal stop). There are other tribes related to the Kwa-kwa'ka-wakw. These include four to the

south—the Le-queɫt-təxw (Lekwiltok) of Cape Mudge, the K'umuks-a-la of Comox, the Wewikim of Campbell River, and the Qualicum of Qualicum. There are also three to the north—the Heiltsuk of Bella Bella, the Owik'inox (Wikeno) of Rivers Inlet, and the Haisla of Kitimat. At one time, there were 25 Kwa-kwa'ka-wakw bands. However, some have amalgamated making fewer bands today.

Boas (1858-1942), one of the earliest and most important ethnographers working in Canada, worked among the Kwa-kwa'ka-wakw and called them the "Kwakiutl." Boas (1938) learned to speak the language, and that ability allowed him to amass great quantities of descriptive information on the myths and traditions of these people whom he described in numerous writings. Thus the Kwa-kwa'ka-wakw became one of the most documented aboriginal people in Canada. Boas worked primarily with the Kwa-kwa'ka-wakw who lived near Fort Rupert. Technically his use of the word "Kwakiutl" to describe these people is limited because only the Kwa-kwa'ka-wakw tribe who lived at Fort Rupert (Tsahis) were known by this name (McMillan, 1988). Some researchers continue to use the term "Kwakiutl" originally coined by Boas as the authentic way to refer to the Kwa-kwa'ka-wakw people (Young, 1994). Despite their diversity, the Kwa-kwa'ka-wakw tribes have similarities that include cultural and spiritual understandings emphasizing traditions, community, and harmony with nature and the natural environment (Seniors Advisory Council, 1996). To respond to the health care needs of the Kwa-kwa'ka-wakw people, it is important to understand the significance of their traditional way of life and its influence on their physical, mental, and spiritual well-being.

Originally the Kwa-kwa'ka-wakw people resided on the northwest coast of British Columbia. Before the arrival of the Europeans to North America, the Kwa-kwa'ka-wakw lived as a distinct and self-sufficient nation having a unique language, a system of law and government, and their own territory (Seniors Advisory Council, 1996). The Kwa-kwa'ka-wakw economy was based on hunting, gathering, and fishing (Miller, 1986). Historically the Kwa-kwa'ka-wakw people lived and roamed throughout British Columbia, but this way of life changed when they were forced to assimilate practices of the newly arrived Europeans, and many were confined to reserves (Miller, 1986). With the confinement to reserves and necessary acculturation, the cultural values of the Kwa-kwa'ka-wakw people began to change. With these changing values and health care practices, their health status began to deteriorate. Further erosion of the values was evident by children being forced to attend residential schools where unique use of the tribal language, spiritual practices, and customs of holistic health began to disappear.

Despite rapid assimilation of Western values, the Kwa-kwa'ka-wakw people hold fast to the belief that because the earth they walk on still contains the bones and the dust of their ancestors the spirits of the ancestors are still present. The presence of the spirit of the ancestors gives the Kwa-kwa'ka-wakw people hope in reviving their dignity, self-esteem, and traditional health. Today it is estimated that there are 4120 registered Kwa-kwa'ka-wakw people with 59% living on reserves (Statistics Canada, 1991; Indian and Northern Affairs, 1996). However, others estimate that there may be as many as 13,000 because some choose not to register and live in backwoods areas (Young, 1994). Stories of the origin of each tribe vary (Rohner, 1967). These stories, legends, and myths depict the values and beliefs of the Kwa-kwa'ka-wakw. In addition, these stories give in-depth insight about the complex societies, health, justice, and resource management of the Kwa-kwa'ka-wakw and have traditionally aided in determining who owned land, crests, dances, and songs (Seniors Advisory Council, 1996). To relate all the tribes' origins is beyond the scope of this chapter; therefore only one will be described. This is the origin of the Dzawada'enox tribe of Kingcome Inlet on the Gwa'yee River.

Kawadilikala with his four children and his younger brother Qwolili lived before there was light on earth. They heard the voice of the Creator (God), who said they were to go and find a place that they could claim. They were in their animal form—wolf. The two brothers and four children came first to Kingcome Inlet. The older brother picked a site up the Gwa'yee river as his own. Qwolili did not want to share the same area as his brother, and so he moved on to look for his own place. He traveled on until he found Wakeman river. He stayed there for a long time before visiting his old brother. Quolili asked Kawadilikala, "What did the birds say at his location?" Kawadilikala said, "The birds say *dzawadali, dzawadali*," and so Qwolili said, "Your people will be called *Dzawada'enox.*" Kawadilikala then asked his brother, "What did the birds of Wakeman say?" Qwolili answered, "They say *ha'hwa-la.*" So, since then, the tribe of Wakeman has been called the *Ha'hua-mis* (modified from Willie, 1962).

This narrative illustrates how the Kwa-kwa'ka-wakw people received their tribal names. It also tells why these people still consider themselves responsible for continuing the stewardship of the land as an important part of their culture (Seniors Advisory Council, 1996).

COMMUNICATION
Language

As previously indicated, the language spoken by the Kwa-kwa'ka-wakw people is *Kwa'kwa-la*. This language has been identified as belonging to the Wakashan linguistic stock. Kwa'kwa-la is a guttural language, making it difficult to enunciate the words unless one has been born into it. Each tribe or area had a slightly different way of saying some words (Ford, 1941). Traditionally, Kwa'kwa-la was not a written language; however, with the arrival of Christianity, the Church of England (Anglican church) translated some of their hymns into the Kwa'kwa-la tongue. This translation provided the first written account of the language. Transcribing the language into a written form was difficult for many reasons including the fact that many of the earlier translators attempted to use the Latin alphabet following English conventions. For many of these earlier translators, use of the English spelling methods to provide a written form of Kwa'kwa-la was an arduous task because the phonetic sounds of many of the words did not appear in English. Various individuals have therefore invented different symbols to signify a sound that is in the Kwa'kwa-la language. Despite the effort to provide a written form of Kwa'kwa-la, the language was nevertheless lost because children were forced to live in residential schools and were not allowed to speak the language. However, today, Kwa'kwa-la is being restored because it is being taught in some classrooms (The Royal Commission on Aboriginal Peoples, 1995).

Silence

Silence among the Kwa-kwa'ka-wakw people is considered a virtue and as such some Kwa-kwa'ka-wakw people do not speak just for the sake of talking. For many of these people speaking is reserved for manners of extreme importance, even in jesting. For example, to say "It's a nice day" would be unnecessary speech because if it were a nice day it would be obvious (Sealy and McDonald, 1990). A nurse may go visit an elder, not even speaking a word, yet the client may say, "Thank you for coming." The presence of a caring person is appreciated more than words.

Touch

Body language is important to the Kwa-kwa'ka-wakw. Hand shakes, hugs, and embraces are practiced. Upon meeting family members, hugs and embraces are given. However, to the visitor or nonfamily member greetings such as *yo* 'hi' or *ki-la-kás-la,* equivalent to 'hello', 'welcome', and 'thank you' are used. *Ha-la-kás-la* is 'good-bye' or 'go in peace'.

Eye contact

Eye contact is very important to the Kwa-kwa'ka-wakw. If eye contact is avoided when someone is speaking, the person will assume that the speaker is hiding something or is not interested. For some Kwa-kwa'ka-wakw people, it is considered disrespectful to not look at the speaker.

Implications for nursing care

For effective communication to occur, the nurse must develop a relationship built on trust with the client that will in time give rise to acceptance and respect. To develop a trusting relationship with the Kwa-kwa'ka-wakw client, it is essential for the nurse to display an acceptance and endorsement of the culture, values, and beliefs of the people. Since some or most of the elders do not write or read English, proficient interpreters are needed to communicate effectively with those who do not necessarily speak English or understand a Westernized written version of the Kwa'kwa-la language. It is important to have interpreters who have a good knowledge of medical terminology and who speak Kwa'kwa-la fluently.

The initial encounter with the client should include introductions and small talk, and during this period a formal assessment can occur. The initial interaction will eventually lead to talking about the needs of the client. The nurse should not begin the relationship by telling the client what to do. The client will respect the nurse who listens. The nurse should not be afraid to touch individuals who are upset in an effort to provide comfort and support. For some Kwa-kwa'ka-wakw, touching will usually be interpreted as a mode of communicating the nurse's genuine concern.

It is important to give simple explanations to the client and the family concerning procedures that are to be done. If a client is illiterate or if the client does not speak the dominant language or if the nurse is unfamiliar with the client's language, it is essential that gestures and demonstrations be used to explain to the client what will be done. For example, The nurse may want to tell a non-English speaking mother to give her child amoxicillin 250 mg tid for her child's bacterial chest infection. After the nurse examines the child, the findings should be relayed to the mother by using gestures. The nurse can describe that the child's chest is full by placing a hand on the throat and making coughing sounds. To give instructions on how to give medication, the nurse can use fingers, a spoon, and a watch or clock. The mother can be shown how to administer the medication appropriately by first shaking the bottle of medication and putting the exact amount in a spoon of the right size and then pointing to the watch or clock the hours of when to give the medication. To communicate to the mother how many times a day the medication is to be given to the child, fingers can used to indicate the number. If fluids need to be forced, the nurse can get a glass of water and show her how many times to give it to the child. Written instructions may be useful if someone else in the household can read. The community health representative who visits the client can use the instructions to reinforce what care is to be given.

It is important to consider the traditional way things have been done for a Kwa-kwa'ka-wakw client if the treatment regimen is to be successful. For example, if Kwa-kwa'ka-kakw clients stop their medication to use a more traditional therapy, the nurse may want to encourage the client to use both methods but only if the tradition method is efficacious (beneficial) or neutral. The key to providing quality care to the Kwa-kwa'ka-wakw is the importance of avoiding telling the Kwa-kwa'ka-wakw that their ways are wrong.

SPACE

Traditionally, the Kwa-kwa'ka-wakw were a nomadic people and were used to wide open spaces. They followed and lived where seasonal foods were available, such as clams, fish, and berries (The Royal Commission on Aboriginal Peoples, 1995). Houses were built in various locations belonging to the tribe. In October or November, during the running of dog salmon, many of the people would move up the river to smoke and dry their year's supply of fish. In the spring when berries were ripe, this became the focus of activity.

Living space was frequently limited, and therefore many of the houses of the Kwa-kwa'ka-wakw people were large communal dwellings with walls and gabled roofs of overlapping cedar planks. Historically a family crest on the roof top identified the clan who lived there (Ford, 1941). The houses were called "big houses" because they accommodated more than one family. The head of the house was the father or chief. When sons with wives and children moved in, they would be given a corner. Another big house would be built to accommodate the other children who got married. There was a fire in the middle of the house where all the cooking was done.

In the old days, the Kwa-kwa'ka-wakw people had no beds, chairs, tables, or other furniture. At meal times, men sat on the floor with their legs crossed while the women squatted on their haunches wrapped in blankets (Ford, 1941). Utensils were made out of stone or wood. Sleeping was done on the floor on softened woven cedar bark pieces and with furs for covering. When cloth became available, mattresses and pillows were made with feathers from birds such as ducks.

Today, there are approximately 13,000 Kwa-kwa'ka-wakw people with about half living on reserves. Even today, Kwa-kwa'ka-wakw people are segregated into bands, assigned to a village, and have restrictions on where to build homes. Family units generally live alone in modern homes with appliances, indoor plumbing, electricity, furniture, beds, sheets, blankets, and store-bought utensils.

Implications for nursing care

To provide culturally competent care, the astute nurse who cares for Kwa-kwa'ka-wakw people should be aware that these people have historically been accustomed to the wide open spaces. Reduction of the space available to these people has created some problems of adjustment where spatial needs are concerned. In the past, communal living made support of family members readily available. However, once again, restricted space has made traditional values virtually impossible. Although the Kwa-kwa'ka-wakw of today have their own homes and possessions, they no longer have the ready availability of an extended family living under the same roof from which to get support. The lack of family support creates additional client concerns for the nurse.

SOCIAL ORGANIZATION
Family roles and structure

The family's support and security are an integral and focal aspect of Kwa-kwa'ka-wakw culture both traditionally and in the present (Seniors Advisory Council, 1996). Many family members rally around a person needing support, whether for illness, an interpersonal problem, or a special occasion. A Kwa-kwa'ka-wakw is never alone when in need of help. White and Jacobs (1992) note that providing a holistic approach of support to extended families is a First Nations people's law. The Kwa-kwa'ka-wakw people value children and believe them to be a precious gift from the Creator (Willie, 1962). When a Kwa-kwa'ka-wakw woman is expecting, the whole family becomes involved in prenatal care. After the birth of a child, the whole family helps raise the child—grandparents, great-grandparents, uncles, aunts, and cousins. Since the Kwa-kwa'ka-wakw people believe that it takes a village to raise a child, the child is considered everybody's child. For many Kwa-kwa'ka-wakw women, postnatal blues occur very infrequently. The Kwa-kwa'ka-wakw family is so traditionally oriented that in the case of the death of a parent a childless couple will often adopt the child or children of the deceased (White and Jacobs, 1992).

The family structure consists of not only the immediate family, but also the extended family, and, as such, first cousins are thought of as brothers and sisters, particularly because there is no word for "cousin" in the Kwa'kwa-la language. In addition, the sisters and brothers of the grandparents are referred to as "grandparents." Grandparents and elders have a positive role to support the younger generation and have the responsibility to pass on the wisdom and wonders of the culture (Seniors Advisory Council, 1996). It is through the grandparents and elders that Kwa-kwa'ka-wakw children learn their cultural roots, values, beliefs, and history of their songs, crests, arts, regalia, and memorabilia. In the past, elders were kept busy and useful, even in their very old age, by tending to the babies while the mothers were busy.

Likewise traditional values dictated that each family member took turns caring for the elderly. The Kwa-kwa'ka-wakw elders were respected, lived long lives, and rarely became confused even though their physical bodies began to weaken (Seniors Advisory Council, 1996). Today, elders are more likely to be put in nursing homes, become confused, and die much younger (Seniors Advisory Council, 1996). However, respect for elders is still practiced at community gatherings, funerals, potlatches, and weddings. The *hamatsas* (the people who hold the highest dance of the Kwa-kwa'ka-wakw people) are served first and then the elders.

The role of the parents in the family has not changed over time. Mothers are usually responsible for the household duties, whereas fathers do the outside heavy work. The spouses help one another, especially if one is ill. A man does not think it is beneath him to wash clothes, cook a meal, or tend to the children when his wife is ill. The wife helps her husband do his work when there is no one else available.

Tribes

Tribes are organized into clans with the head of the clan usually designated as the father, who is the chief, which is relegated to the eldest son upon the death of the chief (Ford, 1941). The only time this position is passed onto the oldest daughter is when the head of the clan has no son or younger brother. Even today, this is the traditional way of passing on the chieftainship in the Kwa-kwa'ka-wakw nation. Personal identity originates from the family name, clan, village, and specific community of origin.

Marriage

Marriages were arranged up to the 1950s. Ninety-nine percent of arranged marriages remained intact until a spouse died. The marriage was arranged by the elders. Often it was the aunt or grandmother of the young man who initiated the talks with the elders of the young girl whom they believed was best suited for their young man. The aunt or grandmother would tell the girl's family what a great hunter and worker their young man was. The man's family would persuade the girl's family that she would never be in need. Once the consent was given the focus was on what the girl would bring to the marriage such as dances, names, and songs. These in turn would be passed onto the children of the couple (Willie, 1962). Both the immediate and extended family assisted in providing a dowry for the bride (Smith, 1957).

Today a marriage still serves to increase the extended family and the number of people to help at funerals, potlatches, weddings, and feasts. The head of the clan is still the official organizer of such events, with all family members providing support either by giving money, dry goods, or food or by helping to make plans.

Education

The Kwa-kwa'ka-wakw people believe that education begins in utero with the communication of a feeling of being wanted and valued. While in utero, the unborn child is sung and spoken to. From the time of birth children were taught that in order to respect one's self one must take care of one's physical, spiritual, emotional, and mental needs (Seniors Advisory Council, 1996).

Young girls were educated about childrearing at their first menses. The girl was put in seclusion, a darkened room with only the wise women of the tribe, for 4 days. She was counseled about her behavior, her conduct now that she had become a woman, and prepared for childrearing. She was fed only nutritious foods. She was told her thoughts must be free of any negative thoughts and not to harbor any bad feelings about anyone or anything. She was taught about spiritual, physical, emotional, and mental health so that she would have healthy children (Robertson, 1957). This process was also believed to prevent gynecological problems after childbirth.

Traditional dress

Historically Kwa-kwa'ka-wakw children wore no clothes. Men and women dressed in an apron and a blanket made out of woven cedar bark or furs and kept in place by a belt made out of cedar string (Patterson, 1972). They wore no shoes or covering on their feet even in the wintertime (Ford, 1941). Ornaments were worn by both Kwa-kwa'ka-wakw men and women, on either their ears or their noses (Ford, 1941). Most of the earrings were made out of abalone shells. Arm bracelets, knee rings, and finger rings were made out of mountain goat wool and yellow and red cedar bark (Ford, 1941). Later on, these ornaments were made out of copper, brass, gold, and silver. Both women and men wore their hair long. Women braided their hair in two plaits that hung on either side of their necks, whereas men tied their hair back. Stringed otter teeth were used as hair ornaments like headbands to keep their long hair in place. On a daily basis men and women covered their faces with tallow, so that paint could be easily removed, and painted their faces with red and black paint (Ford, 1941). Today Kwa-kwa'ka-wakw still paint their faces when performing some traditional dances.

With the arrival of the Europeans and the Hudson's Bay Company, button blankets were made for the Kwa-kwa'ka-wakw and traded for furs. Today the Native clothing has primarily been replaced by store-bought clothes.

Traditional dress for ceremonies Ceremonial dress was a part of each special occasion. The type of robe used in the ceremony depended on the rank of the individual and the event being celebrated (Jensen and Sargant, 1985). The typical ceremonial robes was made out of yellow cedar with a narrow fur border around the blanket and were worn by both men and women (Jensen and Sargant, 1985; Smith, 1985).

A bride was clothed in a blanket covered with abalone shells when she got married. This blanket was then taken off her and put on her new husband after the wedding ceremony was completed (Robertson, 1955).

Today ceremonial blankets are bordered with a red border to represent their sacred red cedar bark, the blood of life, and have a family crest on the center back. Headpieces are frequently made from red cedar bark. Headpieces may be adorned with abalone shells or weasel furs.

Traditional Dances

Dances have been passed on from generation to generation. The origins of dances vary. A person could receive a vision of how a dance was to be done by spending sacred time in the forest meditating and praying. Sometimes the Kwa-kwa'ka-wakw stayed as long as 4 months in the forest, living off the land or fasting. The time of return to the village was celebrated by ceremonies and dances in the big house. Dancers were dressed in full regalia related to an inherited dance or one received in a vision that they would perform. Full regalia included aprons, blankets, and headpieces elaborately decorated and related to the dance. Aprons had designs sewn on them with buttons, sequins, beads, and bells to make a design. Headpieces were used in different dances such as the wolf head for the wolf dance and thunderbird for the thunderbird dance. In the past and even today, the spirit dancers use plain blankets with no designs and have on their heads hemlock boughs that almost cover their faces.

Today the ceremonies are shortened to a day. It used to take months to have a ceremonial dance. The dances are still being done, but new dancers are not taken into the forest for their vision quest or spiritual initiation into the role.

Spirituality

The Kwa-kwa'ka-wakw people, like other First Nations people, used the whole universe to practice their spirituality, such as going into the forest to fast and pray. Traditionally they talked to the Creator all the time (Willie, 1971; Willie, 1962). They prayed to thank the Creator for whatever they did: received, made, or caught food in fishing or hunting (Willie, 1972). For example, after a canoe was made and launched, an elder would thank the Creator for the tree that was used to make the canoe (Dawson, 1996). The bones of fish caught were always put back into the water with a prayer that fish would return the next year (Willie, 1962).

Shamans were the spiritual leaders in the Kwa-kwa'ka-wakw communities. These men or women were referred to as the "healers or technicians of the sacred" and "masters of ecstasy" (Seniors Advisory Council, 1996). They were taught to journey to the spirit world to communicate with the ones who had already crossed over.

After the arrival of the Europeans, many of the First Nations people, such as the Kwa-kwa'ka-wakw people, were forced to abandon their traditional ways of worshiping. Some of the Kwa-kwa'ka-wakw people embraced Christianity and were baptized, confirmed, and married in the Western tradition. The Westernization of the Kwa-kwa'ka-wakw people has left many of these individuals confused and unsettled about their traditional beliefs and spirituality (Seniors Advisory Council, 1996).

The elders taught that death is a part of the life cycle within the sacred realm and that death is actually a form of returning home (Seniors Advisory Council, 1996). However, it is believed that the individual will eventually return as the child of one of hers or his descendants. It is believed that all living things have their place in the fullness of life, and all living things have their roles and functions (Seniors Advisory Council, 1996). Additionally, some Kwa-kwa'ka-wakw people hold the belief that everything in the universe is part of a whole, being interrelated and connected to everything else (Seniors Advisory Council, 1996). Today many Kwa-kwa'ka-wakw people are seeking their identity through their traditional spiritual ways because following the non-

Native religion brought by the Europeans has not worked for them.

Implications for nursing care

The culturally sensitive nurse should appreciate the value of family to the Kwa-kwa'ka-wakw people. When a Kwa-kwa'ka-wakw client is hospitalized, consideration needs to be given not only to the client, but also to the client's need for family support. If visiting hours are restricted to specific times but there is no one to translate for a Kwa-kwa'ka-wakw client, the nurse should modify the rules so that a family member can be present to translate. It is also important to remember that the Kwa-kwa'ka-wakw will adjust more readily to the treatment regimen with family members around all the time. As much as possible the client's need for family visits should be accommodated. According to Voyageur (1989) the presence of family is a precipitating factor that has been known to result in improvement in a client's condition. In addition, the presence of family is especially important if the client is elderly because children are seen as extensions of the elderly who will continue on with their lives when the elders are gone (Willie, 1962; Sealy and McDonald, 1990). The nurse should remember that because the use of silence is a virtue in the Kwa-kwa'ka-wakw culture, children are generally not disruptive while sitting with their relative.

Nurses should encourage family members to bring traditional foods to the hospital if they are efficacious and beneficial to the dietary treatment plan. Some foods such as dog codfish may smell and be offensive to the nurse. Nevertheless, it is important not to show distaste about the smell.

It may be useful for the culturally sensitive nurse to be aware that the number *four* is very significant to all First Nations people and the Kwa-kwa'ka-wakw people would not be an exception to this belief. The number *four* represents the four directions or four winds—south, north, east, and west. Also it represents holistic health—physical, spiritual, emotional, and mental (Willie, 1962). If possible, aspects of client care should be done in fours. For example, assist the client with four aspects of personal hygiene, which consequently might include (1) as-

sisting the client to bathe, (2) assisting the client with oral hygiene, (3) assisting the client to change dressings if present, and (4) assisting the client with foot care.

TIME

Traditionally, Kwa-kwa'ka-wakw were past-time and present-time oriented. Past-time orientation was evident by the desire of the individuals to respect their elders, maintain harmony with nature, and carry on age-old traditions. Likewise, present-time orientation was evident in the earlier society by activities such as the nomadic lifestyle, which included ceasing all other activities to participate in present-oriented activities such as seasonal food gathering. For example, if fish and game were present, fishing and hunting became the important priority, and other activities were dropped. If a person was engaged in a conversation, completing this interaction in an unhurried manner was a way to show respect for the person being communicated with.

Implications for nursing care

It is important to avoid the appearance of being in a hurry when interacting with the Kwa-kwa'ka-wakw people. It is important for the nurse whether she works in an acute or community health setting to take time to get to know the people and the community in order to be respected and accepted. Some Kwa-kwa'ka-wakw people value and appreciate the nurse more when time and effort are given to participation in the community by attendance at traditional Native ceremonies and functions. The nurse should attend and experience potlatches, feasts, and funerals in the Kwa-kwa'ka-wakw community to appreciate and gain sensitivity to the culture. The people will appreciate the nurse who takes time to listen to stories of long ago and to understand the meaning of traditions such as dances. The stories of what happened when the Kwa-kwa'ka-wakw people first met the Europeans will help the nurse understand their cultural heritage and their cultural behaviors, which may have given rise to some of these persons experiencing feelings of low self-esteem (Voyageur, 1989). The nurses should always take time to find out how things are done in the Kwa-

kwa'ka-wakw culture, and these ways should be respected.

ENVIRONMENTAL CONTROL

The Kwa-kwa'ka-wakw people considered the natural environment the source of great power and wisdom for the Kwa-kwa'ka-wakw who were able to gain it (Willie, 1962). Elders believed this was done by contacting the patron beings, often the animals, the birds, or fish, who could bestow gifts of power (Willie, 1962). The Kwa-kwa'ka-wakw people took careful stock of the environment, how many there were of each species, and where they were to be found. Hunting was controlled by this accurate census of animals and a knowledge of how many could be taken without depleting the supply (Willie, 1972). Out of respect for the environment, animals, sea mammals, and fowls, the Kwa-kwa'ka-wakw learned their breeding habits and used only what was needed for food and shelter, and therefore nothing was wasted. Trees were never cut down for the sake of just cutting them down but rather for needs for shelter, warmth, and tools. For some Kwa-kwa'ka-wakw people it is important to communicate with the animals, birds, sea mammals, and all the living things given by the Creator (Willie, 1962).

To keep harmony and balance with nature, after a birth, the afterbirth was buried in a nice grassy, sunny site (Willie, l955). The ancestors believed that this would enable the baby to grow into a well-balanced adolescent and adult. Thus the elders not only honored nature, but also integrated explanations of its dynamics (Willie, 1997).

Today, Kwa-kwa'ka-wakw people are not allowed to practice what they once did with the environment. They are restricted to catch only a few fish, hunt with a permit, and dig clams with permits and are not allowed to strip the cedar bark from the trees. Unfortunately this changed cultural pattern has thrown off the balance of nature that once was present, and although the Kwa-kwa'ka-wakw valued the sanctity of the environment, they nevertheless are often blamed for the extinction of certain species of animals, fish, and fowl (Seniors Advisory Council, 1996).

Illness and wellness behaviors

Before contact with the Europeans, the Kwa-kwa'ka-wakw approached health holistically. This holistic approach for creating a healthful environment encompassed the physical, spiritual, social, and mental well-being of the people (Seniors Advisory Council, 1996). This was done through a traditional diet and the extensive use of herbs and plants (Seniors Advisory Council, l996). Also included in their practice of being one with Mother Earth and holistic health were traditional ceremonies: singing songs, dancing sacred dances, and giving feasts (Willie, 1997). The Kwa-kwa'ka-wakw people practiced health promotion in its truest form (Seniors Advisory Council, 1996). The good health of the Kwa-kwa'ka-wakw people then was attributed in part to physical activities. "Though we never wore shoes, even on cold winter days, and we had no winter clothing, we were never sick, like today" (Willie, 1968).

Today Kwa-kwa'ka-wakw are faced with a number of health-related problems (Acheson, 1995). These are attributed to the old ways being lost, change of diet, and the loss of identity and self-esteem. It has been reported that among many First Nations people, which include the Kwa-kwa'ka-wakw, residing on reserves, 84% have incomes less than $20,000 (Canadian) a year, which by Canadian standards indicates at or below the poverty level. Because many of these individuals live in poverty, they receive some form of social assistance. The economic conditions of some Kwa-kwa'ka-wakw people have necessitated crowded living conditions. Therefore, density-dependent diseases such as tuberculosis are now present (Acheson, 1995).

Although the infant mortality was high in the past and remains higher for the First Nations people (17.1 per 1000 in l984-1988) compared to Canadians in general (7.8 per 1000), it has decreased among the Kwa-kwa'ka-wakw nation (Health and Welfare Canada, 1991). Status Indians population accounted for 221 of the 1946 deaths recorded in British Columbia from 1987 to 1992 (Foster, MacDonald, Tuk, Uh, and Talbot, 1995). The Pacific Coast average crude death rate for 1984-1988 for the registered Indian population is

5.36 compared to 7.2 per 1000 for Canadians in general (Health and Welfare Canada, 1991).

Traditional healing therapies

It is important to appreciate the fact that for some Kwa-kwa'ka-wakw people health is equated with being in harmony with the environment and in accord with all the family (Smith, 1955; Hanley, 1995). Thus healing ceremonies frequently utilized aspects of the environment. Traditional medicine included herbs, roots, decoctions made from tree barks, and hands-on practices such as therapeutic touch (Willie, 1989). A belief in healing is central to the attitudes, beliefs, values, and perceptions of the Kwa-kwa'ka-wakw people.

The *pa-xa-lá* (*x* like *ch* in German *Bach*), or shaman, in the White man's language, was believed to have special healing powers given at birth. The *pa-xa-lá* pray and chant while working over an ill person. The *pa-xa-lá* might utilize a feather, a rattle, or a cedar branch in a healing ceremony. In the old days, the *pa-xa-lá* worked in the Big House. During the ceremony the whole village was invited to watch, sing, and pray (Smith, 1960).

For many years, the First Nations people, including the Kwa-kwa'ka-wakw, did not practice traditional healing because it was outlawed, and therefore this practice appeared to have been lost. However, with the help of the elders who maintained the accurate history of the culture, traditional healing ways are slowly being revived. Now, herbs are being used to treat clients with cancer, respiratory problems, arthritis, and infections. Pitch (glue) from hemlock trees is melted into poultice to apply to painful areas, broken bones, carbuncles, and boils. Today, it is reported that even tuberculosis clients have felt better when drinking the hemlock brew (Seniors Advisory Council, 1996). However, the tradition stressed the importance of being whole in body, mind, soul and actions. Some people are using the herbs, plants, and pitch today without changing their negative habits of smoking, drinking, eating unhealthy foods, and not taking good care of themselves. Without a holistic approach, the Kwa-kwa'ka-wakw believe that traditional therapies will not work (Seniors Advisory Council, 1996).

Implications for nursing care

It is important for the nurse to be aware that there are many stories of effective healing using traditional healing ceremonies and that the culturally sensitive nurse will not discourage use of these remedies if they are efficacious. However, it is also important to appreciate that it is believed that healing will occur only if there is harmony of body, soul, mind, and actions. The nurse should understand the relationship between the Kwa-kwa'ka-wakw and the universe. The Kwa-kwa'ka-wakw people believe that fish, birds, and animals are gifts from the Creator and, as such, can be communicated with by the spoken word. Therefore the culturally sensitive nurse should avoid passing negative judgment if this behavior is observed.

The nurse should learn what herbs and plants are used for and should not stop the clients from using them. When possible, nontraditional medicine should be incorporated into the medical regime (Grypma, 1993). The nurse should promote efficacious (beneficial) health practices that are desired by the client. However, if any practice is harmful to the client and augments the symptoms of a particular illness or disease, this should be carefully explained to the client. It is best to avoid eliminating traditional health practices without providing a rationale in a respectful manner.

It is important for the nurse to value and appreciate the significance of cultural behaviors that give rise to the way and manner particular things are done. For example, in the hospital setting, if a healer has been called, privacy should be provided and, if possible, a large area made available so that the family can be present. The culturally sensitive nurse should delay doing personal care if the healer arrives at the time the care is scheduled.

BIOLOGICAL VARIATIONS
Body size and structure

In the past the Kwa-kwa'ka-wakw people were said to be tall and broad. With the diet changes over the years, the stature of the people has become shorter and less broad. Today there are many overweight Kwa-kwa'ka-wakw persons because of the lack of activity (Sokoloski, 1995). Thompson (1990) notes that a heavy birth weight occurs 50% more frequently in Native persons than in non-Native persons in British Columbia.

Skin color and other visible characteristics

Most Kwa-kwa'ka-wakw people have brown skin. Some have darker complexions than others. Although hair color is generally dark, there are various shades of dark black and dark brown shades found among the Kwa-kwa'ka-wakw. Eye shapes are varied too; for example, some have very slanted and narrow eyes, whereas others have big round eyes (Bailey and Bailey, 1995).

Enzymatic and genetic variations

American Indians have an excessive level of high-activity alcohol dehydrogenase (ADH) and a low level of aldehyde dehydrogenase-1 (ALDH-1). Consequently, alcohol is metabolized to acetaldehyde rapidly, whereas the metabolism to acetic acid is delayed. Because acetaldehyde is toxic and acetic acid is not, the net result is unpleasant effects such as facial flushing and palpitations (Giger and Davidhizar, 1995, Hanley, 1995; Wing and Thompson, 1995). Although there are few data to document this in the Kwa-kwa'ka-wakw, because this is true of the American Indians in general, this may be one explanation for the extreme problem created by alcohol in their lives (Davidhizar, 1997).

Many researchers attribute the problem of drinking as a symptom of what was done to the Kwa-kwa'ka-wakw people when they were forced to give up their traditional lifestyles. It has been suggested that alcohol has become a way of blocking out the pain that is carried inside by many of these people (Dye, 1989; Anon. 1, 1986; Anon. 2, 1986). The introduction of alcohol to the Kwa-kwa'ka-wakw has been destructive to their way of life and caused a dramatic deterioration in their spiritual, physical, and emotional health. Alcohol use by the Kwa-kwa'ka-wakw people has resulted in a loss of physical and mental health, a loss of productivity and jobs, and diverse chronic illnesses.

In addition to broken homes, alcohol has resulted in negative effects on family life. There is a fear of the drinker because of the erratic or inappropriate behaviors associated with alcohol (Wegsceder, 1985). Children fear that their parents will separate, and such a situation will leave them in the care of the Ministry of Housing and Social Services (often MHSS will put apprehended children into foster homes instead of with their extended families). Alcohol also has resulted in an increase in fetal alcohol syndrome (FAS) in First Nations babies born to women drinking during pregnancy (Anon. 3, 1990; Dempster, 1996). The "First Nations" model of the whole family and the "sacred circle of life" to live a creative and positive life has been broken by alcohol use and abuse (Nelson, 1990).

Susceptibility to disease

First Nations people have a high incidence of non-insulin dependent diabetes, tuberculosis, diarrhea, and myocardial infarction. The deaths in the First Nations communities are caused by different reasons. Following is a box excerpted from a study of the First Nations people in British Columbia done by the Medical Service branch for a 6-year period: 1987 to 1992 (A Statistical Report on the Health of the First Nations of British Columbia, 1995). The age-standardized mortality (ASM) for status Indians (100.3) was almost twice the provincial rate (52.0) (Box 11-1).

Tuberculosis The role of socioeconomic factors in the incidence of tuberculosis, which include conditions such as overcrowding, poor nutrition, high alcohol use, and poor self-care, would seem to be a significant factor in the high incidence of tuberculosis among the First Nations people (Hanley, 1995). Canadian aboriginal people accounted for approximately 20% of the cases of tuberculosis in Canada in 1994 (Editorial, 1996).

Diabetes Non-insulin dependent diabetes (NIDDM), or type II diabetes, is on the rise among Native Canadians (Daniel and Gamble, 1995). In fact, for Native Canadians in Ontario prevalence rates of NIDDM are among the highest reported in the world (Harris et al., 1997). In contrast, although diabetes mellitus is the most frequently reported chronic condition in the Pacific region with 343 cases, or 14.64% of the persons surveyed (Health and Welfare Canada, 1991), Young (1990) reports that the prevalence of diabetes among Canadian Indians is actually lowest among those on the West coast including British Columbia, the Yukon, and Northwest Territories. Young (1990, 1993) also notes that prevalence rates vary according to language family, culture area, latitude, longitude, and geographical isolation. The Kwa-kwa'ka-wakw elders say, "Many diseases or illnesses are found among us today. It is because we have lost our wholeness—spirituality, physical activities—and eat foods from the store and rely on tools that we stick into the wall. Our bodies are not being fed correctly; we are too idle because we can no longer hunt, catch fish, or pick berries to our hearts' content" (Smith, 1955). Daniel and Gamble (1985) also note that the high prevalence of NIDDM in Canada's Native communities corresponds with high diabetes prevalence among populations of indigenous peoples that have undergone changes associated with acculturation.

Diarrhea Diarrhea among the First Nations is sometimes caused by water reservoirs not being cleaned. Food poisoning is not very common and is not considered to be a threat. The Kwa-kwa'ka-wakw people have been known to serve large crowds at potlatches for centuries and so appear to know how to prepare food with no danger of causing food poisoning. They have maintained their safe practices.

Myocardial infarction Myocardial infarction has increased among the middle-aged First Nations people, especially in the men. Not only is myocardial infarction increasing, but also ischemic heart diseases (Young, 1994).

Nutritional preferences and deficiencies Before the arrival of the Europeans, food was prepared simply. Meat came from the wild animals—deer, moose, ducks, mountain goats, beavers, and sea lions. These were dried and smoked and then stored for later use. Few meats were not eaten, and therefore dogs, frogs, or snakes were a part of the diet too. Sea gulls were too tough to cook, but their eggs were a delicacy. Porcupine was available but not considered appetizing (Ford, 1941). Available to the Kwa-kwa'ka-wakw are over 50 plant species, which provide essential vitamins, minerals, and fiber while maintaining low sodium intake (Hopkinson, Stephenson, and Turner, 1995). In the past sugar and honey were not available; thus the only sweets eaten were the many wild berries and fruits found in the terrain. To fulfill the need for iodine, they ate many seafoods, which contain salt, which in turn contain iodine. Traditionally, tobacco was unknown to the Kwa-kwa'ka-wakw people. However, gum chewing is an old tradition (Ford, 1941). Gum was made from hemlock pitch after it was refined by being heated over a fire and filtered through a basket. The only fluid intake was from water from the mountain streams (Ford, 1941).

Since the arrival of the Europeans and the introduction to tobacco, smoking was readily adopted. Today no one chews gum from hemlock pitch, but rather gum chewers commercially purchase gum.

The diet of the Kwa-kwa'ka-wakw consists of commercially purchased products. Foods high in sugar such as candy and soda are commonly used. These drastic changes in diet have contributed to various illnesses as well as dental problems that formerly were nonexistent.

Lactose intolerance Lactose intolerance has been found in most First Nations people in Canada (A Statistical Report on the Health of First Nations in British Columbia, 1995). In fact, Gerchufsky (1996) notes that approximately 100% of American and Canadian Indian babies have lactose intolerance. Because of the lack of treatment, babies have died from this condition. Infant who are lactose intolerant generally get bloody stools and do not gain weight as a result.

IMPLICATIONS FOR NURSING CARE

It is important for the nurse providing culturally appropriate health care to the Kwa-kwa'ka-wakw to involve the community in planning health-related interventions. The plan should meet the perceived needs of the people as well as the needs identified by the nurse. Education is an important aspect to include in the plan of intervention, and an ongoing educational plan should be established and conducted regularly. The whole community needs to be reoriented to the traditional beliefs in holism and the need to be involved in the promotion of physical, emotional, and spiritual well-being in activities of daily living. The Kwa-kwa'ka-wakw should be advised that health promotion is congruent with their own traditional values, which emphasize physical, emotional, and spiritual well-being.

It is important for the nurse who wishes to provide culturally sensitive care to incorporate into the dietary plan good nutritional native foods. A report on the First Nations' traditional foods suggests that seafoods and wild meat fats are more healthful than the fats of beef and pork (Medical Services Branch, 1980). In-service education on good nutrition is important to assist the Kwa-kwa'ka-wakw to develop better eating habits. A good teaching strategy might include the preparation of a healthful meal that could be served to the participants to demonstrate how to prepare and serve a menu of foods that promote optimal wellness.

Nurses should promote breast feeding in prenatal classes because breast milk may be more tolerable than cow's milk. In addition, the nurse should give explanations of lactose intolerance and the detrimental effects this condition can have on infants, children, and adults. The nurse needs to help mothers find the right formula for their babies if they do not wish to breast feed and should also make the mothers aware of signs and symptoms of lactose intolerance. Because there is a disproportionately high infant mortality found among First Nations people, it is essential to advise the expectant mother on proper prenatal care.

The nurse should have in-service education on prevention of diabetes as well as classes for clients that have diabetes that needs to be controlled. Signs and symptoms of certain diseases should be described and talked about. For example, tuberculosis may be present if a cough is prolonged or gets progressively worse, if there are night sweats, if there is weight loss, and if blood is seen in sputum. Diabetes may be present if there is ongoing thirst and a dry mouth, if there is the urge to urinate frequently, and if a person fatigues easily. It is important to use terminology in in-service care so that the lay person will understand; for example, avoid medical words such as "urinate" but use instead the word "pee." Pictures, drawings, and demonstrations are useful to promote understanding about the expected treatment protocol.

Ongoing clinical checkups for high-risk people should be conducted so that blood glucose values, blood pressures, and weights are checked. Tuberculosis screening (Mantoux tests, chest x-ray films, and so forth) should be done yearly in schools. Mantoux tests may be given to persons in contact with a new case of tuberculosis to detect active infection.

Classes for children in the schools should include the importance of good diet, personal hygiene, rest, activity, dental hygiene and care, and coping skills. Educating the children is one way of educating the whole community. Education about the high incidence of alcoholism among First Nations people should begin as early as the elementary grades.

SUMMARY

Today the Kwa-kwa'ka-wakw nation is regaining their traditional ways. Language and art are being taught in the classrooms, and children are learning about their heritage. Despite the apparent Westernization of the Kwa-kwa'ka-wakw people, some of these individuals are once again embracing traditional values, beliefs, practices, and customs. Bringing Kwa-kwa'ka-wakw culture into the schools is important if change is to occur within Kwa-kwa'ka-wakw families and communities.

Individuals and particularly nurses throughout Canada need to learn about Kwa-kwa'ka-wakw culture. Knowledge of the culture can enable the nurse to provide culturally appropriate nursing care to the Kwa-kwa'ka-wakw people.

Case Study

Developed by Ruth Shearer, MSN, RN, Assistant Professor, Division of Nursing, Bethel College, Mishawaka, Indiana

A 55-year-old Kwa-kwa'ka-wakw man is admitted to the hospital with diabetic ketoacidosis. His wife and pregnant daughter accompanied him. They explained that he had been losing a lot of weight and strength. Previously he was strong, healthy, and muscular. Lately he had been nauseated and vomiting. He was always thirsty and going to pee. At the time of admission he was disoriented as to time and place. His family attributed these symptoms to his use of alcohol. During this hospitalization he is stabilized with intravenous fluids of saline, 5% dextrose, potassium, phosphate, and bicarbonate. His blood gases, blood glucose, neurological status, intake, output, and vital signs are monitored. Before discharge, the client, his wife, and their daughter attend diabetic classes. The client is withdrawn, noncommunicative, and with depressed facial features as he tells his family to call the *pa-xa-lá*.

CARE PLAN

 Nursing Diagnosis   Spiritual distress related to suffering as evidenced by use of alcohol and request for *pa-xa-lá* (native healer).

Client Outcomes

1. Client will be whole *(synala)* during the healing ceremony.

Nursing Interventions

1. Encourage family to call *pa-xa-la* and provide privacy.
2. Allow family to remain with client because the presence of a caring person is more important than conversation.
3. Maintain eye contact while client or family member talks to demonstrate interest and honesty.
4. Assess spiritual needs by asking the client and family what could be done in the hospital to facilitate wholeness.

 Nursing Diagnosis   Altered health maintenance related to increased alcohol consumption as evidenced by weight loss, mental confusion, and electrolyte imbalance.

Client Outcome

1. Client will eat healthful food to maintain desired body weight.

Nursing Intervention

1. Assess client's preference of foods in each food group. Have client keep food diary to show the community health representative (CHP).

2. Client will follow medical regime on discharge.

2. Encourage use of traditional foods such as fish and wild animals because these are healthful for First Nations people.
3. Discourage use of refined sugars and alcohol because they are detrimental to the diabetic's well-being.
4. Schedule visit with CHR to have client weighed once every week and to determine progress on diet.
5. Explain and demonstrate to client how and when to check blood glucose, administer insulin, and safety measures using daughter as an interpreter.
6. Send written instructions home with client and send copy to CHR.
7. Ask client to repeat back through interpreter what he understands about his treatment of diabetes.
8. Instruct client to go to the clinic each week to have blood glucose checked and to report energy level.

3. Client and family will maintain health.

9. Instruct family members to have health screening for tuberculosis and diabetes done at clinic each year.

STUDY QUESTIONS

1. Describe the metabolism of alcohol among the Kwa-kwa'ka-wakw people and the implications for nursing care.
2. Identify focal themes of religious rites specific to the Kwa-kwa'ka-wakw.
3. Identify at least two other conditions that have a prevalence among the Kwa-kwa'ka-wakw people.
4. Explain the ceremonial rituals for the dead and the dying unique to the Kwa-kwa'ka-wakw people.
5. List at least three reasons why it may be difficult for this client to adhere to the prescribed treatment regimen.

References

A statistical report on the health of First Nations in British Columbia. (1995). Ottawa: Minister of Health.

Acheson, S. (1995). Culture contact, demography and health among the aboriginal peoples of British Columbia. *A persistent spirit: toward understanding aboriginal health in British Columbia.* Victoria, B.C.: University of Victoria.

Anonymous 1. (1986). *Alcoholism in the home.* Daly City, Calif.: Karma's Communication.

Anonymous 2. (1986). *Alcoholism in the workplace.* Daly City, Calif.: Karma's Communication.

Anonymous 3. (1990). *Fetal alcohol syndrome prevention program.* California Urban Indian Council, Inc.

Bailey, E., & Bailey, R. (1995). *Discover Canada.* Oxford: Berlitz Publishing Company.

Boas, F. (1938). *The mind of primitive man.* New York: MacMillan.

Daniel, M., & Gamble, D. (1995). Diabetes and Canada's aboriginal peoples: the need for primary prevention.

International Journal of Nursing Studies, 32(3), 243-259.

Davidhizar, R. (1997). Personal communication. Mishawaka, Indiana.

Dawson, J. (1996). *Canoe launching at Kingcome Inlet.*

Dempster, J.S. (1996). Fetal alcohol syndrome: the nurse practitioner perspective. *Journal of the American Academy of Nurse Practitioners, 8*(7), 343-352.

Dye, A. (1989). *Interview with Miss Dye.* Victoria, B.C.

Editorial. (1996, May). Modest increase in Canadian rate in midst of global emergency. *The Canadian Nurse, 18.*

Ford, C. (1941). *Smoke from their fires.* Hamden, Conn.: The Shoestring Press, Inc.

Foster, L.T., Macdonald, J., Tuk, T.A., Uh, S.H., & Talbot, D. (1995). Native health in British Columbia: a vital statistics perspective. *A persistent spirit: towards understanding Aboriginal health in British Columbia.* Victoria, B.C.: University of Victoria.

Gerchufsky, M. (1996). Milk: does it really do a body good? *Advances for Nurse Practitioners, 4,* 39-41.

Giger, J., & Davidhizar, R. (1995). *Transcultural nursing: assessment and intervention.* St. Louis: Mosby.

Grypma, S. (1993). Culture shock. *Canadian Nurse, 89*(8), 33-36.

Hanley, C. (1995). Navajo Indians. In Giger, J., & Davidhizar, R. (Eds.), *Transcultural nursing: assessment and intervention.* St. Louis: Mosby.

Harris, S., Gittelsohn, J., Hanley, A., Barnie, A., Wolever, T., Gao, J., Logan, A., & Zinman, B. (1997). The prevalence of NIDDM and associated risk factors in Native Canadians. *Diabetes Care, 20*(1), 185-187.

Health and Welfare Canada. (1991). *Health status of Canadian Indians and Inuits 1990.* Ottawa: Minister of Supply and Services.

Hopkinson, J., Stephenson, P.H., & Turner, N.J. (1995). Changing traditional diet and nutrition in aboriginal peoples of coastal British Columbia. *A persistent spirit: towards understanding aboriginal health in British Columbia.* Victoria, B.C.: University of Victoria.

Indian and Northern Affairs, Canada. (1996). *Facts from stats* (Issue No. 11, March-April). Ottawa: Information Quality and Research Directorate.

Jensen, D., & Sargant, P. (1985). *Robes of power, totem poles on cloth.* Vancouver: UBC Press.

McMillan, A. (1988). *Native peoples and cultures of Canada: an anthropological overview.* Vancouver/ Toronto: Douglas & McIntyre.

Medical Services Branch. (1980). *Nutrition in alcoholic rehabilitation.* Regina, Saskatchewan: Medical Services, Saskatchewan Branch.

Miller, V. (1986). In Morrison, R., & Wilson, C. (Eds.), *Native peoples: the Canadian experience* (pp. 324-352). Toronto: McClelland & Stewart.

Nelson, W. (1990). *Enter the sacred circle of life: ADAPT. The longest journey is the journey inward.* Fort Berthold, N.D.

Patterson, P. (1972). *The Canadian Indian history since 1500.* Don Mills, Ont.: Collier-MacMillan Canada, Ltd.

Robertson, D. (1957). *Interview with an elder.* Kingcome Inlet, B.C.

Rohner, R. (1967). *The people of Gilford Island: a contemporary Kwakiutl village.* Ottawa: National Museum of Canada.

Sealy, B., & McDonald, N. (1990). *The health care professional in a Native community: a cross-cultural study guide.* Winnipeg: University of Manitoba.

Seniors Advisory Council. (1996). *Health profile of aboriginal seniors in British Columbia.* Victoria, B.C.: Minister of Health.

Smith, D.S. (1985). Kwakiutl ceremonial blankets. *Robes of power.* Vancouver: UBC Press.

Smith, G. (1955, 1957, 1960). *Interviews with Granny Smith.* Kingcome Inlet, B.C.

Sokoloski, E.H. (1995). Canadian First Nations women's beliefs about pregnancy and prenatal care. *Canadian Journal of Nursing Research, 27*(1), 89-100.

Statistics Canada. (1991). *Profile of Canada's aboriginal population.* Ottawa: Indian and Northern Affairs Canada.

The Royal Commission on Aboriginal Peoples. (1995). *Looking forward, looking back.* Ottawa, CMA Webspinners.

Thompson, M. (1990). Heavy birthweight of native Indians of British Columbia. *Canadian Journal of Public Health, 81,* 443-446.

Voyageur, E. (1989). *A hospital experience.* Victoria, B.C.

Wegsceder, S. (1985). *Family trap.* Minneapolis, Minn.

White, L., & Jacobs, E. (1992). *Liberating our children, liberating our nations.* Victoria, B.C.: Minister of Social Services.

Willie, B.S. (1962, 1968, 1971, 1972). *Tapes of Kwa-kwa'ka-wakw history.* Victoria, B.C.: Royal Museum.

Willie, E. (1997). *Interview with Reverend Willie.* Port Hardy, B.C.

Willie, J. (1955). *My mother's words of wisdom when my first child was born.* Alert Bay, B.C.

Willie, J. (1989). *My mother's words about healing.* Kingcome Inlet, B.C.

Wing, D.M., & Thompson, T. (1995). Causes of alcoholism: a qualitative study of traditional Muscogee (Creek) Indians. *Public Health Nursing, 12*(6), 417-423.

Young, T., Szathmary, E., Evers, S., & Wheatley, B. (1990). Geographical distribution of diabetes among the Native population of Canada: a national survey. *Social Science and Medicine 31*(2), 129-139.

Young, T. (1993). Diabetes mellitus among Native Americans in Canada and the United States: an epidemiological review. *American Journal of Human Biology, 5,* 399-413.

Young, T. (1994). *The health of Native Americans.* New York: Oxford University Press.

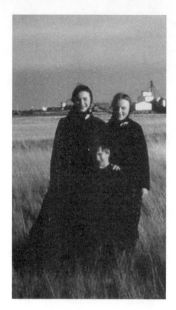

CHAPTER 12
Canadian Hutterites

Howard Brunt

BEHAVIORAL OBJECTIVES

Upon completion of this chapter, the nurse will be able to:

1. Describe the communication patterns unique to the Canadian Hutterites.
2. Discuss the spatial behaviors or needs of the Canadian Hutterite.
3. Describe the social organization of the Hutterite community.
4. Discuss relevant gender-role assignment unique to the Hutterite community.
5. Describe the time orientation of the Hutterite client.
6. Identify environmental control issues relevant to care of the Hutterite.
7. Identify common susceptible diseases unique to the Hutterite.

OVERVIEW OF NORTH AMERICAN HUTTERITES

The Hutterian Brethren, or Hutterites, as they are more commonly known, is the single largest rural ethnic group in Canada. At the present time, two thirds of the estimated 35,000 Hutterites reside in the prairie provinces of Canada with the remainder spread across the states bordering these provinces (Evans, 1985). Theologically related to both the Amish and the Mennonites, Hutterites are a Christian Anabaptist group whose distinctiveness lies in its agrarian-communal way of life based on religious precepts drawn from the New Testament. North American Hutterites are subdivided into three genetically distinct sects, the *Dariusleute, Lehrerleute,* and *Schmeideleute,* all with similar lifestyles and virtually identical religious beliefs and practices. In- and out-migration from the three endogamous sects is relatively rare, and when this is combined with their high fertility, the genetic expression of health

and illness in this population is a important factor. Hutterite life can be summed up in the phrase "all things in common," which reflects the deeply held belief that they have about the importance of living a simple communal existence on large farms called "colonies." Unlike their Amish "cousins," Hutterites use the latest in agricultural technology and take full advantage of modern medicine.

One of the longest existing and most successful communal societies known, the Hutterian Brethren emerged during the period of the Radical Reformation (1520s) at a time when they were violently persecuted by the existing nobility and the Roman Catholic church (Hostetler, 1968). Indeed, persecution has been one of the historical hallmarks of Hutterian existence that helps shape their world view. Jakob Hutter, the group's founder and namesake, had become an influential and charismatic leader of a group of Anabaptists who lived a communal life in South Tyrol, an area in southern Austria. Hutter and his group were ruthlessly pursued by the authorities, and, in 1536, Jakob Hutter was executed at Innsbruck. Hutter's followers then spent a turbulent period of time in which they were either forced to hide in the forest or to go "underground" and rejoin society. However, by the 1550s the persecutions had eased and Hutterite colonies were established in Moravia, and by 1621 there were 102 colonies (*Bruderhöfe*) in Moravia with 20,000 to 30,000 members. This period of relative prosperity came to an end with the Thirty Years War largely because of the Hutterites' refusal to participate in it.

Over the next 150 years the Hutterites went through brief periods of resettlement in eastern Europe, punctuated by frequent persecution and forced migration. For much of this time, communal living was not possible. In 1770 a group of Hutterites immigrated to Russia, and over the next 100 years colonies and the communal lifestyle were reestablished, though a large number of Hutterites continued to live noncommunally. Once again, war interceded, and in 1874 many Hutterites who refused to participate in the war effort left Russia, with just over 400 moving to the Dakota territories of the United States. The three major sects were formed during this period, and each had approximately 100 founding members. Another 100 or so of the original immigrants chose not to live on the colonies, and they became known as the *"Prairieleute."* Although small breakaway groups have formed from time to time in other locations, the western North American groups are far and away the major representations of Hutterian society.

Although Hutterites began to immigrate to Canada from America before the First World War, immigration greatly increased because of persecutions related to their Germanic origins, pacifist beliefs, and refusal to be conscripted into the war effort. Over the intervening decades, colonies were established in the Canadian provinces of Manitoba, Saskatchewan, Alberta, and British Columbia, with the highest concentration found in Alberta. As late as the 1960s, discriminatory laws that sought to restrict the free expression of Hutterite life were still in force in some Canadian provinces (Saunders, 1964). Although state-sanctioned persecution is a thing of the past for the Hutterites, because of their distinct cultural beliefs, appearance, and lifestyle, they continue to be a target of ethnic discrimination.

Communication

Linguistically most present-day Hutterites are trilingual. Their everyday language on the colony is medieval in origin, representing an unwritten form of an early, Upper High German dialect originally spoken in the Tyrolean and Carinthian provinces of Austria. This Huttrish dialect is peppered with phrases and words that have been added over the centuries as they migrated across Europe and, more recently, North America (Claus-Peter, 1972). Once in school, Hutterite children learn both modern German in their German school and English in their regular school. German is the language used in religious services, and every Hutterite is prepared to understand enough German to comprehend the sermons they attend on a daily basis. Excellent penmanship is highly prized in German school, and those most adept at writing German are given the important task of copying in longhand the sermons that have been handed down from minister to minister over the last five centuries. More recently, photocopying has become more frequent on the colonies, and it remains to be seen if rote learning and writing of German will be adversely affected. In many ways, English is really the second language to the Huttrish dialect for Hutterites because they are more adept at using it than modern German during their regular contacts with non-Hutterites. Hutterite children attending English school are mainly taught by non-Hutterite teachers who use the standard provincial or state curriculum. However, some *Schmeideleute* colonies are beginning to send a few of their college-aged young adults for teacher certification. Despite the relative isolation of the colonies, from an early age most Hutterites come into regular contact with English-speaking non-Hutterites (that is, during visits to town), and so they have ample opportunity to use the language of the mainstream North American culture in their region. The one caution to the above discussion of language is that a small proportion of Hutterites who are now in their seventies or older are less facile with English than the younger colony members. The Hutterites' English accent is quite similar to what one hears when listening to a person who has German as a first language, and although there is a range in the degree of accent, it is very easy to understand and poses little problem for non-Hutterites.

As a rule, Hutterites are no more laconic or loquacious than one might expect in the general North American culture. They are good conversationalists and enjoy sharing stories and jokes in social settings and are very business-like and direct in everyday conversation. Many Hutterites display a tremendous sense of warmth, humor, and "presence" during conversation. Hutterites are good questioners and listeners and are not reticent in asking for clarification if they are uncertain about what has been said. At the same time, it is important to use a variety of approaches if the nurse is trying to describe an idea or ask a question that deals with unfamiliar content. The body language of Hutterites during communication conveys neither overt formality nor excessive familiarity.

Reading comprehension of English is generally quite good, and virtually all Hutterites, except for a small proportion of the elderly, are literate to the eighth-grade reading level. Upon completion of formal schooling at 15 years of age, Hutterites are exposed to a variety of reading materials, including books, newspapers, and magazines; however, this varies greatly among colonies. Some of the more conservative colonies strictly enforce rules against reading "worldly" print materials, whereas others are less restrictive. Generally speaking, most Hutterites would be expected to keep up with the latest technical farming information found in industry publications and agribusiness journals and newspapers. On most colonies, other forms of communication such as radios and televisions are officially forbidden. Nevertheless, it is possible to find radios in some of the vehicles and apartments, though this varies from colony to colony.

Given the communal nature of Hutterite life, most conversations are done in the presence of others. In many cases, "private" interaction is generally unexpected or unfeasible, even when topics that would generally be thought of as confidential are being discussed. Just as small towns often have no secrets, colonies are designed to make almost everything a matter of public record and open to communal scrutiny.

Implications for nursing care

It is important for the nurse to remember that Hutterite clients are in most ways no different from other clients encountered in the health care delivery system. In this regard, Hutterites appreciate receiving education about their health and therapeutic communication from their nurse. Health professionals are well respected as a rule by Hutterites, and any verbal communication should be done in a straightforward manner with a minimum of jargon and "nursespeak." Augmentation of verbal communication with written materials is entirely appropriate, if they are written at a level appropriate for the general public. More often than not, interaction with a Hutterite client is generally done with other family members present, and although this may seem counter to notions of individual privacy and confidentiality, it is culturally expected. It is also important for nurses to consider the family as the unit of interaction, and sessions on health teaching and discussions about procedures or care should ideally take place when other family members are present unless the client specifically requests otherwise.

It is essential to recognize that Hutterite clients may be quite interested in hearing about the caregiver's life and experiences (that is, many are interested in learning about someone from another culture). It is important to remember that many Hutterites communicate with the same set of people everyday; thus the nurse from another culture may be viewed as a novelty and can expect to be "interviewed." Although the Hutterian world view is strongly held, they do not believe in proselytizing, and many enjoy conversations with people holding other religious and lifestyle beliefs.

SPACE

In a colony, everything of the material world is shared and there is really no such thing as a concept or expectation of "personal space"; indeed, this is counter to the religious dictum "all things in common." All meals are eaten communally in the dining hall, daily church services are conducted for the entire colony, and most of the regular work is done in small groups. Trips to town are well coordinated so that groups go together, saving both fuel and time. Free time is spent with family and friends, and in the course of a typical day there is little time to oneself. Colonies are designed so that immediate family (parents and children) all live in one large apartment, often with between six and eight bedrooms. Given the large extended kinships on colonies, it is not uncommon to have an entire colony of 100 people made up of just one or two large families ranging over four generations. Thus one is hardly ever alone and is always surrounded by family and close friends.

Hutterite behavior is directed by a high moral code of conduct based on an interpretation of biblical teaching that includes careful prescriptions about appropriate activities for and between men and women. Much of the space within the colony is either explicitly or implicitly defined as being for males or females. For example, one half of the dining room is for the men and the other half for women; children eat separately with the German teacher, usually in a separate dining area. Similarly there is a place set aside for males, females, and children in the chapel. Monogamy is strictly enforced, and the maintenance of the sanctity of one's sexual being is expected.

It would be impossible to discuss Hutterian culture without briefly describing the way the land and the layout of the colony help to support the sense of "spiritual space" and a deeper personal connection with God. Just like the early colonies, called *Bruderhöfe*, present-day colonies are designed to help remove Hutterites from the earthly distractions that impede their spiritual practice and devotion. Thus colonies are typically well removed from cities and comprise between 10,000 and 20,000 acres of land. The basic layout of colonies follows a time-tested formula, though there are variations between colonies. Generally each colony is made up of groups of "row" living apartments, a central kitchen and dining hall, a school building, a chapel, laundry facility, and a variety of agribusiness buildings including garages, barns, silos, meat-processing plants, and an assortment of other outbuildings. Most family apartments have a livingroom area, bedrooms, bath-

rooms, and a small "snack" kitchen and dining area for between-meal snacks. To minimize the reliance on the outside world, most of the food, clothing, furniture, and everyday needs of Hutterites are produced right on the colony. Things that cannot be grown or manufactured on the colony are usually bought in large bulk orders as both a way to reduce costs and a way to minimize the need to make frequent trips to purchase necessities. Virtually all the maintenance and construction on the colony is done by colony members. Specialty trades such as electricians, plumbers, carpenters, and even computer technicians are all represented. Visits to town, or even hospitalizations, can engender a great deal of interest and excitement because they afford Hutterites the opportunity to take a brief break from the regularity of colony life and to see new and different things.

Implications for nursing care

Nurses working with a Hutterite client in an institutional setting will undoubtedly find that there will be a large number of colony members visiting on a regular basis. It is important to talk with the hospitalized Hutterite client about his or her personal preferences about visitation, and, to the degree possible, visitation policy should be modified to recognize the important role the family plays in meeting the Hutterian spiritual and material needs. Keep in mind that most colonies will be quite distant from larger urban centers with highly specialized tertiary-level hospitals, and so everything that can be done to help accommodate visitors should be given priority. In terms of Hutterian "personal space," it should be respected in the same way as any client in the hospital setting. During procedures or examinations, it is entirely appropriate to ask family members to leave the room if privacy is required. On the other hand, family members are often eager to assist and to stay and learn about postdischarge care (that is, wound care or rehabilitative exercises). It is important for the nurse to talk with the client about how to best accommodate their spiritual needs during their stay. This may include making time and space available for visits from the colony preacher to be with the client and his or her family.

It is not uncommon for public or community health nurses to work with groups of people milling about, even if the focus is on a particular individual. Nurses visiting colonies during mealtime can expect to eat with the colony and will usually be seated in the area reserved for their gender. Although clinics are often held in communal areas such as the dining room or school, it is also a common practice for the nurse to be invited into family apartments for more personal examinations or consultations. Nurses who will be working regularly with a particular colony should take the time to tour all the facilities so that they can better understand the environmental factors affecting the health of their clients.

SOCIAL ORGANIZATION

The social order and lives of Hutterites are strictly governed by a series of principles that have changed little over their 500-year history (Boldt, 1978). The elders of the colony, all baptized men, are charged with the responsibility of maintaining the Hutterian vision of a proper spiritual and secular life. There is a well-ordered and prescribed hierarchy on the colony, with the minister and farm manager given the greatest responsibility. From the Hutterite perspective, those in positions of authority are not seen as being "powerful"; rather they are considered to be the "servants" of the colony who carry the greatest burden. Work on the colony is strictly organized along gender lines, with males taking responsibility for the economic and agribusiness roles and females taking responsibility for childrearing and the domestic needs of the colony. Typically there is a "senior" minister and a "junior" minister on each colony who are charged with maintaining the spiritual health of the colony. The farm manager handles the secular administration of the colony and the various farm operations each have a "boss." Although there are variations between colonies, most are mixed farming operations with dairy and beef cattle and a variety of other meat-producing animals such as chickens, sheep, and hogs. Crops such as corn, barley, oats, and canola* are grown for both commercial and colony use, and a large garden area

supplies the colony with vegetables and fruits. Many colonies also produce manufactured goods such as furniture and specialty agricultural equipment, but these are generally small-scale operations. Women run the communal nursery and kindergarten and often are in charge of the garden and milking operations of the colony. One of the most important jobs on the colony is that of head cook, and this job is typically held for several years by just one woman. The cooking is done communally by the women who work on a rotational basis in small groups. Although men usually continue working at their jobs for as long as they are physically able, with many gradually moving into more supervisory positions, most women are "retired" from the usual communal cooking and other domestic duty rotations as early as their late forties.

The Hutterian view of males and females and their appropriate roles and responsibilities are deeply rooted to their religious beliefs. These beliefs often stand in stark contrast to the notions of gender equity and equality that now predominate in North American culture, and it is important for the nurse to approach these differences in a culturally sensitive way. Women on the colony do wield a considerable amount of power and exert control both in an informal and formal sense over many aspects of colony life. In term of most health-related matters, female Hutterites provide the leadership on the colony; however, they do so at the discretion and under the ultimate control of the minister and elders. It is this facet of Hutterite society that has most tested my personal mettle when it comes to practicing nursing in a culturally sensitive way. It is important for each nurse working with Hutterites to reconcile his or her personal views with the Hutterian vision of gender in a way that permits the provision of care in a way that is as free of ethnocentricity as possible.

The socialization process on the colony is carefully monitored by the elders; however, every Hutterite is charged with the responsibility of helping to maintain the spiritual environment. Neonates stay with their mother until 4 weeks of age, and then they are placed under the care of the older women in the communal nursery. Beginning in kindergarten and then more formally in German school, young Hut-

---

*Canola is a genetically engineered variety of rapeseed with 7% saturated fat; *Can*ada, *o*il, *l*ow *a*cid, 1978.

terites learn about their history and become familiarized with the religious foundation of their lives (Hostetler, 1968). Although the process of socialization and religious training continues throughout life, a major turning point occurs at the time of baptism. Adult baptism is the defining precept for Anabaptists, and the decision to become a fully responsible member of the Hutterian faith usually occurs in the midtwenties. Only baptized adults can marry and hold positions of responsibility in the colony.

Marriage in Hutterite society is based on patrilocality, with the wife moving to the husband's colony for the remainder of her life. Thus women are uprooted from their friends and family and must learn to adapt to an entirely new colony. Offsetting this potential isolation, trips back to their birth colony are taken fairly regularly during vacation time by female Hutterites, and it is not uncommon to find women from one colony marrying into the same colony (Hostetler, 1975).

It is not possible to gain an appreciation of the Hutterites' world view and socialization process, particularly in relation to their views on health, without a brief overview of some of the key religious beliefs that inform their every decision. In addition to the belief in adult baptism that was described above, communalism, *Gelassenheit* ('imperturbability'), shunning worldliness, personal responsibility and moderation in all things are factors that help inform Hutterian life.

Communalism is the central feature of Hutterite life that sets it apart from all the other Anabaptist groups. The practice of communalism is based on the biblical quotation: "And all that believed were together, and had all things common and they sold their possessions and goods and distributed them to all, as any had need" (Acts 2:44). The Hutterites have reaped virtually all the benefits of communal life, including a highly efficient means of production to meet their basic needs, with relatively few of the destructive elements that have historically made communal life a temporary arrangement (Hostetler, 1968).

At the heart of the success of communalism is the shared spiritual belief in *Gelassenheit*, the aspiration to live a live on earth that is based on selflessness.

Virtually every act, emotion and thought can be measured against the ideal of *Gelassenheit*. Stephenson has described the experience of *Gelassenheit* as representing a bit of heaven on earth characterized by a calmness, resigned composure, and deliberate patience. The powerful socializing influence of *Gelassenheit* lies in the way it serves to act as the benchmark against which all changes can be judged. That is, modification of the status quo is sanctioned only to the degree that it positively supports selflessness and strengthens the communal nature of colony life.

Shunning of worldliness has led to what Stephenson (1991) called the "doctrine of two worlds" in which Christian values are inextricably confronted by the banal and sinful "ways of the world." The geographic isolation of colonies is a powerful manifestation of this doctrine, as is the distinctive attire of Hutterites, which is characterized by simple black coats, hats, and pants for the men and dark ankle-length dresses and simple scarf head coverings for the women. Although there is some variation between the three major Hutterite sects, all of them use a wide range of colors and patterns for men's shirts and women's aprons. Nevertheless, Hutterite appearance is designed to be plain and effectively sets them apart from the world (Stephenson, 1991).

In contrast to the deterministic perspective that obtains in the Old Testament Bible, Hutterites take the New Testament view that they must exercise free will to live a spiritual life, as represented in Ezekiel 10:27: "And when the wicked turneth himself from his wickedness, which he hath wrought, and doeth judgment, and justice, he shall save his soul." Thus Hutterites are expected to take responsibility for their choices and to struggle to lead a good Christian life. Closely aligned with self-determinism is the belief that there should be moderation in all things, as represented in this quote, "Do not join those who drink too much wine or gorge themselves on meat, for drunkards and gluttons become poor and drowsiness clothes them in rags" (Proverbs 23:20-21).

Implications for nursing care

It is important to appreciate the particular roles that the Hutterite client fulfills on the colony to better understand the context of life. For example, the illness of a farm manager or a head cook may be quite disruptive to colony life by virtue of the social and work-related roles they fill within the communal order. At the same time, because of the high degree of social cohesiveness of Hutterite society, many of the duties that may be performed by colony members can be relatively easily transferred to others. Thus a young mother who must be away from the colony is secure in the knowledge that her children are being well tended by close family and friends.

Hutterites are well grounded in their world view, and nurses should feel comfortable working with them in ways that are essentially no different from the way of anyone else. There can be a tendency to "tiptoe" around people from other cultures out of a desire to not appear disrespectful or to do something culturally inappropriate. However, Hutterites are tolerant of others' views and do not expect the nurse to fully understand their habits and customs. The key is to be respectful, and if the nurse is unsure of what might be appropriate in a given situation, it would be best to ask the clients what they expect. Again, Hutterites are quite used to modern health care and will appreciate and expect the nurse to treat them with the same professional care as any other client. Because of the professional status that most nurses are accorded, there are usually no problems with female nurses caring for males and male nurses working with female Hutterite clients.

The religious perspectives on "moderation in all things" and taking personal responsibility provide nurses with options during health education to fashion messages so that they are congruent with the Hutterian world view. For example, one researcher designed an educational booklet about the prevention of heart disease that uses the concept of moderation when discussing diet and exercise patterns (Brunt, 1996). In contrast, educational teaching that focuses on the need for an individual to be treated differently by colony members must be carefully considered in light of the concept of *Gelassenheit* and the emphasis Hutterites place on selflessness and not asking for or expecting special

treatment. For example, in cases where it is important for a Hutterite to be provided a special diet because of a particular health problem (such as diabetes or lactose intolerance), knowledge of the social order on the colony is important to consider so that the elders and head cook can be included in planning for dietary change. In most cases, colonies are very accommodating to special needs; however, simply telling someone to change their diet in isolation from their cultural reality is almost guaranteed to fail.

Public and community health nurses who are interested in setting up health programs, introducing health-related changes, or even conducting clinics on the colony must respect the Hutterian decision-making process. Typically the first step in gaining acceptance of a health program is to sit down with the head minister and the colony manager to discuss ideas. It is essential that a nurse have a well-thought out and detailed plan to present that clearly indicates the resource implications and the costs and benefits for the colony.

TIME

The concept of time in Hutterite society is closely connected to their sense of history, the growing seasons, and the regimentation of daily life. Virtually every Hutterite can trace his or her particular lineage back from anywhere between three and four centuries. Beyond the personal sense of connection to the past, there is also a rich oral and written tradition that details the history of the Hutterites and the struggles they have endured throughout the latter part of this millennium. This deeply rooted embeddedness in time permeates the Hutterian experience, and they can draw upon countless examples of how others responded to similar circumstances when they face new personal challenges. The Hutterites' experience of historical time provides a grounding and situatedness in the world that has a profound effect on their sense of and confidence in who they are as a people.

It is only natural that, being so closely tied to the land and the agrarian life, Hutterite society is synchronized with the diurnal and seasonal cycles. Because most colonies are in the northern growing regions of North America, their crops follow a single yearly cycle that require mostly planting in the spring and harvest in the early to midfall. Similarly, many of the animals are born and eventually sold or slaughtered at specific times of the year. This means that everyone pitches in to work extra-long hours at various points in the annual cycle. Most marriages, baptisms, and visits to other colonies are timed so that they occur in the interval between spring and fall; thus summer is a time of great excitement and activity when many of the rituals and meaningful events in a Hutterite's life take place. Winter is time for repairing broken equipment, fixing up the interior of the various buildings, making crafts, and running the farm operations that are less dependent on weather (such as eggs and hogs). The winter also provides the colony with more time to spend with family and friends and to rest up for the coming cycle of hard outdoor labor.

Each colony has a system of marking time throughout the day, often the ringing of a large bell outside the dining hall or electric bells in the residences and main work areas. Although there are alterations in the schedule that happen between the seasons, each day is highly regimented with set times for the three main meals and three snack periods, school, work and church services. Most Hutterites wear wristwatches, and clocks are scattered throughout the colony. As one might expect, in contrast to cultures that are not concerned with "real" time, Hutterites are highly conscious of time and most events start and end punctually. Meals are not taken leisurely because they are seen as being times to replenish the body to continue God's work, not to socialize or relax. As regimented as the workday is, evenings are usually a time to relax, visit with family and friends, and engage in more personal interests such as craft making.

Implications for nursing care

Probably the most important factor related to time that nurses both in hospitals and the community need to consider when working with their Hutterite clients is the season, particularly as it relates to farming. Depending on the role clients play, their absence from work may have a greater or lesser effect on the day-to-day running of the colony. Similarly the ability of family and friends to visit an ill relative will be affected by their ability to be away from their work and the vagaries of winter weather. Community and public health nurses who are planning to conduct clinics or make colony visits must take the season into account, and the harvest season is usually too busy to plan any special health-related visits or events. On the other hand, because of the regimentation of the Hutterian daily schedule, it is usually relatively easy to work with the colony to schedule a colony visit at a convenient time. Your hospitalized Hutterite clients will appreciate knowing as much as possible about the daily schedule and routine so that they can plan for visits and times to pray.

ENVIRONMENTAL CONTROL

Concept of health and use of health services. The Hutterite concept of health is primarily considered in spiritual terms and is closely aligned with the concept of *Gelassenheit.* Good physical, mental, and emotional health are considered gifts from God, though ill health is not necessarily considered a punishment. Rather, ill health is considered a burden that one must bear, in part, as a test of faith as expressed in Romans 5:3-5: "We rejoice in our sufferings, because we know that suffering produces perseverance; perseverance, character; and character, hope." Thus Hutterites do not consider it appropriate to pray for good health, instead they pray for the wisdom to know how to either live a healthy life or to bear their suffering without complaint. As previously discussed, Hutterian religious beliefs emphasize the personal responsibility required to make personal lifestyle choices that influence their health. Next to baptism, death is considered the most important moment in a Hutterite's life because it marks the entry into eternal life in heaven and provides the colony with an important social occasion. Thus death *per se* is an unlikely stimulus for risk modification. However, the sudden disability of a colony member in his or her prime has a largely negative effect on the colony as a whole, requiring replacement of the affected individual in the work force and, in some cases, the provision of care. An ideal death in the Hutterite culture is one that is relatively slow and drawn out, permitting the dying person to socialize other Hutterites into the acceptance of death and to prepare for entry into heaven (Stephenson, 1983).

Physical illness is considered to be a normal part of human existence, and the treatment of health problems is thought of in a straightforward, pragmatic way. Thus all the modern allopathic remedies, including medicines and surgery, are sought out, and Hutterites make full use of social medicine in Canada and private health care in the United States. Because of differences in the health care systems between Canada and the United States, there is some evidence that Canadian Hutterites make greater use of prevention and treatment services (Converse, Buker, and Lee, 1973; Hostetler, 1985). Hutterites also utilize the full complement of health professionals in their treatment, including nurses, physiotherapists, chiropractors, nutritionists, and occupational therapists. In addition to "mainstream" health care, 80% of Hutterites we recently surveyed also seek out the services of both colony and non–colony based alternative therapies including herbalists, acupuncturists, reflexologists, naturopaths, and homeopaths (unpublished data). Indeed, the Hutterites have a long history of providing skilled care to themselves and their neighbors by means of midwives, bonesetters, dentists, and herbalists (Hostetler, 1975; Sommer, 1953).

Disorders of what is known as "mental health" are understood in ways that are congruent with the prevailing allopathic view (that is the biological basis of manic depression requiring medical intervention) and are expressed in more spiritual terms. An extreme form of spiritual *Angst*, called *Anfechtung*, is based on the belief that one has sinned and is beyond redemption. Hutterites suffering from *Anfechtung* are withdrawn, appear depressed, and continually ruminate on their religious unworthiness (Kaplan and Plaut, 1956). The treatment of *Anfechtung* is largely the responsibility of the minister and, like the way other mental disorders are dealt with by the colony members, the afflicted are given as much support as possible on the colony. The person with a mental disorder is neither socially isolated nor stigmatized for life (Hostetler, 1975).

A notable exception to the Hutterites' use of modern health care is their practice of noninstitutionalization of severely handicapped individuals and the infirm elderly. Hutterites believe in the sanctity of all life and take their role as "thy brother's keeper" literally when it comes to long-term care. Elderly parents are nursed and given skilled care on the colony, usually either by their daughters or their daughter-in-laws (Longhofer, 1994). Similarly, handicapped children are taken care of on the colony within the context of the extant communal child care system, or, in cases of profound need, special care may be provided by the immediate family. Health professionals, such as home care nurses, are used to augment the care of the infirm and are often called upon to teach the Hutterian care providers on how to administer more technical care (such as catheter care).

Although Hutterites mainly hold modern views of health and illness, they also have maintained some beliefs with ancient biblical roots that are more closely linked to the spiritual causes of disease and the battle between good and evil. For example, Stephenson (1979) describes the belief that Hutterites have about the "evil eye" *(Pschrien)*, the ability of a person to use an intense gaze while holding destructive thoughts to cause harm to others. Any evil eye is believed to be able to cause sudden unexplainable illness and even death. Children are considered particularly susceptible to the ill effects of *Pschrien,* and they are believed to be protected by wearing a piece of red cloth either as a ribbon in the hair or around the wrist. The color red is not considered to carry any magical power; rather it serves as a reminder of the suffering and sacrifice of Christ and is a mnemonic link with faith (Stephenson, 1979).

Hutterite lifestyle and health. The approximately 35,000 Hutterites now in North America are descended from just 300 founding members. When this strong founder effect is combined with their practice of endogamy, marriage within one's own sect *(Leute)*, it is not surprising that they have one of the highest known population coefficients of inbreeding known. It has been estimated that every Hutterite spouse is genetically related at the level of a second-cousin (Hostetler, 1985). Surprisingly this genetic concentration has not led to an overall rate of genetic disorders any higher than that found in the general population. However, certain genetic disorders, such as cystic fibrosis, are overrepresented. Because Hutterites practice patrilocality at the time of marriage, the males on any given colony are more closely related than the females (Brunt, Reeder, Stephenson, Love, and Chen, 1994). When males are approaching the age of marriage, they are often sent to work on other colonies so that they have the opportunity to meet eligible females. Marriages are not arranged, but the opportunity to meet potential spouses is strongly affected by the culture of "summer visits." Details about genetic factors and health are detailed in greater depth in the section of Chapter 7.

Modernization of farming practices, such as reliance on sophisticated combines in the fields and automated bread kneaders in the kitchen, has greatly reduced the routine physical exercise traditionally associated with colony life. Although some strenuous physical labor is still required, it is usually performed by the younger colony members (Stephenson, 1985). The opportunity to engage in non–work related exercise is also limited by the belief that adults should not engage in anything that would be regarded as childish or playful, such as sports. The Hutterite diet is high in both fat and caloric content because there is a cultural tradition of "eating what you grow," in this case a large quantity of meat and dairy products (Rukusek-Kennedy, Parry, and Schlenker, 1987). Deep frying in animal lard is a common practice, and fried potatoes are one of most ubiquitous components of meals on many the colony. Smoking is strictly forbidden, and our research has found that less than 4% of male Hutterites report having ever tried a cigarette; this is usually restricted to young males who want to see what it is like (Brunt and Love, 1993). Although alcoholism is rare, consumption of alcohol, usually wine made on the colony, is common (Brunt and Love, 1992).

Implications for nursing care

Overall, Hutterite clients are very interested in their health, and they will require the same level of care and health education as would be provided to anyone else encountered in practice. Interestingly, Hut-

terian beliefs about death and disability do not provide the same motivating factors often used in more traditional health education (Brunt, Lindsey, and Hopkinson, 1997). Both health and illness are considered to be gifts from God that provide the individual with opportunities to experience *Gelassenheit*. Although a disability is not to be feared by the individual, it does have an effect on the operation of the colony, and this approach may be useful in explaining the importance of engaging in activities that will hasten recovery or prevent further deterioration of a health condition (such as exercise in diabetes).

Because many of the lifestyle factors associated with Hutterite health are governed by cultural and religious norms, problems with diet and exercise are relatively difficult to work with at the level of the individual client. Rather, community-based programs that are congruent with Hutterian beliefs and the blessing of the elders have a better chance of making incremental changes in lifestyle factors. We are presently engaging with the Hutterite community on a program of health promotion development that is focusing on dietary modification. An unpublished dietary pilot project that focused on changing existing meal-preparation methods was conducted with two colonies. Nutritionists worked with the cooks to find substitutes, such as vegetable oil for lard, that would help lower the intake of saturated fats. Because change diffuses rapidly between colonies, we are hoping to establish several colony "test kitchens" where new preparation methods and new foods can be tested and then shared with neighboring colonies.

The sacred nature of death also carries with it some particular implications for nurses and other health care professionals who are caring for a dying Hutterite. Stephenson (1983) has outlined several recommendations for treating a Hutterite with a terminal illness: (1) if at all possible, return the Hutterite to his or her colony to die, (2) visitation policies should be modified to permit as many colony members to be with the dying person as possible, and (3) as much care should be performed on the colony as is possible, minimizing the need to be away from family and friends. Because children are considered to be pure in the Hutterite culture, their death assures them a place in heaven, and thus health care providers should not be surprised if the death of a child is not met with a great outpouring of grief . . . it is considered a blessing (Stephenson, 1983).

BIOLOGICAL VARIATIONS
Genetics

The genetic isolation of each of the three sects (*Leute*) of Hutterites, when combined with the relatively homogeneous inter-*Leute* lifestyles, makes this population uniquely situated for increasing our understanding of the role nurture and nature play in health (Hegele, Brunt, and Connelly, 1995a; Hostetler, 1985). As previously mentioned, Hutterites mainly marry within their own *Leute,* and this practice has led to a highly concentrated gene pool that increases the likelihood of finding otherwise rare genetic conditions but does not appear to increase their overall risk for genetic disorders (Hostetler, 1985). Three factors contribute to the potential for increased expression of otherwise rare recessive genetic disorders in the Hutterites: (1) *founder effect:* the relatively few original founders of the present three *Leute* increases the chances that a relatively large number of contemporary Hutterites carry a particular recessive gene; (2) *consanguinity:* the average relationship between Hutterite spouses is that of second cousin who share $1/32$ of their genes; and (3) *fertility:* Hutterite families are large (8 to 12 children), and so the chances of at least one child in a family carrying a rare gene is increased (Bowen and Lowry, 1982). Cystic fibrosis, dwarfism, and albinism, along with a host of other known but exceedingly rare genetic disorders, have been reported in the Hutterite population (Hostetler, 1975). The Hutterites have contributed greatly to our understanding of a variety of health-related genetic factors such as the regulation of blood pressure (Hegele, Brunt, and Connelly, 1994, 1996), body fat distribution (Hegele, Brunt, and Connelly, 1995a), and blood lipids (Hegele, Brunt, and Connelly, 1995b, 1995c; Hegele, Gandhi, Brunt, and Connelly, 1995).

Physical and mental health

Over the years, Hutterites have been extensively surveyed to determine their physical characteristics. Goldbarg, Kurczynski, Hellerstein, and Steinberg (1970) reported that the age- and sex-specific mean cholesterol, anthropometric measures (height,

weight, and so on), blood pressure, and electrocardiograms were similar to those found in non-Hutterite populations. However, more recent studies have determined that Hutterites have a higher prevalence of obesity, elevated blood pressure, and elevated blood lipids than non-Hutterites (Brunt, Reeder, Stephenson, Love, and Chen, 1994; Schlenker, Parry, and McMillan, 1989); however, these differences are more pronounced in some *Leute* than in others. Because a body mass index (BMI) elevated above 27 kg/m^2 has been shown to carry an increased risk for health problems such as diabetes and hypertension, it is noteworthy that approximately 30% to 75% of Hutterites (depending on age and gender) have an elevated BMI (Brunt et al., 1994). As in non-Hutterite populations, blood pressure increases with age and the overall prevalence of diastolic hypertension (>90 mm Hg) among Hutterites has been found on colony-wide screening to be as high as 58% in males and 30% in females. Blood cholesterol above 5.2 mmol/L has been associated with an increased risk for heart disease, and the prevalence of levels above this range in the Hutterites falls between 47% and 67%, depending on gender and age (Brunt et al., 1994).

The life expectancy of Hutterites has been found to be approximately 10 years less than in the general population and, in sharp contrast to other Western populations where females outlive males by 6 to 8 years, males and females have approximately the same life expectancy (Schlenker et al., 1989). Of the two major known causes of premature death in Western cultures (cancer and heart disease), studies have largely ruled out an increased incidence of cancer among Hutterites as the likely cause of their reduced life expectancy (Morgan, Holmes, Grace, Kemel, and Robson, 1983). Using detailed cancer register data, Morgan et al. found that the overall incidence of cancer was significantly less than expected among Hutterites, particularly in relation to uterine cancer in women and lung cancer in men. Males were found to be at a small increased risk for stomach cancer and leukemias. Martin et al. (1980) have hypothesized that the low rates of smoking and the lack of promiscuity combine to reduce the risk for some of the major forms of cancer among Hutterites, most notably lung and cervical cancer. Although the absence of heart disease registries do not allow such detailed studies, the combination of elevated coronary risk factors such as hypertension, hyperlipidemia, and obesity makes it likely that heart disease is the leading cause of premature death in adult Hutterites. The similar life expectancies between male and female Hutterites may result from the effects of multiple births on women (Eaton and Mayer, 1953) or from the high levels of coronary risk factors in both sexes. However, Stephenson (1985) has questioned the role of any specific disease cause in the similar life expectancies of males and females. He has hypothesized that the forced retirement of female Hutterites at a relatively early age may, in a culture that views death as a blessed event leading to eternal life, hasten their death through unknown mechanisms that are deeply rooted in their culture.

Neurological disorders such as dementia, Parkinson's disease, multiple sclerosis, and major psychoses do not appear to be major problems in the Hutterite population. My own research on approximately 100 colonies failed to uncover a single case of dementia or Parkinson's disease. However, it is possible that cases were either missed or the lower life expectancy of Hutterites precludes them from expressing this disorder to any great degree. Recent research has revealed that the prevalence of multiple sclerosis is significantly less than that in non-Hutterite populations (Ross, Nicolle, and Cheang, 1995), though the few cases that do exist may be related to a genetic predisposition (Hader, Seland, Hader, Harris, and Dietrich, 1996). Eaton, Weil, and Kaplan's (1951) mental health studies found extremely low rates of major psychoses (that is, schizophrenia) in the Hutterite population.

Modern farm life comes with its own set of unique health risks related to repeated exposure to mechanical and chemical agents from an early life. Hutterites have been found to have a high prevalence of respiratory symptoms that are related to exposure to molds, dust, endotoxins, animal dander, grain dust, and animal excrement (Rylander, 1986). Male Hutterites have been found to be more affected by exposure to farm-related agents than females, though both sexes experience more symptoms (cough, sputum production, fever, and skin irritation) than the general population (Parry and

Schlenker, 1994). Accidents related to farm machinery are all too common and represent a significant cause of premature death and disability in the farming community in general and in the Hutterite population specifically (Farthing, 1994).

The high birth rate of Hutterites has gradually declined over the past few decades, in large part attributable to the later age of marriage (Laing, 1980). The use of birth control methods is forbidden on the colonies unless they are required for very specific health reasons. The total fertility for Hutterite women 15 to 49 years of age has declined from 9.83 in the years 1946 to 1965 to 6.29 between 1981 and 1985; it is estimated that the age-specific fertility in the period 1981 to 1985 declined by 50% as compared to the rates in the period 1951 to 1955 (Nonaka, Miura, and Peter, 1994). The reduction of the fertility is largely related to the decline in the rate at which colonies grow and split into daughter colonies (Peter, 1980). Normally, when a colony has close to 100 residents, the elders begin planning for a new colony. As the price and availability of quality agricultural land has increased and decreased respectively during the past few decades, it has become more difficult to create new colonies (Evans, 1985). This makes it harder for the colony to provide opportunities for work and advancement through the labor ranks for the young men, and so the age of marriage has increased. As the age of marriage has grown steadily older, the number of years a woman is fertile has declined, thus the lowering in fertility.

Implications for nursing care

In relation to genetic disorders, Hutterites are well versed in the role genetics play in their lives, and they actively discourage marriages between first cousins and take lineage into account when making marital choices. Colonies are entirely receptive to genetic counseling, and many community health agencies are regularly contacted to provide education about the treatment and prevention of genetic problems (Bowen and Lowry, 1982). Nurses who do care for newborns with genetic anomalies need to be aware that the family will be the primary care provider for the infant, and so they will need appropriate teaching.

The combination of a high prevalence of elevated BMI, blood pressure, and cholesterol places the Hutterite population at an increased risk for heart disease and stroke. Community and public health nurses should encourage their agencies to set up ongoing blood pressure clinics on the colonies and provide educational materials about lifestyle risk factors to their Hutterite clients. Similarly, nurses caring for Hutterite clients in the hospital setting should provide education about lifestyle risk reduction. My own work on the colonies in Alberta has shown that Hutterites are interested in reducing their risk for heart disease and stroke and respond well to screening for both hypertension (Brunt and Love, 1992) and cholesterol (Brunt and Sheilds, 1996). There is also a great need for prevention education on the colonies related to the exposure risk they have to chemical, biological, and mechanical agents. Community and public health nurses should work closely with occupational health specialists to help the colonies develop and implement work safety plans.

Regardless of the nature of chronic illness, whether it be mental or physical in its expression, Hutterites will seek out the most up-to-date treatments including specialized care at large tertiary care hospitals. As previously discussed, mental illness does not carry the same stigma in the Hutterite community as it does in North American culture as a whole. Individuals affected by psychoses may be hospitalized during acute episodes, but they will mainly be taken care of by members of the colony. Thus the need for education about postdischarge care is crucial, and the family should be included in the discharge process as much as possible.

SUMMARY

The Hutterites are the single largest rural ethnic group in Canada and comprise a significant proportion of the rural ethnic population in many of the northernmost midwestern states. Their agrarian and communal way of life, based on the Christian religious precepts of anabaptism, provides them with a unique set of both health-risk and health-promoting factors that nurses must understand when providing care to their Hutterite clients. Although Hutterites are firmly rooted in maintaining their sense of religious tradition, they are very interested in discovering new ways and new ideas to help them live healthier lives. Many of the risks to Hutterite health are identical to those facing other rural agrarian populations including exposure to chemical, biological, and mechanical agents, an increase in sedentary work, and the stress and strain of farm life. Their traditional diet, high in fat and caloric intake, was entirely appropriate when farm life was characterized by heavy physical labor. However, mechanization has changed the opportunity for regular physical exercise for all but the youngest Hutterites, and this has led to the serious health problems associated with obesity, hypertension, and hyperlipidemias, which are unfortunately also so highly prevalent in North American society. The spiritual dimension of Hutterian life provides them with enormous strength and resilience, and this asset is a critical health-promoting factor that must be considered when working with this population. Despite the rigors of colony life, each Hutterite has a strong sense of belonging and community, which can teach us all something about the true meaning of health.

Case study

Developed by Ruth Scherer, MSN, RN, Assistant Professor of Nursing, Bethel College, Mishawaka, Indiana

Joseph Hofer, a Canadian Hutterite, age 63, suffered a massive stroke while delivering a load of chickens to the nearby town approximately 3 weeks ago. Mr. Hofer is the farm manager for his colony, which is approximately 100 kilometers from the tertiary care hospital where he was air lifted after the stroke. His medical history includes hypertension (20+ years), non-insulin dependent dia betes (10 years), and an elevated body mass index of 30 kg/m². He is married and has three grown sons, who also reside on his colony, and two grown daughters, one of whom has married and moved out of the province to another colony. Mr. Hofer has remained in a deep coma since his stroke and is not expected to recover. He was extubated 2 days ago, and the family has requested that he be transported back to the colony as soon as arrangements can be made.

CARE PLAN

 Nursing Diagnosis   Knowledge deficit related to care of the unconscious client.

Client Outcomes

1. Client will receive adequate care from family members and colony.

Nursing Interventions

1. Teach family members how to care for unconscious client in the colony.
2. Involve family members in care of client before discharge.
3. Have family members return to demonstrate such things as tube feeding, turning and positioning, oral care, catheter care, glucose monitoring, and medication administration.
4. Encourage use of alternative therapies that client has found helpful in the past such as herbal therapy, acupuncture, and reflexology, spiritual rituals.

Client Outcomes

1. Client or family will express satisfaction with spiritual condition and their opportunity to experience *Gelassenheit.*

Nursing Interventions

1. Modify visitation policies to permit colony members to visit in hospital.
2. Encourage any colony members who are experiencing spiritual *Angst,* called *Anfechtung,* in which they believe they have sinned beyond redemption, are depressed or withdrawn, and are ruminating religious unworthiness, to seek the support of the colony minister.
3. Support family's decision to care for client in the colony where the client can die slowly because this is the ideal death in the Hutterian culture.

 Nursing Diagnosis   Anticipatory grieving of family members related to Joseph's stroke and deteriorating condition.

Client Outcomes

1. Family and colony members will acknowledge changes in role expectations.
2. Family and colony members will discuss the grief process as experienced by Hutterites.

Nursing Interventions

1. Assess family and colony members regarding changes in role expectations since Joseph's stroke.
2. Ask family or colony members to describe the stages of grief that have been observed in their colony when a member dies.
3. Explain grief work as a normal response to loss even though death is sacred. Grief work involves accepting the reality of loss, experiencing the pain of grief, adjusting to an environment from which the lost person is missing, and reinvesting in another relationship (Carpenito, 1995).

STUDY QUESTIONS

1. Describe the cultural significance of religion for the Hutterites.
2. Describe role expectations by gender for the Hutterite client.
3. Discuss the role of community in the social organization of the Hutterite client.
4. Identify at least two diseases or conditions with high prevalence among the Hutterites.
5. Discuss the unique communication needs of the Hutterite client.

References

Acts 2:44. (1984). *The Holy Bible: the international version.* Grand Rapids, Michigan: Zondervan Corporation.

Boldt, E.D. (1978). Structural tightness, autonomy, and observability: an analysis of Hutterite conformity and orderliness. *The Canadian Journal of Sociology, 3,* 349-363.

Bowen, P., & Lowry, R.B. (1982). Genetic disorders in Hutterites. *Bulletin of the Hereditary Diseases Program of Alberta, 1*(4), 9-10.

Brunt, J.H., & Love, E.J. (1992). Evaluation of hypertension screening in the Hutterite population. *Research in nursing and health, 15,* 103-110.

Brunt, J.H., & Love, E.J. (1993). Hypertension in the Hutterite community of Alberta. *Canadian Journal of Public Health, 83,* 362-364.

Brunt, J.H., Reeder, B., Stephenson, P., Love, E.J., & Chen, Y. (1994). A comparison of physical and laboratory measures between two Hutterite *Leute* and the rural Saskatchewan population. *Canadian Journal of Public Health, 85,* 299-302.

Brunt, J.H. (1996). *Hutterite heart health guide.* Victoria, B.C.: the author.

Brunt, J.H., & Sheilds, L. (1996). Preventive behaviours in the Hutterite community following a nurse-managed cholesterol screening program. *Canadian Journal of Cardiovascular Nursing, 7*(2), 6-11.

Brunt, J.H., Lindsey, L., & Hopkinson, J. (1997). Health promotion in the Hutterite community and the ethnocentricity of empowerment. *Canadian Journal of Nursing Research, 29*(1), 17-28.

Carpenito, L.J. (1995). *Handbook of nursing diagnosis* (ed. 6). Philadelphia: J.B. Lippincott, p. 413.

Claus-Peter, C. (1972). *Anabaptism: a social history.* Ithaca, N.Y.: Cornell University Press, p. 271.

Converse, T.A., Buker, R.S., & Lee, R.V. (1973). Hutterite midwifery. *American Journal of Obstetrics and Gynecology, 116,* 719-725.

Eaton, J.W., & Mayer, A.J. (1953). The social biology of a very high fertility among the Hutterites: the demography of a unique population. *Human Biology, 25,* 206-264.

Eaton, J.W., Weil, R.J., & Kaplan, B. (1951, January). The Hutterite Mental Health Study. *Mennonite Quarterly Review,* 47-65.

Evans, S.M. (1985). Some developments in the diffusion patterns of Hutterite colonies. *The Canadian Geographer, 29,* 327-339.

Farthing, M. (1994). Health education needs of a Hutterite colony. *The Canadian Nurse, 90*(7), 20-26.

Goldbarg, A.N., Kurczynski, T.W., Hellerstein, H.K., & Steinberg, A.G. (1970). Electrocardiographic findings among the total adult population of a large religious isolate. *Circulation, 41,* 257-269.

Hader, W.J., Seland, T.P., Hader, M.B., Harris, C.J., & Dietrich, D.W. (1996). The occurrence of multiple sclerosis in the Hutterites of North America. *Canadian Journal of Neurological Science, 23,* 291-295.

Hegele, R.A., Brunt, J.H., & Connelly, P.W. (1994). A polymorphism of the angiotensinogen gene associated with variation in blood pressure in a genetic isolate. *Circulation, 90,* 2207-2212.

Hegele, R.A., Gandhi, S., Brunt, J.H., & Connelly, P.W. (1995). Restriction isotyping of the premature termination variant of lipoprotein lipase in Alberta Hutterites. *Clinical Biochemistry, 29,* 63-66.

Hegele, R.A., Brunt, J.H., & Connelly, P.W. (1995a). Multiple genetic determinants of variation of plasma lipoproteins in Alberta Hutterites. *Arterioscleroses, Thrombosis and Vascular Biology, 15,* 861-871.

Hegele, R.A., Brunt, J.H., & Connelly, P.W. (1995b). Genetic variation on chromosome 1 associated with variation in body fat distribution in men. *Circulation, 92,* 1089-1093.

Hegele, R.A., Brunt, J.H., & Connelly, P.W. (1995c). A polymorphism of the paraxonase gene associated with variation in plasma lipoproteins in a genetic isolate. *Arteriosclerosis, Thrombosis and Vascular Biology, 15,* 89-95.

Hegele, R.A., Brunt, J.H., & Connelly, P.W. (1996). Genetic and biochemical factors associated with variation in blood pressure in a genetic isolate. *Hypertension, 27,* 308-312.

Hostetler, J.A. (1968). Communal socialization patterns in Hutterite society. *Ethnology, 7,* 331-355.

Hostetler, J.A. (1975). *Hutterite society.* Baltimore: Johns Hopkins University Press.

Hostetler, J.A. (1985). History and relevance of the Hutterite population for genetic studies. *American Journal of Medical Genetics, 22,* 453-462

Kaplan, B., & Plaut, T.F.A. (1956). *Personality in a communal society.* Lawrence, Kansas: University of Kansas Press.

Laing, L.M. (1980). Declining fertility in a religious isolate: the Hutterite population of Alberta, Canada, 1951-1971. *Human Biology, 52*(2), 288-310.

Longhofer, J. (1994). Nursing home utilization: a comparative study of the Hutterian Brethren, the Old Order Amish, and the Mennonites. *Journal of Aging Studies, 8*(1), 95-120.

Martin, A.O., Dunn, J.K., Simpson, J.L., Olsen, C.L., Kemel, S., Race, M., Elias, S., Sarto, G.E., Smalley, B., & Steinberg, A.G. (1980). Cancer mortality in a human isolate. *Journal of the National Cancer Institute, 65,* 1109-1113.

Martin, A.O., Kurczynski, T.W., & Steinberg, A.G. (1973). Familial studies of medical and anthropometric variables in a human isolate. *American Journal of Human Genetics, 25,* 581-593.

Morgan, K., Holmes, T.M., Grace, M., Kemel, S., & Robson, D. (1983). Patterns of cancer in geographic and endogamous subdivisions of the Hutterite Brethren of Canada. *American Journal of Physical Anthropology, 62,* 3-10.

Nonaka, K., Miura, T., & Peter, T. (1994). Recent fertility decline in Dariusleut Hutterites: an extension of Eaton and Mayer's Hutterite fertility study. *Human Biology, 66,* 411-420.

Parry, P.R., & Schlenker, E. (1994). Respiratory, atopic, and serological characterization of Hutterite farmers in South Dakota. In McDuffie, H.H., Dosman, J.A., Semchuk, K.M., Olenchock, S.A., & Senthilselvan, A. (Eds.), *Supplement to agricultural health and safety: workplace, environment, sustainability,* pp. 1-6. Saskatoon, Sask.: Centre for Agricultural Medicine.

Peter, K.A. (1980). The decline of the Hutterite population growth. *Canadian Ethnic Studies, 12*(3), 97-110.

Ross, R.T., Nicolle, L.E., & Cheang, M. (1995). Varicella zoster virus and multiple sclerosis in a Hutterite population. *Journal of Clinical Epidemiology, 48,* 1319-1324.

Rukusek-Kennedy, C., Parry, R.R., & Schlenker, E.H. (1987). The nutritional status of Hutterites in South Dakota. *Federation Proceedings, 46,* 1157.

Rylander, R. (1986). Lung diseases caused by organic dusts in the farm environment. *American Journal of Industrial Medicine, 10,* 221-227.

Saunders, D.E. (1964). The Hutterites: a case study in minority rights. *The Canadian Bar Review, 42,* 225-242.

Schlenker, E.H., Parry, R.R., & McMillan, M.J (1989). Influence of age, sex, and obesity on blood pressure of Hutterites in South Dakota. *Chest, 95,* 1269-1273.

Sommer, J.L. (1953, April). Hutterite medicine and physicians in Moravia in the sixteenth century and after. *Mennonite Quarterly Review,* 111-227.

Stephenson, P. (1979). Hutterite belief in evil eye: beyond paranoia and toward a general theory of invidia. *Culture, Medicine and Psychiatry, 3*(3), 247-265.

Stephenson, P.H. (1983). He died too quick! The process of dying in a Hutterian colony. *Omega, 14,* 127-134.

Stephenson, P.H. (1985). Gender, aging, and mortality in Hutterite society: a critique of the doctrine of specific etiology. *Medical Anthropology, 9,* 355-365.

Stephenson, P.H. (1991). *The Hutterian people: ritual and rebirth into the evolution of communal life.* Lanham, Md.: University Press of America.

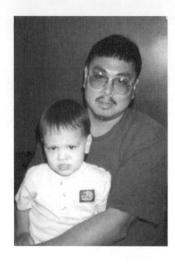

CHAPTER 13

The Newfoundland (Labrador) Inuit

Paula Didham and Maggie Angnatok

BEHAVIORAL OBJECTIVES

After reading this chapter, the nurse will be able to:

1. Describe the communication patterns unique to the Newfoundland (Labrador) Inuit.
2. Describe the time orientation of the Newfoundland (Labrador) Inuit.
3. Describe the social organization structure of the Newfoundland (Labrador) Inuit.
4. Identify major biological variations found among the Newfoundland (Labrador) Inuit.
5. Discuss the spatial needs of the Newfoundland (Labrador) Inuit.

OVERVIEW OF NEWFOUNDLAND

Newfoundland is the tenth largest island in the world with 10,625 miles of deeply indented coastline off the east coast of Canada. Adjacent to Labrador and Quebec on the mainland of Canada, Newfoundland is surrounded by the Atlantic Ocean (Johnson, 1997; Walz and Walz, 1970). Newfoundland and Labrador, the provincial capital of which is Saint John's, has over 500,000 people (Johnson, 1997; Statistics Canada, 1996). Newfoundland is the largest of the four Canadian Atlantic provinces with a total area of 405,720 square kilometers (156,647 square miles). Most of the population is concentrated on the island in the cities of St. John's and Corner Brook and in the towns of Gander and Grand Falls. The Labrador towns of Goose Bay and Happy Valley, Wabush, and Labrador City are also growing.

Newfoundland is noted for Viking settlements, which date back to A.D. 1000 (Bailey and Bailey, 1995). Viking settlements were discovered in New-

foundland's northern peninsula in 1960 by a Norwegian archeological team led by L'Anse aux Meadows (Bailey and Bailey, 1995). The Italian-English explorer John Cabot is said to have arrived on St. John's day in 1497 and thus named the port St. John's (Fodor's staff, 1987). For a century the "newfound land" remained unknown in Europe except to a handful of Bristol merchants and fisherman employed by them. The British west-country men carried back the rich harvest from the Newfoundland fishing banks, even establishing seasonal colonies from which to support the fishery. For years, the fishermen west of England sought to conceal their profitable voyages from the scrutiny of a tyrannical crown in order to avoid payment of oppressive taxes. But the trade became too large and too prosperous to be hidden for long.

In 1583 Sir Humphrey Gilbert claimed the land for Elizabeth I and set up a trading stall on what is now the St. John's waterfront. Sir Humphrey also distinguished himself by bringing from England the first professional dancers and musicians to play in the New World; they were the "hobby horses and Morris dancers and many like conceits" who performed on shore at St. John's on Aug. 5, 1583 (Fodor's staff, 1987). Gilbert's claim for Britain ended the *laissez-faire* days of international fishing off the coast of Newfoundland by 30,000 fisherman from half a dozen nations in relative peace and began the infamous era of the "fishing admiral." The fishing admiral was the first captain to sail into any Newfoundland harbor each year. This distinction allowed the fortunate skipper to set himself up as a total despot for the season, thereby creating unceasing turmoil between permanent settlers and English adventurers. In 1711, the colony was placed under the rule of naval governors and the fishing admirals' "empire" was dissolved. However, after ongoing dispute, in 1763 the Treaty of Paris gave Newfoundland to Great Britain. The province retained its independence until 1949, when it belatedly joined the Dominion of Canada (Bailey and Bailey, 1995).

Cod have always been plentiful in the waters off Newfoundland, and for many years it was known as the fishing outpost of Europe. Mining is another industry that has contributed to the economy (Bailey and Bailey, 1995). The province's dense forests provide lumber for the paper mills that supply much of the world's newsprint. In recent years Newfoundland has become famous for its skiing. It is also known for the number of whale species to be found around its shores, including pilot whales and killer whales, and for its birds, particularly seabirds. Whale watching, bird watching and iceberg watching are all pastimes of residents and visitors to Newfoundland. Labrador's main appeal is fishing and a limited amount of hunting. Salmon, arctic char, trout, and northern pike are fished.

OVERVIEW OF NEWFOUNDLAND INUIT

The earliest known inhabitants of Newfoundland were Maritime Archaic Indians, whose burial mounds date back to 7500 years ago (Walz and Walz, 1970). However, about 4000 years ago, a group of arctic people appeared in northern Labrador and as far south as Newfoundland. These arctic people reached the Atlantic coast as a part of their expansion across Canada's north (McMillan, 1988). A variant of the arctic people termed the "Paleo-Eskimos" and later referred to as the "Dorset people" spread farther than any other Eskimos did and were the only such people to occupy a subarctic environment. In Newfoundland the Dorset were typically a coastal people and left sites encircling Newfoundland but did not penetrate far inland. The abundance of sea mammals allowed the Dorset to settle in large villages, such as the one near Port au Choix, where more than 35 rectangular depressions mark where houses once stood. Each house had sod walls, with timber rafters supporting a roof of hide and sod, and was dug slightly into the ground. Also in Newfoundland, the Dorset people quarried a soapstone cliff to carve their distinctive bowls and rectangular lamps fueled with seal blubber (McMillan, 1988; Simons, 1976). Burial remains from several small caves indicate a physical type similar to the prehistoric Eskimo of the Arctic and quite distinct from the Indian populations of Atlantic Canada. The Dorset people were gradually replaced by more recent arrivals, the Thule, who are generally considered to be the direct ancestors of the present Inuit who reside in this area (McMillan, 1988). However, the cultural practices of the Dorset can be found in the customs practiced by the Eskimos living in Newfoundland when the Europeans arrived and can still be noted in practices today (McMillan, 1988). These Inuit also share common cultural practices and beliefs with the Inuit living in the northernmost regions of Canada and with the Eskimos in Alaska.

The Thule arrived in the coast of Labrador around 1450. The waters of this eastern region were richly stocked with sea mammals, which were pursued by Inuit hunters (McMillan, 1988). Walrus, seal, and whale were harpooned from *kayak*s, or *umiak*s in the case of the large whales, and in winter from the ice edge. Whaling required ritual preparation, involving observation of taboos, magical treatment of implements, and shamanistic consultation with spirit helpers for information in planning the hunt. Such rituals strongly resemble those performed by Inuit whalers in Alaska. Caribou hunting was practiced in the fall when hides were needed for winter clothing.

Today, Eskimos living in Newfoundland are called the *"Inuit"* (singular *Inuk*, 'man, person'; dual *Inuuk*). This change in name was officially made by the Canadian government at the request of the Canadian Eskimo in the 1970s. When the Europeans were encountered, the Canadian Eskimo took exception to the definition of "Eskimo" in the Algonquian language, which was said to mean 'eaters of raw meat' and requested to be called instead *"Inuit,"* which in Inuktitut means 'people.' It is now assumed that "Eskimo" was a Montagnais word for 'Micmacs of the Gaspé Peninsula' because it meant 'speaking the language of a foreign land' (Mailhot, 1978).

At the time of the 1986 census it was estimated that some 34,000 Inuit lived in Canada with approximately 2380 (7%) living in Newfoundland (Labrador) (Health and Welfare Canada, 1991; Young, 1994). In 1991 some 6675 persons in Newfoundland indicated that they had Inuit origin, though only 70 were registered under the Indian Registration Act. Of this group 3220 were male and 3240 were female (Statistics Canada, l991).

The Inuit culture, like the various Canadian Indian cultures, has been prey to the incursions of Europeans into Canada, resulting in cultural disruption and the introduction of infectious diseases (Dobson, 1991). The population dropped dramatically as unknown diseases were encountered and health-promoting cultural practices were abandoned to take on the new practices that were introduced. Early contact between the Inuit in Labrador often took the form of battles and trade. The Inuit eagerly sought the iron tools and other goods of the foreign invaders, yet through mutual misunderstanding and suspicion the encounters often ended in bloodshed. The earliest continuous contact was with Moravian missionaries, familiar with the Inuit language from Greenland, who helped negotiate peace with the Inuit in 1765. The Moravians established the first mission in Nain in 1771. As well as a church, each mission contained a trading post to supply goods upon which the Inuit had come to depend. The Inuit settled in permanent wooden houses at these self-contained communities. Although many elements of their culture were lost under the Moravian influence, they enjoyed a lengthy period of near-isolation from other outside influences (McMillan, 1988).

In the 1950s the Canadian government took a more active role in Inuit administration. Services formerly provided by missionaries, fur traders, or police were transferred to government administrators, who became a permanent feature of the community. Schools were built at many Inuit settlements. Family allowances, welfare, and old-age pensions were extended to the Inuit on the same basis as other Canadians. Inuit abandoned their hunting camps for government-subsidized housing and towns with shopping malls, hotels, hospitals, regular air service, and other amenities of Canadian life.

COMMUNICATION

Several Eskimo languages are spoken in Alaska and Siberia. However, only one, Inuktitut, is spoken across the entire Canadian Arctic. An even larger number of Inuktitut speakers exists in Greenland (McMillan, 1988; Szathmary, 1984). This common language origin has had the resulting effect that the Inuit can understand each other wherever they are in Canada when they use their native language (Simons, 1976).

Inuktitut is a difficult language because one word is often used to express a whole sentence. Inuktitut is also described as an agglutinative language, where individual meanings are strung together into much longer words. The complication arises from the rules of such joining. What may be regarded as a sentence when translated into English may be one long agglutinative "word" (Simons, 1976). Originally Inuktitut had no written forms; thus the recounting of events in story form and in dance provided the only record of Eskimo life. Today there is a phonetically written form of Inuktitut that was developed by missionaries to Alaska (Lefever and Davidhizar, 1995). The Europeans who came to Canada, however, demanded that the Inuit children learn English, which has now become the primary language of the younger generation of Inuit. Many children are unable to speak their original native tongue. This has resulted in problems communicating within families where the elderly who speak only Inuktitut may be unable to speak to their grandchildren who speak only English. However, whereas around 1980 this was more of a problem, today there are only small numbers of the very elderly left in the Newfoundland Inuit communities who cannot speak English and even they can often speak a few words. In fact, although 825 indicate they know Inuktitut, only 479 of the registered Inuit in Newfoundland indicate that Inuktitut is their mother tongue, whereas the rest are English speaking (Statistics Canada, 1991).

The language spoken by the Inuit is very descriptive of dominant concerns and interests related to the culture. Certain words take on more significant meanings than other words. For example the Inuit have some 20 separate words for snow (to distinguish "crusted snow" from "blowing snow" and by the snow's consistency, texture, and so forth) (Boas, 1938). There is a variety of separate words for skins of caribou, the animal that has played an important part in their livelihood. The word for "seal" depends on whether it is in or out of the water (Simons, 1976).

Nonverbal communication

In the Inuit culture, silence is valued and is often a communication of respect. Interactions are often started with a period of silence, which may be followed by small talk before getting to the main point of concern. It is important for the health professional to avoid starting a conversation immediately with verbal questions related to data collection. The health profession should be aware of subtle meanings in nonverbal communication. For example, the Inuit may nod and say yes when they do not understand completely what is being spoken rather than to admit that they do not understand English. In addition, the Inuit will often avoid asking questions in order to clarify something they do not understand. They are unlikely to assert themselves in saying, "I'm sorry; I really don't understand what you are saying." Rather, they are more likely to nod and agree even though they do not understand or have the right information.

Respect and courtesy for others has always been highly valued by the Inuit. Historically it was a matter of courtesy for the Inuit to lend wives to guests. However, unauthorized wife borrowing was subject to killing (Simons, 1976). Today the value of sharing is still present and may be evidenced by the behavior of sharing food with others. Even if there is little food for tomorrow, the small amount food present today is freely shared with guests. This can present problems for the client with diabetes who may need to be on a regular diet and whose blood glucose level can be significantly harmed when food present today is shared and there is none left for tomorrow. O'Neil (1989) studied dissatisfaction with care from Westerners by Inuit clients and noted that the Inuit found the Westerners to be paternalistic and to show disregard for cultural factors. Disregard for cultural factors was also a significant barrier to care.

Implications for nursing care

Because of their cultural heritage with agglutinative words, the nurse may find that Inuit persons speak in unusually long sentences. It may be necessary to ask the Inuit to repeat statements or for the nurse to ask for clarification to fully comprehend what the Inuit client is saying.

When elderly Inuit are in need of health care, it is important for the nurse to remember that they may understand little English and require a translator. When doing health teaching with an Inuit family, the nurse must assess who can speak English and who needs an interpreter and who can understand only part of what is said in English. Because it may be embarrassing for individuals to admit they don't understand English very well, the nurse should carefully assess the Inuit client for adequate comprehension. In a family setting the grandparents may understand little English, the parents may understand both English and Inuit, and the children may understand only English. Therefore it is important to give explanations in detail, to repeat instructions, and to seek clarification rather than take for granted that all the Inuit in a family group being taught will understand the meaning of what is being said after one explanation. Even if Inuit clients speak English, it is important for the nurse to be aware that vocabulary may be limited and medical terms and English jargon may not be understood. An Inuit client is more likely to go ahead and let the health care professional do a procedure rather than to ask why it is being done. The nurse may find that even though the client has had a procedure done before, the client still may not understand the purpose or steps of the procedure, and so a careful explanation is important to provide culturally appropriate care and to increase the client's comfort level. A thorough explanation of care is particularly important when the health care professional does an invasive procedure such as a Pap smear. The health care professional must allow time for the client to fully understand what is to be done before privacy is invaded. It may be helpful for the health care professional to say, "This is a invasive procedure. I'm going to do it as quickly as I can so that you are not too uncomfortable for too long, and I'm going to be as gentle as I possibly can." It is helpful to tell the client when the professional is ready to start and then to explain each step of the procedure so that there are no surprises. It is reassuring for the professional to say, "I told you I was going to do this, and now I am going to do it," while continuing with the procedure.

SPACE

In the historic Inuit culture, individual space was often shared with other family members because of the need to stay warm during the cold parts of the year (Lange, 1988). What was perceived as crowded living conditions by individuals in Western society was viewed by the Inuit as a necessity for survival. Labrador Inuit lived for up to 6 months of the year in large, permanent, semisubterranean structures, similar to those of the Thule period. The walls were made of sod or stone, with a sod-covered roof supported on rafters of whalebones or timber. A long covered entrance passage led to the house, and a skylight of translucent seal intestine was set into the roof over the entrance. Skin tents were the summer dwellings (McMillan, 1988). On the other hand, Inuit value space. Although living occurred in a crowded space, there was always the opportunity to enjoy the wide open spaces while hunting, fishing, or doing other outdoor activities. Today's Newfound-

land Inuit value space. They are not a "touching and feeling" kind of people. Although a handshake distance between two people is considered the acceptable space for socialization on a daily basis, closer approaches without permission are perceived as threatening.

Implications for nursing care

Because of the value of personal space, some Inuit may feel uncomfortable with close personal contact in the course of medical and nursing care. It is important for the nurse to provide a careful and detailed explanation before physical contact with a client and to provide an ongoing explanation of what is happening during the steps of a procedure that require personal contact. Even routine procedures for the nurse such as giving a bed bath or providing oral care may be considered invasive by the Inuit client and cause discomfort (Lefever and Davidhizar, 1995).

SOCIAL ORGANIZATION

Historically the Inuit lived in small living spaces with extended family members. There could be as many as three generations living in the same household. As in other Indian cultures, elders were respected and held in high regard. Today with improvements in housing, families and individuals have more space and are more likely to live separately in houses of their own. In fact, 4775 persons of Inuit origin in Newfoundland indicate that they live in single detached houses (Statistics Canada, 1991). As Inuit life increasingly takes on the ways, expectations, and technologies of Western society, the traditions of former years are not always the ways of the young, nor is today's lifestyle always seen as so satisfying (Dobson, 1991). There is a large number of unmarried mothers in many Inuit communities. This is particularly true in Labrador. McGillivray (1988) noted that in one northern Labrador community the birth rate for the age group 15 to 19 years was 416 per 1000 population from 1981 to 1985. Most of the teen-aged mothers were single, but McGillivray concluded that the babies were wanted. Within Inuit lone-parent families, in 1991 women constituted the head of the family in 79.9 % of cases, a substantial increase over the 1986 figure of 73.4 % (Indian and Northern Affairs, 1995). In 1991, 4286 of the persons in Newfoundland of Inuit origin indicated that they were single, whereas 1810 indicated that they were married (Statistics Canada, 1991). There is an increasing number of homes for women to live together with their children. Nevertheless, although not so much as historically, extended family support is still apparent, and it may be the mother, father, or grandparents who bring sick children into a clinic.

The structure of the Inuit population is characterized by a large youthful component. In both the 1991 and 1986 census, the cohort under the age of 25 represented about six tenths of the entire Inuit population (Indian and Northern Affairs, 1995). Among Inuit persons 15 to 24 years of age, mobility levels reported for 1991 were only slightly higher than those occurring for the entire Inuit population. In 1991, 58.9 % of the 15 to 24 years cohort were classified as movers, a substantial expansion over the 1986 figure of 53.2 percent (Indian and Northern Affairs, 1995). However, although many move to find a more satisfying lifestyle, this is not always the case because many Inuit have little access to regular and satisfying wage employment (Anoee, 1979). Change has made it difficult to maintain the cultural ways and a sense of Inuit identity. Without the enjoyment of life on the land and pride in their heritage, many Inuit are unhappy and are struggling to fit into the Westernized world that surrounds them (Anoee, 1979). Unlike the more western provinces, Newfoundland no longer has communities classified as remote and isolated, and adjustment to Western culture has become a necessity for the Newfoundland Inuit (Health and Welfare Canada, l991).

Gender roles

Historically activities for the Newfoundland Inuit have, for the most part, been divided by gender. Men primarily assumed the roles of hunting, fishing, whaling, and catching seals. Women were involved with berry picking, food preparation, sewing furs to make parkas and mukluks (sealskin food coverings), and child rearing. Most Newfoundland Inuit men are not involved with the woman's care during pregnancy. Women generally go to the clinic alone for their monthly checks during pregnancy. However, when it is time to actually have the baby, the father will usually accompany the mother to the hospital for the delivery. Taking care of children is seem primarily as woman's work by the traditional Newfoundland Inuit though this is changing as the Inuit are becoming Westernized.

Economy

Traditionally items such as whale tusks and codfish ear bones were used for jewelry and ornamental items. Today Newfoundland Inuit, both men and women, may be involved in reproducing traditional artifacts to sell to tourists including labradorite jewelry (labradorite is a quartzlike rock that takes a high polish), earrings of codfish ear bones, sealskin products, art prints, sculpture, carvings, and other handicrafts (Walz and Walz, 1976; Fodor's staff, 1987; Bailey and Bailey, 1995). Inuit soapstone sculptures have a raw power and vitality that makes them attractive to southern art collectors (McMillan, 1988). The subjects of modern art of the Inuit commonly depict Arctic animals or hunting and domestic scenes, though spirit beings from the legends also occur. The success of soapstone carving led to experiments with print making (McMillan, 1988). Flamboyant depictions of fantasy birds are among the most famous Inuit works of art.

Until recently, many Inuit were able to supplement their income through the sale of sealskins. However, outrage against the clubbing of infant seals along Canada's east coast led to a European boycott of all seal products in 1982. This boycott destroyed the market for skins of the adult ringed seal traditionally taken by the Inuit, causing considerable hardship in areas with few other sources of income.

Employment

Some 1460 persons of Inuit origin in Newfoundland have gone beyond grade 13 educationally. The postsecondary occupation most frequently held by 440 males of Inuit origin is engineering and applied-science technologies and trades. The postsecondary occupations and the occupations most frequently held by 239 females are commerce, management, and business administration (Statistics Canada,

1991). Men and women of Inuit origin in New-foundland are primarily employed in the labor force though the unemployment rate is high: 36.6% for males over 15 years of age and 28.6% for females over 15, with an overall unemployment rate of 31.2% (Statistics Canada, 1991). The average income in Canadian dollars for Newfoundland Inuit males is $16,059, whereas for Inuit females it is $10,901, with an average income of $13,480. (Statistics Canada, 1991).

Political negotiation

On the political level, the Inuit Tapirisat of Canada was formed in 1971. Its mandate is to promote Inuit culture and identity and to present a common front on political, economic, and environmental issues concerning the Inuit. Its role is national, with six regional affiliates, from Labrador to the Mackenzie river delta, to deal with local concerns. A major item of business has been negotiation on land claims for all traditional Inuit territory (McMillan, 1988).

Religious beliefs

The Inuit in Canada belong to a variety of churches, with 850 identifying themselves as Catholics and 3020 identifying themselves as Protestants (Statistics, 1991). Many Newfoundland Inuit are Moravian as a result of the early Moravian German missionaries (McMillan, 1988; Dobson, 1991). The Moravian mission built a church and mission house in 1830 at Hebron on the shore of Kanershutsoak Bay (officially now Kangiqsujuak, 'bay-big'). This is said to be the oldest wooden building in eastern Canada. It stands at the water's edge in a bleak, windswept terrain and was finally abandoned in 1959. It was designated a National Historic Site in 1970. The Moravian church is a Christian denomination that holds pacifism as a central doctrine. Church services are held on Saturday evening, Sunday morning, and Sunday evening. Today, although the Church in Nain is well filled with Inuit on holidays like Easter, religious rituals do not fill a central role in the life of the Inuit.

Implications for nursing care

The nurse should be aware of the role many young Inuit women are assuming as single parents. Al-though studies have shown that babies are desired, the young woman may lack experience and knowledge of good parenting techniques and need education concerning childrearing. Additionally, it is important that social support systems be activated so that extended family involvement and financial resources are available to assist in providing stability for the children as well as in helping the young women to gain the skills necessary to be self-supporting. It may be helpful for the nurse to share that the infant mortalities are very high for Inuit babies as is the likelihood that the Inuit baby will be born with a low birth weight (Aboriginal Peoples Output Program, 1989; Silins et al., 1985). Thus, prenatal care is paramount to ensure that a healthy baby is born. It is important that personal values of the nurse about unwed pregnancy not be shared with the client because communication of acceptance and the feeling of support are essential if a therapeutic nurse-client relationship is to be developed.

TIME

Traditionally the Newfoundland Inuit have been present-time oriented. During peak times for hunting and fishing, food gathering was the focus of all efforts. Children would be taken out of school, and the whole family would move to a fishing or hunting camp for several months, such as moving in the spring before the ice broke and coming back in the summer when boat travel was possible. This is less common now, though it still may be done on weekends. For example, the family may go ice fishing during weekends in the spring. Some Inuit elders regard these trips out to the "bush" where there is fresh air and "living off the land" with fresh meat and berries as having a positive influence on health and encourage them to continue. However, some Inuit have jobs in the community and do not have the flexible schedule or the desire to go back to living off the land.

Implications for nursing care

Although Newfoundland Inuit today generally come to the nursing station or clinics on their scheduled appointments, the nurse working in a community setting may be given an excuse that something else was going on and that seemed more important. In some cases a reality-orienting approach, said in a positive caring way, can increase the focus on the importance of health care particularly for children; for example, "What's more important, your housework, or your child's health?" It is important for the nurse to remember that cultural values about time orientation change very slowly and increasing an individual's focus on health care can usually be obtained only when the individual respects the health care provider and understands the importance of preventive health care and health provided in a timely manner.

ENVIRONMENTAL CONTROL

Traditionally the Inuit have believed that they were primarily controlled by the spirits of nature (Ekoomiak, 1988). Famine, bad luck, and failure in hunting meant that the spirits were displeased, whereas success in hunting and times of plenty meant that the spirits were pleased. Although to some extent the Inuit regarded their situation as a matter of fate, they also believed that living in harmony with nature was important if the spirits were to be pleased. Today, most Inuit believe spiritual beliefs and being in harmony with the spiritual world is important (Mitchel and Patch, 1986).

Illness-wellness behaviors

The nurse working in a community setting may experience frustration because persons who are sick do not come for help until they are quite ill, such as having a severe chest infection or otitis media. The nurse may be told, "I thought I was going to get better" or "The child wasn't that sick" (even though the child was really sick).

Implications for nursing care

The nurse who works with the Inuit people should be actively involved in teaching about healthful living habits and proper health care (IINC, 1985). This may occur in the clinic on a one-to-one basis. A nurse who sees the same client repeatedly for the same problem may provide individual teaching to try to prevent this problem from recurring. The relationship of the nurse with the Inuik client and the manner in which teaching occurs is very important

for optimal success of teaching. The client who feels comfortable and reassured will come back again. The Newfoundland Inuit clients appreciate a gentle caring respectful approach by the nurse, and if this is perceived by the clients, they are likely to return to the clinic. It is very important for the nurse to communicate genuine concern for the people if teaching about health is to be effective (Cardenas and Lucarz, 1985).

The nurse working in public health should assess the community for health care needs and should talk with the villagers about what they beleive their needs are (Mardiros, 1987). Classes related to specific community needs, such as prenatal classes, planning a healthy diet, and classes to stop smoking, should be available to persons in the community All teaching should be done in simple communication that can be understood and with the use of visual helps to facilitate understanding (England, 1986). Classes should also be held in the schools to emphasize the importance of taking care of one's health on subjects like good hygiene, diet, AIDS, and good mouth care. Messer (1988) reported that although Newfoundland Inuit are responsive to dental intervention strategies in the schools, additional strategies still need to be utilized for optimal effect. Based on surveys carried out in 1969 and 1986 the prevalence of dental caries declined dramatically in coastal communities in Labrador after educational programs were instituted in the schools. When predominantly Inuit populations were compared with a community with a mainly settler or White population, it was found that although the caries prevalence had declined in Inuit communities, the prevalence was still almost twice the rate found in the non-Inuit community. It has been noted by MacDonald and Mcmillan (1988) that Inuit children entering the school system in the Northwest Territories already had at least half of their deciduous teeth decayed, missing, or filled because of caries. In this case, intervention for good hygiene was needed at an earlier age.

BIOLOGICAL VARIATIONS
Body size, structure, and color

Genetic studies have related the origin of the Inuit to a population living on Asiatic Beringia that are believed to have crossed on a land bridge between Asia and Alaska and to have originated from the mongoloid race (Szathmary, 1984). The mongoloid racial traits seen in the Inuit include a short muscular body, large oblong skull with a definite occipital protuberance, well-developed lower jaw and maxillary bone, epicanthal folds, little or no body hair, dark-pigmented skin, and lumbar mongolian spots (Banks, 1956; Zegura 1985).

Early medical research noted the short stature and heavier weight per height of the Inuit, which was greatly different from that of Europeans and other circumpolar people, such as Icelanders and Finns (Milan, 1980). Three theories were proposed to explain this difference: (1) a genetic inheritance, (2) a combination of genetic and environmental adaptation, and (3) a condition of long-term nutritional deficiency. Part of this weight difference was attributed to the Inuit's thicker skeleton and muscular chest and arms (Milan, 1980). Muscular development resulting from an active lifestyle and genetic inheritance contributed to the early Inuit's body structure.

The Inuit have a "tanned" complexion that becomes deep brown to black with continuous exposure to the sun. This pigmentation is part of the mongoloid heritage. However, evolutionary selection may also explain this feature. Skin cancer research indicates that deeply pigmented skin has some natural protection from the ultraviolet rays of the sun. Therefore the evolutionary conclusion is that the Inuit are more protected from skin cancer because of their deep skin pigmentation (Young, 1986).

Other visible physical characteristics

Mongoloid heritage among the Inuit is reflected in the lumbar pigmented spots and the epicanthal eye folds. However, neither of these characteristics gives rise to significant health problems. The nurse who cares for Inuit children needs to be able to distinguish between mongolian spots and those bruises that might be associated with child abuse. Child abuse may be reported to health care providers by well-meaning Westerners who notice "bruises" on an infant's arms and buttocks when these are only mongolian spots. However, during physical assessment it is important for the nurse to remember to document unusual placement of mongolian spots on areas such as the wrist, legs, and chest.

Enzymatic variations

The races of man have adapted to specific kinds of environmental stress. For the Inuit it has been to the cold. The Inuit people resist the cold by having a high basal metabolism that burns a high-calorie diet (Simons, 1976).

Drug interactions and metabolism

Some studies have documented that drug metabolism differs among Inuit. For example isoniazid is a drug commonly used to treat tuberculosis. Vessell (1972) noted that rapid inactivation of the drug occurred among 60% to 90% of Inuit studied. Fenna, Schaefer, Mix, and Gilbert (1971) reported a study where alcohol was intravenously administered to determine its metabolic rate. Findings from this study indicate that the Inuit had a slower rate of disappearance of blood alcohol than that of Whites. Succinylcholine is a muscle relaxant used during surgery. One out of 135 Inuit is unable to metabolize this drug normally (Vessell, 1972).

Susceptibility to disease

Hepatitis B Baikie (1988) studied the epidemiology of hepatitis B virus infection in five communities in northern Labrador. Findings from the study indicate that the Inuit had the highest overall prevalence at 26.5% with an HbsAg carrier rate of 7.1%. The prevalences by ages reached a peak for the Inuit in the 41- to 50-year age group with an 89% rate.

Blood variations The Inuit as an ethnic group have a distinctive blood group variation; specifically, the Rh-negative factor is absent in the Inuit (Overfield, 1985). Although the Rh-negative factor is apparently absent among the Inuit, as more interracial marriages occur, it is essential for the nurse to not exclude the possibility of infant Rh incompatibility.

Nutritional and lifestyle preferences Caribou, seals, polar bears, mussels, sea urchins, arctic chars, birds, bird eggs, berries, and other plant life have long provided a source of food for the Newfoundland Inuit. Still today much of the Inuit diet comes from the rivers, ocean, and woods. Newfoundland has some of the best fishing in North America. Brook trout can be found in most streams, and salmon populate many of the larger rivers. In saltwater, codfish, sea trout, flounder, tuna, mackerel, and capelin can be caught. Deep-sea tuna fishing is also done. Moose and bear are available in the woods. However, with Westernization more and more Newfoundland Inuit are purchasing food in cans from stores rather than living off the land.

Psychological characteristics

Responding to an increasing awareness of the importance of mental health for the welfare of Canadian indigenous people, in November 1987 the Medical Services Branch appointed a special advisor for mental health and also started a working group that included regional representatives from the Indian and Inuit Nurses' Association, the Labrador Inuit Health Commission, the Northern Affairs Region Social Development Branch, and others (Working Group, Mental Health, 1989). This group identified that a high rate of depression appeared to exist in Native communities and identified the need to develop culturally appropriate, community-based responses to mental health problems. Also identified as an important area of need are self-help projects among Inuit groups that aim at alcohol control and "culture-congenial" programs to reintegrate the young and provide them with a useful role in their community (Jilek-Aall, 1988).

Implications for nursing care

It is important for the nurse providing care for the Newfoundland Inuit to be particularly concerned with implementation of vaccination programs, particularly for hepatitis B. Health care providers have found that initial discussion of the need for vaccinations that precede the actual vaccination program has increased vaccination rates in Inuit communities (Larke, 1988). Education of the prospective mother about Rh factors and the need for good prenatal and postnatal care should be another priority of care.

SUMMARY

Where formerly the indigenous people were the sole proprietors of Newfoundland, today Indians and Inuit share the land with a variety of European and British immigrants. No longer do the Inuit live in isolated communities but increasingly are intermarrying with the nonaboriginals with whom they share the land. Western ways are being adopted and the traditional culture is increasingly commercialized as Inuit crafts are sold and historic sites and museums provide a record of the way things once were. The Inuit are struggling to adjust to Westernization and to become part of a more industrialized and technological society. This adjustment has been problematic for many and can be facilitated by a culturally competent nurse who appreciates the struggle of this transition.

Case Study

Developed by Ruth Shearer, MSN, RN, Assistant Professor, Bethel College, Mishawaka, Indiana

Lulu Anicvak, a pregnant 17-year-old Newfoundland (Labrador) Inuk comes to the clinic with her 2-year-old child and her mother. She is single and lives with her mother, aunt, and cousins. They are happy about this pregnancy but lack knowledge regarding prenatal and child care. Her first child weighed less than 5 pounds at birth and had to stay in the hospital because of yellow skin. She had no prenatal care and was taken to the hospital by the baby's father when she started bleeding and having constant pain. She brought the baby back to the clinic several times but missed several appointments because she has been too sick vomiting since getting pregnant.

Ms. Anicvak is 5 feet tall and weighs 122 pounds, which is her usual weight even though she is 5 months pregnant. She states that she has not been eating much because everything makes her sick.

CARE PLAN

 Nursing Diagnosis Nutrition, altered: less than body requirements; related to anorexia secondary to early pregnancy as evidenced by insufficient weight gain during pregnancy; remains at prepregnant weight of 122 pounds while 5 months pregnant.

Client Outcomes	*Nursing Interventions*
1. Client will gain appropriate weight during pregnancy of 25 to 30 pounds.	1. Teach client about weight-gain curve of pregnancy.
	2. Obtain weight and graph on standard prenatal chart. Client can weigh and chart each week at home. Instruct her to return to clinic in 1 month to be weighed.
2. Client will meet daily nutritional requirements.	3. Encourage client to eat small meals every 2 hours with dry carbohydrates to begin the day if still nauseated. Explain the food pyramid using a visual aid and sending a copy home with her. She needs an increase in protein (1 meat serving) and increased vitamins A, B, C from fruits and vegetables and 30 to 60 mg of iron from meat or supplement.
	4. Provide a food diary for her to complete at home keeping a record of what she eats. Instruct her to compare what she eats with the food pyramid each day.
	5. Instruct her to bring her food diary to the clinic in 1 month. Assess nutritional intake.
3. Client will understand safety measures.	6. Provide client with prenatal vitamins and instruct her to take one each day. Explain that it will cause her stools to be black because of the iron but that it is important for her to have this iron and vitamins in order to have a healthy baby.
	7. Instruct mother to keep multiple vitamins out of the reach of children to prevent them from developing iron toxicity from taking an adult dosage.

 Nursing Diagnosis Knowledge deficit regarding prenatal care as evidenced by lack of prenatal care with first pregnancy.

Client Outcomes	*Nursing Interventions*
1. Client will describe what she needs to do to have healthy baby.	1. Assess causative factors for client's lack of prenatal care.
	2. Assess client's understanding of pregnancy, labor, and delivery.
	3. Teach client the importance of prenatal care as well as what to expect during visit and subsequent visits.
	4. Assess client's use of alcohol and other environmental hazards.
2. Client will describe her understanding of danger signs during pregnancy and what she should do in each situation.	5. Assess client's understanding of danger signs during pregnancy and her expected response.
3. Client will describe reasons for returning to clinic for prenatal care and what care she will receive.	6. Ask client to state reasons to return for prenatal care and what she expects to have done.
4. Client will describe her understanding of labor and delivery and things that were helpful during her first delivery.	7. Teach signs and symptoms of true labor and what client can do in response to each stage of labor.
5. Client will receive optimal prenatal, perinatal, and postnatal care.	8. Assess blood pressure, pulse, respirations, progress of pregnancy, health of baby; determine Rh factor, CBC, blood glucose. Screen mother and baby for harmful conditions.

Nursing Diagnosis   Knowledge deficit regarding child care as evidenced by not completing immunizations and high incidence of dental caries in Inuit children of preschool age.

Client Outcomes	*Nursing Interventions*
1. Client will describe understanding of child care.	1. Assess client level of understanding.
	2. Encourage client to breast-feed infant.
	3. Provide information regarding breast-feeding before and after delivery, such as benefits and techniques.
2. Client will describe which of the suggestions given by the nurse she plans to incorporate during the next month	4. Teach oral care and child tooth care.
	5. Teach the importance of having immunizations completed.
	6. Provide mother with nutritional requirements of infants, children, and adolescents. Give her written information to take home with diagrams of food pyramid.
	7. Encourage client to use natural foods rather than candy and sweetened gum, baked goods, and canned food.

STUDY QUESTIONS

1. List at least two communication differences that may be noted by the nurse from a different culture when interacting with this client.
2. Describe the social organization roles of this client.
3. Identify at least three environmental control issues relative to the care of this client.
4. Discuss the normal nutritional habits of this population.
5. List at least two other diseases that this client may have a high susceptibility for developing.

References

Aboriginal Peoples Output Program. (1989). *A data book on Canada's aboriginal population from the 1986 census of Canada*. Ottawa: Statistics Canada.

Anoee, M.P. (1979). Remembered childhood. In *Ajurnarmat* (Special edition: The Education Issue No. 4). Eskimo Point, NWT: Inuit and Cultural Institute.

Baikie, M.J. (1988). The epidemiology of hepatitis B virus infection in northern Labrador, Canada. *Arctic Medical Research, 47*(suppl. 1), 714-716.

Bailey, E., & Bailey, R. (1995). *Discover Canada*. Oxford: Berlitz Publishing Company.

Banks, T. (1956). *Birthplace of the wind*. New York: T.Y. Crowell.

Boas, F. (Ed.). (1938). General anthropology. Boston: T.Y. Crowell.

Cardenas, B., & Lucarz, J. (1985). Canadian Indian health care: a model for service. In Stewart, M., Innes, J., Searl, S., & Smillie, C. (Eds.), *Community health nursing in Canada*. Toronto: Gage.

Dobson, S. (1991). *Transcultural nursing*. London: Scutari Press.

Ekoomiak, N. (1988). *Arctic memories*. Toronto: NC Press (New Canada Press, distributed by the University of Toronto Press).

England, J. (1986). Cross-cultural health care. *Canada's Mental Health, 34*(4), 13-15.

Fodor's staff. (1987). *Fodor's Canada, 1988*. New York: Fodor's Travel Publications.

Fenna, D., Schaefer, O., Mix, L., & Gilbert, J. (1971). Ethanol metabolism in various racial groups. *Canadian Medical Association Journal, 105*, 472-475.

Health and Welfare Canada. (1991). *Health status of Canadian Indians and Inuit, 1990*. Ottawa: Minister of Supply and Services.

IINC (Indian and Inuit Nurses of Canada) (n.d., c. 1985). *Tenth anniversary. The story of the Indian and Inuit nurses of Canada*. Ottawa: IINC.

Indian and Northern Affairs, Canada. (1995). *Highlights of aboriginal conditions, 1991, 1986. Demographic and economic characteristics*. Ottawa: Minister of Public Works and Government Services, Canada.

Jilek-Aall, L. (1988). Juvenile alcohol use and self-destructive behavior in northern populations: a cross-cultural comparison. *Arctic Medical Research, 47*(suppl. 1), 604-610.

Johnson, O. (Ed.). (1997). *Information please almanac atlas and yearbook 1997* (ed. 50). Boston & New York: Houghton Mifflin Company.

Lange, B. (1988). Ethnographic interview: an occupational therapy needs assessment tool for American Indian and Alaska-Native alcoholics. *Occupational Therapy in Mental Health, 8*(2), 61-80.

Larke, R. (1988). Initiation of a hepatitis B vaccination program in the Northwest Territories of Canada. *Arctic Medical Research, 47* (suppl. 1), 719-722.

Lefever, D., & Davidhizar, R. (1995). American Eskimos. In Giger, J., & Davidhizar, R. (Eds.), *Transcultural nursing: assessment and intervention.* St. Louis: Mosby.

MacDonald, L., & MacMillan, R. (1988). Dental caries experience of Inuit children in the Keewatin region, Northwest Territories 1983-1984. *Arctic Medical Research, 47*(suppl. 1), 557-561.

Mailhot, J. (1978). L'´etymologie de revue et corrigée. *Études Inuit Inuit Studies 2,* 59-69.

Mardiros, M. (1987). Primary health care and Canada's indigenous people. *The Canadian Nurse, 83*(8), 20-24.

McGillivray, S. (1988). Teenage pregnancy in northern Labrador. *Arctic Medical Research, 47*(suppl. 1), 498-499.

McMillan, A. (1988). *Native peoples and cultures of Canada: an anthropological overview.* Vancouver/Toronto: Douglas & McIntyre.

Messer, J. (1988). Changing patterns in dental caries and treatment needs in Labrador school children. *Arctic Medical Research, 47*(suppl. 1), 554-556.

Milan, F. (Ed.). (1980). *The human biology of circumpolar populations.* Cambridge, Mass.: Cambridge University Press.

Mitchell, W., & Patch, K. (1986). Religion, spiritualism, and the recovery of Native American alcoholics. *IHS Primary Care Provider, 11,* 129.

O'Neil, J. (1989). The cultural and political context of patient dissatisfaction in cross-cultural clinical encounters: a Canadian Inuit study. *Medical Anthropology Quarterly, 3*(4), 325-344.

Overfield, T. (1985). *Biologic variation in health and illness.* Reading, Mass.: Addison-Wesley.

Silins, J., Semenciw, R.M., Morrison, H.I., et al. (1988). Risk factors for perinatal mortality in Canada. *Canada Medical Association Journal, 133*(12), 1214-1219.

Simons, B. (Ed.). (1976). *The volume library.* Nashville, Ten.: The Southwestern Co.

Statistics Canada. (1991). *Profile of Canada's aboriginal population.* Ottawa: Indian and Northern Affairs Canada.

Statistics Canada. (1996). *Canada at a glance.* 1996 Communication Division of Statistics, Ottawa, Canada.

Szathmary, M. (1984). Tuberculosis in the north: a lifestyle issue. *The Canadian Nurse, 80*(1), 41-43.

Vessell, E. (1972). Therapy-pharmacogenetics. *New England Journal of Medicine, 287*(18), 904-909.

Walz, J., & Walz, A. (1970). *Portrait of Canada.* New York: American Heritage Press.

Working Group, Mental Health. (1989). *Final report.* Ottawa: Medical Services Branch, Indian and Northern Health Services.

Young, T. (1986). Epidemiology and control of chronic disease in circumpolar Eskimo/Inuit populations. *Arctic Medical Research, 42,* 25-47.

Young, T. (1994). *The health of Native Americans.* New York: Oxford University Press.

Zegura, S. (1985). The initial peopling of the Americas: an overview from the perspective of physical anthropology. *Acta Anthropogenetica, 8*(1-2), 1-21.

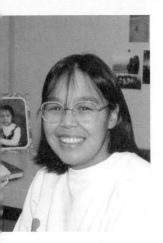

CHAPTER 14
The Inuit of Nunavut

Nancy Edgecombe

BEHAVIORAL OBJECTIVES

After reading this chapter, the nurse will be able to:

1. Describe communication patterns that are used by the Inuit in Nunavut.
2. Appreciate the traditional importance of space for the Inuit in Nunavut.
3. Relate the practices utilized in social organization by the Inuit in Nunavut.
4. Appreciate the present-time orientation of the Inuit in Nunavut.
5. Discuss the traditional ways that the Inuit have related to the environment.
6. Describe unique biological variations of the Inuit.

OVERVIEW OF THE NORTHWEST TERRITORIES

The Northwest Territories of Canada is a large and diverse geographical and cultural area. It makes up approximately one third of the land mass of Canada covering 1.3 million square miles, about the size of India (Jepson, Lee, and Smith, 1995). It covers 2400 kilometers east to west and 2700 kilometers north to south. Some 45% of the land mass extends across the northern portion of Canada's mainland, with the balance "distributed throughout a large archipelago of hundreds of islands" (Loken, 1997). Just three roads nibble at the edges of this vast area, which is primarily accessed by airplane. The capital of the Northwest Territories is Yellowknife, which serves as the hub of the flight network servicing the area's widely dispersed communities (Jepson, Lee, and Smith, 1995).

Winters are long and extend well into spring and start in early fall. Summer is limited to July and Au-

gust, and snow may occur even then. During the winter months the sun appears low on the horizon for short periods and fails to rise at all for several weeks. Winter temperatures across the Northwest Territories range from −20 to −37 degrees Celsius and can drop even further with the wind chill (Price, 1979; Dewdney and Arbuckle, 1975). In contrast, in the summer months it is daylight 24 hours a day, and for short periods the sun never sets. Summer temperatures range from +10 to +2 degrees Celsius. This results is a distinct winter-summer dichotomy that affects not only the inhabitants of the territories but also the resources available to them (McMillan, 1995).

Snow remains on the ground well into summer, and the permafrost never leaves the land. This limits the variety and quantity of vegetation able to survive this environment. For the most part, however, vegetation is limited to heather, moss, grass, and tiny flowering plants (Jenness, 1922). Several edible varieties of plant life, such as crowberries, cloudberries, bearberries, and sorrel, exist in limited amounts. The restrictions on plant life influences the disposition of wildlife in the area. Caribou migrate across the terrain to the north in the summer when there were plants for grazing but back to the south in the winter when plants are not available. The caribou remain constantly on the move because they deplete the local growth. Polar bears and musk-oxen can also be found in this area. Smaller grazing animals, such as lemmings and Arctic hares, thrive (McMillan, 1995). This small game allows small carnivores such as the fox and wolf to survive. This area is the summer nesting ground for a variety of birds, such as falcons, snow buntings, hawks, snowy owls, swans, sandpipers, plovers, gulls, terns, ducks, and loons (Udvardy, 1977) A few birds, such as the ptarmigan, stay in the area year around (O'Leary and Levinson, 1991).

The terrain is varied. Baffin Island is part of the Canadian Shield, resulting in mountains, fjords, and rocky outcroppings. In the far north, there are areas where the sea ice never melts, and the icebergs from the Greenlandic ice fields are common. In the winter months, many straits and gulfs are covered by a continuous sheet of ice from October or November until sometime in July preventing access to marine life (Damas, 1984). Seals remain throughout the winter maintaining holes for breathing. In the spring, they converge at the floe edge where they lay at the edge of the ice basking in the sun (Kehoe, 1981; Morrison and Wilson, 1995).

The Northwest Territories has a population of only 64,000 people (Government of the Northwest Territories, 1997). The population is divided among 56 communities and numerous outpost camps. Most communities are small with populations between 250 and 2000 people, and the largest community is Yellowknife with a population of 16,000 (Government of the Northwest Territories, 1997). Most communities are accessible only by air or by sea for a brief period each year. Although small, the population is diverse. There are nine official languages (seven of which are aboriginal) and at least 10 others that have not obtained official status. With each language is a corresponding cultural group, that is, Inuktitut (Inuit language), North Slavey (Sahtu, 'bear-lake'), South Slavey, Dogrib, Gwich'in, Chipewyan (Dene, or Déné SoNlhine), and Cree.

The Inuit represent 37% of the population of the Northwest Territories and reside primarily along the Arctic coasts and the eastern portion of the Northwest Territories (Statistics Canada, 1991). For the most part the Inuit live in isolated regions and do not have access to higher education. In 1991 some 6% of the Inuit population had university degrees, 18% had college or university diplomas, and 15% had some other type of post secondary school education (Government of the Northwest Territories, 1997).

The life expectancy has dramatically increased over the past 50 years. The life expectancy of the Inuit in the Northwest Territories more than doubled between the periods 1941-1950 and 1978-1982, when it was 66 years (Robitaille and Choinière, 1985). More recently the life expectancy of the Inuit was 68.3 compared to the Canadian national average of 77.95 (Government of the Northwest Territories, 1996).

The central and eastern portion of this area is referred to as Nunavut, which is an Inuktitut word for 'our land'. In 1976, the Inuit Tapirisat of Canada (ITC), a national organization of Inuit, proposed that a new territory in northern Canada be created (Indian and Northern Affairs, 1996). In April 1999, the area referred to as "Nunavut" will become its own territory with Inuit self-governance (Pollick, 1997). It is the Inuit who live in Nunavut who are the focus of this chapter.

The historic origins of the Inuit people

The Inuit in Canada were historically referred to as "Eskimo." The name was changed to "Inuit," which means the 'people' in preference to the Algonquian word "Eskimo," which was long assumed to mean 'eaters of raw meat', but this name has been found to have been first applied to the Algonquian Micmacs of Gaspé Peninsula and properly means 'speaking the language of a foreign land' (Mailhot, 1978). Although the term "Eskimo" is still used in Alaska, Canadian Inuit consider it a derogatory term. The Inuit were preceded in Canada by a series of ancient migratory groups from Asia. It is believed that the first inhabitants of the Arctic were the Paleo-Eskimo who crossed the land bridge from Siberia approximately 4000 years ago (Morrison and Wilson, 1995). They spread rapidly across the Canadian Arctic coast and then on to Greenland. Although not direct ancestors to the modern Inuit, they brought an "Eskimo way of life," which is evident by sites littered with finely crafted miniature implements of stone (McMillan, 1995). They disappeared after several centuries.

Approximately 300 years later the Pre-Dorset people similarly migrated out of Alaska across the Canadian Arctic replacing the earlier people. The Pre-Dorset people, like the Inuit, were nomadic hunters and gatherers who eventually concentrated around the Foxe Basin and Hudson Strait north of Hudson Bay (McMillan, 1995). Here the culture evolved and adapted as they developed more sophisticated tools for Arctic survival such as the snow knife. The Pre-Dorset people occupied regions of the Arctic until about 800 B.C. leaving remains that indicated that they harpooned sea mammals and used bows and arrows for hunting land animals (McMillan, 1995).

Between 1000 and 1600, the Thule people arrived from Alaska. As Inuktitut speakers, the Thule appear to be the direct ancestors of the present Inuit. During a period of general environmental warming the Thule culture advanced the Dorset technology with methods for navigating open water. Thule whale hunters traveled in skin boats and dogsleds. The Thule brought the *kayak* (a small, single-person hunting boat) and the *umiak* (a large, open, hide-covered boat), which are still used today in the Arctic. The Thule sites yield toggles and buckles used in harnessing dogs. The Thule brought the Alaskan practice of manufacturing pottery, lamps, and other vessels. Small sculptures include humans (usually female) in wood, bone, and ivory and flat-bottomed ivory figures of swimming birds, often with a woman's head and torso. The latter were likely tossed in a game but may have had a mythological basis, representing the Inuit belief in an association between women and sea animals (McMillan, 1995). *Ulus*, the semicircular "women's knives," with ground-slate blades and wooden or bone handles and a major

tool for cutting meat and preparing hides, are also still found in use today by some Inuit.

The Thule built substantial winter houses, which offered much greater comfort than the Dorset enjoyed. Although the style was Alaskan, in the wood-scarce Canadian Arctic, they had to substitute whale ribs and jaws for driftwood logs as construction materials. The entrance tunnel sloped downwards, trapping cold air below the level of the house. Inside, the floor was paved with flat stones, which were also used to construct a sleeping platform, elevated to take advantage of the warmer air (McMillan, 1995). There is evidence that they used stowhouses as temporary camps. However, in the summer the Thule were more mobile, camping in hide-covered tents (Morrison and Wilson, 1986).

When Martin Frobisher arrived by ship in 1576 through the fabled Northwest Passage, historical accounts described natives who were more likely the Thule, yet they had features of the nineteenth-century Inuit (Swayze, 1960). When later explorers encountered the Inuit, they described a culture less complex than the Thule. A "Little Ice Age," which lasted from about A.D. 1600 to 1850, significantly affected the food distribution the Inuit were dependent on: living off whale meat was no longer possible because of sea ice blocks, and their diet became dependent on locally available foods, usually some combination of seal, walrus, small whales, caribou, and fish. Virtually no vegetation was available to them. Although heather and brush were used as fuel in summer, the seal oil lamp was the most important source of heat and light for most of the year (O'Leary and Levinson, 1991). Seals provided hides that could be made into boots, summer clothing, harpoon lines, and dog harnesses. The walrus provided meat and blubber, ivory from their tusks, and tough hides, which could be used for various purposes, including covering boats.

With the onset of the "Little Ice Age," permanent homes had to be abandoned for temporary shelters of skin tents in the summer and snowhouses in the winter as the Inuit migrated to where they could find food. Tents were made from caribou skin or sealskin and could be a tipi or rigid form. Although the Inuit continued many aspects of the Thule culture, not all the lifestyle customs survived the colder climate.

Life in the Northwest Territories has resulted in the Inuit being a group of people who are distinct from all other Canadian Native peoples (Morrison and Wilson, 1995). Throughout the Northwest Territories the Inuit and their predecessors survived on whatever resources were available. The economy was based on a combination of hunting land and sea mammals and fishing. Caribou and seals were the essential resources. If the hunt were not successful, starvation was an ever-present threat (Stefansson, 1913). The limited resources supported a population density much lower than that of Alaska, Greenland, or the rest of Canada (Kehoe, 1981). For the Inuit in the Northwest Territories contact with Europeans was fleeting. Diamond Jenness (1992) studied the Inuit in a Canadian Arctic Expedition (1913 to 1918) as Rasmussen, Mathiassen, and Kaj Birket-Smith (Price, 1979) did in the Fifth Thule Expedition (1921 to 1924).

With the dawning of the nineteenth century and encounters with commercial whalers in Hudson Bay, traditional customs of the Inuit gradually began to change. The Inuit were used as crew on the whaleboats and as hunters to provide fresh meat for the crew, and their services were paid with goods including firearms, iron tools, metal pots, kettles, woolen clothing, beads, and tobacco. Kerosene lamps and canvas tents became common among the Inuit. Whaleboats replaced the *umiak*. The whalers hastened the erosion of traditional Inuit culture in the eastern Arctic but had even more devastating effects in western Canada where whalers liberally dispensed alcohol, interacted sexually with the women, and introduced diseases foreign to the Inuit. The seasonal cycle of migration for meat dramatically slowed with the introduction of rifles, nets, steel traps, and small wooden boats.

When the demand for whales ended after 1910, the fur traders began to fill the void in the Inuit economy left by the whalers. The Hudson Bay Company built many posts across the north, and the Inuit supplied furs including white fox and muskrat in exchange for goods. Arctic fox furs could be traded for hunting and fishing tools as well as tea,

tobacco, and flour, commodities that became necessities by the 1920s (Damas, 1984; Jenness, 1922; Rasmussen, 1932). With the fur trade came the spread of the missionaries, both Roman Catholic and Anglican, which introduced education and medical assistance. Missions often existed alongside the trading stations. Major change and new economic opportunities came with World War II in northern Canada. The Inuit found jobs assisting American and Canadian military personnel in construction of roads, airfields, hangars, barracks, and other facilities. However, exposure to White workers also brought exposure to disease. In Chesterfield Inlet, Northwest Territories, 8% of the Inuit contracted poliomyelitis from White workers and 2% died (Adamson, Moody, Peart, et al., 1949). In 1952, a measles epidemic swept through Bafffin Island with an attack rate of 99% and a mortality between 2% and 7%. This was traced to Inuit visitors to the armed forces bases (Peart and Nagler, 1954). In the following cold-war era construction of radar installations stretching across Canada brought another opportunity for employment.

Increased attention on the north also exposed the neglect of the Native peoples and forced increased government involvement in their welfare. Thus, in the 1950s and 1960s, government-sponsored building programs provided oil-heated, insulated, wooden houses for some Inuit. Larger groups of Inuit were encouraged to live in settlements in permanent communities that were equipped with schools and nursing stations. Family allowances, welfare, and old age pensions began to be provided on the same basis as that available to other Canadians. Attempts were initiated to assist the Inuit to be self- supporting by development of local craft industries and fox-skin and fish export (O'Leary and Levinson, 1991). However, although the benefits of life in settlements were evident, unemployment, idleness, and readily available alcohol created social problems. The government attempted to intervene by relocation. Inuit from many smaller settlements were relocated to larger centers for administrative convenience and economy. Some Inuit were induced to settle in remote areas where seals and other game were abundant. Only recently, in 1996, a $10-million compensation package was finalized for Inuit who were relocated from northern Quebec to the high Arctic in the 1950s. The Inuit maintained that the federal government had wanted to populate the north to assert sovereignty but instead had resulted in their personal hardship, suffering, and loss (Canada Notes, 1996).

Today, many Inuit communities lack any real economic base, and unemployment is high. Many of the few available jobs are part time or seasonal. Government assistance is required by most families in order to live (McMillan, 1995). Trapping and hunting can provide a supplemental income and put meat on the table but cannot take care of the high cost of fuel and ammunition.

Nunavut

In the 1970s Canadian Inuit began pressuring the national government to divide the Northwest Territories into two regions, allowing the natives in the eastern half to govern themselves. An Ottawa-based Inuit group that proposed the eastern territory would be known as "Nunavut" ('our land' in Inuktitut) and would be controlled by a unique form of Native government. Since the Inuit account for about 84% of the population (18,017 in 1991) in the sparsely populated eastern Arctic, it was the dream of the Inuit people that the new government would enable focusing on Inuit priorities such as issues of language, wildlife management, education, and restoration of their cultural heritage (Government of the Northwest Territories, 1997; Pollick, 1997).

In 1991 a land-claim agreement guaranteed the Inuit $1.1 billion over 14 years as well as outright ownership of about 140,000 square miles of land. The agreement made the Inuit the single largest private landowners in the world (Jepson, Lee, and Smith, 1995). This agreement gave back to the Inuit their homeland. They, in return, renounced their claim to the remainder of the Northwest Territories (Jepson, Lee, and Smith, 1995).

It was further decided after a plebiscite, or popular vote, that on April 1, 1999, a fifth of Canada, more than 733,000 square miles—1.25 times the size of Alaska—will become Nunavut, a land to be governed by the First Nation people who live there. In the minds of many of the people, Nunavut already exists (Pollick, 1997). Of the 773,000-plus square miles in the territory, the Inuit already own 140,000 as a part of the Native land-claims settlement in 1991 (Pollick, 1997). Many Inuit hope that Nunavut will rekindle an interest in heritage among the younger generations (Pollick, 1997). Although the Inuit population is small, it is rapidly growing. Some 58% of the population in this region is under 24 years of age (Government of the Northwest Territories, 1997) compared to 33% for the population of Canada (Government of Canada, 1991).

The Inuit of the Nunavut area were initially made up of six groups, the Copper, Netsilik, Iglulik, Caribou, Sallirmiut (Coral Harbour), and Baffin Inuit (Morrison and Wilson, 1995). The Sallirmiut were wiped out by an epidemic of unknown origin in 1902-1903 after contact with whalers (McMillan, 1995). Each group was separated geographically. Although they have a shared culture, there are variations between the five remaining groups. This is illustrated in the unique clothing design worn by members of each group (Houston, 1997).

Iqaluit ('many-fish'), on Baffin Island in the east, will be the capital of Nunavut. This community of 4000 is the only community in the area with more than 2000 people (Pollick, 1997). Nunavut is composed of 28 communities with only one hospital in the entire area. Transportation between communities is by air, and the distance between communities and the nearest hospital ranges from several hundred kilometers to over 1000 kilometers. Health services in the other communities is provided by nurses functioning in an expanded role at health centers. These nurses provide primary care, emergency care, and community health services for the population in consultation with physicians located in the larger centers. Physicians visit the communities on a regular basis, and clients are referred out in between visits and for specialist referrals. When an emergency situation occurs, nurses work to stabilize the client, and the client is then air lifted to the nearest hospital for more intensive health care. However, because the weather sometimes prohibits air travel, nurses sometimes need to provide advanced care for longer periods.

There has been opposition to a governmental separation of Nunavut and to the whole concept of division (Pollick, 1997). Yellowknife, a city that is home to thousands of territorial and federal civil servants, many of them non-Natives, fear the loss of jobs and a reduction in federal funding for services for territorial residents (Bergman, 1992). Some Inuit fear that the government in Ottawa will not allow the Inuit to mold democracy in their own image and likeness in Nunavut (Pollick, 1997). Others however, support the concept of "community" and believe that having a "home" will give the Inuit a new sense of identity, curtail the eroding of Inuit cultural tradition, keep alive cultural roots, and facilitate the development of real jobs (Ryan, 1992). Most agree that the new land will need help in developing mining and tourism to make the country economically feasible (Pollick, 1997). Some believe that the Inuit did not get enough. In fact, the Inuit have mineral rights to only 14,000 square miles though they have unrestricted rights to hunt, fish, and trap over a far greater area.

COMMUNICATION

Some 79 languages can be found in Canada today (Internet on Canada, 1997). The native language spoken by the Inuit, Inuktitut, is one of three native languages spoken by large enough numbers of speakers that it is not threatened with extinction (Young, 1994).

The Inuit linguistic stock is termed Eskimo-Aleut, or "Eskaleut," which has two major branches. The Aleut live on the Aleutian islands of Alaska. The other branch, the Eskimo, is divided into five separate language groups and includes persons living in eastern Siberia, central and southern Alaska, and across northern Canada to Greenland, including all of arctic Canada. Throughout their vast distribution, the Inuit speak the same language, Inuktitut, though the dialects vary significantly. Eastern Canadian Inuktitut is spoken by some 14,000 speakers out of a population of 17,500 Inuit in eastern Canada and the eastern Arctic (Internet on Canada, 1997). North Alaskan Inuktitut is spoken by 2500 total speakers out of some 8000 Inuit in the Mackenzie River Delta region to Norton Sound, Alaska. In

addition, each of these branches of the Inuktitut language contains additional dialects (Internet on Canada, 1997). Some 20,000 of the Canadian population with aboriginal origins identify Inuktitut as their home language, and 26,120 persons in Canada claim knowledge of the Inuktitut language (Statistics Canada, 1995).

There is an Eskimo sign language (ESL) that is used near the Arctic Circle by the deaf. This is distinctly different from the Canadian and French-Canadian sign languages, but there is little literature to describe it (Internet on Canada, 1997).

As the official language of the Inuit, Inuktitut will be the official language of Nunavut. This language is both verbal and nonverbal in nature. Within the language there are several dialects in both written and oral language. However, the spoken language has less variation than the written. The Inuit word for an 'arctic squirrel' is *silsik* in the eastern Baffin dialect and *hikhik* in the western Innuniqtun dialect. Eighty-nine percent (89%) of the Inuit population identify Inuktitut as their mother tongue and first language. In many communities it is the language used in primary school grades, with English being introduced gradually until about grade 5, when it becomes the working language. The language depending on the dialect is made up of 16 to 18 basic phonemes (Collis, 1990)

With the coming of the whalers, traders, and the goods and technology that accompanied them new words needed to be introduced into the language. Often the names for these items were adopted into the Inuktitut language with slight variation to reflect the phonemes of the language. 'Sugar' became *sukaq*, 'tea' became *ti*, and 'paper' became *paipaq*. Similarly when Inuit gave their children English names, the names changed slightly because of the differences in phonemes; for example, Elizabeth became Elisapee, Rebecca became Repecca, and Adam became Adamee.

Inuktitut has two forms in the way it is written—using roman orthography (with Latin letters) or using a syllabary (syllabics, syllabic letters). Roman orthography is a phonetic representation of the spoken word and has in part been responsible for some of the variation in this form of writing. Now, however, the writing has been standardized; for example, traditional "skin boots" is written as singular: *kamik*, dual: *kamiik*, and plural: *kamiit* (with English plural *kamik*s). The syllabic system was developed by Rev. James Evans for the Cree in Norway House, Manitoba, where with possible help from the Native assistants and Native design elements he published a Cree hymn book in syllabics in 1841 (Murdoch, 1984). The system was adapted for the Inuit by Edmund Peck. Its symbols are fashioned after secretarial shorthand (Hanson, 1997), with each symbol representing one phoneme. The symbol ⟨ represents the phoneme *pa*, and the symbol ⟩ represents the phoneme *pu* (Collis, 1990). Although most Inuit speak one form of Inuktitut, they remain a verbal and nonverbal people.

There is also a strong nonverbal component in the Inuit language system. Although words exist today for yes and no, these responses are first learned in their traditional nonverbal forms. A raising of the eyebrows indicates 'yes' and a squinting of the eye indicates 'no'. Most older children and adults have learned to answer verbally; however, young children commonly answer in this manner. The Inuit are a quiet people who are not uncomfortable with silences in conversation. In fact, to fill a silence with chatter is considered unmannerly (Brody, 1975).

Because Inuktitut remains the first language of the people and the comfort level of some Inuit with English varies at times, communication takes place through interpreters. This creates its own problems because concepts are not always easily translated. The words used for "bacteria" and "virus" are very similar in Inuktitut. At times this is confusing for the Inuit who are told that they need an antibiotic one time and not the next to what they see as the same type of infection.

Implications for nursing care

Nurses working with the Inuit people often are not familiar with Inuktitut both in its verbal and nonverbal form. Working through a translator is often difficult, since precise meanings can be lost in translation. Nurses unfamiliar with the nonverbal expressions of the language often miss responses. It is not unusual for a health care professional who has not worked with an Inuik client to be frustrated at what is perceived as a failure to answer a question because the nonverbal answer is not recognized by the health care professional (Hodgson, 1980; Smith, 1979).

It is also important for the nurse to understand the social context of the language. This understanding is closely related to the development of a relationship with the client. Within the culture there are acceptable ways of presenting a problem and in responding to questions. Often clients with vague nonspecific complaints are actually concerned about a social or personal problem but hesitate to volunteer the nature of the problem directly. In this case, indirect questioning may be more appropriate. Instead of asking, "Is there anything else bothering you?" the nurse might state, "Sometimes when things are bothering a person symptoms like the ones you have occur."

The Inuit respect expert knowledge. Because the nurse is usually considered an expert, the nurse is usually viewed with a certain degree of respect and as an authority. This in combination with the desire to avoid conflict has implications for nursing care. Clients may not feel comfortable directly questioning the nurse or challenging the nurse's evaluation of the situation. Thus, even if the clients or their family disagree with the nurse, they may say nothing. This makes it essential for the nurse to develop a trusting relationship where the Inuk client feels free to express true feelings. The nurse must also recognize that other "experts" both within the family and in the community at large may be giving advice based on their knowledge. A mother may bring her child with a cold to the clinic after hours not so much because she is overly worried about the cold or believes she cannot manage the illness but because some considered to have "expert" knowledge and or with more authority in the family unit such as an elder advised her to do so.

The nurse should know that reading does not have the same emphasis in the Inuit culture as speaking and watching do. Therefore, whenever possible, information should be provided in oral or pictorial form. The use of videos, audio tapes, and posters are more appropriate than information pamphlets for health promotion. When pamphlets are used, they should be graphic in nature (Irvine, 1987).

SPACE

Traditionally, through much of the year the Inuit lived in close quarters where sharing space was essential. Today, partly because of housing shortages and partly for social reasons, they continue to live in proximity to each other. Parents often share their bedroom with infants for the first year or longer. Siblings share beds. In some groups the oldest son has special status and will have a room of his own. Visiting and socializing is an important part of daily life. It is expected that individuals will share their personal property and resources with the extended family and in some cases with the community at large.

The acceptable space between adults and adults and between adults and children varies significantly among the Inuit. Infants and young children are given constant physical contact. They are carried nestled against their mother's back either in the traditional woman's coat, the *amonti*. However, as they get older, public displays of physical closeness become less and less. As adults, Inuit seldom show affection publicly, and physical contact is limited to handshakes. The handshake is considered to be the acceptable way of greeting. This is related to the traditional way of approaching a potential enemy with arms outward demonstrating the absence of weapons. The acceptable space for adults who are socializing is at handshaking distance. This is in strong contrast to the acceptable space for relating to children, which is much less.

Implications for nursing care

It is important that the nurse be aware that close physical contact between adults may be perceived as invasion of personal space even in a nursing care situation. If personal space is to be invaded, it is important to explain carefully to the client what is going to be done and why. If the Inuk client understands the reason for the physical contact, it will usually be accepted. When nursing the Inuit, the nurse needs to recognize that the Inuit may be more comfortable with others and at home than on their own. The ability to see and visit with other Inuit is important to them. For this reason there are mechanisms for Inuit in common referral centers to stay in Inuit boarding homes when out for referral and for Inuit staff to visit with them while they are in the hospital. It is not usual for the Inuit to have numerous visitors at one time, but when possible, this should be accommodated.

In visiting an Inuit home the nurse should remember that the Inuit are use to living in proximity to each other. On the one hand, sleeping arrangements may seem overcrowded by the nurse's standards, but unless there is a health concern, it should be accepted. On the other hand, the nurse should be aware that most Inuit feel no need to be in a private space to speak to the health care provider. On the other hand, the nurse should not feel uncomfortable if the client appears to be having a private conversation with other family members in front of the nurse. Although the opportunity for privacy should be offered, this often is not valued by the Inuit client.

SOCIAL ORGANIZATION

The basic social unit for the Inuit family has traditionally been the nuclear family, consisting of a man and a woman and their descendants. In the average family four or five children were born, three of which were likely to survive. When a family could not support a child, it would be either adopted by another family or alternatively killed by suffocation or abandonment. Children adopted into a family held full membership, but the previous relationships were also recognized. In other words, the individual had two sets of families. When a twin birth occurred, one infant was killed because it was not possible to provide for both infants (Jenness, 1922).

Upon marriage, children formed a new and distinct family of their own living separately from other family members, but in most groups they stayed closely affiliated with other family members. Although there was no formal arranging of marriages, if the bridegroom were going to move away with his new bride, a small payment was made to the girl's parents. If the couple remained in the area, they simply moved into their own home. Marriage by capture was common but usually involved women who had already been married. During the initial period of the marriage it was common for the marriage to be dissolved by either party. However, once children were born marriages were relatively stable. Polygamy occurred on occasion but was not the norm (McMillan, 1995). Under special circumstances wife sharing or exchanging did occur. Such exchanges served to create a lasting bond between a visitor and the group being visited. Similar bonds are also formed when couples became "dancing associates" or "seal-flipper associates" with someone in the group. In case of divorce a woman returned to her kinsfolk (Jenness, 1922).

The Inuit gender roles are clearly identifiable. Traditionally most tasks were clearly identifiable as either male or female in nature. Their roles complemented each other, and in general men had responsibility for tasks related to travel, hunting, shelter, and related equipment, whereas women were responsible for tasks related to clothing, food, and childrearing. During migrations men were responsible for the preparation and operation of the dogs and the sled. Women were responsible for dressing of skins and the maintenance of the shelter once it was built. This included the gathering of fuel and the maintaining of seal lamps. Everyone participated in fishing both with rod and line; however only men used spears for fishing.

Social groups varied with the seasons (McMillan, 1995). Several families, generally related through males, remained together throughout most of the year. When food was abundant or more people were needed, people lived in larger groups. For example, the winter sealing camps of the Central Inuit required many hunters to watch the breathing holes, resulting in communities of about 100 people. Similarly the caribou hunt among the Caribou Inuit and whaling among the Mackenzie River Delta Inuit brought together large numbers.

Property was distinguished as being either personal, family, or communal. Personal property consisted of anything used by the individual in daily life, such as tools (weapons for a man or lamps and sewing kit for a women). In the case of divorce or marriage such personal property belonged to the individual. However, it was not unusual for friends and relatives to borrow from each other. When an owner died, a portion of his or her property was laid on the grave. The remaining articles were distributed among the kinsfolk based on group discussion with no priority to any one individual.

Traditionally all food and skins acquired by family members were considered to be family property, though some must be shared with neighbors, depending on the abundance of food in the community at that time. Land was considered the possession of the community, which used it as hunting and fishing grounds. Visitors were restricted from using local natural resources unless they established a bond with the community.

In the traditional Inuit communities leadership was flexible based on the characteristic of the individual who earned respect from other community members. "A man acquires influence by his force of character, his energy and success in hunting, or his skill in magic. As long as these last he will increase his influence, but when they fail, his prestige and authority vanish" (Jenness, 1922). There is no organized council to oversee the conduct of community members. Competition over women sometimes occurred when Inuit lived closely together. Without any strong position of leadership methods of social control were limited. One technique to resolve conflict was a song duel, where a singer publicly ridiculed the behavior of another. Another way of dealing with unacceptable behavior was for the band to move and leave behind the offender. Murder was one form of coping with anger, which often resulted in feuds between families and additional deaths.

The Inuit spiritual system was animistic. Birds, animals, and even land forms were considered to have supernatural power. Spirits of the dead may also affect the living. Water or oil was poured into the mouth of killed animals to quench their thirst. Oil was rubbed into the skins of killed birds. Offerings were also left beside the larger animals such as polar bears when they were killed. The Copper Inuit made clear distinctions between animals of the land and those of the sea, and the products of the two were kept and used separately. Caribou, a land food, could not be cooked or new clothes sewn while the people were living on sea ice. At no time were caribou and seal meat to be cooked in the same pot. Similarly sealskin was not to be tanned or sewn while fishing was taking place at a freshwater site. Failure to follow the rules of this land-sea dichotomy was believed to cause storms, famine, or other misfortune (O'Leary and Levinson, 1991).

Some control over an uncertain world came from the *angakok* ('shaman'). Both men and women could obtain spirit power, enabling them to communicate with the supernatural realm and mediate and intercede between the Inuit and the world of shades and spirits. The shaman was attributed with powers to cure the sick, prophesy the future, and summon supernatural aid when the animals could not be found or storms kept the hunters trapped in their homes. In the fall the shaman conducted an important ceremony before winter sealing in which the shaman went into a trance, visited the sea goddess, Sedna, in the spirit world to appease her of any wrath for any taboo violations. Part of this ceremony included pairing off men and women for a brief spouse exchange, which was believed to be pleasing to the sea goddess (Jenness, 1922). Although many of these traditions are no longer practiced by the young Inuit, for many older Inuit, whether practiced or not, the traditions are still very much a part of their thinking and influence actions. Because many of the Inuit still live in isolated communities, many of the old cultural patterns are still practiced. For many Inuit it is memories of the old way of life that have prompted the dream of Nunavut and once again having personal autonomy to follow cultural traditions. For many Inuit living in Nunavut, having a decent income and a job are pressing social problems. The unemployment rate for the Inuit living in Nunavut was 22% in 1991, and the average income was $21,715 (Government of the Northwest Territories, 1997).

Implications for nursing care

The nurse who works with the Inuit needs to be aware of how the social organization affects the behavior and beliefs of the people. In most Inuit groups the needs of the individual are considered secondary to the groups. Because of the proximity in which they have lived, they have developed the ability to avoid conflict, since disharmony could affect survival.

The nurse should be aware that an adopted person may have two nuclear families, that is, both the biological family and the family in which they were raised. Both families need to be treated as family by the nurse and the treatment team.

The Inuit have adopted some beliefs from both the Christian religions and medical science. However, the nurse should be aware that this does not mean that traditional beliefs have been rejected. In fact, after years of silence concerning these beliefs rather than avoidance of conflict with the clergy and health practitioners, there is now a beginning openness to express traditional ideas that may still be believed. The nurse needs to be careful to respect expression of traditional beliefs and when possible should incorporate them into the treatment plan (Edgecombe, 1994).

It is important for the nurse to appreciate that the Inuit approach to childrearing and discipline is very different from that held by most other cultures in Canada. Many Inuit do not discipline their children and grant them great independence. Children are seldom refused anything or forced to do things they do not want to do. Small children are permitted to play alone out of doors and to roam quite far from the village. Children may eat at whatever house they wish, and because mealtimes and bedtimes are irregular, it is unusual to hear a parent express concern about where a child is at a particular time. Children are allowed to judge their own needs. The nurse should appreciate that this attitude toward childrearing represents a traditional belief that a child should be reared in freedom rather than a lack of concern or neglect on the part of the parents (Brody, 1975). There is also a belief that a child may be the reincarnation of someone who has recently died. Because of this, the child may actually be an elder and therefore treated with respect rather than with a judgmental attitude (Browne, 1995).

When a child needs to take medication at home on a regular basis, the nurse should be aware that if the child refuses the medication, the parents may hesitate to encourage compliance. If a certain dietary regimen is required, the parents may also hesitate to use an authoritarian approach. The culturally competent nurse needs to be sensitive to this culturally oriented parenting style and to work with the parents to appreciate the importance of adhering to a treatment plan.

The nurse needs to be aware that some developmental milestones may be reached slightly later in Inuit children because these children tend to be carried until a later age and therefore may crawl and walk slightly later. Developmental testing may have to be adapted in some areas. For example, because they have different play activities, riding a tricycle may not be an appropriate developmental milestone. An Inuk child may not be able to identify a picture of a horse but would be able to identify a picture of a musk-ox.

Primary health care for prenatal Inuit clients includes routine prenatal care and prenatal health teaching. Health care professionals have attempted to routinely evacuate women in rural areas to communities with hospitals between 36 and 38 weeks of gestation. Because there is only one hospital in Nunavut, for some this means going quite a distance. The perception of this practice can create a cultural conflict. To the health professional this evacuation is necessary to provide modern medical technology and reduce neonatal death. The Inuit also want a healthy infant but are more accepting of the possibility of neonatal death. In the period 1956 to 1960 the Inuit in the Northwest Territories had the highest infant mortality of any group, 223 of 1000 live births. Although this rate has dramatically declined (28 of 1000 in the period 1981 to 1985), it is still higher than that in any other group (Young, 1994).

Some women do not want to be separated from their families for 2 to 6 weeks and are concerned about the burden to their family because of their absence. To many Inuit women the risk of delivery in the settlement at a health center is more acceptable than leaving their family alone for this period of time (Qinuajuak, 1996). Male and female roles are clearly defined, and the women may hesitate to see her husband the object of jokes about performing domestic duties that are clearly women's work in her absence (Brody, 1975). Similarly males are hesitant to assume a woman's role while she is out having a baby and may also object to her being taken away (O'Neil et al., 1991).

The nurse providing prenatal education should also be aware that there is a decreasing prevalence to breast feed among Inuit mothers. Presently the number of women who breast feed to 1 week is 70%, to 3 months is 32%, and to 6 months is 22% (Daviss, 1966).

The nurse should be aware that the total fertility rate (TFR) for the Inuit had dramatically dropped since the 1960s. At that time the Canadian TFR was 2.5 children per woman compared to 9.2 for the Inuit. By the early 1980s the TFR was 1.7 for Canadian women and 4.1 for the Inuit (Norris, 1990). This is related to an increase in family planning programs (Young, 1994).

TIME

The Inuit perspective of time is highly influenced by where they are located in relation to the sun. Living along or above the Arctic Circle means that for one period of the year there is no or little darkness whereas for another period there is no or little light. In many areas of Nunavut the sun disappears for weeks below the horizon in winter and in summer never sets. The farther north, the longer these periods are, and so in the high Arctic it is dark for a month in midwinter. With no regular cycle of day and night there is no external cue to trigger activities such as eating, sleeping, and waking. This has resulted in a tendency by the Inuit to sleep when they are tired rather than in relation to the actual time. It is interesting to observe that in the summer when it is always light Inuit appear to function well on very little sleep whereas in the winter many Inuit sleep much more than other Canadians (Jenness, 1922).

The environment influences the Inuit's perception of time in other ways as well. Weather in the Arctic is unpredictable and harsh. When a storm occurs, especially in the winter, there is little one can do but settle down and wait. Similarly the availability of resources has a tentative nature to them. There will be food if the weather holds and if the caribou migration does not change. If breakup of the sea ice is late, there won't be any char until they return to spawn in the river in the fall. As a result there is always a tentative nature to the future, one can plan only for today with any certainty. Where people in other cultures say "when" in relation to time, the Inuit say "if."

Implications for nursing care

It is important for the nurse to be aware of the philosophy of time of the Inuit people and to recognize that it will affect their behavior and response to the health care system. The Inuit are most likely to respond to illness and treatment in a reactive way rather than a proactive way. Preventive measures are unlikely to be a priority. This time orientation also results in a higher emphasis on requesting and expecting immediate action and treatment response. This can lead to conflict based on a difference between the health care professional's and the client's expectations. Understanding the Inuit perspective may decrease the frustration experienced by the health care professional (Irvine, 1987).

Similarly clients and families may fail to make plans about discharge ahead of time. Understanding the present-time orientation can allow the nurse to be more proactive for Inuit clients regarding discharge planning. The nurse should be prepared for problems in establishing regular clinic hours in remote stations. Traditional Inuit do not regulate their actions by the clock and do not understand that a nurse may want to have certain hours for the clinic to be open and certain hours for personal time. The Inuit client in the Arctic may not understand why a nurse cannot be available anytime. "After all, why shouldn't a nurse want to nurse at any time? Isn't that her job and her life? If hospitals provide around the clock care, shouldn't the nurse's station do the same?" (Hodgson, 1980). To understand the Inuit people and their unique perspectives and to be an effective caregiver it is important for the nurse to make friends with the Inuit clients and to gain their trust. Inuit people will find medical services psychologically unsatisfying and socially alienating unless they can establish ties with the caregivers and vice versa (Hodgson, 1980).

ENVIRONMENTAL CONTROL

Traditionally the Inuit have held strong beliefs in the spirit world and in the powers of supernatural beings such as the sea goddess (known, depending on the group, as *Sedna, Nuliajuk, Arnapkapsaluk, Takanakapsaluk* or 'the terrible one down there', and *Arnarkuagsak*), the deity of the air, *Hilap Inua* (or *Silap Inua*), and other powerful dieties. The use of a shaman, religious ceremonies, and special rituals that enabled the supernatural to come to the aid of the individual were an important part of the culture. Illness was frequently combated by rituals believed to enable supernatural intervention. The Copper Inuit believed that headaches could be treated by bleeding (Damas, 1984). However, the ability of the Inuit to adapt to the harsh environment of the Arctic has also played an important role in survival. One of the most important of the cultural adaptations was the use of caribou skin for clothing. Caribou skins were used for winter clothing as well as mattresses and coverings on sleeping platforms. The insulation of the caribou skins allowed the Inuit to function in a cold environment. As discussed by Stenton (1989) the use of caribou skins more than any other cultural feature allowed them to brave the elements to move camps in order to follow sources of food and to hunt. These skins were so important to the functioning and health of the population that their scarcity resulted in a fall in the birth rate and an increase in susceptibility to disease (Stenton, 1989).

The traditional habitat of the majority of the Inuit was the igloo, or snowhouse, in the winter and a skin tent insulated with moss in the summer. Both were effective in providing an environment that, with the use of seal-oil lamps, was considerably warmer than the external environment. The Inuit were also accustomed to the cold Arctic winters. They avoided travel and remained inside their shelters during periods of extreme cold and winds thus minimizing exposure to cold when possible (Foutch and Mills, 1988).

Implications for nursing care

It is very important for the nurse caring for Inuit clients to appreciate the Inuk client's perspective on environmental control and to appreciate that the client may feel little control over powerful elements the client believes may account for an illness or disease. Assisting the client to feel personal control and to see a correlation between both personal actions and preventing illness as well as treating illness is a significant challenge for the nurse working with the Inuk client. The nurse needs to appreciate that the Inuit client's attitude toward the cause of the illness can play a large part in how successful treatment or taking any action directed at treatment will be (Hodgson, 1980).

BIOLOGICAL VARIATIONS

The major causes of death for the Inuit are injury, suicide, respiratory disease, and cancer. Injuries are a major cause of death in Inuit children, adolescents, and young adults (Government of the Northwest Territories, 1996; Koglin, 1977). The causes of death are related to their unique susceptibility to disease and to factors in the environment.

Body structure and visible physical characteristics

The Inuit differ from all other Native Canadians in their physical features, which are decidedly Asiatic. All Eskimos and Aleuts are classified with eastern Siberian native peoples in a category known as "Arctic mongoloids" (Price, 1979). The Inuit have straight black hair. Physical growth of the Inuit is different because of evolutionary adaptation to the Arctic environment in which they live. The two basic theories regarding climate and physical adaptation are the Allen and Bergmann rules. Bergmann's rule, according to Ruff (1991), states that the cooler the climate the heavier the individual in relation to height. The result is that the proportion of mass to surface area is increased, and this condition results in an increase in the amount of heat retained. Allen's rule, as described by Ruff (1991), is that in colder climates the length of appendages will be reduced in relation to trunk size. Similarly Jong, Tigchelaar, and Godwin

(1996) noted that the growth of Inuit children tended to be shorter and heavier in comparison to National Center for Health Statistics (NCHS) percentages. The result is a decrease of surface area and therefore less heat loss from that surface area. Both Bergmann's rule and Allen's rule serve to decrease the ratio of surface area to mass. This reduction retards the heat loss by the individual.

Jamison (1990) studied growth in arctic populations of North America from data collected in the 1960s and 1970s. This study used the NCHS percentages as a baseline value for comparison. He found that the Inuit/Eskimo population was between the 5th and 25th percentile for height and between the 25th and 50th percentile for weight. The relationship between height and weight was between the 75th and 90th percentile, an indication of a higher weight per unit of height than the NCHS standard. The percentage of body fat was determined by use of triceps skinfold measurements, and the percentage of body fat was found to be below the 50th percentile for all Eskimos and below the 5th percentile for Canadian Inuit. This study supports physical adaptation of the Eskimo population in accordance with Bergmann's rule. Jamison (1990) also reports that in earlier studies it was demonstrated that the proportion between body height and limb length in the Eskimo populations supports Allen's rule.

Similar findings to support Bergman's and Allen's rules are reported by Johnston and his colleagues (1982) on recent measurements of Eskimo children and youths. In addition, they (Johnson et al., 1982) studied the lean body mass of their subjects and found a higher lean body mass per unit weight than that in other populations. They concluded that this higher lean body mass is a physical adaptation that provides an increased amount of heat-producing tissue.

Enzymatic and genetic variations

Hepatitis B prevalence has been studied in various Inuit communities in the circumpolar region. Many studies have documented the prevalence of serological markers (Young, 1994).

Susceptibility to disease

Botulism Botulism has special significance in certain Native populations and can be considered a "culture-bound" disease. In Canada between 1971 and 1984, 61 outbreaks involving 122 cases and 21 deaths were reported. Ninety-three percent of the cases were Inuit. All Native cases belong to type E (Hauschild and Gauvreau, 1985).

Respiratory disease The rates of death from respiratory disease in the Inuit population, especially women in the Northwest Territories is 2.5 times the Canadian rate (Government of the Northwest Territories, 1996). Death was primarily attributable to chronic obstructive pulmonary disease (COPD), likely related to heavy cigarette smoking. Tobacco was first introduced by whalers and traders and became a staple consumable and trade item and an integral part of Inuit lifestyle. Bjerregaard (1983) found elevated rates of respiratory infections among Greenland Inuit related to poor housing and being in the lowest social class.

Acute rheumatic fever The incidence of acute rheumatic fever has been declining in the developing countries since the 1920s, even before the advent of antibiotics. This disease however, persists in low-income inner-city neighborhoods and certain minority populations of Native Americans. A study among Indian and Inuit children in the Northwest Territories and Manitoba in the 1970s indicated that the Native incidence rate was 125 of 100,000 compared to 29 of 100,000 among non-Natives (Longstaffe, Postl, Kao, Nicolle, and Ferguson, 1982).

Hydatid Disease Hydatid disease is caused by various species of the *Echinococcus* cestode (a small tapeworm). In communities where dogs live in proximity to human beings, poor domestic hygiene increases the likelihood of human infections. A large number of cases have been reported in northern Canada and Alaska. With the decline of the dogsled in transportation, this disease has declined substantially. A recent survey in northern Quebec found that only 1% of Inuit have diagnostic titers (Tanner, Staudt, and Adamowski et al.,1987).

Cancer The overall cancer incidence in the Northwest Territories is 20% higher than for the rest of the general population of Canada. The most common cancers found in the Inuit population are lung cancer, cancer in situ of the cervix, and bowel cancer. Although there has not been a high incidence of breast cancer in the past, this trend seems to be changing as the life expectancy increases and may also be related to changes in the Inuit diet (Government of the Northwest Territories, 1996). Of particular interest is the extremely high risk of several cancers in the Eskimo/Inuit that are relatively rare in other populations: nasopharyngeal, salivary gland, and esophageal cancer (Hildes and Schaefer, 1984).

Sexually transmitted diseases Sexually transmitted disease (STD) is the most common of the reportable diseases (Government of the Northwest Territories, 1996). Seroprevalence surveys of antibodies to *Chlamydia, Cytomegalovirus,* and *Herpesvirus* organisms in the Canadian Inuit population have shown higher levels than that in other non-Native residents in the same settlements (Nicolle, Minuk, and Postl, 1986). *Chlamydia* antibodies have been identified in 80% of Canadian Inuit in one community (Kordov′a, Wilt, Sekla, et al., 1983). Because there has been a high rate of STDs in the Northwest Territories, there has been concern about HIV being introduced. As of March 1996, only 28 residents with HIV in the Northwest Territories including all ethnic groups have been reported.

Tuberculosis Because the 1920s tuberculosis has been a problem for aboriginal people of the Northwest Territories including the Inuit. Bergmen (1996) reports medical surveys of tuberculosis on the *C.D. Howe,* a ship that brought mail and supplies to hunting camps and settlements in the 1940s and the attempts to reunite Inuit families in the Arctic who were separated in the 1950s in an attempt to control a tuberculosis epidemic. The current incidence is seven times the overall Canadian rate (Government of the Northwest Territories, 1996). In the 1960s the Inuit had a dramatically high rate of tuberculosis compared to other groups. These cases seemed to be related rather to inadequate treatment in the 1960s and 1970s resulting in reactivation though for a while it was believed that tuberculosis must be a "racial characteristic" of the Inuit. Unlike tuberculosis cases in other parts of North America the tuberculosis present in the Northwest Territories has not been drug resistant and the rate among the Inuit is now less than that of Indians (Young, 1994).

Meningitis The high case rate of meningitis appears to be associated with a high carriage rate of the organisms in the general population in Inuit communities. In a 1980 survey of nasopharyngeal carriage of meningococci and *Haemophilus influenzae* in Baker Lake in the central Arctic, 32% of the Inuit were found to carry the former and 16% the latter (Nicolle, Postl, and Kotelewetz, et al., 1982).

Nutritional preferences and deficiencies Although nutritional patterns vary from one Inuit to the next and one community to the next, a dietary analysis of 366 Inuit in a Baffin Island community provides some data on dietary patterns. Traditional foods contributed 30% to 40% of the average daily energy intake, with sea mammals providing the greater quantity and variety of traditional food, followed by land animals, fish, birds and eggs, berries, and shellfish. Traditional food intake varied by season, gender, and most importantly age. Younger people tended to eat less traditional food than their elders and conversely more market food. Sucrose intake in the younger age groups was high, as well as tea and coffee consumption in all age and gender categories (Kuhnlein, Soueida, and Receveur, 1995, 1996). Laghi (1997) reported that contaminants are being found in seal and whale blubber in the Arctic and they could increase the risk of subtle memory and learning impairments among unborn Inuit children. However, it is noted that despite the potential health problems the nutritional advantages of a traditional Inuit diet outweigh any potential health problems.

Psychological characteristics Death by suicide in the Northwest Territories is 5.7 times the Canadian national rate. It is of particular concern to the Inuit because most suicides in the Northwest Territories occur among the Inuit, with 80.8% occurring among males who hang themselves (Health and Welfare Canada, 1991). It has been suggested that the high suicide is related to the home situation and deteriorating childrearing practices. Parents, frustrated by the overwhelmingly rapid culture change, involved in alcohol abuse, and suffering from frequent family disasters, have little time or emotional resources to give to their children. Frequent experience of bereavement and exposure to pain through neglect, hunger, physical abuse, and disease cause many Inuit children to grow up scared and depressed with few inner resources to deal with stress (Health and Welfare Canada, 1991).

Implications for nursing care

In caring for the Inuit client the nurse needs to recognize that the Inuit stature is unique and that growth and development may differ from the norms set by White-based growth and development. Therefore behavior that might be considered an "abnormality" must be evaluated by comparison with other Inuit.

The Inuit have evolved to survive in an Arctic environment, and as a result consideration should be given to this particularly if it is necessary for them to travel to southern Canada for medical treatment. They are used to temperatures that do not go above 15 degrees Celsius and a humidity that is very dry. Being in Ottawa in August especially when the Celsius temperature is often in the 30s with high humidity can be unbearable, especially for the old. Efforts should be made to avoid elective referrals in summer months, and when they do occur, every effort should be made to minimize the effect of the change in climate.

SUMMARY

The Inuit have long held a fascination for southern Canadians (McMillan, 1995). This group of people has truly lived on the fringe of the habitable world. Through centuries of habitation in the Arctic, the Inuit have learned ingenious methods of survival against formidable odds in the Arctic's harsh environment (Morrison and Wilson, 1986). Working with the modern Inuk client presents a challenge to the nurse to demonstrate cultural sensitivity and creativity in meeting the culturally influenced health care needs of these unique clients.

Case Study

During a home visit the nurse notes that James, a 4-year-old Inuk, has a perforated right tympanic membrane with a small amount of purulent discharge. The left tympanic membrane shows scar tissue consistent with previous tympanic perforations. According to his chart he had visited the clinic 5 days ago because of a fever and was diagnosed as having right otitis media. The treatment included an antibiotic to be taken four times a day. When asked, the mother stated that James had not liked the medicine and took it only three times. She admits that since James was a baby he has had numerous ear infections and that she seldom gave him the entire bottle of medicine because he did not want it or because he seemed better. James is on the 50th percentile for weight and the 5th percentile for height. The nurse notes that his language skills are below normal using the Denver Developmental screening. James has significant dental decay of his front teeth. The mother is unable to provide basic information about his diet or sleeping habits, and when asked specific questions, she asks James for the answers.

CARE PLAN

 Nursing Diagnosis   Effective management of individual therapeutic regimen, related to cultural attitude that gives the child great independence as evidenced by not forcing the child to take a medication that he does not like.

Client Outcomes

1. Client will take entire amount of prescription as ordered.

Nursing Interventions

1. Explain to James and his mother using a video, diagram, or audio recording the importance of taking the entire bottle of antibiotic each time James gets an earache.
2. Use pictures of a clock, the bottle of medication, a teaspoon, calendar, face of boy with earache, smiling face of boy when his ear is better, and smiling face when the medication is all used up.
3. Encourage James to be responsible for medication regardless of where he is eating or sleeping. Thus he can carry it with him at all times. He must watch the clock and take his medication each time it is due.

 Nursing Diagnosis   Altered health maintenance related to insufficient knowledge of dental hygiene as evidenced by James having significant dental decay of his front teeth.

Client Outcomes

1. Client will state his understanding of good dental hygiene.

Nursing Interventions

1. Explain basic tooth-brushing technique to James and his mother using a toothbrush, toothpaste, and a glass of water.
2. Ask James to demonstrate in turn how to brush his teeth.
3. Explain when to brush teeth using pictures of child eating, getting up from sleep, and going to bed.
4. Encourage the mother to breast-feed her future infants as a basis for good tooth formation. Tell story of how putting the baby to bed with a bottle can cause tooth decay. Explain that giving a bottle of water would rinse out the mouth to lessen the bacteria.

5. Ask mother to explain how she plans to feed her next infant.
6. Inform James and his mother of the importance of having teeth examined and repaired. Regular dental care will prevent future toothaches and loss of permanent teeth.
7. Ask James and his mother to explain their understanding of dental checkups.

 Nursing Diagnosis Impaired communicaton related to frequent ear infections as evidenced by below-normal language skills.

Client Outcomes	*Nursing Interventions*
1. Client will be assessed for hearing, speech, and IQ.	1. Arrange to have professional assessment of hearing, speech, and IQ at next clinic visit.
2. Client will be treated and referred for assistance with language skills.	2. Refer client for language development based on needs.
	3. Teach mother activities that will promote language development in James. The Inuit are not very verbal; therefore James may be developmentally slow because of lack of verbal stimulation. Small physical size is the average normal for this culture.

STUDY QUESTIONS

1. Describe reasons for the needed adjustment to the environment for the Inuit of Nunavut.
2. Discuss one reason suicide has such a high prevalence among the Inuit of Nunavut.
3. Identify at least three diseases that the Inuit of Nunavut have a high susceptibility to contract.
4. List at least two barriers to communication for the nurse who does not speak the Inuit language in the care of the Inuk client.
5. Discuss the historical significance of the new territory set aside for the Inuit (Nunavut) and identify possible health care concerns.

References

Adamson, J., Moody, J., Peart, A., et al. (1949). Poliomyelitis in the arctic. *Canadian Medical Association Journal, 61,* 339-348.

Bergman, B. (1992). A test of will. *Maclean's, 105*(18), 20.

Bergman, B. (1996). Dark days for the Inuit. *Maclean's, 109*(10), 66.

Bjerregaard, P. (1983). Housing standards, social group, and respiratory infections in children of Upernavik, Greenland. *Scandinavian Journal of Social Medicine, 11,* 107-111.

Brody, H. (1975). *The people's land: Whites and the eastern Arctic.* Markham, Ont.: Penguin Books.

Browne, (1995). The meaning of respect: a First Nations perspectives. *Canadian Journal of Nursing Research, 27*(4), 95-109.

Canada Notes. (1996). Compensating the Inuit. *Maclean's, 109*(15), 25.

Collis, R.F. (1990). *Arctic languages: an awakening.* Paris, France: Inprimerie des Presses Universitaires de France, Vendôme.

Damas, D. (1984). Copper Eskimo. In Sturtevant, C. (Ed.), *Handbook of North American Indians* (vol. 5, pp. 397-414). Washington, D.C.: Smithsonian Institution.

Daviss, B. (1996). Heeding warnings from the canary, the whale, and the Inuit: a framework for analyzing competing types of knowledge about childbirth. Part 1. *Midwifery Today and Childbirth Education,* (40), 45-53.

Dewdney, S., & Arbuckle, F. (1975). *They shared to survive: the native peoples of Canada.* Toronto: Macmillan.

Edgecombe, N.A. (1994). *Value orientation of the Copper Inuit.* Unpublished master's thesis, University of Alberta, Edmonton, AB.

Foutch, R.G., & Mills, W.J. (1988). Treatment and prevention of cold injuries by ancient peoples indigenous to arctic and subarctic regions. *Arctic Medical Research, 47*(suppl. 1), 286-289.

Government of Canada. (1991). *Statistics Canada: age composition.* Ottawa: Statistics Canada.

Government of the Northwest Territories. (1996). *Health and health services in the N.W.T.* Yellowknife, N.W.T.: Department of Health and Social Services.

Government of the Northwest Territories. (1997). *Health and health services in the N.W.T.* Yellowknife, N.W.T.: Department of Health and Social Services.

Government of the Northwest Territories. (1997). *Nunavut/Western NWT fact sheet.* Yellowknife, N.W.T.: Bureau of Statistics.

Hanson, A.M. (1997). *The Nunavut handbook.* Iqaluit, NT.

Hauschild, A.H., & Gauvreau, L. (1985). Food-borne botulism in Canada, 1971-84. *Canadian Medical Association Journal, 133*(11), 1141-1146.

Health and Welfare Canada. (1991). *Health status of Canadian Indians and Inuit 1990.* Ottawa, Ont.: Department of National Health and Welfare.

Hildes, J., & Schaefer, O. (1984). The changing picture of neoplastic disease in the western and central Canadian arctic (1950-1980). *Canadian Medical Association Journal, 30,* 25-33.

Hodgson, C. (1980). Transcultural nursing: the Canadian experience. *The Canadian Nurse, 76*(6), 23-25.

Houston, J. (1997). *Confessions of an igloo dweller: memories of the old Arctic.* Boston: Houghton Mifflin.

Internet on Canada. (1997, September 11). *Canada.*

Irvine, R. (1987). Nursing education moves to the north. *The Canadian Nurse, 93*(2), 16-18.

Jamison, P.L. (1990). Secular trends and patterns of growth in arctic populations. *Social Science and Medicine, 30,* 751-759.

Jenness, D. (1922). *Report of the Canadian arctic expedition 1913-1918* (vol. XII). Ottawa: F.A. Acland.

Jepson, T., Lee, P., & Smith, T. (1995). *Canada.* London: The Penguin Group.

Johnston, F.E., Laughlin, W.S., Harper, A.B., & Ensroth, A.E. (1982). Physical growth of St. Lawrence Island Eskimo: body size, proportion, and composition. *American Journal of Physical Anthropology, 58,* 397-401.

Jong, M., Tigchelaar, T., & Godwin, M. (1996). *Growth parameters of Inuit children in coastal Labrador.* Presentation at International Congress for Circumpolar Health, June 1994, Anchorage, Alaska.

Kehoe, A.B. (1981). *North American Indians: a comprehensive account.* Englewood Cliffs, N.J.: Prentice-Hall.

Koglin, O.H. (1997, February 26). Report says Blacks, Indians live shorter lives in Oregon. *The Oregonian,* p. B1.

Kordová, N., Wilt, J.C., & Sekla, L. et al. (1983). High prevalence of antibodies to *Chlamydia trachomatis* in a northern Canadian community. *Canadian Journal of Public Health, 74,* 246-249.

Kuhnlein, H.V., Soueida, R., & Receveur, O. (1995). Baffin Inuit food use by age, gender and season. *Journal of the Canadian Dietetic Association, 56*(4), 175-183.

Kuhnlein, H.V., Soueida, R., & Receveur, O. (1996). Dietary nutrient profiles of Canadian Baffin Island Inuit differ by food source, season, and age. *Journal of the American Dietetic Association, 96*(2), 155-162.

Laghi, B. (1997, June 1). Inuit children may be at risk from fatty diet. *Toronto Globe and Mail, 5.*

Loken, O. (1997). *The Nunavut handbook.* Iqaluit, NT.

Longstaffe, S., Postl, B., Kao, H., Nicolle, L., & Ferguson, C. (1982). Rheumatic fever in native children in Manitoba. *Canadian Medical Association Journal, 127,* 497-498.

Mailhot, J. (1978). L'étymologie de «Esquimau» revue et corrigée. Études Inuit— Inuit Studies, 2, 59-69.

McMillan, A.D. (1995). *Native peoples and cultures of Canada* (ed. 2). Toronto: Douglas & McIntyre.

Morrison, R.B., & Wilson, C.R. (Eds.). (1986). *Native peoples: the Canadian experience.* Toronto: McClelland & Stewart.

Morrison, R.B., & Wilson, C.R. (1995). *Native peoples: the Canadian experience* (ed. 2). Toronto: McClelland & Stewart.

Murdoch, J. (1984). A bibliography of Algonquian syllabic texts in Canadian repositories. Montreal: Gouvernement du Québec, Ministères des Affaires culturelles, Direction régionale du Nouveau Québec et service aux autochtones.

Nicolle, L.E., Minuk, G.Y., & Postl, B. (1986). Cross-sectional seroepidemiologic study of the prevalence of cytomegalovirus and herpes simplex virus infection in a Canadian Inuit (Eskimo) community. *Scandinavian Journal of Disease, 18,* 19-23.

Nicolle, L.E., Postl, B., & Kotelewetz, E., et al. (1982). Emergence of rifampin-resistant *Haemophilus influenzae. Antimicrobial Agents and Chemotherapy, 21,* 498-500.

Norris, N. (1990). The demography of aboriginal people in Canada. In Hall, S.S., Travato, F., & Driedger, L. (Eds.), *Ethnic demography: Canadian immigrant, racial and cultural variations* (pp. 33-59). Ottawa: Carleton University Press.

Nowak, Elke. (1998, Feb.) Personal communication, Stuttgart, Germany.

O'Leary, T.J., & Levinson, D. (Volume Eds.). (1991). *Encyclopedia of world cultures* (vol. 1). Boston: G.K. Hall & Co.

O'Neil, J.D., Gilbert, P., Kusugak, N., St. John, C., Kaufert, P.L., Moffat, M.E., Brown, R., & Postl, B. (1991). Obstetric policy for the Keewatin region, N.W.T.: results of the childbirth experience survey. In Postl, B.D., Gilbert, P., Goodwill, J., Moffat, M.E.K., O'Neil, J.D., Sarafield, P.A., & Young, T.K. (Eds.), *Circumpolar Health 90: Proceedings of the 18th International Congress on Circumpolar Health* (pp. 572-576). Winnipeg: The Canadian Society for Circumpolar Health.

Peart, A., & Nagler, F. (1954). Measles in the Canadian arctic 1952. *Canadian Journal of Public Health, 45,* 146-157.

Pollick, S. (1997, June 18). *Our Land will seek identity.* Toledo, Ohio: The Blade.

Price, J. (1979). *Indians of Canada: cultural dynamics.* Scarborough, Ont.: Prentice-Hall.

Qinuajuak, L. (1996). Inuit birth traditions. *Midwifery Today and Childbirth Education,* (40), 56.

Rasmussen, K. (1932). *Intellectual culture of the Copper Eskimos. Report of the fifth Thule expedition, 1921-1924* (vol. 9). Copenhagen: Gyldendalske Boghandel.

Robitaille, N., & Choinière, R. (1985). *An overview of the demographic and socio-economic conditions of the Inuit of Canada.* Ottawa: Research Branch. Corporate Policy, Indian and Northern Affairs, Canada.

Ruff, C.B. (1991). Climate and body shape in hominid evolution. *Journal of Human Evolution, 21*(2), 81-105.

Ryan, J. (1992). Eroding Innu cultural tradition: individualization and communality. *Journal of Canadian Studies, 26*(4), 94.

Smith, S. (1979). Coming to terms with reality. *Canadian Nursing Journal,* 11, 20-21.

Statistics Canada. (1991). *Statistics Canada information.* Ottawa: Department of Health and Social Services.

Statistics Canada. (1995). *Profile of Canada's aboriginal population.* Ottawa: Industry, science and technology, 1991 Census of Canada. Catalogue number 94-325.

Stefansson, V. (1913). *My life with the Eskimo.* New York: Macmillan Publishing Co.

Stenton, D.R. (1989). *Terrestrial adaptation of neo-Eskimo coastal-marine hunters on southern Baffin Island, NWT.* Unpublished doctoral dissertation, University of Alberta, Alberta.

Swayze, N. (1960). *The man hunters: famous Canadian anthropologists.* Toronto: Clarke, Irwin.

Tanner, C.E., Staudt, M., Adamowski, R., et al. (1987). Seroepidemiological study for five different zoonotic parasites in northern Quebec, *Canadian Journal of Public Health, 78*(4), 262-266.

Udvardy, M. (1977). *The Audubon society field guide to North American birds, western region.* New York: Knopf.

Young, T. (1994). *The health of Native Americans.* New York: Oxford University Press.

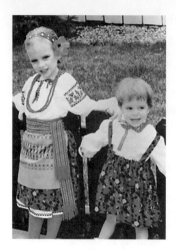

CHAPTER 15
Ukrainian Canadians

Marjorie Linwood

BEHAVIORAL OBJECTIVES

After reading this chapter, the nurse will be able to:

1. Appreciate the pride experienced by Canadians of Ukrainian heritage.
2. Demonstrate sensitivity and understanding to verbal and nonverbal communications of Canadians with Ukrainian heritage.
3. Appreciate the role of space for traditional Ukrainians.
4. Recognize the influence of social organization and religious heritage on current practices by Canadians of Ukrainian heritage.
5. Recognize the past and future time orientation of many Canadians of Ukrainian heritage.
6. Describe the cultural health practices of Canadians of Ukrainian heritage in relation to health-seeking and illness behaviors.
7. Identify the relationship between cultural practices and behavior within the health care system.
8. Describe nutritional preferences of Canadians with Ukrainian heritage.

OVERVIEW OF THE UKRAINE

The Ukraine (meaning 'border, edge') is the third largest autonomous country to emerge from the collapse of the Soviet Union (USSR) in 1991 (The New Encyclopaedia Britannica, 1997). As of 1991 it is now officially called "Ukraine." With a land mass of 233,100 miles, Ukraine is slightly smaller than the province of Alberta (World Almanac, 1997). The Ukraine is located in the southwest corner of the former USSR. Its southern border forms the larger part of the north shore of the Black Sea and the Sea of Azov. To the west of Ukraine is Romania and Moldova, Hungary, Slovakia, and Poland; to the north Belarus; and to the north and east the Russian Federation. Ukraine is situated between northern latitude 44 degrees to 52 degrees, roughly comparable to Windsor, Ontario, and Calgary, Alberta, respectively. The southernmost point of Ukraine, which juts out into the Black Sea and provides a warm, resort climate, is Crimea, which is on a peninsula. The climate in Ukraine is continental with cold winters and hot summers except where tempered by the Black Sea and proximity to the Mediterranean.

Ukraine consists almost entirely of level plains at an average elevation of 574 feet above sea level (The New Encyclopaedia Britannica, 1997). However, Ukraine has mountainous areas on two borders, the Ukrainian Carpathian mountains in the extreme southwest and the Crimean mountains in the south.

Additionally, on the west, the Dnieper Upland is abutted by the rugged Volyn-Podolsk Upland, which rises to 1549 feet at its highest point, Mount Kamula. The Dnepr, or Dnieper, is a river that bisects the country flowing south and emptying into the Black Sea. In Ukrainian song and poetry the Dnieper is a favorite subject. Immediately to the west and to the east of Ukraine's borders and also emptying into the Black Sea are the rivers of the Danube and the Volga, also made famous in song.

Ukraine has fertile soil that supports the growth of fruits, vegetables, and grains and cattle production for domestic use and export. Ukraine's crop production is highly developed. Its grain output rivals that of Germany, its potato output is among the highest in Europe, and it is the world's largest producer of sugar beets. Fishing occurs in the seas and rivers but is declining because of pollution. Pollution increased significantly during the Soviet period. In fact, lack of pollution controls has resulted in serious effects on the environment. Today Ukraine is recognized for having some of the most polluted areas in the world (The New Encyclopaedia Britannica, 1997).

Ukraine has rich natural resources, especially huge deposits of hard coal, iron, oil, and gas. There is industrial development especially in the Dnieper valley, but mining and industry suffer from outmoded practices and outdated machinery, and industrial casualties are frequent. Ukraine has five nuclear power stations. In April 1986, the world's worst nuclear power plant disaster occurred in Chernobyl when the plant was destroyed by an explosion and fire. The disaster was later discovered to be attributable to the fault of substandard materials (Moynahan, 1994).

Today, more than 50 million people live in Ukraine, of which 11 million are Russians (World Almanac, 1997). Ukrainians and Russians are Eastern Slavs, Kiyiv, or Kiev, is the capital and largest city of the Ukraine with 2.6 million people (World Almanac, 1997). Other large cities are Kharkov, Donetsk, Odessa, and Dnepropetrovsk. The republic of Ukraine is divided into 25 subdivisions (Edwards, 1993).

The life expectancy for the average Ukrainian (1996) is 62 for males and 72 for females with an infant mortality of 23 per 1000 (World Almanac, 1997). This is in contrast to the general life expectancy in Canada of 76 for males and 83 for females with an infant mortality of 6 per 1000 (World Almanac, 1997). The Ukrainian per capita gross domestic product (GDP) is $3,650 dollars (World Almanac, 1997).

The present constitution specifies Ukrainian as the state language but allows for use of several alternative languages in communities where a large ethnic population predominates including Russian, Romanian, Polish, Belarussian, Bulgarian, and Hungarian (Lindheim and Luckyi, 1996; The New Encyclopaedia Britannica, 1997). For example, Russian is the language taught in the Russian-speaking area in the Crimea (The New Encyclopaedia Britannica, 1997). The freedom to speak Ukrainian or Russian has not always been present. Under Soviet domination, the use of the Ukrainian language and the publication of books in Ukrainian was suppressed, and Russian was the required official language (The New Encyclopaedia Britannica, 1997).

Ukrainians take pride in their cultural tradition, which is part of a broader Slavic culture but retains a distinctive national flavor In the countryside, outdoor festivals feature brightly colored folk costumes, dance, and traditional music. Urban life is enriched by a large number of performing arts facilities and other cultural institutions (The New Encyclopaedia Britannica, 1997). Through years of political oppression, the song, dance, folklore, and literature have helped to maintain unique Ukrainian customs and cultural folkways.

The role of women is evident to outsiders in the beautiful symbolic and colorful cross-stitch embroideries for costumes and table and church linens. In Pysanka the art of Easter-egg decorating is passed on from mother to daughter or grandchild just as the baking of braided breads, poppy-seed or honey cakes, borshch, pierogi (*pyrohy*), and cabbage rolls. However, women have traditionally also been almost equal partners in tending the farm and land and have been socially, politically, and culturally active (Rudnytska, 1934). As early as the 1880s there was a distinctive women's movement, organized to promote day care, education, and liberation of women (Lindheim and Luckyi, 1996).

In the present Ukrainian Constitution, every citizen has a right to general and free access to elementary through vocational and secondary education. The literacy rate is 98% (World Almanac, 1997).

During some periods of occupation in Ukrainian history, religion was strongly discouraged. Today the most predominant religion is Ukrainian Orthodoxy with the second most prevalent being Ukrainian Catholicism (World Almanac, 1997). The Ukraine has a rich and turbulent history. Ukrainians have repeatedly struggled for independence. The ancient ancestors of the Ukrainians, the Trypilians, flourished along the Dnieper from 6000 to 1000 B.C. The Slavic ancestors of the Ukrainians inhabited modern Ukrainian territory well before the first century of our era. In the ninth century the princes of Kiev established a strong state called "Kievan Rus'," which included much of present-day Ukraine. A strong dynasty was established with ties to virtually all major European royal families. St. Vladimir the Great, ruler of Kievan Rus', accepted Christianity as the national faith in 988. At the crossroads of European trade routes, Kievan Rus' reached its zenith under Yaroslav the Wise (1019-1054). Internal conflicts led to the disintegration of the Ukrainian state into principalities by the time of the Asian invasion of Europe in the thirteenth century. Mongol rule was supplanted by Poland and Lithuania in the fourteenth and fifteenth centuries. The Black Sea coast and Crimea came under the control of the Turks in 1478 (World Almanac, 1997).

Ukrainian Cossacks, starting in the late sixteenth century, waged numerous wars of liberation against the occupiers of Ukraine—Russia, Poland, and Turkey. During the years of subjugation of the Ukraine by the Russian Tsarina (Empress) Catherine II (1762-1796), German Mennonite farmers were invited to settle in the Ukraine. Between 1789 and 1840 many Mennonites found this opportunity for land attractive and energetically promoted agricultural, industrial, and business development (Dyck and Dyck, 1991). At the beginning of the 1800s, the Ukraine was occupied by Russia and Austria-Hungary.

Although most of the Ukraine was rich in natural resources and some Mennonite landowners were prospering, many other Ukrainians had little benefit in the presence of Russian empire policies. It was at this time that Ukrainians from the western region provinces of Galicia, Bukovina, and Transcarpathia, which were considered among the poorest and overpopulated regions of Europe, began to emigrate to Canada (Subtelny, 1991). The basic cause of poverty of the peasants was the use of them as cheap labor in a system of serfdom. In 1848, even though serfdom was abolished and the peasants could buy land, the landlords maintained their ownership of the forests and pastures, and the peasants had to pay for pastures to feed their stock, for wood to build their homes, and for firewood. Because of the Ukrainian custom of dividing land among the children, farms grew smaller and even less self-supporting. By 1902 80% of the peasants were desperately poor (Kostash, 1992). Health care was almost nonexistent. A morbidity of 50% for children was in part attributable to epidemics of communicable disease but mostly to malnutrition. The life expectancy of a male Ukrainian was 13 years less than that of an Englishman (Subtelny, 1991). For many Ukrainians the only prospect for improvement and life for their children appeared to be emigration. The offer of free land in Canada for farmers was very attractive.

The independent Ukrainian People's Republic was proclaimed in 1918. In 1922, Ukraine became a constituent republic of the USSR as the Ukrainian SSR. During the five-year plan that Stalin used to control the economy, private farms, especially in the Ukraine, were taken over to produce state-owned and state-controlled collective farms in which former landowners, many of them Mennonites, were forced to become cheap labor (Dyck and Dyck, 1991). Before 1917 about 75,000 Mennonites lived in the Ukraine (The Mennonite Encyclopedia, 1959). However, when communist rule eliminated private land ownership, they fled, were killed, or were exiled to Siberian work camps (The Mennonite Encyclopedia, 1959). In 1932 and 1933, when the Ukrainian peasantry resisted, the Soviet government engineered a man-made famine in the eastern Ukraine, resulting in the deaths of as many as 10 million Ukrainians (World Almanac, 1997; Edwards, 1993; Times Atlas, 1996). During this time many Ukrainians and the formerly German Mennonites living in the Ukraine saw emigration as an opportunity to remain alive.

In March 1939, independent Carpatho-Ukraine was the first European state to wage war against Nazi-led aggression in the region. During World Ward II, the Ukrainian nationalist underground and its Ukrainian Insurgent Army fought both Nazi German and Soviet forces. The restoration of Ukrainian independence was declared in June 1941. Over 5 million Ukrainians lost their lives during the war. However, with the reoccupation of the Ukraine by Soviet troops in 1944 came a renewed wave of mass arrests, executions, and deportations of Ukrainians. Again, some Ukrainians attempted to emigrate to avoid Soviet rule, and ethnic Germans who had moved to the Ukraine saw it as a way to stay alive because they were now associated with the enemy.

Ukrainian independence was restored in December 1991 with the dissolution of the Soviet Union. However, in the post-Soviet period Ukraine has been burdened with a deteriorating economy and almost nonexistent health care (Johnson, 1994). Subsequent to its change in status Ukraine has had some internal strife, with the west of it being more nationalistic and land based and the east being more industrialized and influenced by Russia in language and outlook (Moynahan, 1994). Some of the controversy with Russia centered on the Crimea. In 1991 and 1992 the Crimean Tatars took part in unsuccessful ethnic uprisings against Russian minorities. The peninsula city of Sevastpol is home port of the Black Sea fleet, to which Ukraine and Russia each laid claim, whereas Yalta has been the winter haven for Muskovites. However, in 1995, Russia and Ukraine reached an agreement on the disputed Black Sea fleet at Sevastopol. After a 1994 accord with Russia and the United States, Ukraine's large nuclear arsenal was deactivated in June 1996. A new constitution was approved by parliament in June 1996 legalizing private property and establishing Ukrainian as the sole official language of the Ukraine (World Almanac, 1997).

Ukrainians left for Canada in three waves. Most of the Ukrainians who left their homes during the late 1800s did so for socioeconomic reasons. Whereas eastern Ukrainians were moved to the Russian empire in the Asian territories, the Ukrainians from the west emigrated to Canada in the late 1800s and early part of the twentieth century. Immigration into Canada began with two peasants from the Kalush district of Galicia who traveled to Canada in 1891 to inspect opportunities for securing free homestead land reported from emigrated ethnic Germans from the same district. A year later a slow trickle of Ukrainians, almost all from the village of Nebyliw in Kalush and mostly related by blood or marriage, began to settle in Alberta around Star (Lehr, 1992). However, in 1896 the number of immigrants dramatically increased in volume to include emigrants from the province of Bukovina. Guided by officials of the Department of the Interior, some chose lands in Saskatchewan and Manitoba, laying the foundation of the distinctive geography of Ukrainian settlement, which had clearly emerged by 1900 (Lehr, 1992).

The immigrants before 1914 were mostly peasant farmers bent on securing land. A high proportion were illiterate, and the majority were poor. They were by no means a homogeneous group but rather included members of many ethnographic Ukrainian subgroups (Lehr, 1992). By 1914 some 170,000 Ukrainians occupied thousands of square miles of agricultural land, virtually all obtained under the homestead and preemption provisions of the Dominion Lands Act, whereby homestead spaces were spread out across the prairie in a deliberate plan to keep the density of the population low (Darcovich and Yusyk, 1977).

Later in the 1930s an additional wave of Ukrainians fled Soviet Russia for political and economic reasons in relation to Stalin's Five-Year Plan. Finally, in the 1940s a third wave of emigrants left to avoid the hazards of reoccupation by the Soviets.

Today in western Canada there are 406,645 people who describe themselves as Ukrainians (Statistics Canada, 1996). Ukrainians rank fifth in size as an ethnic group (Subtelny, 1991). Although most of these Canadians have assimilated themselves into the general population, they still view themselves with self-defined characteristics and a unique cultural heritage. It is important for the nurse providing care to the Canadian client with a Ukrainian heritage to understand Ukrainian customs and traditions in order to provide culturally competent care (Masi, Mensah, and McLeod, 1995; Burch, 1990).

COMMUNICATION

The language spoken by most of the original immigrants from the Ukraine is Ukrainian. Some persons who immigrated to Canada in the 1930s have maintained Ukrainian as their first language although approximately 75% speak some degree of English (Statistics Canada, 1991, Table 2.4). Today most persons of Ukrainian descent speak both Ukrainian and English. Many churches have their services in both Ukrainian and English to satisfy all Ukrainian Canadians and to respect the language needs of those members of intermarriage. The Ukrainian accent in the English language is now considered by some to be a dialect of English (Kostash, 1992).

Ukrainian immigrants to Canada tended to continue to speak and write in Ukrainian. Early settlers established over 400 schools where Ukrainian was the language in the classroom These schools were eliminated in 1916, but private Ukrainian organizations have provided opportunities for later generations to learn the language in heritage schools in special sessions after public school (Kostash, 1992). Today, 166,830 Ukrainian Canadians have Ukrainian as their first language. Over 70,500 of these are in the 65 and over age group (Cipywnyk, 1997; Statistics Canada, 1991, Table 4). In Canada, the Ukrainian language is the fifth most frequent mother tongue following English, French, German, and Italian (Statistics Canada, 1991, Table 2.4).

Ukrainian belongs to the East Slavic language family, which also includes Russian and Belorussian. Ukrainian uses the Cyrillic alphabet. It is closely related to Russian, and the two languages are mutually intelligible (The New Encyclopaedia Britannica, 1997). The cadence of the language is described as lyrical (J. Jurdyga, personal communication, February 19, 1997).

Gestures are frequently used as an aspect of body language to emphasize the verbal message. Touch is important between family members and friends. A handshake is considered a sign of respect and may be used to seal a contract

Ukrainian Canadians are generally polite in actions and in their speech. This is particularly true for the older generation who tend to maintain the manners they were taught to use as children and are often very socially correct. Older Ukrainians are often very proud of their Ukrainian heritage and seek to preserve it when possible.

Implications for nursing care

The nurse should appreciate that use of the Ukrainian language has been helpful in maintaining religious beliefs, customs, values, literature, poetry, and crafts of Canadians with this cultural heritage and is often spoken with pride (Silverthorne, 1991). However, the nurse who does not speak Ukrainian may find that the client who speaks Ukrainian may also speak English when the client understands that this language is required for communication. The majority of Canadians of Ukrainian descent enjoy conversing with their friends and relatives in both Ukrainian and English. They may introduce a Ukrainian word or expression into an English sentence when the Ukrainian term better identifies their thoughts or feelings. Some Ukrainian words have been Anglicized. For example, the word 'ball' should be pronounced *halka* but has changed to *balka*. The health care worker may be assisted in communicating with the client who speaks limited English by recognizing that the word for 'pain' sounds like *beel'*; 'good' sounds like *dobry*; 'thank you' like *dyákooyoo;* 'please' like *próshoo*, and asking 'where does it hurt?' by saying *dǎ boláyt?* (modified from Masi, 1989, Part IV). These clients may be stoic and not readily report pain or may be extremely demonstrative overemphasizing the pain. The Canadian of Ukrainian descent may identify where the pain is located by touching the area of discomfort.

Ukrainian Canadians may be either open and verbal with their thoughts and feelings or more reserved with what they think and feel. If the client is hesitant to readily express information, the nurse may want to verify the extent of the client's complaints, such as how long the symptoms have been present, with a family member who may know the client better and be more likely to provide accurate information.

The nurse should be aware that in the health care setting a person of Ukrainian descent will likely interpret touch as an expression of warmth. Thus it is usually appropriate for the health care worker to touch the client while conversing. Eye contact can generally be maintained with Canadians of Ukrainian ancestry once a trusting relationship and familiarity has been established.

Canadians of Ukrainian descent are usually more comfortable with being addressed more formally by health care givers. Thus the use of "Mr." or "Mrs." is more likely to be accepted than a surname. However, if the client is unresponsive, the use of a first name may help the client gain consciousness.

SPACE

An estimated 91% of the original immigrants from the Ukraine settled on free homestead land in the prairies that stretched across Manitoba, Alberta, and Saskatchewan, which together were over twice the size of the entire Ukraine (Subtelny, 1991; Noble, 1992). Unlike some groups such as the Mennonites and Doukhobors, who settled on land reserved specifically for their tightly organized groups, the Ukrainians arrived as independent settlers and were given individual blocks of land to homestead. However, they sought out homesteads adjacent to friends, kinfolk, and compatriots and thus created a remarkable degree of ethnic integrity within Ukrainian block settlements in the provinces (Lehr, 1992). Over time the block settlements grew into villages and towns and are today a distinct characteristic of western Canadian Ukrainian life (Subtelny, 1991). Today, the Ukrainian Cultural Heritage Village in Edmonton provides a settlement of restored buildings that resembles a turn-of-the-century Ukrainian Canadian community (Bailey and Bailey, 1995). The Ukrainian

Culture Museum in Winnipeg also provides information on what early life was like. The annual National Ukrainian Festival in Manitoba provides demonstration of traditional artwork, dancers in authentic costumes, and Ukrainian food (Walz and Walz, 1970; Berton, 1984).

Although living in a different geographic space and on the wide open prairie, the Ukrainian immigrants built farmsteads dramatically resembling the living spaces left in the Ukraine. The first Ukrainian immigrants faced the pressures of survival. Many lived in temporary shelters, often a sod-roofed dugout termed a *zemlyanka*, or a small one-room long hut, a *buda* (Lehr, 1992). The latter were strongly reminiscent of the chimneyless *chorna khata* ('black house') that had been common in the Carpathian region in the eighteenth century. The dugout was similarly modeled upon the largely defunct form of the Carpathian mountain hut, or *staya*, of the Hutsul shepherds (Zvarych, 1962). Occasionally these temporary dwellings were occupied for several years and with many homeless relatives until a more substantial house could be built. The second dwelling constituted the first major element of Ukrainian material culture to be placed on the new landscape and emerged with other western Ukrainian features including the farm layout, fence types, water drawing arrangements, design of animal shelters, and hay storage The family dwelling proved to be the most enduring and most obvious element of Ukrainian material culture in the pioneer landscape. The house was made of rough logs, rough hewed and chinked with a mortar made of clay and straw. Inside, some were plastered, but almost all were limewashed to a dazzling whiteness (Elston, 1915). The house and outbuildings faced south and were low browed and usually thatched (Elston, 1915). Within the variation of building detail that reflected the settler's region of origin, these pioneer homes had a unity of form, design, and decorative element, of which the most evident were a southward orientation, a single-story rectangular plan, a basic two- or three-room configuration, a central chimney, a gable, hipped gable, or hipped roof, and very frequently an exterior both plastered and limewashed (Lehr, 1992).

Although there are 406,645 persons who see themselves as Ukrainian Canadians, there is a total of 650,000 people who see themselves as part Ukrainian Their populations are now clustered in Ontario, Alberta, Manitoba, Saskatchewan, and British Columbia (Statistics Canada, 1997, Tables 1A and 2A). These are the provinces where most of their ancestors originally settled at the turn of the century (Statistics Canada, 1991). Examples of cities where population clusters exist are Edmonton, Winnipeg, Toronto, Windsor, Vancouver, Calgary, Saskatoon, Montreal, Hamilton, and Regina (Statistics Canada, 1991, Tables 1B and 2B).

Feelings of prejudice by other European-derived settlers toward the Ukrainians contributed to a tendency for some to avoid relating to persons from other nationalities. Thus, social interaction outside the block was sometimes limited (Kostash, 1992). Some of these tendencies of social isolation are still present among the elderly who prefer and are more comfortable socializing in Ukrainian with other Ukrainians. Today the reverse appears to be true as successive generations have integrated into the political, business, and educational systems and mingle with ease with those outside of their ethnic community (Kostash, 1992). Multiculturism passed as an act in parliament in 1971 has provided a continuing vehicle for the preservation of their culture (Masi, 1988).

Implications for nursing care

It is important in caring for the Ukrainian-Canadian client to appreciate the need of the client to adhere to traditional Ukrainian customs and to be in a living space surrounded by familiar material objects. Not only are objects important, but being surrounded by family and familiar people is also highly significant. The Ukrainian-Canadian client appreciates being with people whether they are familiar or are strangers. This is particularly true when illness occurs and in the health care setting. However, the nurse should be aware that because some older Ukrainian immigrants grew up in poverty they may be hesitant to relate to persons who they know are financially better off (M. Parchewsky, personal communication, April 25, 1997).

SOCIAL ORGANIZATION
Family

The traditional nuclear family has been the foundation for Ukrainian family structure. The early settlers who arrived with their families wanted desperately to obtain land to establish themselves (Lehr, 1992). The arrangements with the Canadian government gave 160 acres for a homestead for any Ukrainian settler able to pay a $10 entry fee, build a house however humble, cultivate 30 acres within 3 years, and reside on the land for 6 months each year. If these provisions were met at the end of 3 years, a final title would be given for the land, and Canadian citizenship could be applied for (Richtik, 1975).

Typically the entire Ukrainian immigrant family unit worked very hard in the cultivation of the homestead in the wilderness regions of the Canadian prairies (Kostash, 1992). Developing a productive farm in the virgin land over the short farming season meant overcoming immeasurable hardships. There was always a shortage of money, and so the father usually left home for seasonal work, generally on the railway, leaving the wife in charge of the family and homestead. The survival of these Ukrainian-Canadian pioneers fostered a closeness to family and friends that is the subject of family stories passed on from generation to generation by oral historians (Kostash, 1992). The stories of survival promoted an awareness of how hard work and opportunity enables improvement of status and ultimate success. Even though family roles traditionally placed the wife in a subservient role to her husband, within the home the wife was the authority. This provided a measure of protection from acculturation by adherence to esthetic traditions based squarely on the deep-set patterns of Old World peasant society (Lehr, 1992).

Most Ukrainian homesteaders suffered from abject poverty up to World War I when they began to sell their crops for profits. They have progressed monetarily and socially since that time. The first generation sacrificed to ensure that their children would have a better life. Each successive generation demonstrated their ability to assist relatives and friends to improve their lot in life. From the first days of immigration, Ukrainians have been active culturally, professionally, and politically in Canada. Newspapers were developed in the Ukrainian language. The Ukrainian Canadian Committee oversees numerous organizations that continue the maintenance of cultural traditions. Writers, painters, and architects of Ukrainian-Canadian heritage are world famous. There has been a proliferation of Ukrainian Canadians in politics, from mayors of municipal governments up to the governor general (Noble, 1992).

As early as World War I, the younger generation of the immigrants were beginning to adapt to the ways of their non-Ukrainian neighbors and to move away from the Ukrainian settlements (Subtelny, 1991). However, even then, the customs, dances, music, literature, and characteristics of their culture have not been lost but are still maintained and practiced on certain occasions, and the importance and value of family as well other values of parents and grandparents still remains.

Burch (1990) noted that on the average Ukrainian Canadians tend to have 2.6 children, 7.8 relatives, and 7.4 close friends. Of the number of Ukrainian children who had left home, 44% saw their mothers at least once a week and 40% saw their fathers. In the study 22.4% saw their siblings at least once a week. The total adult kin was 14.3. There were 9.6% men and 24.4% women living alone. Today in many families of Ukrainian descent the father and the mother have shared responsibilities and power in the home. However, the mother is generally the leader in relation to care for the children and as the health care provider for the family. The family members remain close to one another though they have settled away from the parental home. There is a strong sense of family. In-laws are considered relatives, and even a cousin fourth removed is still referred to as a cousin. Many do remain geographically close to the parental home. Older Ukrainian Canadians tend to remain extremely independent. Many stay in their own homes as long as possible. Trovato and Halli (1990) noted that Ukrainian Canadians tend to stay within the province of their origin.

Religion

Early immigrants to Canada quickly established churches, and the Ukrainian immigrants followed this pattern in establishing Ukrainian Greek Catholic and Ukrainian Greek Orthodox churches. Once in Canada, the Ukrainians believed that they had more ability to influence how the churches should be managed than they had in the Ukraine, and they exercised this ability. Initially there were no Greek Catholic priests in western Canada. American priests came to the prairies from time to time to celebrate mass. The French-Canadian priests attempted to fill this gap but were rejected. The Russian Orthodox church sent missionaries who were eventually ousted.

In 1912 the need for a Ukrainian Catholic bishop for Canada was finally recognized by the pope. Pius X created the Ukrainian Ordinariate of Canada with Nykyta Budka as first bishop. Budka was established at St. Nicholas Church in Winnipeg in 1912 but found he had 75,000 faithful and 80 parishes scattered across Canada. In 1913 Budka effected the incorporation of Ukrainian parishes by an act of parliament. Under Budka's direction, the Greek Ukrainian rite continued to grow and establish parishes, missions, parochial schools, and institutions (New Catholic Encyclopedia, 1967).

In 1918 the Ukrainian Greek Orthodox church was formed in Canada. There was great difficulty in establishing the Ukrainian Orthodox church because it had been nearly extinct for hundreds of years in the Ukraine, but at its initiation in Canada it held solid Ukrainian identification. Initially the legitimacy of the church was questioned because initially there was no bishop. A bishop did arrive from the Soviet Ukraine in 1924. The new Orthodox church attracted many former Greek Catholics, and such interest seemed to ferment ongoing disputes, lawsuits, and actual face-to-face challenges by members of the two denominations throughout the 1920s. The battles continued until 1931 when the Russians dissolved all churches within its borders. Despite these difficulties, the church continued to grow supported by the Ukrainian Self-Reliance League, the Ukrainian Women's Association, and the Canadian Ukrainian Youth Organization. The new

Ukrainian intelligentsia in Canada and the Orthodox Bukovinians joined this church providing a
broader base. The group that expanded the church
were known as the Ukrainian Orthodox Brother-
hood. By 1941 nearly 30% of the Ukrainian Canadians belonged to the Orthodox church (Subtelny,
1991; Ohienko, 1986).

The Ukrainian Greek Catholic church and the
Ukrainian Greek Orthodox church are the recognized churches of the Ukrainian people in Canada.
The term "Greek" in the title of both churches was
later dropped in the 1970s. In the early pioneer days
churches were very simply constructed. However, as
soon as expertise, capital, and time became available,
the churches got more elaborate. Today, Ukrainian-
Canadian churches are distinctive with a bulb for a
dome and a cross indicating the rite, or ornate pear-
shaped *banya*s (Byzantine cupolas) and a separate
bell tower (Lehr, 1992). Alongside the older churches
lies the graveyard where weathered wooded crosses
with Cyrillic lettering mark the faith of the graves of
the pioneers, whereas glossy slabs of black granite
with Latin lettering mark those of their descendants
(Lehr, 1992). Inside, an iconostasis, or screen with
icons, separates the congregation from the taber-
nacle. Beautiful hand-painted screens and hand-
embroidered altar cloths provide color (Trosky,
1968). Until the sense of national consciousness began to fade in the Ukrainian-Canadian community,
building a church in accordance with Anglo-
Canadian tastes was unthinkable (Lehr, 1992).

Whether Catholic or Orthodox, the Ukrainian
Canadians focus many of their cultural and social
activities around the church (Ohienko, 1986). The
church functions as the guardian of cultural and
ethnic identity, fulfilling the role of a national state
in promoting ethnic heritage, linguistic survival, and
spiritual awareness (Lehr, 1992). Some of the important feasts in the church are Christmas, New Year's
Day, Lent, and Easter and are celebrated by the Orthodox Ukrainians on Julian calendar dates. The
Catholics observe the Gregorian calendar celebrating the Christian festivities as celebrated by most
Canadians. Celebration of these religious events is
what made and makes one a Ukrainian Canadian.
Christmas is characterized by weeks of food prepa-

ration and religious activities. Lent, the 6 weeks leading up to Easter, was and is a time of spiritual purification, of fasting and abstinence from pleasures,
and of penance and forgiveness (Holowachuk,
1994). Easter, the most celebrated religious holiday,
is identified with fasting and food brought to the
priest for blessing. Easter is also characterized by the
preparation of *pysanke*, eggs painted with intricate
patterns and given to guests as treasured gifts. They
were and are a symbol of spring and rebirth. Green
Sunday is a day in May when prayers are said for a
good crop (Kostach, 1992). Children are included in
church activities as are the elderly. Ukrainian Canadians are firmly attached and loyal to their churches.

Most Ukrainian Canadians hold the perception
that religious beliefs affect their health. Many rely on
prayer to maintain health (Masi, 1988, Part III).
There is a religious orientation in daily living practices in their homes. For example, they do not eat
meat the day before Christmas

Festivals and customs

Essentially, in Canada, the traditional customs and
festivals have been maintained, with minimal
change, from generation to generation. The desire to
continue cultural traditions has been strongly supported by a variety of Canadian-Ukrainian organizations. For example, the Ukrainian Women's Association of Canada collected folk art and founded
museums to house it. Church choirs, amateur theatrical groups, music, orchestras, poetic recitations,
dances, and commemoration of national heroes assist to maintain the cultural heritage (Bailey and
Bailey, 1995). Ukrainian festivals that welcome persons of any culture background are held across
Canada. These festivals include Ukrainian dance en-
sembles in colorful cross-stitched authentic custom.
There are hundreds of such dance groups across
Canada, composed of primarily young men and
women. Ukrainian music and food are always high-
lighted in these joyous, exuberant occasions.

Education

Although many early settlers were illiterate, education has been highly valued by Ukrainian-Canadian
immigrants. The first Canadian-born generation,

particularly the boys, attended school. Female illiteracy was not considered unusual because their role was considered in the home, but soon girls too were sent to school, and their education opened opportunities for them outside of the home (Kostash 1992).

Implications for nursing care

The nurse should be aware that support from the family is very important for the Ukrainian-Canadian client. It is also important for the nurse to recognize that the client may want and need the involvement of other family members. This may be especially true for the male family member who is closest geographically when a health care decision is being made. In the delivery room, most Ukrainian-Canadian fathers wish to be present and to assist their partners in the delivery of their children (Bohay, 1991). The nurse should be aware that many Ukrainian Canadians rely on prayer and rituals of their faith to assist in maintaining health and recovering from illness. The nurse should incorporate the client's religious faith in the provision of culturally competent care, and participation in religious events should be facilitated even if the client is hospitalized.

TIME

Ukrainian Canadians have a close relationship to the earth and are bound by seasons. Because the society has been strongly agrarian, the focus has been both present and future oriented. However, there is also a strong relationship with the past in relation to cultural activities and appreciation for heritage. Ukrainian Canadians tend to take pleasure in each season; for example, spring is enjoyed for gardening and summer for the harvest.

Ukrainian Canadians tend to be cognizant of both the clock and the calendar. They are generally punctual and expect others to be the same. The Julian and Gregorian calendars of the Orthodox and Catholic churches serve as an important time orientation for Ukrainian Canadians because religious holidays provide an important role in family activities and preserving cultural heritage (New Catholic Encyclopedia, 1967).

Implications for nursing care

The nurse should be aware that Ukrainian-Canadian clients will generally be on time and be compliant with appointments for health care activities. The nurse should also appreciate the importance of ethnically and religiously related activities on the client's calendar when making health care appointments. When a client is hospitalized, it is important to plan time for the client to take part in events related to their religious faith because such planning is often of great personal significance.

ENVIRONMENTAL CONTROL
Locus of control

Ukrainian Canadians may demonstrate evidence of belief in both internal and external locuses of control. Persons in an agrarian society may feel a sense of helplessness in relation to the weather and the growing of crops. On the other hand, historically the Ukrainian-Canadian people have been able to overcome great difficulties in conquering the wilderness, and such success is evidence of the power of hard work. This triumph over nature is present even today in family stories.

Folk medicine

Appreciation for the environment is fundamental for most Ukrainians. Since the first Ukrainian settlers arrived in Canada, gardening has been an activity held in high esteem. Today the Green Holiday festivals celebrate the growth of plant life. Not only has the environment been the source of food and livelihood, but also stories passed from one generation to the next have acted as a report of medicinal properties in specific flowers and herbs. Upon immigration many Ukrainian Canadians grew poppies in their gardens. In folklore poppies are reported to have medicinal properties and to represent hope and contentment. The heads of the plant were used to produce a milk used as a pain killer, the juice was good for lung inflammation, the green seeds were used as a sedative, and the flowers were ground to a powder to be used for gastric disorders and as a sleeping potion (Kischuk, 1984). Folklore also reports female healers who could *strakh zlovete*, that is, cure fears as well as other ills. For example, a child was taken by her mother to her grandmother, a female healer, to cure her nightmares about bantam roosters chasing her. The grandmother held a dish of cold water over the child's head, poured hot wax into it, and told her the nightmares would go away. The child never had another nightmare (R. Fedoruk, personal communication, February 20, 1997). There is a small group of *vorozhkĕ*, or female healers, popularly 'fortune tellers', still practicing in some Ukrainian communities (Kischuk, 1984).

Folk medicine, including cupping for coughs and applying mustard packs for fever, is still practiced by some Ukrainian Canadians. A stuffy nose is treated by the wrapping of boiled potatoes in a towel and holding them to the nose. Nose drops of honey and water are used. Drinking vodka is a commonly used cure to restore health (Spector, 1996).

Illness-wellness beliefs

Even today many Ukrainians believe that health can be maintained by drinking vodka, eating chicken soup, and eating healthy food (Spector, 1996). Health can be protected by bundling up in cold weather (Spector, 1996). However, most modern Ukrainian-Canadian clients believe in a biomedical model of illness and will be compliant with examinations and treatment and a medical treatment plan. They do believe that blessing from the church and having faith are important in preventing and treating illness (Masi, 1988, Part III).

Death

Ukrainian Canadians have many traditions related to their religious faith in relation to death. After death there will be a prayer service at the church followed by the funeral the next day. The casket will be present at both services and may be open. Forty days after the funeral a special memorial service is held when the deceased has ascended into heaven. One year later another memorial service is held with a regular church service or separately. Each spring the grave is blessed by the priest. Food is taken to the grave site for blessing and returned home to be eaten. In the year after a death no dancing is allowed, and some older people wear dark clothes (Cowles,

1996; Latimer and Lundy, 1995; Trosky, 1968). A loss is deeply mourned (Trosky, 1968).

Implications for nursing care

It is important for the culturally sensitive nurse to be aware that some older Ukrainian Canadians may come for health care only after other folk healing methods have been exhausted. For example, clients with arthritis may have tried a combination of honey and vinegar to reduce the pain and stiffness. As part of the initial assessment the nurse should question what has already been tried to reduce presenting symptoms. The nurse should be aware that some older clients may have beliefs that illness has been caused by an evil eye being placed upon them (Masi, 1988, parts II and III).

Ukrainian-Canadian clients value when health care professionals take time with them and communicate caring. Some Ukrainian Canadians are critical of physicians if they believe that not enough attention is given to them or that a complete physical assessment and history has not been done by the physician (Dimou, 1995). Most Ukrainian-Canadian clients prefer to be given medical information that is available even when a negative prognosis is present (Korb, 1996).

The nurse who provides care for a Ukrainian-Canadian client in the hospital should be aware that although families want to be involved in health care decisions they generally prefer to limit care they may provide to help with feeding. When a Canadian-Ukrainian client is dying, the family usually sits in vigil.

BIOLOGICAL VARIATIONS

Ukrainian Canadians have average Canadian statures. Men are taller than women and may be overweight. Older women also tend to be obese though this is not considered to be a personal problem. The younger generations are generally within the average Canadian weight for height and age. Ukrainian Canadians take pride in being industrious and strong, that is, good physical workers (Stechishin, 1995). Ukrainian Canadians generally have skin color that is swarthy or light tan. Some have a slight oriental shape to their eyes and high cheekbones characteristically Slavic.

Early settlers had a high incidence of tuberculosis. Presently this threat for Ukrainian Canadians is the same as the general Canadian population (Lloyd, 1995; Rieder and Raviglione, 1993). Hypertension, cancer, and cardiovascular problems are within the national average. Some Ukrainian Canadians exhibit somatic complaints (Brod and Heurtin-Roberts, 1992).

Nutritional preference

Over many centuries, Ukrainians have developed their own distinctive and original cooking. Rich foods are the order of the day. They enjoy fresh food, particularly from their own gardens, but are often tempted to add rich sauces and sour cream. Ethnic dishes are made with recipes brought by the first settlers and include *holubtsi* (or cabbage rolls), *paska*, or *babka* (an Easter bread), *pyrohy* (dumplings made from dough with a filling of cottage cheese), *borshch* (the national beet soup of Ukraine), *shashlýk* (a barbecued lamb), *lokshýna* (or homemade noodles), and delicious desserts (Stechishin, 1995; Holowachuk, 1994).

Large quantities of food are prepared for special events, and family and guests are expected to overeat to enjoy. Festivals, religious holidays, and celebrations have two foci: first the church ceremony and then the feast. Dieting is not favored by the older generation.

Daily diet usually consists of a variety of breads, meat dishes, vegetables, soups, and desserts. To the Ukrainian, bread is one of the most holy of foods. Leftover bread is often fed to the birds or burned. It is disrespectful to throw food out. The most sincere form of welcome to guests is to meet them at the door with a plate holding a loaf of bread and a mound of salt. Today this ritual is used to greet important people. Each kind of bread has its own specific shape, name, decorative dough ornaments, and a symbolic meaning. Meat has always been an important food item, primarily beef and then veal and pork in that order. Meat is prepared in the North American styles with the addition of sour cream used in the accompanying sauces. Poultry is prepared in a variety of recipes. Boned, stuffed chicken and chicken breasts are favorites as is stuffed goose, which is preferred over turkey. Fish has been a favorite dish for many Ukrainian Canadians. During Lent they use fresh fish or pickled herring. Vegetables are a welcome part of the meal. Cucumbers are the favorite vegetable, followed by corn on the cob. Cooked vegetables are generally served with browned butter or browned crumbs or a thickened sauce. Potatoes are considered to be a staple. Soup is essential to a meal. There is a great variety of soups ranging from vegetables, broth, cereal, cream, milk, and fruit puree. Borshch is an everyday soup and chicken broth is for special days. On very hot days Ukrainians prefer to serve their soup cold. Fruit soups are common in Ukraine but are less popular in Canada. Soups may be accompanied by *pěrizhkě*, a pastry. A variety of fancy desserts are essential for serving guests. For everyday meals, a fruit dish is adequate. Ukrainian desserts are limitless in their variety and the pride of the woman preparing the meal.

Ukrainians have served appetizers along with wine for centuries to relax and whet the appetites of guests. This is known as *zákuska*, a time for pleasure and relaxation. Formerly numerous foods were served. However, today in Canada an appetizer is usually limited to one or two dishes.

Alcohol use

Alcohol is generally included in celebrations (Masi, 1989, Part V). Adrian, Dini, MacGregor, and Stoduto (1995) found that 48% of Ukrainian/Polish-Canadian women had a greater use of alcohol than women in other ethnic groups did, and that percentage placed them in the moderate to high range of alcohol use. The Ukrainian/Polish-Canadian women in the study tended to use drugs and tobacco less than the average. Today there is a definite alcohol problem for residents of Ukraine possibly related to their living circumstances (Duncan and Simmons, 1996). Adrian, Dini, MacGregor, and Stoduto (1995) suggested that the longer an ethnic group remained in Canada the less alcohol, drugs, and tobacco they consumed.

Implications for nursing care

It is important for the nurse to be aware that for some immigrants, who have come to Canada but have been relatively isolated from their social group, there has been a problem with depression associated with isolation and assimilation. For many Ukrainians, family members have remained in proximity. However, depression is always a possibility for a person whose spouse dies and who may be hesitant to reach out to family, friends, and health professionals. Sue (1977) identified that there was general underutilization of health services by individuals who did not regard themselves as being in the ethnic majority. It is particularly important for health care professionals to be aware of emotional distress among clients from diverse cultural backgrounds who may feel uncomfortable relating to health professionals of a different ethnic group. In some cases finding a health care professional from the same ethic group is important to enable the sharing that will enable proper treatment (Short and Johnston, 1994).

SUMMARY

One of Canada's most flamboyant ethnic groups, Ukrainians first trickled into the country with the Mennonites and other German immigrants in the 1870s (Bailey and Bailey, 1995). However, they did not arrive in significant numbers until after 1896 when Canada began to seek agricultural immigrants from eastern Europe.

As nurses enter the health care system with their own cultural upbringing, they must prepare themselves to recognize, understand, and respect the diverse cultures of clients they may encounter (Rajan, 1995; Giger and Davidhizar, 1995). This is particularly important in Canada where the population is significantly multicultural and the nurse will likely encounter clients from diverse cultures on a regular basis (Masi, 1988, Part I). Nursing programs in Canada are becoming increasingly sensitive to the need to prepare students to relate to clients with an understanding of cultural differences and with techniques and nursing approaches that will bridge the cultural gap that may exist (Kikuchi, 1996; Cipywnyk, 1993; Hennen and Blackman, 1992; Culley, 1996; Habayeb, 1995; Rosenbaum, 1995). It is only with this increased awareness and appreciation that nursing care can become truly culturally sensitive.

Case Study

Mrs. Mary Boychuk is an 88-year-old lady who has lived all her life within a 60-kilometer radius of the western Canadian city where she now resides. She speaks English with a pronounced Ukrainian accent. She is a small, wiry individual with a decided stoop to her posture. Mrs. Boychuck has been brought by her son to a rehabilitation outpatient clinic for reassessment. He tells the nurse his mother has had arthritis for years but now she seems to be having more pain and moving more slowly with the aid of a cane and appears to be in pain when she walks. When the nurse asks how she is, Mrs. Boychuk tells her that she is O.K. but needs pills so that she is not so still. She goes on to say that she wants to get her garden planted or she will not have a good crop. Mrs. Boychuck lives in a small comfortable home in the same city as her son and his family. She has been a widow for over 35 years and is fiercely independent. She enjoys her own home with all her belongings surrounding her. Her children and grandchildren visit regularly and frequently. She tells the nurse she has been taking a mixture of vinegar and honey for her arthritis, but it no longer relieves her discomfort as in the past.

CARE PLAN

 Nursing Diagnosis   Pain related to arthritis.

Client Outcome

1. Decrease pain as verbalized by the need for less pain medication.

Nursing Interventions

1. Encourage client to to take medications as prescribed.
2. Explain home pain management.
3. Assist client in self-reporting of changes in pain and whom to notify.
4. Make appointments for reassessment in 6 months.

 Nursing Diagnosis   Inability to maintain usual routines related to arthritis.

Client Outcome

1. Will maintain routine.

Nursing Interventions

1. Offer assessment and independence by home care team to identify services that may be provided to reduce barriers.
2. Support concern for maintaining independence and future-oriented thinking.
3. Encourage family members to assist with physical tasks.

STUDY QUESTIONS

1. Identify cultural themes relevant to the time orientation of this client.
2. Identify at least three diseases or illnesses Ukrainian clients may have a high susceptibility to contract.
3. Describe the communication barriers that may be encountered by the nurse who does not speak Ukrainian but is assigned to care for a client who speaks only Ukrainian.
4. Identify the social organization of the family system for the Ukrainian client.
5. Describe the religious orientation of the Ukrainian client.

References

Adrian, M., Dini, C.M., MacGregor, L.J., & Stoduto, G. (1995). Substance use as a measure of social integration for women of different ethnocultural groups into mainstream culture in a pluralist society: the example of Canada. *The International Journal of Addictions, 30*(6), 699-734.

Bailey, E., & Bailey, R. (1995). *Discover Canada.* Oxford, England: Berlitz Publishing Co.

Berton, P. (1984). *The promised land.* Toronto: McClelland & Stewart.

Bohay, I.Z. (1991). Culture care meanings and experiences of pregnancy and childbirth of Ukrainians. In Leininger, M.M. (Ed.), *Culture care diversity and universality: a theory of nursing* (pp. 203-229). New York: National League for Nursing, Press Pub. No. 15-2402.

Brod, M., & Heurtin-Roberts, S. (1992). Cross-cultural medicine a decade later. *The Western Journal of Medicine, 157*(3), 333-336.

Burch, T.K. (1990). Family structure and ethnicity. In Halli, S.S., Trovato, F., & Driedger, L. (Eds.), *Ethnic demography* (pp. 199-212). Ottawa: Carleton University Press.

Cipywnyk, D. (1993, June). *Multiculturalism and medicine.* Paper presented at the 8th Annual Alumni Reunion Conference, Saskatoon, SK.

Cipywnyk, D. (1997, January). Coping with trauma. In Ship, S.J., Tarbell, R., Eapen, S., & Cipywnyk, D. (Eds.), *Our nation's elders speak* (pp. 65-67). Kahnawake, Quebec: Government of Canada.

Cowles, K.V. (1996). Cultural perspectives of grief: an expanded concept analysis. *Journal of Advanced Nursing, 23,* 287-294.

Culley, L. (1996). A critique of multiculturalism in health care: the challenge for nursing education. *Journal of Advanced Nursing, 23,* 564-570.

Darcovich, W., & Yusyk, P. (Eds.). (1977). *A statistical compendium of Ukrainians in Canada 1891-1976.* Edmonton: University of Alberta Press.

Dimou, N. (1995). Illness and culture: learning differences. *Patient Education and Counselling, 26,* 153-157.

Duncan, L., & Simmons, M. (1996). Health practices among Russian and Ukrainian immigrants. *Journal of Community Health Nursing, 13*(2), 129-137.

Dyck, P., & Dyck, E. (1991). *Up from the rubble.* Waterloo, Ont.: Herald Press.

Edwards, M. (1993). After the Soviet Union's collapse: a broken empire: Ukraine. *National Geographic, 183*(3), 42-53.

Elston, M. (1915). *The Russian in our midst.* Philadelphia: Westminster Press.

Fedoruk, R. (Feb 20, 1997). Personal communication to Marjorie Linwood. Saskatoon, Sask.

Giger, J.N., & Davidhizar, R.E. (1995). *Transcultural nursing: assessment and intervention.* St. Louis: Mosby.

Habayeb, G.L. (1995). Cultural diversity: a nursing concept not yet reliably defined. *Nursing Outlook, 43,* 224-227.

Hennen, B.K., & Blackman, N. (1992). Teaching about culture and health in Ontario medical schools. *Canadian Family Physician, 38,* 1123-1129.

Holowachuk, M. (1994, March). Bread symbolic of Easter message (p. C19). *The Star Phoenix.* Phoenix, Az.

Johnson, M. (1994). From so much to so little. *The Canadian Nurse, 90*(10), 58-59.

Jurdyga, J. (Feb. 19, 1997). Personal communication to Marjorie Linwood. Saskatoon, Sask.

Kikuchi, J.F. (1996). Multicultural ethics in nursing education: a potential threat to responsible practice. *Journal of Professional Nursing, 12*(3), 159-165.

Kischuk, M. (1984). *The veneration of flowers and herbs in Ukrainian folklore: rituals and beliefs.* Unpublished manuscript.

Korb, M.D. (1996). Expectations in giving and receiving help among nurses and Russian refugees. *International Journal of Nursing Studies, 33*(5), 479-486.

Kostash, M. (1992). *All of Baba's children.* Edmonton: Hurtig Publishers Ltd.

Latimer, E., & Lundy, M. (1995). The care of the dying: multicultural influences. In Masi, R., Mensah, L. & McLeod, K. (Eds.), *Health and culture* (vol. 2). Oakville: Mosaic Press, Ontario.

Lehr, J. (1992). Ukrainians in western Canada. In Noble, A. (Ed.), *To build a new land: ethnic landscapes in North America.* Baltimore, Md.: Johns Hopkins Press.

Lindheim, R., & Luckyi, G.S.N. (1996). *Toward an intellectual history of Ukraine: an anthology of Ukrainian thought from 1710 to 1995.* Toronto: University of Toronto Press in association with the Shevchenko Scientific Society, Inc.

Lloyd, N. (1995). Tuberculosis: the threat lingers. *The Canadian Nurse, 91*(10), 33-37.

Masi, H. (1988). Multiculturalism, medicine, and health. Part I: Multicultural health care. *Canadian Family Physician, 34,* 2173-2177.

Masi, H. (1988). Multiculturalism, medicine, and health. Part II: Health-related beliefs. *Canadian Family Physician, 34,* 2429-2434.

Masi, H. (1988). Multiculturalism, medicine, and health. Part III: Health beliefs. *Canadian Family Physician, 34,* 2649-2653.

Masi, H. (1989). Multiculturalism, medicine, and health. Part IV: Individual considerations. *Canadian Family Physician, 35,* 69-73.

Masi, H. (1989). Multiculturalism, medicine, and health. Part V: Community considerations. *Canadian Family Physician, 35,* 251-254.

Masi, R., Mensah, L., & McLeod, K. (Eds.). (1995). *Health and cultures* (vols. 1-2). Oakville, Ontario: Mosaic Press.

The Mennonite encyclopedia. (1959). Scottdale, Pa.: Mennonite Publishing House.

Moynahan, B. (1994). *The Russian century: a history of the last hundred years.* New York: Random House.

New Catholic encyclopedia. (1967). Washington, D.C.: The Catholic University of America.

The new encyclopaedia britannica. (1997). Chicago: Encyclopaedia Britannica, Inc.

Noble, A. (1992). *To build a new land: ethnic landscapes in North-America.* Baltimore, Md.: Johns Hopkins Press.

Ohienko, I. (1986). *The Ukrainian church* (O. Ferbey, Trans.). (Original work published 1942). Winnipeg: Kromar Printing Ltd.

Parchewsky, M. (April 25, 1997). Personal communication.

Rajan, M.-F.J. (1995). Transcultural nursing: a perspective derived from Jean-Paul Sartre. *Journal of Advanced Nursing, 23*, 450-455.

Richtik, J. (1975). The policy framework for settling the Canadian west 1870-1880. *Agricultural History, 49*, 613-628.

Rieder, H., & Raviglione, N. (1993). *World Health, 46*(4), 20-21.

Rosenbaum, J.N. (1995). Teaching cultural sensitivity. *Journal of Nursing Education, 34*(4), 188-189.

Rudnytska, M. (1934). Ukrainian reality and the task of women. In Lindheim, R., & Luckyi, G.S.N. (1996). *Toward an intellectual history of Ukraine: an anthology of Ukrainian thought from 1710 to 1995.* Toronto: University of Toronto Press in association with the Shevchenko Society, Inc.

Short, E., & Johnston, C. (1994). Ethnocultural parent education in Canada: current status and directions. *Canadian Journal of Community Mental Health, 13*(1), 43-54.

Silverthorne, J. (1991). *Made in Saskatchewan: Peter Rupchan.* Regina: Brigdens Printers.

Spector, R. (1996). *Guide to heritage assessment and health traditions.* Stamford, Conn.: Appleton & Lange.

Statistics Canada. (1991). *Table 1A. Population by ethnic origin and sex, for Canada, provinces and territories, 1991 census 20% sample data.* (Statistics Canada Cat. No. 93-315, The nation). Ottawa: Government of Canada.

Statistics Canada. (1991). *Table 1B. Population by ethnic origin and sex, for census metropolitan areas, 1991 census—20% sample data.* (Statistics Canada—Cat. No. 93-315, The nation). Ottawa: Government of Canada.

Statistics Canada. (1991). *Table 2A. Ethnic origin and sex, showing single and multiple responses for Canada, provinces and territories, 1991 census—20% sample data. (Statistics Canada—Cat. No. 93-315, The nation). Ottawa: Government of Canada.*

Statistics Canada. (1991). *Table 2B. Selected ethnic origins and sex, showing single and multiple responses for census metropolitan areas, 1991 census—20% sample data.* (Statistics Canada—Cat. No. 93-315, The nation). Ottawa: Government of Canada.

Statistics Canada. (1991). *Table 2.4. Most frequent mother tongues for the Canadian-born and immigrants, Canada, 1991.* (Statistics Canada—Cat. No. 96-311E, Canada's changing immigrant population). Ottawa: Government of Canada.

Statistics Canada. (1991). *Table 4. Population by mother tongue and sex, showing age groups, for Canada, provinces and territories, 1991—100% data.* (Statistics Canada—Cat. No. 93313). Ottawa: Government of Canada.

Stechishin, S. (1995). *Traditional Ukrainian cooking.* Winnipeg: Trident Press Limited.

Subtelny, O. (1991). *Ukrainians in North America.* Toronto: University of Toronto Press.

Sue, S. (1977). Community mental health services to minority groups. *American Psychologist, 32*, 616-624.

Taptich, B.J., et al. (1994). *Nursing diagnosis and care planning* (ed. 2). Philadelphia: W.B. Saunders Co.

The Times atlas of the twentieth century: the definitive account of our century. (1996). London: Times Books.

Trosky, O. (1968). *The Ukrainian Greek Orthodox church in Canada.* Winnipeg: Bulman Bros. Ltd.

Trovato, F., & Halli, S.S. (1990). Ethnicity and geographic mobility. In Halli, S.S., Trovato, F., & Driedger, L. (Eds.), *Ethnic demography* (pp. 75-89). Ottawa: Carleton University Press.

Walz, J., & Walz, A. (1970). *Portrait of Canada.* New York: American Heritage Press.

World Almanac. (1997). Mahwah, N.J.: World Almanac Books.

Zvarych, P. (1962). *On the problem of development and progress of material culture of Ukrainian settlers in Canada.* Paris: Zapysky Naukovoho Tovarystva im. Shevchenka.

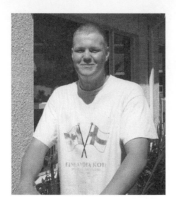

CHAPTER 16
Finnish Canadians

Heather Jessup-Falcioni

BEHAVIORAL OBJECTIVES

After reading this chapter the nurse will be able to:

1. Describe attitudes and beliefs of Finnish Canadians that relate to health and illness.
2. Recognize cultural factors that affect the health-seeking behaviors of Finnish Canadians.
3. Identify at least two health problems unique to Finnish Canadians.
4. Identify the importance of family and community to Finnish Canadians.
5. Explain how Finnish Canadians use space as a part of communication.
6. Identify future-oriented values for Finnish Canadians.
7. Describe specific characteristics of the Finnish language.

OVERVIEW OF FINLAND

Suomi, the Finnish word for 'Finland', is the most northernmost state in Europe and the second most northerly country in the world, second to Iceland. The Republic of Finland, or Finland for short, is bounded by Sweden to the northwest, Norway in the north, Russia along the entire eastern border, and the Baltic Sea to the west and south. Its southern point falls north of Churchill, Manitoba, and one third of its length lies north of the Arctic Circle (Lindstrom, 1992). Finland is a long narrow country covering an approximate area of 130,558 square miles and is exceeded in size in Europe by France, Spain, Sweden, and Russia. The population of Finland is estimated at over 5,100,000, with Helsinki being the capital city with an estimated population of over 515,000 residents (Johnson, 1997). The ethnic groups of Finland are Finns, Swedes, Lapps (Samis), Gypsies, and Tatars (Colombo, 1997).

Ice has been dominant in the formation of the Finnish landscape as evidenced by granite, huge boulders, and hollows gouged in the rock that are currently filled with water. These formations give Finland the extensive lake and river systems that are estimated to constitute 9% to 10% of the surface area of the country. About 76% of the land area is covered in forests. The thin but fertile layer of earth over the primeval rocks explains the immense woods: only pines and spruce thrive in such thin soil and Finland's national tree, the birch tree. Wood is a raw material of great importance. The forests have been called Finland's "green gold." Finland is one of the biggest timber, pulpwood, and paper suppliers in the world. Metal production and engineering are Finland's second most important export followed by chemicals and consumer goods such as clothing, footwear, furniture, glassware, and jewelry (Lander and Charbonneau, 1990). Finland's natural resources are timber, copper, zinc, iron ore, and silver (Colombo, 1997).

Largely because of the influence of the Gulf Stream, Finland's climate is not so severe as that of other areas on the same latitude. During the long cold winter, days are short with about 6 hours of daylight. The summers are brief and warm, and in June and July the sun sets for only 2 or 3 hours before rising again. In the far north, the sun does not set at all for about 73 days during the summer. The most unpleasant time of the year is autumn, when the brief days are accompanied by rain, sleet, or snow.

Over the years, the Finnish people have struggled to survive. For more than 650 years (1157 to 1809) Finland was controlled by Sweden. During that time Sweden was a strong military power. Wars were waged continuously on Finnish soil. In the 1808-1809 war between Sweden and Russia, the Swedes lost, and Finland was ceded to Russian sovereignty. For the years 1809 to 1917, the Finnish people lived under the Russian tsar. On November 7, 1917, a second revolution occurred in Russia with a revolt among the Russian soldiers wanting to put an end to the war. The war resulted in leadership of the Lenin and the Bolshevik party. One of the first diplomatic moves was to grant Finland independence on December 6, 1917, and Finland became a constitutional democracy in 1919 (Tester, 1986).

Political power in Finland tends to be scattered among a wide variety of political parties. Currently Finland is attempting to realign its domestic and foreign policies to reflect changes caused by the breakup of the Soviet Union. Finland is divided into 12 provinces, each of which is headed by a presidentially appointed governor. The provinces are further divided into municipalities led by elected councils. The voting age is 18 years for all persons (Lander and Charbonneau, 1990). Elections occur every 6 years. Finland has recently weathered a recession, and the economy is slowly recovering. Approximately 16.7% of the work force are unemployed, and inflation was at 0.7% in April 1996 (Colombo, 1997). Today, many Finnish Canadians are far removed from the political changes that have occurred in Finland. However politics can be a topic of heated debate and is probably best to be avoided by the older Finnish immigrants.

IMMIGRATION TO CANADA

Most Finns who prepared to emigrate were dissatisfied with the political situation in Finland and were looking for a freer political climate. In fact, many of the Finnish population who immigrated to Canada as adults have retained their political views. Mostly immigrants were young single men, healthy and full of optimism. Finnish women often came alone and became employed as domestic workers in Canada (Lindstrom-Best, 1981).

The Finnish immigrants came to the United States and Canada in series of waves. Finnish immigrants initially migrated to the United States. The first wave was settled between 1641 and 1655 in what is now Wilmington, Delaware (Sillanpää, 1988). In Canada, the migration of Finns can be traced back to the nineteenth century. The first Finnish immigrants to Canada came by way of the United States rather than directly from Finland (Saarinen, 1981). Before 1900, there were probably no more than 1000 Finns in Canada; however by 1911 there were approximately 15,000 Finns (Engle, 1975). Finnish Canadians settled as pioneers in and around Thunder Bay, Sudbury, Kirkland Lake, Timmins, and Sault Ste. Marie. Before World War I, some Finns settled in Toronto, and their numbers increased after World War II (Sillanpää, 1988).

The second wave of immigrants arrived in Canada in the 1920s with about 37,000 Finns arriving in Canada, with Ontario being the most favored destination (Lindstrom, 1996). Since the 1920s there has been an active Finnish community in Montreal, but few settled elsewhere in Quebec. Alberta and Saskatchewan have a few small rural Finnish communities (Sillanpää, 1988). Many came without any formal schooling because Finland had no compulsory education until 1922, and many were landless with very little if any economic prospects in Finland. They were largely unskilled with most of the men employed in lumbering, mining, railroad work, and farming whereas the women worked as domestics (Sillanpää, 1988). By the depression, over 40% of the Finnish Canadians were women (Engle, 1975). An important factor in drawing so many Finns was the phenomenon of "chain migration," which was the encouragement and assistance of friends and relatives to immigrate into a new country by those friends and family already settled there (Sillanpää, 1988).

A third wave arrived between 1950 and 1960 after the years when Finland's borders were closed because of war. The postwar immigrants were considerably different from earlier arrivals because they generally had a higher level of education, came as families, settled in urban areas, and tended to be politically conservative (Lindstrom-Best, 1981). In the 1960s, immigration policy changed and the number of immigrants declined to about 200 a year. Unskilled workers no longer met the entrance requirements to Canada. Those who came to Canada were highly skilled and professional. For the skilled and professional Finnish people emigration is less attractive, and good opportunities are available in their homeland (Lindstrom-Best, 1985).

Since the beginning of Finnish immigration to Canada, Ontario has been the preferred destination with British Columbia the second preferred destination. The Finnish Canadians were among the first pioneers in northern Ontario communities where they found work in the resource industries and in building the railroads. In the 1920s the lumber industry had become the most important source of livelihood for Finnish-Canadian men (Lindstrom-Best, 1985).

According to the Canadian 1991 census, there were 39,230 Finnish Canadians with approximately 65% living in Ontario, 22% living in British Columbia, 7% living in Alberta, 3% living in Saskatchewan, and others living in the remainder of the provinces. The Finnish make up 0.1% of the Canadian population by mother tongue statistics. The largest number of Finnish Canadians using Finnish as their home language live in Thunder Bay, followed by Toronto, Vancouver, and Sudbury (Statistics Canada, 1993).

COMMUNICATION

The Finnish Canadians are bound together by their distinctive language Finnish which bears no resemblance to the Romance, Slavic, or Germanic languages of Europe. It does have similarities to Estonian and Hungarian and is referred to in the 1993 Statistics Canada language listings under the category Finno-Ugric. The language survived despite being ruled for over 600 years by Sweden and over 100 years by Russia. Finland's two official languages are *suomi*, or *suomen kieli* (Finnish) and *svenska* (Swedish). All students must learn both Finnish and Swedish in school and may elect to learn English or German, or both. Finnish is spoken by over 93% of the population in Finland with Swedish being spoken by just over 6%. A small number of people also speak Russian and Lapp, or *Saami* (Geissler, 1994).

Some features of the Finnish language are that it uses many vowels and few consonants; some words are very close, such as *tuli* means 'fire', *tuuli* means 'wind', and *tulli* means 'customs'; it does not distinguish feminine, masculine, or neuter in pronouns or nouns, as many languages do; words are formed by adding endings to the stem; it does not have separate articles, prepositions, and pronouns; and it has a relatively free word order (Lander and Charbonneau, 1990). Words, even common words, can be very long. It is also an unusually expressive language. Depending on the words used, one can talk very harshly, using abrasive *k*'s, *s*'s, and rolled *r*'s. The language is also descriptive. For example, June is *Kesäkuu*, or 'summer moon', and September is *Syyskuu*, or 'autumn moon'. One Finnish Canadian, upon returning to her homeland, dropped by to visit her cousin at his home. The cousin was not at home, and she left him a note indicating that she had stopped in to meet him. The word for 'meeting' is *tapaamassa* [or in better Finnish *tapaamisiin* 'let's meet soon']; however, she wrote *tappamassa*, which means 'killing'! Many a misunderstanding can be blamed on the language.

Few Finns retain the dialect of their parents or of their region. In Finland, one cannot detect a person's social background from the way in which he or she speaks because the differences do not show in the pronunciation of different words. Finnish is a phonetic language that is written largely as it is spoken (da Costa, 1987). The Finnish spoken in Canada is not so pure as the Finnish in Finland, which tends to be more proper and to be less of a dialect.

The Finnish language was a stumbling block for the early immigrants because it bears no resemblance to English. The Finns were among the slowest European immigrants to learn to speak English (Lindstrom-Best, 1985). Many of the Finns of the pre-1930 period were of working age and spoke only Finnish. Several significant Finnish-language newspapers were established in Canada, such as the independent *Vapaa Sana* ('free word') (1931), published in Toronto; *Vapaus* ('freedom'), published in Sudbury from 1917 to 1975; and the independent Canadian *Uutiset* ('news'), published in Thunder Bay since 1915 (Sillanpää, 1988). Two other papers are the *Länsirannikon Uutiset* ('West Coast news') published in Port Coquitlam; and the *Todistaja* ('witness'), published in Vancouver (Corpus Almanac, 1997). Presently there are Finnish-language courses offered in Canada in most of the major Finnish settlements for adults and youth wishing to learn the language. This is a result of a growing cultural consciousness and support from various government agencies in the 1970s (Sillanpää, 1988). By the 1970s, ethnic Canadians persuaded the federal government to introduce a new policy of multiculturalism that recognized them as full and equal partners in Canadian society and affirmed their right to decide for themselves whatever part, if any, of their ethnic heritage, affiliations, and identities they might choose to retain (Sillanpää, 1994).

Nonverbal language is an important communication modality to the Finnish-Canadian people because most Finns touch infrequently. Younger couples tend to touch more frequently (Geissler, 1994). When greeting each other, Finnish Canadians usually shake hands with very few bowing in the formal greeting of the earlier Finnish Canadians.

The Finnish Canadians use direct eye contact. However the eye contact is usually intermittent (Geissler, 1994).

Some Finnish Canadians can be described as quiet, meditative, bashful, or rigid, whereas others may be described as laughing or quick witted. Because of these variations, it is difficult to describe the typical Finnish character, but it can be said that they are rugged individualists, when it comes to likes and dislikes, work and achievement. They are the strong silent types and are a very reflective people. They are proud of their heritage and their freedom, which was fought so hard for (Ojakangas, 1964).

There is an important cultural trait of people of Finnish origin that is best described by the word *sisu,* which is defined in English as 'enduring energy', 'possessing guts', or the trait of 'sticking to it'. For many it appears to be a cultural trait related to ethnic origin. Finnish Canadians generally seem to have the physical energy or special strength and mental endurance or stubborn determination to complete any job well and not to give up. They have a strong work ethic. This may be the reason why Finnish Canadians seem to exceed in individual sports rather than team sports and possibly why they are known for being good workers (Ojakangas, 1964). Schneider (1986) describes her father as having said that in the melting pot of America the last immigrant, holding on to the edge and struggling to keep out of the stew, was sure to be a Finn.

Implications for nursing care

It is important for the nurse to remember that when caring for the Finnish-Canadian client they may not speak anything but Finnish. They may avoid verbal communication because of not being understood and may become hostile or uncooperative or may withdraw. It is important not to isolate these clients. It is important to use an interpreter whenever possible. According to Spector the use of interpreters is preferred over the use of translators because interpreters are usually professionally trained and interpret the meanings of words and phrases. Using family members as translators is least effective because they may filter or change the information in an attempt to protect the client from some health information or not convey some information from the client that they may deem necessary as well as violate confidentiality for the client. When using an interpreter, the nurse should speak directly to the client and be aware of his or her body language (1996). For community health nurses practicing in the client's home there may be a greater tendency to use the family as translators, and the aforementioned regarding interpreters needs to be seriously considered, particularly for complex health care issues. The family should be encouraged to participate in the client's care in other ways such as providing comfort measures or some of the client's favorite foods (if permitted). Spector (1996) further emphasizes that, whether translators or interpreters are used, the nurse should speak slowly, avoid excessive medical terminology, and allow for the client to ask questions and return-demonstrate any material that was taught. In addition, Andrews and Boyle (1995) have a section of suggestions for overcoming language barriers when there is no interpreter available, and they also discuss how to use an interpreter.

The nurse will need to assess the comfort measures preferred by Finnish Canadians with particular attention to the area of touch. It is a common practice of Canadian nurses to touch their clients as a comforting measure, particularly when the client may be in pain or is grieving, stressed, or upset. Many Finnish Canadians may prefer being talked to or read to while having a cup of coffee. It is important for the nurse to be attentive to signs of fear, anxiety, and pain because the Finnish-Canadian client may not verbalize or demonstrate these signs. Nursing actions should be continually evaluated for effectiveness and modified as needed.

SPACE

Personal space refers to people's attitudes and behaviors toward the space surrounding them (Spector, 1996). According to Andrews and Boyle the perceptions of appropriate space, or distance zones, vary widely among cultural groups, with people of the same culture usually acting similarly with some individual variations. The authors describe four distance zones, which are the intimate zone (0 to 1½ feet), personal distance (1½ to 4 feet), social distance (4 to 12 feet), and public distance (12+ feet) (Andrews and Boyle, 1996).

Many Finns like their space and distance, and they do not like to have their space intruded on. They prefer to speak and work in the social or public zone. According to Spector (1996) White European immigrants are noncontact people and may be described as aloof and distant.

Implications for nursing care

Nonverbal communication techniques according to Cookfair (1996) should be used by the nurse while taking cues from the client. In some instances touching the client may be an invasion of personal space, whereas in other instances touching may signify caring. The most effective nursing action should be guided by the client's response because these behaviors are not culture bound (1996). Consequently, when interacting with the Finnish-Canadian client whom the nurse is not familiar with, the nurse should try to establish the client's trust and respect his or her space-zone distance using the client as the nurse's guide to acceptable interaction in reference to space zones.

SOCIAL ORGANIZATION

The family has been and still is the basic unit of society in Finland and consequently for the Finnish Canadians. Traditionally Finns raised large families with several generations living together. It was common for a young man about to be married to bring his bride home to live in his parent's house. Currently, young people are moving away from home and are finding their own accommodations because they want to live their own lives and be independent. Urbanization, occurring mostly in the 1960s, has decreased the need for large families that once were needed to help with farming chores, and it is also a rarity for extended families to be living together (da Costa, 1987).

About 15% of families are single-parent families. The average Finnish family has less than two children, with families with four or more children being infrequent. More than half of all families have only one child. This may be attributed to more women furthering their studies and developing a working career before having children. It is becoming common for women to delay parenthood, with over half of women having their first baby in the 25 to 34 year age group (Runeberg, 1983). This is also the case for Finnish-Canadian families. Family size is usually one or two children. Many Finnish Canadians have extended family in Finland and will frequently travel to Finland to visit relatives.

Finland government family policy formerly focused on health policy. More recently family policy emphasis shifted to child care and concentrates on effective leveling out of family expenses and day care and improving family guidance and counseling. There are family allowances, maternity allowances, housing allowances, and child care allowances. Family allowances was one of the first important achievements of family policy in Finland, and it came about in the 1940s for all children under 16 (Runeberg, 1983). Finnish Canadians also benefit from Canada's social programs, which closely mirror those of Finland.

Recently, in Canada, it has come to be that when older people are no longer able to care for themselves they rarely move in with family as was the case in the past. The tendency is to move to a senior's home or to a rest home. Several rest homes that have a significant number of Finnish residents have been organized in Canadian communities. They are usually called "Finnish rest homes" and often are incorporated to provide for fund-raising efforts to contribute to building other rest homes or nursing homes that could provide more skilled health care services and continuity of care in a Finnish cultural environment.

Presently, in Finland, class distinctions are not so evident except for differences in lifestyle rather than income. Developments in health care, social services for families with children, unemployment benefits, pensions, and so forth have reduced the evidence of poverty in Finland (da Costa, 1987).

There is great respect for education in Finland, and the level of education is generally a more important criterion than salary. Some professions that are respected by Finnish people are judges, doctors, and teachers. Finnish people do not refer to someone as "Mr." or "Mrs." but may use the person's academic or professional title (da Costa, 1987). In Canada, Finnish Canadians often do not question professionals. They are viewed as having the knowledge required for their position, and this knowledge is respected and may accord the professionals a class distinction because of their recognized and respected position.

Women's rights came earlier in Finland than in the rest of Europe. Women in Finland got the right to vote in 1906 and were the first in the world to run for office (Lander and Charbonneau, 1990). Many women began to take jobs outside of the home along with the growth of industry in the 1960s. Development of day-care facilities became a necessity.

In Finland children start school when they are 7 years of age. This has been the age for starting school in Finland since the compulsory education act passed in 1921, affecting 7 to 16 year olds, who are provided free general education. Finland's late school-starting age, compared to that of other European countries, is largely attributable to Finland's size and composition of large areas with very sparse settlement and great distances for traveling to school coupled with severe northern winters (Runeberg, 1983). A basic level of literacy was achieved throughout Finland because all Finnish children were required to attend confirmation classes. The doctrine of the Evangelical Lutheran church of Finland was that all Christians must be able to read the Bible (Sillanpää, 1994).

Very few families have domestic help. Housework and child care are divided between the parents, and usually the women carry most of the responsibility for the home and children (da Costa, 1987). Husband and wife usually share responsibility for making health care decisions for the children (Geissler, 1994). Domestic care is a rarity for Finnish-Canadian families. Family responsibilities are shared among family members. Most Finnish Canadians are very clean, neat, and organized, and generally a thorough cleaning by scrubbing and airing items outside and so forth is done in the home twice a year, usually before Christmas and in the spring.

In the Finnish countryside young women practice the Scandinavian custom of "night courting." During the summer months a young woman would sleep in a cabin or hut apart from the main farmhouse, and she might be visited by local young men. These suitors would court her by singing or reading and so on, trying to persuade her to allow him to spend the night. The decision was hers, and there was no stigma if she said yes (Lander and Charbonneau, 1990). This is not a custom that has been practiced in Canada.

In Finland the average age at which people get married is 25. Traditional Finnish wedding rings are two plain matching gold bands—one being the engagement ring and the other the wedding ring. Common-law partnerships, or open union, are frequent with almost the same status as a marriage. Open union is not officially sanctioned like marriage but is widely considered its equivalent. Divorce is becoming more common because it is no longer morally condemned, and women can better afford to remove themselves from an unsuccessful marriage. Some of these customs are also followed by Finnish Canadians. However, marriages are more common than open unions.

Religion in Finland is predominantly Evangelical Lutheran for approximately 89%, Greek Orthodox 1%, none 9%, and other 1%. Children are baptized in church, and couples are usually married in a church ceremony (da Costa, 1987). As in Canada, religious celebrations such as Christmas and Easter are very commercialized.

The Finnish immigrants were exclusively Lutheran on their arrival in Canada, and in 1893 the first two Finnish Lutheran congregations were organized. The Finnish-Canadian Lutheran church began to prosper somewhere in the 1930s. Before the 1930s Finnish immigrants often joined the Presbyterian church, the United Church of Canada, and various independent Lutheran congregations (Lindstrom-Best, 1981). The Lutheran churches constitute the largest of all Protestant churches and are exceeded only by the Orthodox and Roman Catholic churches in the worldwide Christian community (Bishop and Darton, 1988). Religion usually holds an important place in the life of Finnish Canadians, with religion being a personal and often private experience. The Finnish-Canadian churches are usually very practical and are usually not highly decorated with religious symbols.

The Finnish Canadians celebrate 12 national holidays. Every holiday is usually celebrated with a fiddle tune, a dance, or a church service. A very important holiday is the one associated with the Midsummer Day (*Juhannus*), which is the nearest Saturday to

June 24, and one that emphasizes Finnish values. *Juhannus* is the biggest event of the year next to Christmas. Usually families travel long distances to be together, and houses are decorated inside and out with young birch branches and flags. Many couples plan their wedding on this day. During *Juhannus* Finnish Canadians wear a national costume that is usually handmade and reflects one of the 12 provinces, which have a style different from each other. Boys' and men's costumes often consist of long pants and vests with wide lapels and narrow, stand-up collars as well as full-sleeved shirts and skull caps. The girls' and women's outfits consist of wide full skirts that might be striped or a solid color and laced, sleeveless vests of a matching or contrasting design. Unmarried girls wear colored ribbons in their hair, whereas married women wear small caps. The Finnish Independence Day is celebrated on December 6, and many Finns burn a candle in a window to commemorate the day. This practice is celebrated by traditional Finnish Canadians. Christmas Eve is also special because that is the day that the Finnish celebrate the Yuletide. On Christmas Eve there may be a traditional meal of glazed ham, vegetables, possibly a sweet turnip casserole spiced with nutmeg, rice pudding with a whole almond (any woman getting the almond would be the next bride or mother), and a dessert of prune whip with mounds of whipped cream on top. Gifts are usually opened on Christmas Eve, and there is singing of Christmas carols (Schneider, 1986). Christmas Day is usually treated as a quiet occasion with the emphasis on church and family (Sillanpää, 1994).

Finnish Canadians are great music lovers of all music and singing and usually have annual music festivals. Many have well-stocked musical libraries, and folk music is very important to them. They also enjoy the theater and are avid readers of magazines, books, and daily papers often utilizing library facilities and having quite an extensive library of their own. According to Schneider (1986), there is a saying that when two Finns get together they build a sauna, but when three get together they build a stage and put on amateur theatrical productions.

In 1940, some Lutheran churches and clubs organized the first Finnish Grand Festival to raise funds for Finland during World War II. These festivals have continued as an annual event and feature track and field, gymnastics, folk dancing, choirs, dramas, and a wide range of social activities (Sillanpää, 1988). The 1997 Grand Festival was held in Sault Ste. Marie. In the year 2000 Canada and the United States are having a joint festival to be held in Toronto.

A lot of the craft leisure activities are of useful crafts that are not superfluous or impractical "for decoration only" items. Some Finnish Canadians make the traditional *rya* (properly *ryijy*) rugs, which date back to the fourteenth and fifteenth centuries and can be used for bed covers or for rugs on boats or on sleighs. Other crafts are knit goods or crocheted items or any useful item made from wood. To achieve the feeling of a Finnish-Canadian home would mean including plants, books, and handmade items.

Many Finnish Canadians spend leisure time participating in sports such as gymnastics, swimming, Finnish baseball, and downhill and cross-country skiing. Finns have been called a sports-mad population (Lander and Charbonneau, 1990). Finland has a network of bicycle paths that lead to forests where there are trails for hiking, biking, or cross-country skiing. Skiing is the national pastime, and currently Finns ski for enjoyment rather than for necessity as in the past. The school system is geared for sports and exercise such that after 45 minutes of lessons there is a 15-minute recess. There are various sports organizations in Finland, and this trend has come along with some of the immigrant Finns. In 1902 a sports club was organized in Toronto, and a myriad of sport clubs were formed in remote Canadian localities where Finnish immigrants were often the majority of the work force (Tester, 1986). Hiking, walking, and cross-country skiing are very popular activities for Finnish Canadians, and many are very involved in building and maintaining hiking and ski trails.

The sports clubs, churches, clubs for dances, drama troupes, choirs, bands, and folk dancing met the Finns' need for community and culture. Many of the Finns of the pre-1930 period were of working age and spoke only Finnish; consequently, there was a real need for these social activities, and a close bond linked the members. The Finnish Canadians greatly respect and cherish their family and friends. In 1911 the Finnish Organization of Canada (originally the Finnish Socialist Organization of Canada) was established and is the oldest Canadian nationwide cultural organization for Finns currently located in Toronto (Sillanpää, 1988).

Implications for nursing care

Andrews and Boyle (1995) indicate that a mutually respectful relationship is established with appropriate introductions and that nurses should introduce themselves as they prefer to be called and ensure that they understand how the client prefers to be called. This gesture will help to establish a better rapport with clients, particularly in the client's home environment, which is where most Finnish Canadians prefer to remain for as long as possible. It is always appropriate to explore the preferred form of address with the client even when working with a client from the same cultural group.

According to Andrews and Boyle (1995) Europeans generally are much more willing to discuss private and family matters quite freely with friends, acquaintances and even strangers. As a result obtaining health care information should not be a problem.

It is important for the nurse to consider that even though Finnish Canadians are usually very literate and well educated this may be applicable only for the Finnish language, and the nurse may need to adapt techniques that are usually used for clients with low literacy skills. Information should be short, direct, and specific and be supplemented by visual cues. As previously mentioned the use of an interpreter is highly recommended.

The Finnish-Canadian family is usually important, and it is encouraged that any health care education be provided to all members whenever possible. When referring to a client's partner, the word "partner" is preferable to "spouse" particularly if the relationship is an open union and not marriage.

Most Finnish Canadians prefer to be as independent as possible. Activities should be encouraged that will allow them to be as active as possible. Recreational activities that may involve crafts such as knitting or social activities such as playing cards could be provided. Reading and music are important activities, and these should be encouraged and supported. The nurse needs to keep in mind that Finnish Canadians enjoy their family and friends, and so the nurse should be somewhat flexible in interventions with the client when visitors are present, provided that there are no potential harmful client outcomes.

TIME

Finnish Canadians are usually very punctual and may be irritated by tardiness (Geissler, 1994). The Finnish Canadians are generally present and future oriented in that they work and play hard in the present but also work to achieve future goals.

Implications for nursing care

The nurse should consider the circumstances of the current situation with the Finnish-Canadian client. The future may be influenced by the current situation. According to Spector (1996) people who are future oriented are usually focused on long-term goals and with health-care measures in the present that may prevent the occurrence of illness in the future, and they usually prefer to plan ahead. Health care planning may include primary and secondary measures such as care being taken regarding diet and health.

ENVIRONMENTAL CONTROL

Preventive health care is very important in Finland, and these services are available free to all families. All mothers of newborn babies receive a maternity gift pack that contains such items as basic clothing and bedding as well as other baby items, or the mother may choose money in lieu of the gift pack. The gift pack is usually worth more than the money and often is the choice of mothers. Dental care is free for all school children.

Finnish Canadians are hard working, self-reliant, and independent. When ill, they will usually try to remain in their own home for as long as possible and will utilize the services of home care.

Cultural values

Study of the literature indicates that the cultural values of Finnish Canadians are family closeness, individualism with an internal locus of control, education, hard work and industriousness, conscientiousness, thriftiness, cleanliness, good use of natural resources and living in harmony with nature, endurance and perseverance, and pride and emphasis on a continuation of their language and culture (Lindstrom, 1992; Ojakangas, 1964; Schneider, 1986; Sillanpää, 1994; Vahtola, 1994).

Cultural health practices Vahtola's literature search found many cultural health practices that were traditionally practiced in Finland and sometimes in Canada; for example, healing would often take place at sites of supernatural significance such as lakes, high rocks, or saunas; treatments were varied and included charms, magic potions, herbal treatments, hot baths, physical manipulation, use of fire and water for healing, bloodletting, and cupping, which was used usually in the spring and fall to remove bad blood and was performed in the sauna by using cups or horns (1994).

In 1967 a survey of Thunder Bay Finns and existing folklore was conducted by M. Salo as cited by Vahtola. Salo found that immigrants who had resided in Canada for 50 to 60 years talked of the mythical legends or tales that appeared to have survived because of their ease of telling and brevity. Salo concluded that plentiful folk cures and folk medicines were still in use but that supernatural practices such as incantations, spells, and charms were no longer believed to be in existence. Proverbs and riddles were also found to be abundant (Vahtola, 1994).

Salo conducted field research with Finnish immigrants in the Sudbury district of northern Ontario. Salo found that traditional beliefs and practices existed and were preserved because of the clustering of Finns in communities. Traditional healing was found to be more of a concealed activity and existed despite the general Finnish community's having limited belief in the supernatural. The first-generation immigrants were more familiar with the healing traditions, but the second generation acquired fragments of some of the first generation's practices. Antagonism toward medical doctors was found in the Sudbury area Finns who preferred their own remedies and healers (1973). Vahtola also found that many Thunder Bay Finns preferred their own remedies or alternative therapy such as herbal remedies, naturopathy, chiropractic, acupuncture, massage, and nutritional supplements rather than seek medical attention unless it would be absolutely necessary because being ill and needing care may be perceived as a sign of personal failure (1994).

The *sauna* (pronounced sów-nah) was the original and still is the most common bathing form in Finland. It seems to be uniquely Finnish and has spread in popularity to other Scandinavian countries and throughout Europe. Almost every Finnish home has a sauna in Finland and in Canada. Physical benefits from the sauna are cleanliness and a sense of well-being and relaxation.

Sauna practices vary from region to region. In some areas the entire family bathes together, whereas in other areas men may bathe first, in the hottest heat, followed by the women and children. In Canada the men usually bathe separately from the women and children. The sauna was usually the first building erected by the Finnish immigrants, and often they would live in the sauna while building their house.

A sauna is usually a small low room containing benches for sitting on and a wood-burning firebox and chimney, unless it is a modernized heat source such as electricity. There is usually a separate change room that is adjacent to the sauna, and normally it contains a shower. All saunas have a basket of rocks, preferably granite from the seacoast of Finland, heated by the stove on which water is thrown to increase the humidity, which increases the feeling of heat and makes a person sweat. Traditionally the walls of the sauna were made of pine and firs because they absorb the moisture of steam with rapidity and leave behind the dry, savory heat. The sauna is usually heated with birch logs because birch gives off a dry, sharp heat, a powerful fire with no soot or resin, and a distinctive aroma. The sauna in a Canadian home is often heated with electricity; however,

the sauna at a Finnish-Canadian cottage or camp is built as close to the traditional type of Finnish sauna as possible, preferably adjacent to a lake.

Before taking a sauna, the bathers remove all clothes, and a shower is taken. A small towel is placed on the bench for hygienic reasons and because the bench may feel hot. During the sauna one's body can be scrubbed with brushes or loofah sponges or could be massaged or lightly beaten with birch branches that are fully leaved and cut between June 24 and the beginning of July so that the foliage will remain. In the sauna the birch branches are dipped in lukewarm water and are used to whisk the body to stimulate the circulation and open up the pores and to rid oneself of the "bad" influences of previous days. Whether in summer or in winter it is customary to jump into a freshwater lake to cool off or to roll in snow that is preferably fresh and powdery rather than old and icy, which may feel like sandpaper. These customs are practiced by Finnish Canadians, and the sauna has become popular with other Canadians who enjoy this practice.

The previous Finnish generations may have been born in a sauna, and the elderly were often brought to the sauna to die. Some reasons were that the sauna could be warmed up quickly, there was water available to bathe a newborn and mother or dying person, the afterbirth could be burned in the fire, and it was considered to be a very clean environment (Lindstrom, 1992). Evidence of these customs currently being practiced in Canada has not been found.

According to Kauppinen, sauna baths are indicated for maintenance of good health and relief for general tension, anxiety, or irritability (1996). Kauppinen's research and review of the literature indicate that sauna baths are well tolerated and pose no risk to healthy people of all ages including healthy pregnant women. It was further noted by Kauppinen that the sauna bath does not pose any circulatory risk to healthy people and that stable cardiovascular patients may also take sauna baths without undue risk (1996).

Vahtola reports from Edelswaard's master's thesis on the *Sauna as Symbol* that the steam of the sauna, called *löyly,* is a distinguishing factor of the sacredness of the sauna because the soul is cleansed in the steam and the body is cleansed through perspiration. Along with cleansing the sauna functions as a place of purification, healing, and renewal. Edelswaard indicated that there is a recognized code of behavior in the sauna, that being that one should be quiet and should behave as one should in church. The sauna is a social event that promotes contact and closeness for participants and plays a social role with the Finns. In Salo's 1967 literature he spoke of Finnish proverbs regarding the sauna with one being that "the sauna is a poor man's doctor" (1994).

Some Finnish Canadians have their own remedies to treat some common illnesses. For a sore throat a cold wet cloth is wrapped around the neck and then this is covered with a wool sock or wool scarf. Another sore-throat practice is to drink hot milk that contains chopped onion. For an earache tobacco smoke is blown into the affected ear and then a cotton ball is inserted to keep the smoke in the ear (T. Koskela, personal communication, June 13, 1997). Some folk remedies according to Salo (1973) are plantain leaves put over wounds, balsam pitch for colds and cough, sugar in the eye for cataracts, and Labrador tea baths for rheumatism.

Definition of health and illness Vahtola found in reviewing the literature and in her own study of some Thunder Bay Finns that the elements of health, illness, and healing beliefs that appeared repeatedly were the idea of mind-body unity; the importance of self-care; prevention; use of alternative medicine; nutrition—described as consuming only whole natural foods without additives; fresh air, which included airing of home and bedding and being outdoors daily to ensure some exposure to the sun, which is seen as healthful and life giving; exercise preferably outside and vigorous enough to sweat; the sauna; and the emphasis on cleanliness usually achieved in the sauna because baths are perceived by many as not cleansing (1994).

It was also found by Vahtola (1994) that Finnish Canadians take a great deal of pride in remaining healthy, and the key to health is prevention by staying dry and warm, dressing appropriately in the winter with the head covered and the feet warm, and avoiding drafts. Balance was mentioned frequently as important for a healthful life, which was identified as not doing things in excess but moderately. Proverbs dealing with health and illness were widely remembered.

Illness-wellness behaviors

According to Runeberg, Finland's national health care system is one of the best in the world, and public health issues were first legislated in 1879. In the early 1900s there was high infant mortalities and highly infectious diseases. In the 1920s a private advisory service for health care information and inoculations was initiated. The government assumed responsibility for these services in the late 1940s and established maternity and child health clinics. Currently the infant mortality in Finland is one of the lowest in the world, and a large number of children's infectious diseases have been completely eliminated as a result of immunization (1983). According to Lindstrom-Best, the infant mortality of the early Finnish Canadians was lower than the national average with cleanliness and diet contributing to the lower rate. Additionally the Finns had a tendency of caring for themselves at childbirth or when ill and preferred using their own midwives and home remedies that they trusted, with women generally having responsibility for these practices (1988). According to Geissler (1994) Finns believe in active involvement and believe that health promotion is important.

Folk medicine

In the early 1800s a collection of narrative poetry, called the *Kalevala* (the 'clan of Kaleva') was published by Elias Lönnrot. These poems have been part of the Finnish folklore for centuries, and the *Kalevala* connects the past for Finns, including the origin of the world, advent of Christianity, myths, rituals, and Finnish symbols. Vahtola indicates that according to Middleton (1967) anthropologists agree that myths are conscious elaborations of cultural beliefs (1994). In Vahtola's review of the literature shamanism was found to be a strong component in Finnish folklore, and the *Kalevala* has been described as shamanic poetry. A shaman practices folk remedies, and the word for shaman in Finnish is *tietäjä*, which means the 'knower' (1994). Salo refers to the *tietäjä* as a person who possesses supernatural powers or who knows more than ordinary humans do and uses magic and natural means to heal the sick and to assist people with various other problems. Some roles assumed by the *tietäjä* are those of bloodletter, cupper, bonesetter, masseuse, and midwife (1973). Shamanism still exists in Canada according to Vahtola. She indicated that Lakehead University Professor of Anthropology Raija Warkentin would soon have a published article in the *Journal of Finnish Studies* titled "A Modern Finnish Shaman in a Northwestern Ontario City," which discusses the practice of shamanism in and around Thunder Bay (M. Vahtola, personal communication, July 23, 1997).

Implications for nursing care

Some Finnish Canadians are perceived as having an internal locus of control, which is reflected in their preference for self-care and independence. The nurse should recognize these traits as strengths and utilize them by encouraging and supporting positive health behaviors that will facilitate adaptation to health changes. Families are important to Finnish Canadians, and they should be included in as many aspects of the client's health program, with the nurse keeping in mind that the client will ultimately make his or her own health care decisions. These decisions will probably be based on reading and consultation with others. The nurse should recognize the Finn's level of literacy and education and be prepared for the possibility of being asked for health care literature and resources that could assist the client in the planning or intervention phases of care. Finnish Canadians place a lot of emphasis on prevention, and the nurse could utilize this by devising a teaching plan that emphasizes the importance of preventive techniques.

Because the primary level of intervention for an illness for some Finnish Canadians may be folk practices before seeking medical attention, it is important for the nurse to ascertain through assessment what the client's health beliefs and practices are and what each has tried before seeking medical attention. It is important for the nurse to determine which of the practices could be incorporated into the plan of care and which should be discouraged, and such a determination will require the nurse to educate the client about the harmful practices and to avoid them, with the nurse supporting this avoidance and encouraging the family to do the same.

Cleanliness for many Finnish Canadians is a very important component of their beliefs and practices, with the sauna being the preferred choice for cleanliness. The nurse needs to be aware of the Finnish Canadian's need for as clean an environment as possible as well as a clean person. An unclean physical space may diminish the client's confidence in the health care facility or space. The nurse can try to ensure that environmental cleanliness is maintained, and the nurse should try to ensure for personal cleanliness. The client should be given the choice of a bath or a shower, and the nurse should offer to assist the client with achieving optimal cleanliness.

BIOLOGICAL VARIATIONS

Giger and Davidhizar (1995) indicate that even with the introduction of transcultural nursing concepts the nursing literature existing among various racial groups remains scanty. This has been the case with the literature on Finnish Canadians, which was found to be sparse to nonexistent, particularly regarding biological variations, with much of the information being the result of anecdotal notes.

The Finn is very fair skinned with high cheekbones, and most commonly Finns have blue eyes with blond hair coloring that darkens with age. Stature and skin color among Finnish Canadians are quite similar to that of other White European immigrants (Spector, 1996).

Ethnic specific disease risks

Disorders that are present in the Finns in relatively high frequency are congenital nephrosis, generalized amyloidosis syndrome, polycystic liver disease, cardiovascular diseases, and cancer (Geissler, 1994).

Nutritional preferences and deficiencies

In general, food in Finland has its own character. Crops are limited because of the paucity of fertile land. Principal crops are those that form the staple foods of potatoes and cauliflower and other vegetables such as carrots and cucumbers, and a variety of grains including rye, oats, barley, and wheat (Barer-Stein, 1979). Potatoes are usually served at the table unpeeled, boiled in their skins. Many traditional Finnish dishes are molded or jellied veal, sour rye bread (the mainstay of the Finnish diet and their favorite bread), a hearty hot soup or stew as a main course called *keitto*, ('cooking') fish, Karelian pot roast, Finnish meat balls, cabbage rolls, pork gravy (which usually contains pieces of salt pork), various butter cakes and cookies, sweet breads, whipped berry puddings, porridge, and fruit soups. A buffet table in Finland would vary depending on the region or area. In eastern Finland some of the traditional foods are various pastries, some filled, and foods made of sour milk. In east central Finland, where there are more than 50,000 lakes, fish dishes are common such as *kalakukko*, meaning 'fish baked in a crust', or 'fish-pasty'. In the western provinces the traditional dishes center around dairy foods, whole-grain cereals, and saltwater fish such as herring (Ojakangas, 1964). Many Finns are almost addicted to milk products. Milk, cream, and cheeses are used generously. They like cream in their coffee, disliking the canned milk substitute often used by Canadians, and also enjoy various types of sour milk such as buttermilk and yogurt, often making their own yogurt. Because of the short growing season, fruits and vegetables are prized. Preserved fruit and berries are served often with meals. Finland has a wide variety of berries, of which many are found in Canada such as blueberries, raspberries, cranberries, and strawberries. Citrus fruits are imported. Finnish Canadians are keen berry pickers often freezing or preserving the berries for winter usage.

The Finns usually have their morning coffee, possibly with a couple of open-faced sandwiches or a Finn bun. Sometime between 11 o'clock and 1 o'clock a dish of cooked cereal, such as oatmeal, is eaten. Later on they might have more coffee and perhaps another sandwich. The evening meal is usually a casserole such as *maksalaatikko* ('liver-box'), which is a liver-rice casserole. Coffee is not served with the meal but may be served later in the evening whenever anyone wants it. If there were guests, the coffee

may be served with pound cake, butter cookies, spice cake, buns, or slices of cheese. The Finns make a special occasion of drinking coffee and consume more coffee per person than any other people in the world (Lander and Charbonneau, 1990). Coffee is best when made in a copper coffee pot in which the coffee grounds are boiled in the water. Finnish immigrants rarely immigrated without their copper coffee pot. Coffee drinking requires sitting down, preferably with someone else, and taking a break in the day. Few people drink tea; most adults are coffee drinkers or milk drinkers, or both. The Finns are not great sweet eaters and prefer fruit soups or fresh berries. They rarely sweeten their food. Eggs are consumed mostly as an ingredient in other dishes. Much fat is consumed in the form of whole milk, butter, cheeses, cream, and sour cream. Butter is the main cooking fat. Finns prefer natural flavors and seasonings, and smoked meats are very abundant (Barer-Stein, 1979). The above-stated food preferences and deficiencies are also applicable to the Finnish Canadians. One of the first businesses opened by Finnish immigrants was a bakery. Some of the Finnish immigrants did not believe that the bread in Canada was bread at all but merely "white fluff" (Schneider, 1986). Coffee is still highly consumed and may also be served with the meal but will probably be accompanied by a dessert after the meal. If Finnish Canadians offer guests coffee at a time other than mealtime, the guests may be served some food, and extra effort will be taken by the Finnish Canadians to use their fancier plates and cups rather than their everyday dishes or mugs. Coffee time is a social activity.

Psychological characteristics

Vahtola reports from Edelswaard's thesis that among the Finns, self-control is important. Edelswaard found that emotions are kept hidden, and independence and the ability to cope alone is a virtue with some keeping silent even from family and friends. Vahtola found that some elderly Finns, particularly men, were reluctant to verbalize pain and often refuse medication (1994).

Use of controlled substances

In Finland cigarettes and tobacco may not be sold to anyone under 16, mild alcoholic drinks are not sold or served to anyone under 18, and strong liquor to anyone under 20 (Runeberg, 1983). In Canada cigarettes and tobacco may not be sold to anyone under 16, and alcoholic drinks and strong liquor are not sold or served to anyone under 19 (Addiction Research Foundation, 1994).

Sillanpää indicates that alcoholism was a severe problem in Finland and was made worse for the Finnish immigrants in Canada because of the harsh conditions and sense of alienation that they often experienced in their new environment. The temperance society emerged as one of the earliest organizations in the Finnish-Canadian community, with the earliest one being organized in 1890 in British Columbia and the last being dissolved in 1920 (1994).

In 1995, in Finland, the alcohol consumption was 6.6 (7.7 in 1991) liters of absolute alcohol per capita compared to Canada's 6.2 (7.4 in 1991) liters per capita, France's 11.5 (12.6 in 1991) liters per capita, Denmark's 10 (9.9 in 1991) liters per capita, and Sweden's 5.3 (5.5 in 1991) liters per capita (NTC Publications Ltd, 1996). The use of alcohol is viewed as the modern urban way of life, and consumption is highest in the cities, with the countryside traditionally being dry, with abstinence being preferred. Beer constitutes over 50% of all consumption, and Finns continue to drink for intoxication. Only about 1% of Finns use beer or wine with meals. Since 1985 alcohol consumption has been rising until 1991 when an 8% increase in prices and an economical depression caused a decrease in consumption. Young people are included in this increase, with women representing only one fifth of the total intake (Addiction Research Foundation, 1994). Equivalent information on Finnish Canadians has not been collected because ethnic origin questions are not usually asked of survey participants and these questions may be perceived as discriminatory (B. Williams, Addiction Research Foundation, personal communication, July 24, 1997).

Mortality and leading causes of death

Infant mortalities in Finland for both sexes in 1996 was 4.9 deaths per 1000 live births, and the life expectancy at birth (years) for both sexes in 1996 was 75.5 years (Johnson, 1997). Current rates for Finnish Canadians were not found.

Lindstrom writes about the health and welfare of Finnish immigrant women and their children. She shares many stories of the early immigrants' struggle to survive the problems encountered in a new homeland where alienation and isolation claimed some of the Finnish immigrants. Children were particularly vulnerable dying of natural causes, and some succumbed to stomach ailments, pneumonia, tuberculosis (contracted from the mother), various fevers, influenza, and accidental deaths from drowning, gunshot wounds, or poisoning (from eating the lye used to whiten clothes). Many Finnish-Canadian immigrants were living in remote location settlements, and the journey to a physician may have been impossible or treacherous. Women were less likely to suffer an unnatural death (many were affected by tuberculosis), whereas many men's lives ended by accidents or violence. For Finnish-Canadian immigrant women suicide, tuberculosis, and then childbirth were the most common causes of death followed by influenza, fever, and pneumonia (1994).

Lindstrom indicated that the Finns had a tendency to commit suicide, often exceeding the national average in Canada by seven times. The primary motive for female suicide was illness because they did not want to be a burden to their family, and the secondary motive was poverty. Suicide in Finland was seen as a private independent decision, and suicide victims received a normal burial in a consecrated graveyard. The heroines and heroes of Finnish folklore often killed themselves. Four times more Finnish men than women committed suicide, with possible reasons being the abnormality of immigrant life, poverty, illness, alcoholism, and loneliness. In Thunder Bay there used to be a tree that became known as the "last stop" because that is where the Finns hanged themselves (1994). According to folklore the hanging tree was a birch tree, and because of the number of suicides, a Finnish-Canadian chief of police had the tree cut down in an attempt to discourage suicide (M. Vahtola, personal communication, July 23, 1997).

During Finnfest USA '96 there was a Finnfest forum I, which was an examination of linkages between ethnicity and health for Finnish Americans. Aspects of heart disease, diabetes, alcoholism, and mental health were presented by Finnish-American health practitioners from doctors to social workers, utilizing stories through their own practices and families. Written notes from this forum are not currently available: however videotape footage is available for some of the proceedings. According to Jean McKinney, a nurse who is currently writing a master's thesis on certain aspects of the Finnish-American cultural group, the tapes are not all inclusive of the forum, and the material leads one to believe that the cultural inheritance of health practices is understudied and undocumented for the Finns (J. McKinney, personal communication, August 12, 1997). The topics of the Finnfest forum are strongly suggestive that these are areas of concern for this ethnic group. These topic areas also were evident in many personal interviews with Canadian health care practitioners and non health care practitioners; however research and documentation of these identified areas are lacking.

One very useful article was found dealing with the exceptionally high coronary heart disease rates for Finns. According to Puska et al. (1994) Finland was in the 1960s and early 1970s a country that had extremely high mortalities of coronary heart disease, with middle-aged Finnish men having the highest mortality from cardiovascular disease in the world. Researchers demonstrated the central role of elevated serum cholesterol as a risk factor, its close links with diet, and the high blood cholesterol level and saturated fat intake of the Finns. In 1972 the North Karelia Project was launched to reduce the great burden of exceptionally high coronary heart disease mortalities. The 20-year project included implementation of comprehensive, community-based strategies to change the main coronary risk factors, which are the serum cholesterol concentration, blood pressure, and smoking. The results indicated that the mortality from ischemic heart disease declined between 1972 and 1992 by 55% in men and 68% in women. It was also found that cancer mortality was also significantly reduced (1994).

Dietary factors determining diabetes and impaired glucose tolerance were examined over a 30-year period with Finnish and Dutch cohorts. The results indicated that a high intake of fat, especially that of saturated fatty acids, contributes to the risk of glucose intolerance and non insulin dependent diabetes mellitus (Feskens et al., 1995).

Jacono et al. (1996) indicated that there has recently been an increased interest in differences between cultures in relation to specific illnesses but that results of these studies have been variable and are suggestive of the need for continuing research. Jacono et al. completed a retrospective analysis of client charts in an attempt to investigate differences between four cultural groupings in rheumatoid arthritis. The four groupings were Canadian aboriginals, Finnish Canadians, Italian Canadians, and other White Canadians. The findings were similar to those from previous research. In reference to Finnish Canadians the researchers found that there were twice as many Finnish Canadians suffering from rheumatoid arthritis as Italian Canadians (1996). According to Jacono et al. this finding supported research by Isomäki et al. (1978), who suggested that Finns suffered from rheumatoid arthritis more frequently than other Europeans did (1996).

Implications for nursing care

Andrews and Boyle write extensively on transcultural perspectives in mental health. In summary, the authors' key points for a nurse to care for clients with psychological health concerns are to promote a feeling of acceptance by suggesting illness-prevention and health-maintenance practices as well as treatment regimes that compliment or reinforce a client's cultural beliefs and practices; establish open communication by utilizing appropriate salutations, use of space and eye contact, avoidance of jargon, and utilizing open-ended questions; anticipate diversity and emphasize positive points and strengths of health beliefs, and practices as well as being respectful of values, beliefs, rights, and practices; learn what care means to the client; and understand a client's goals and expectations (1994). These points should be considered when a client with all health concerns is being cared for.

Because pain may not be expressed by Finnish Canadians, the nurse should continually assess the client for pain. The nurse should ensure that as many as possible comfort measures, along with other interventions, are offered to the client and should encourage the client to have as much individual control over pain medication as possible, such as through a self-administered medication pump.

The Finnish-Canadian diet is high in fat. This high fat consumption increases the risk of developing heart disease and cancer as well as increases the risk for high blood pressure and diabetes (Smolin and Grosvenor, 1994). The nurse should thoroughly assess the client's diet, specifically how the foods are prepared to determine frying versus baking or broiling. The use of saturated or unsaturated fats, which will have a great effect on the client's cholesterol consumption, should be less than 250 mg daily. The nurse should educate the client about things that can be done to reduce the total intake of fat and cholesterol such as selecting lean poultry and removing the skin before cooking; avoiding fried foods and breaded foods; preparing foods by baking, broiling, boiling, or microwaving rather than frying; selecting skim or low-fat milk products including cheese; selecting monounsaturated or polyunsaturated fats and oils; removing all visible fat from meat before cooking; checking labels for fats and selecting low-fat products; limiting eating foods from fast-food restaurants; and skimming the fat from stews or soups before serving (Bruess and Richardson, 1992).

Finnish Canadians are heavy coffee drinkers, and caffeine can cause toxic effects such as anxiety, respiratory and cardiovascular stimulation, and stomach upset. In one cup of regular coffee there is 139 mg of caffeine compared to 3 mg of caffeine in one cup of decaffeinated coffee (Smolin and Grosvenor, 1994). According to Edelman and Mandle (1998) reports indicate that caffeine increases the blood level of lipids and glucose and the elevated serum fat levels act on the cardiovascular system in such a way that heavy coffee users, rather than moderate users, may have a higher incidence of angina and myocardial infarction. Clients should be encouraged to cut down on their coffee consumption and switch to the decaffeinated type. The nurse needs to keep in mind that coffee time is a social activity and the client will need support in making adjustments to this activity.

Of all the chronic diseases, cardiovascular diseases seem to have the most potential for primary prevention because of the knowledge there is about the risk factors (Bruess and Richardson, 1992). Consequently the nurse should educate the Finnish-Canadian client about the risk factors and interventions. The major risk factors are smoking, hypercholesterolemia, lack of exercise, diabetes mellitus, hypertension, obesity, and excessive stress (Bruess and Richardson, 1992). Most Finnish Canadians have an internal locus of control. This means that they believe that their behavior reduces the chances of developing a health problem. The nurse needs to be aware of the appropriate "teachable moment" and to utilize every opportunity possible to provide the appropriate health care information about each of the cardiovascular risk factors. The client should also be encouraged to take the recommended daily requirement of calcium and drink at least 8 glasses of water daily, if not contraindicated, to reduce the possibility of renal calculi.

The nurse should assess the client's employment and leisure activities to determine the Finnish-Canadians exposure to the sun. Because most are fair skinned and blue eyed, they are at increased risk for skin cancer and should be educated about the preventive measures for skin cancer and other cancers, which would include education about cancer and diet, weight, alcohol consumption, and the use of tobacco.

SUMMARY

Most of the Finnish Canadians currently in Canada are of the second or third generation. Some may not have maintained their language, but many have maintained the Finnish customs. Finnish Canadians vary in their degree of acculturation and may demonstrate a variety of behaviors that are dependent on factors such as generational, regional, and individual differences. It is important for the nurse to assess the unique strengths of each individual. Knowledge of the culture and acceptance of health care beliefs will assist the nurse in providing culturally sensitive and individualized care.

Case Study

Laila Mäki, is a 65-year-old Finnish Canadian who has just moved into a Finnish rest home in northwestern Ontario. The initial assessment of Laila by the nurse in the rest home revealed the following about Laila. Laila immigrated to Canada in 1950 when she was 18. She had been born on a farm in Finland and had just completed her high school education. Her oldest brother had arrived in Canada 2 years earlier and was working in an all-Finn lumber camp as a lumberjack. Laila came over to work as a cook in the camp in the hopes of making enough money to live in Toronto and become an actress or dancer. Shortly after her arrival she met Toivo, a lumberjack friend of her brother, and they were engaged to be married and built a log home together close to the lumber camp. A few weeks before their marriage Toivo was killed when a tree fell on him. Laila continued to live in their home and stayed on as the camp cook.

The months turned into years, and she followed the lumber crew from camp to camp as their cook. The workers thought that she was a good cook, and most of the meals were often traditional Finnish dishes. In the long winter evenings coffee was plentiful, and on occasion she would also have an alcoholic drink. She didn't smoke, but roughly 80% of the camp workers smoked. They had become her Canadian family. She would often send money home to her parents in Finland and would go home each summer when the camps were closed down because of the high-risk fire season. She would pass the time in the camp preparing meals, picking berries, swimming, doing crafts, reading, and writing in a daily journal. She had several male friends but never married.

Two weeks before her moving into the rest home Laila had just returned from Finland having been home to attend her elderly father's funeral. She had found the trip very tiring and experienced headaches, shortness of breath, and chest pain. Laila had always treated herself with home remedies in the past whenever she had felt ill, which was not often. Her symptoms continued, and before returning Laila to camp the foreman insisted that she seek medical attention. She was admitted to hospital for investigation and was diagnosed with coronary artery disease. She was told that she was severely hypertensive because her blood pressure was 180/120. She had hypercholesterolemia and was morbidly obese because she weighed 185 lb and was only 5′ 1″. She was put on a low-fat, low-salt and calorie-reduced diet with an antihypertensive medication, an antianginal medication, and lovastatin, a medication to reduce her blood cholesterol. The physician strongly advised her to quit her job because she was at high risk for a heart attack and to move into a larger center where she would have access to medical care. She was also referred to a cardiac rehabilitation program. With the encouragement of her brother and his family and her extended family of lumber-camp friends she decided to relocate. She was accepted into a Finnish rest home quite quickly because of her medical condition as well as the fact that she spoke limited English and that there happened to be a new vacancy.

The rest home nurse, who was Finnish, managed to encourage Laila to attend the cardiac rehabilitation program with another rest-home resident. There was a Finnish-speaking nurse at the program and the other rest-home participant would drive Laila to the sessions.

Laila found living in the rest home stressful at times because she had been accustomed to having more time and space to herself as well as more autonomy, and she missed her former lifestyle and friends. She would spend hours outside planting and caring for a garden or walking, which she enjoyed now that she had more time. She also took advantage of the indoor swimming pool to exercise in an attempt to lose weight. She didn't eat in the main dining lounge often because she prefered her own cooking and was better able to control her diet.

CARE PLAN

 Nursing Diagnosis   Actively seeking knowledge about medical treatment or disease process (adapted from Stolte, 1996).

Client Outcomes

1. Asks questions about treatment or disease process.
2. Seeks written material about treatment or disease process and reads it.
3. Describes relationships between disease process and treatment as appropriate.
4. Discusses activities specific to disease that will improve health.

Nursing Interventions

1. Reinforce knowledge and provide specific information.
2. Reinforce asking questions.
3. Provide language materials if requested and available.
4. Provide information about treatment or disease process in written or audiovisual format in language of choice.
5. Discuss ways that client can improve health.
6. Encourage participation in a support or interest group.

 Nursing Diagnosis   Beginning acceptance of role change (adapted from Stolte, 1996).

Client Outcomes

1. Describes effect of illness on relationships with others.
2. Expresses feelings of loss.
3. Discusses ways client can accommodate to illness by substituting other activities, hobbies, or interests for those that must be given up.
4. Differentiates between those things that can be controlled and those that cannot.
5. Lets go of those things that cannot be controlled.

Nursing Interventions

1. Encourage ventilation and expression of feelings.
2. Provide empathic listening and build on the positive.
3. Explore alternatives to previous activities, hobbies, or interests that fit within physical limitations.

4. Discuss ways to maintain control and ways to let go of control.

Nursing Diagnosis   Compliance with prescribed diet (adapted from Stolte, 1996).

Client Outcomes

1. Describes prescribed diet.
2. Able to make appropriate substitutions among allowed food items.
3. Has appropriate food items in home.

Nursing Interventions

1. Clarify misunderstandings
2. Reinforce compliance and provide appropriate cultural alternatives.
3. Identify ways to make diet more flexible

STUDY QUESTIONS

1. What would be appropriate interventions by health care providers for clients who do not verbally express pain, discomfort, or stress?
2. What contributing factors predispose Finnish Canadians to cardiovascular disease?
3. What cultural values determine health practice behaviors in this cultural group?
4. How will the nurse keep Laila motivated toward self-help and self-care?
5. How might Laila's attitudes toward self-learning and lifelong learning enhance nursing care strategies?
6. What nursing interventions can be implemented to facilitate communication between Laila and health care practitioners?

References

Andrews, M.M., & Boyle, J.S. (1994). *Transcultural concepts in nursing care* (ed. 2). Philadelphia: J.B. Lippincott Co.

Addiction Research Foundation. (1994). *International profile: alcohol and other drugs.* Toronto: the Foundation.

Barer-Stein, T. (1979). *You eat what you are: a study of ethnic food traditions.* Toronto: McClelland & Stewart Ltd.

Bishop, P., & Darton, M. (1988). *The encyclopedia of world faiths.* New York: Facts on File, Inc.

Bruess, C., & Richardson, G. (1992). *Decisions for health.* Dubuque, Iowa: W.C. Brown Publishers.

Cookfair, J. (1996). *Nursing care in the community.* Toronto: Mosby.

Colombo, J. (1997). *The Canadian global almanac.* Toronto: MacMillan Canada.

Corpus Almanac 1997 Canadian Sourcebook (1996). Don Mills, Ont.: Southam Magazine & Information Group.

da Costa, R. (1987). *Facts about Finland.* Helsinki, Finland: Otava Publishing Company Limited (Otava Kustannusosakeyhtiö).

Edelman, C.L. & Mandle, C.L. (1998). *Health promotion throughout the lifespan.* Toronto: Mosby.

Engle, E. (1975). *Finns in North America.* Englewood Cliffs, N.J.: Reward Paperbacks (Prentice Hall).

Feskens, E.J., Virtanen, S.M., Räsänen, L., et al. (1995). Dietary factors determining diabetes and impaired glucose tolerance. *Diabetes Care, 18*(8), 1104-1112.

Geissler, E. (1994). *Pocket guide: cultural assessment.* Toronto: Mosby.

Giger, J., & Davidhizar, R.E. (1995). *Transcultural nursing: assessment and intervention* (ed. 2). St. Louis: Mosby.

Jacono, J., et al. (1996). An epidemiological study of rheumatoid arthritis in a northern Ontario clinical practice: the role of ethnicity. *Journal of Advanced Nursing, 24*: 31-35.

Johnson, O. (1997). *Information please almanac.* New York: Houghton Mifflin Company.

Lander, P., & Charbonneau, T. (1990). *The land and people of Finland.* Philadelphia: J.B. Lippincott.

Lindstrom, V. (1992). *Defiant sisters: a social history of Finnish immigrant women in Canada.* Toronto: Multicultural History Society of Ontario.

Lindstrom, V. (1996). Finnish women's experience in northern Ontario lumber camps, 1920-1939. In Kechnie, M., & Reitsma-Street, M. (Eds.), *Changing lives: women in northern Ontario* (pp. 107-122). Sudbury, Ont.: Institute of Northern Ontario Research and Development.

Lindstrom-Best, V. (1985). *The Finns in Canada.* Ottawa: Canadian Historical Association.

Lindstrom-Best, V. (1981). Finns in Canada. *Polyphony: The Bulletin of the Multicultural History Society of Ontario, 3*(2): 3-14.

NTC Publications Ltd. (1996). *World drink trends.* Oxfordshire, Lincolnwood, Ill.: NTC Publications Group.

Ojakangas, B. (1964). *The Finnish cookbook.* New York: Crown Publishers.

Puska, P., et al. (1994). Changes in risk factors explain changes in mortality from ischemic heart disease in Finland. *British Medical Journal, 309*, 23-27.

Runeberg, T. (1983). *Childhood in Finland* (D. Tullberg, Trans.). Helsinki: Central Union for Child Welfare in Finland.

Saarinen, O. (1981). Geographical perspectives on Finnish Canadian immigration and settlement. *Polyphony: the Bulletin of the Multicultural Historical Society of Ontario, 3*(2), 16-22.

Salo, M. (1973). *Roles of magic and healing: the* tietäjä *in memorates and legends of Canadian Finns.* Ottawa: National Museum of Canada.

Schneider, A. (1986). *The Finnish Baker's daughters.* Toronto: The Multicultural Historical Society of Ontario.

Sillanpää, V. (1988). The Canadian encyclopedia 2. Edmonton: Gale Research Publishers.

Sillanpää, N. (1994). *Under the northern lights.* Hull, Quebec: Canadian Museum of Civilization.

Smolin, L., & Grosvenor, M. (1994). *Nutrition: science and applications.* Montreal: Saunders College Publishing.

Spector, R. (1996). *Cultural diversity in health and illness.* Toronto: Prentice Hall Canada, Inc.

Statistics Canada: ethnic origin (the nation). (1993). Ottawa: Minister of Industry, Science and Technology.

Stolte, K. (1996). *Wellness: nursing diagnosis for health promotion.* Philadelphia: J.B. Lippincott.

Tester, J. (1986). *Sports pioneers: a history of the Finnish-Canadian Amateur Sports Federation 1906-1986.* Sudbury: Alerts AC Historical Society.

Vahtola, M. (1994). *Health, illness, and healing beliefs among the Thunder Bay Finns.* Unpublished thesis, Department of Anthropology, Lakehead University, Thunder Bay, Ontario.

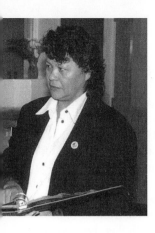

CHAPTER 17
The Mi'kmaq

Cynthia Baker

BEHAVIORAL OBJECTIVES

After reading this chapter the nurse will be able to:

1. Describe elements of the traditional Mi'kmaq culture and Mi'kmaq history that influence their culture today.
2. Delineate potential barriers to communication between nurses and Mi'kmaq clients that may hinder the development of a therapeutic relationship.
3. Discuss the symbolic significance that dimensions of the spatial environment may have to Mi'kmaq clients.
4. Explain the formal structure and functioning of Mi'kmaq bands and its relationship to social organization.
5. Describe norms and values that guide Mi'kmaq social relationships.
6. Discuss Mi'kmaq spirituality and its relationship to health.
7. Describe the significant effect that time has on cultural behavior and adherence to protocols necessary to maintain optimal wellness.
8. Describe the traditional Mi'kmaq orientation to time.
9. Describe Mi'kmaq beliefs about illness and health and their effects on health-seeking behaviors.
10. Describe biological variations germane to the Mi'kmaq that augment susceptibility to selected diseases.

OVERVIEW OF THE MI'KMAQ

The *Mi'kmaq* (English: Micmac) have inhabited Eastern Canada for over 2000 years (Whitehead, 1991). Indeed, archeological evidence indicates that Paleo-Indian hunters had reached Nova Scotia 10,600 years ago (McMillan, 1988). These people continue to have a distinct cultural identity some 500 years after contact with European settlers. The various spellings *Mi'kmak*, *Mi'kmac*, and now properly *Mi'kmaq* represent the pronunciation /meeg(e)makh/ (with *akh* sounding like German

Bach), which, in the older spelling *migmac*, was believed to mean 'allies' because according to oral tradition it was supposed to be the Mi'kmaq name for the early French settlers with whom they developed a strong alliance. However, in reality, according to Bernard Francis (1998), a fluent Mi'kmaq speaker, the word means '(Mi'kmaq) people (in general)' and there is no word in Mi'kmaq for "allies." The word for 'man' is either *lnu* or *nnu*, and its plural is *lnu'k* or *nnu'k* 'men, persons, Indians, people'. The singular of *Mi'kmaq* is *Mi'kmaw*. The Mi'kmaq are culturally very similar to the Maliseet (or Malecite), who have also been living in the Atlantic region of Canada since the precontact era (McMillan, 1988).

Because the Mi'kmaq are one of Canada's aboriginal people, several legal definitions are involved in determining their population size. A person who defines herself or himself as Mi'kmaq may be a status Indian. This refers to a person registered or entitled to be registered as an Indian according to the Indian Act. Status Indians are treaty Indians, that is, persons who are affiliated with an Indian body or band that was signatory to a treaty with the Crown. The Department of Indian and Northern Affairs is responsible for providing certain services to status Indians. A nonstatus Indian is a descendant of an aboriginal person who has lost the right to be registered as Indian. Before June 1985, this group included Indian women who married non-Indian men. With the passage of Bill C-31, however, this regulation was changed, and persons who had formerly lost their status were reinstated (Indian and Northern Affairs Canada, 1995).

In 1992, there were 36,297 registered Mi'kmaq in Canada with 67% of this population living on land designated as reserves (Indian and Northern Affairs, Canada, 1992). The largest number of Mi'kmaq are located in Nova Scotia. In fact, in 1992, there were 9,811 Mi'kmaq people living on 13 Nova Scotian reserves. New Brunswick has eight Mi'kmaq and seven Maliseet reserves. The reserve population of Mi'kmaq in this province numbered 6582 in 1992. There are two Mi'kmaq reserves in Prince Edward Island whose combined population totaled 854. Newfoundland, with one reserve, numbered 960. Two reserves in Quebec, Restigouche and Gesgapégiag, had respective populations of 2538 and 885. In addition to these communities, there is also a population of Mi'kmaq residing in New England and particularly in Boston, where individuals migrated to work in construction (Wien, 1991). The overall population of the aboriginal people decreased to 23% in 1986, as compared with the nonaboriginal population who had no signficant change in census for the same time period (Wien, 1991).

Registered Canadian Indians are a more youthful population than the nonaboriginal population. The 1991 census indicated, for example, that nearly 6 out every 10 registered Indians living on reserves were under 25 years of age compared with less than 4 out of every 10 nonaboriginal Canadians (Indian and Northern Affairs, Canada, 1995). By the same token, registered Indians 65 years and over accounted for a smaller segment of the population than their nonaboriginal counterparts did. In fact, among the on-reserve population, the proportion in this 65 years of age and older cohort actually fell from 4.8% in 1986 to 3.9% in 1991, compared with their nonaboriginal counterparts who actually increased from 10.2% in 1986 to 11.8% in 1991. These demographic patterns for registered Indians as a whole are evident among the Mi'kmaq. For instance, data retrieved from the 1991 census on the aboriginal population for Atlantic Canada indicate that 53% of registered Indians in Nova Scotia, New Brunswick (which includes the Maliseet), and Prince Edward Island were under 25 years of age. Only 2% of the aboriginal population of these provinces were 65 years of age or over (Royal Commission on Aboriginal Peoples, 1996).

Historical origin

When Europeans first arrived in the sixteenth century, the Mi'kmaq were living in what is now Nova Scotia, New Brunswick, Prince Edward Island, and the Gaspé penninsula. Over time, the Mi'kmaq gradually expanded their settlements to Newfoundland, where they replaced the Beothuk whose population was decimated (McMillan, 1988). A picture of Mi'kmaq culture at the time of arrival of the first Europeans has emerged from extensive seventeenth-century accounts (McMillan, 1988). This provides a useful base for understanding their society today. The Mi'kmaq were a seminomadic group of hunters and gatherers who moved seasonally from coastal regions to the rivers and then to the forests in the interior to exploit different food resources in their environment (McMillan, 1988). The most important part of their diet came from the sea. Their method of transportation depended on the season. They traveled in birchbark canoes in the warmer months and on snowshoes, sleds, and toboggans in the colder part of the year. Their housing reflected the need for mobility and consisted of bark-covered wigwams, which were light and portable. They wore robes of furs or hide, leggings, and moccasins and decorated their clothes with paint and porcupine quills (McMillan, 1988).

Historically the size of Mi'kmaq communities varied with the season. In the summer, several hundred individuals would come together forming a band under a sagamore, whose power was limited because society was essentially an egalitarian one. In the winter, they would disperse into small camps consisting of several related families (Bock, 1991; McMillan, 1988; Miller, 1989). The concept of land owernship was alien to the Mi'kmaq though they did respect assigned hunting and fishing territories. According to traditional accounts, there were seven named districts within their territory and a band habitually hunted within a given distict (McMillan, 1988; Augustine, 1992).

Although lacking the political unification normally associated with tribes, the Mi'kmaq perceived themselves to be a common people and paid nominal allegiance to a grand chief located in Cape Breton Island whose position was an inherited one (McMillan, 1988; Bock, 1966). There was also a grand council, which included the chiefs of the seven Mi'kmaq districts. The grand chief and grand council allocated hunting areas to each district, settled disputes, and arranged marriages. Decision making was based on consensus (Bock, 1991; McMillan, 1988).

Contact with Europeans

Sporadic contact with Europeans began shortly after Columbus crossed the Atlantic, and the contacts intensified early in the seventeenth century with French colonialization. The Mi'kmaq were soon partners with the French in the fur trade. This newly formed allegiance appeared to fit with their traditional seasonal nomadic pattern of life and did not have an effect on their independence. Nevertheless, the introduction of European alcohol, epidemics of European diseases, and later warfare with the French against the British took their toll. It appears that as early as 1616 the population, estimated to be over 3000, had already begun to decline, and by the mideighteenth century it had dropped to below 2000 (Brock, 1991).

Despite a series of treaties with the British, the decline of the fur trade and the British conquest combined had an enormous effect on the traditional Mi'kmaq way of life, which culminated in reserve lands being set aside for this seminomadic aboriginal population. The Royal Proclamation of 1763, issued in the name of the king, specified that aboriginal people were not to be molested or disturbed on lands that had not been ceded or purchased by the Crown and that transactions would be conducted between the Crown and assemblies of Indians. After confederation, administrative responsibility for First Nation peoples in Canada was shifted to the federal government. In 1876, the Canadian government passed the Indian Act. Indian agents, who were White men employed by the government, enforced the provisions of the act on reserve lands. The Indian Act established elections for chiefs and band councils by assigning them limited powers.

In 1969, the federal government introduced the "White Paper" on Indian policy, which proposed to abolish the Indian Act and establish a special relationship between aboriginal peoples and the government of Canada to create equality. First Nation communities were nearly unanimous in their rejection of this and began to argue for the continuity of aboriginal peoples as nations within Canada. (Royal Commission on Aboriginal Peoples, 1996). A dozen years later, the existing aboriginal and treaty rights were recognized and confirmed in the Constitution Act of 1982. Section 35 of this act recognized the inherent right of self-government as an existing right. Consultations with First Nation communities have been conducted since 1995 to negotiate self-government in areas such as health care, child welfare, education, and housing (Irwin, 1995).

COMMUNICATION
Language spoken and its origin

The Mi'kmaq language belongs to the Algonquian family along with such individual languages as Cree and Ojibwa (McMillan, 1988). Mi'kmaq was spoken widely until the middle of the century, and now being replaced by English (Wallis and Wallis, 1974; Davis, 1991). Nevertheless, it continues to be the major language spoken on some reserves.

The decline of their native language has been a source of concern for members of the Mi'kmaq community (Pritchard, 1991). Some Mi'kmaq attribute the loss of their language to the Shubenacadie ('wild potato place') residential school where children were forcefully forbidden to speak anything other than English. A poignant poem by Rita Joe, a Mi'kmaq poet, captures the profound effect of this experience. It begins by saying: "I lost my talk, The talk you took away, When I was a little girl, At Shubenacadie school." And concludes with the following: "So gently I offer my hand and ask, Let me find my talk, So I can teach you about me" (Royal Commission on Aboriginal Peoples, 1996). Today efforts are being made to preserve the Mi'kmaq language. One example is a 6-week course on the Big Cove Reserve that teaches Mi'kmaq people to read and write their language. It was developed by Mildred Milliea, a grandmother of 12 who has spent many years researching her native tongue (Gray, 1976). Mi'kmaq has also been included in some schools as an immersion course for Mi'kmaq students.

Dialect

Although Mi'kmaq is a single language, there are some differences in how it is spoken from one community to another. Accents and pronunciation vary; for example, syllables such as *bach* found in the middle of a word in the Eel Ground dialect are pronounced with the *ch* dropped or swallowed in Big Cove (Pritchard, 1991).

Style

Traditionally, the Mi'kmaq have been guided by a philosophy of noninterference that is based on a belief that everyone must discover his or her own path in life (Wallis and Wallis, 1974). There has also been a strong emphasis on showing respect to others. Even today, these values are still present in Mi'kmaq communities and are evident in some existing norms concerning how one should communicate with others (Ellingsen, 1989). For example, a Mi'kmaq resource book developed by the Native Council of Nova Scotia for the Department of Education contains a list of formerly unwritten Mi'kmaq rules

of conduct. These include such norms as not criticizing others, keeping disappointment in others to oneself, and not telling others what they should or should not do. Another unwritten social rule that appears to be common among Mi'kmaq people is listening to what someone has to say without interrupting. Typically, Mi'kmaq do not interrupt one another when conversing and consider such behavior as disrespectful (Ellingsen, 1989).

The Mi'kmaq style of speaking may also be influenced by a long-standing storytelling tradition (Augustine, 1992). It is not uncommon for Mi'kmaq to tell a story to make a point. Often the style of Mi'kmaq speaking is more illustrative, metaphoric, and less direct than the speech pattern commonly found among English and French Canadians.

Volume

Many but not all Mi'kmaq speak more slowly than is common among the nonaboriginal population. It may be that the person's speaking rhythm is influenced by the amount of time spent living among nonaboriginals. It may also reflect the extent to which a person is translating from Mi'kmaq internally when speaking English The Mi'kmaq also tend to allow more periods of silence when conversing than either English Canadians or French Canadians do. The list of unwritten rules of conduct clearly illustrates that it is customary to allow periods of silence in a conversation to permit reflection and time to refresh one's thoughts.

Emotional tone

The Mi'kmaq conversational tone tends to be somewhat more subdued than the pattern of speech of English Canadians or French Canadians. Many of the Mi'kmaq speak more softly as well. Despite this subdued softness in conversational speech, conversations are often punctuated by a wry humor and by laughter. For some Mi'kmaq deeply felt feelings may be expressed if the time seems right. Some Native ceremonies being revived among the Mi'kmaq actually provide a forum for people to speak from the heart. In a "talking circle," for example, people sitting in a circle pass a symbolic object such as an eagle feather from one person to the next in a clockwise fashion. People may speak only when they have the symbol. When in possession of the symbol, however, they may talk frankly about concerns that they would normally keep to themselves. Ellingsen (1989) studied the meaning of health for Mi'kmaq women and noted that feelings are often not voiced. The reason given is that in the Mi'kmaq language to talk about feelings involves discussing the context in which they occurred and this indicates a lack of respect for the privacy of others involved.

Kinesics

English Canadians tend to gesture less when they speak than French Canadians do, and Mi'kmaq tend to gesture less than English Canadians. Mi'kmaq may maintain a motionless stance and minimize the use of gestures when speaking. To show respect, the Mi'kmaq may avoid direct eye contact with those who are in authority or for their elders.

Implications for nursing care

Nurses caring for Mi'kmaq clients need to be aware of potential barriers to communication. For example, some Mi'kmaq speak virtually no English and feel isolated in the hospital or health care environment (Baker and Cormier Daigle, 1996). To communicate effectively with a client who is not fluent in English, the health care providers should utilize an interpreter. However, it is essential to avoid using children or other family members to communicate with the clients. When children are used as interpreters for parents, a generational role reversal occurs (Gold, 1992). The interpreter should be fluent in both Mi'kmaq and English and should attempt to establish a relationship built on trust. The establishment of this trusting relationship will enable the nurse to communicate more effectively with the client in an effort to provide culturally competent care.

Subtle differences in communication patterns of the Mi'kmaq may create misperceptions. For instance, a nurse's questions, interruptions, and attempts to analyze a situation hastily may seem disrespectful to some Mi'kmaq. On the other hand, a Mi'kmaq client's slower and more elliptical style of talking may be confusing to the nurse who may possibly erroneously dismiss the comments as irrelevant and try to refocus the conversation. Similarly, nurses may either misinterpret a Mi'kmaq client's silence or find the silence disconcerting without realizing that their own discomfort is related to inability to understand the meaning of the silence. By the same token, Mi'kmaq clients may feel somewhat intruded upon if their silence were interrupted more quickly than would be the case in their community.

Another potential communication barrier is the tendency for many Mi'kmaq clients to refrain from voicing their needs, expressing complaints, or asking staff questions about treatments and procedures (Baker and Cormier Daigle, 1996). Because many Mi'kmaq have lived on reserves, there is a tendency for these persons to feel uncomfortable when relating to persons outside of their community. It is essential for a nurse to be aware that Mi'kmaq clients may have many concerns or questions even though they say little.

SPACE

Space is a significant dimension among the Mi'kmaq. As a people, they have always identified with the land they occupied. Over time, their territory was steadily encroached upon by immigrant populations who ended up surrounding and dominating them. Rights to land have been a central cultural issue among the Mi'kmaq since the beginning of the eighteenth century. The Mi'kmaq pursued these rights through treaties and political negotiations and more recently through the court system.

A dominant cultural theme among the Mi'kmaq is their spiritual relationship to the land. Their legends reflect the world view of a hunting and gathering people who were acutely aware of, sensitive to, and respectful of the space around them (Miller, 1989). Today, cultural symbols that are still important illustrate this reciprocal relationship between spatial needs and the environment (Whitehead, 1991).

Distance and cultural zones

Perhaps the most important abstract symbol among the Mi'kmaq is the circle. It is the organizing form for ceremonies and for formal social functions. Social activities of many kinds, for example, are conducted in a circle. Its significance rests on the Mi'kmaq's beliefs that the universe is fundamentally interconnected. The circle also represents the value these persons place on harmony with the universe and the notion of the cyclical nature of life.

Objects of spiritual significance that continue to be meaningful to many Mi'kmaq today include the eagle feather, sweetgrass, sage, and tobacco. These natural objects figure prominently in sacred legends (Pritchard, 1991; Augustine, 1992). The eagle feather is a medium for identifying with the Creator, and its symbolic function is to energize. It is used in celebrating events or in ceremonies. Sweetgrass, which is gathered in June and July, has purplish roots and is easy to pick out from the other wild grasses of the region. It is also used to make traditional basketry. Sage and tobacco also have ceremonial functions. Tobacco is smoked in a ceremonial pipe, or it may be sprinkled freely into an open fire.

Proximity to others and comfort level

There may be less need for a permanent area of personal space among the Mi'kmaq. Territoriality traditionally represented a collective right to use an area of land rather than individual ownership of property. Additionally, the Mi'kmaq migrated seasonally, and in a sense this pattern continued into the twentieth century because many were involved in the work force as a rural proletariat of migrant workers (Wien, 1987). Reserve membership is a fluid concept, and it is not uncommon for Mi'kmaq to move from one reserve to another.

In addition to a flexibility about personal territory, the Mi'kmaq may also tend to be more comfortable when in proximity to family members. They have lived in confined quarters with a group of kin throughout their history. The wigwam, in which they were still living in the first half of the nineteenth century, was a small enclosure shared by family members (Gilpin, 1974). These wigwams were replaced by small permanent huts with a wood floor provided to sleep on rather than spruce bushes on the ground. Later in the twentieth century, small frame houses replaced the huts, and beds replaced

the floors for sleeping, but families were large, and people have continued to live in proximity to one another (Wallis and Wallis, 1974). When it is necessary to be isolated from kin and from the community, for example, during hospitalization, this can be a difficult experience for many Mi'kmaq (Baker and Cormier Daigle, 1996).

Implications for nursing care

When taking family histories from Mi'kmaq clients, it is helpful for nurses to appreciate that for the Mi'kmaq spatial mobility is common (Ellingsen, 1989). The cultural emphasis on the interconnectedness of people to their environment, to their family, and to their community can make hospitalization a particularly difficult experience for Mi'kmaq people. It is important for them to have family members present throughout a hospitalization (Baker and Cormier Daigle, 1996).

SOCIAL ORGANIZATION

As a First Nation people, the social organization of Mi'kmaq communities is embedded in a formal band structure. The Indian Act identifies a band as a group of Indians who are recognized by the federal government as a political unit. A reserve is a tract of Crown land that has been set aside for the exclusive use and benefit of members of a band (Bock, 1966). One band, however, may have more than one reserve under its jurisdiction.

With revisions to the Indian Act over the years, reserves are administered today by a band chief and council elected every 2 years instead of a federally appointed Indian agent. One councillor is elected for every 100 registered band members. All band members who are 18 years of age or older and who ordinarily reside on the reserve are eligible to vote for the chief and the councillors. A grand chief and grand council symbolically unite the individual bands, and they meet two or three times a year. This is no longer a decision-making body, and the grand chief position, traditionally inherited, is now filled through a consultative process. The grand chief and grand council continue to be highly respected and focus today on the spiritual needs of the community (McMillan, 1988).

Family systems and family roles

Traditionally the family has been the central social group within Mi'kmaq communities. Historically, bands were composed of groups of kin. The household family unit, however, has tended to be somewhat fluid and is flexible. Although divorce was banned by Catholic priests, ethnographic evidence is suggestive that separations and liaisons between nonmarried people were common (Wallis and Wallis, 1974; Miller, 1989). Today the family composition may be single-parent families, blended families, nuclear families, and extended families (Ellingsen, 1989). However, the significant family group tends to extend beyond the household unit including three generations and a wide range of relatives on both sides of the family. It is the extended family that tends to be the meaningful social group for individuals of this culture (Ellingsen, 1989).

Roles among the Mi'kmaq were largely determined by age and sex. Men hunted, fished, and made items such as shelters, bows, arrows, lances, shields, axes, knives, weirs, fish traps, snowshoes, canoes, cradleboards, and tobacco pipes. Women and girls carried game back to the camp, transported all camp equipment, and moved and set up the wigwams. They also prepared and preserved the food, made birchbark dishes, wove mats from rushes, made clothing, corded snowshoes, fetched water, and took care of children (McMillan, 1988). Social rules dictated that for a first marriage the groom would provide service to his prospective father-in-law for a period of time. Divorce was a part of this culture, and in the case of a second marriage the groom was not expected to work for the bride's family (Bock, 1991).

Although there are differences in the extent that people are guided by traditional Mi'kmaq norms, childrearing in many families is still influenced by traditional values, which emphasized the importance of noninterference and display of respect by children. It is believed that children learn better by discovering things for themselves (Baker and Cormier Daigle, 1996; Ellingsen, 1989, Wallis and Wallis, 1974). Although parents keep an eye on their children, they consider it important to refrain from intervening, questioning, or prying into their actions. Showing others respect tends to be inculcated in children by their family at an early age. Children are not allowed to interrupt an adult's conversation or to speak disrespectfully to adults. In turn, however, parents will not interrupt conversations between children and believe in showing them respect.

Age-related family roles were linked to the cycle of life, and these are still present to a varying extent among Mi'kmaq today. Children were highly valued as the future of the community. Seniors, on the other hand, were respected as the keepers of the community's traditions and were valued for their wisdom and experience. This was particularly important in a culture in which the accumulation of knowledge was transmitted orally from one generation to the next. At social functions, a custom that is still practiced among some Mi'kmaq individuals is to serve seniors and children first to honor symbolically their representation of the past and the future.

The respect given to seniors within the family is extended to members of the community who are known as "elders." These persons have a special place among the Mi'kmaq. The nature of an elder's wisdom varies; for instance, some may have extensive knowledge of herbal remedies, others may be healers during a sweat lodge ceremony, and others may be able to interpret dreams. Their knowledge is passed from elder to elder in an oral tradition.

Before the arrival of the first Europeans, male and female roles were clearly differentiated, but the relationship between the genders was fairly egalitarian (McMillan, 1988). At the present time, women appear to play an important role in the social organization of the community as elders and as members of Band Councils (McMillan, 1988).

Religious views and cultural significance

The Mi'kmaq believed in a supreme being. Some sources indicate that they identified this creator as the sun (McMillan, 1988). Others suggest that they believed in an invisible creator, known as *Gisoolg* (*kisu'lkw* 'he or she created us'), who could make its presence felt in the sun, moon, and heavens (Augustine, 1992; Pritchard, 1991). The term for "God" is now *Niskam*, based originally on 'my-grandfather' (Francis, 1998). Besides the Creator, the Mi'kmaq believed in lesser deities that had supernatural powers. The most important of these was a culture hero called *Glooscap*, who appears in many Mi'kmaq legends. Deities could bestow supernatural powers on people, and certain individuals were identified as having special abilities in forseeing events or interpreting dreams. Such a person was known as a *buoin* (*puwowin*), or 'shaman' (plural *puwowinaq*) (Bock, 1991).

The number seven is meaningful to the Mi'kmaq and figures prominently in a well-known creation legend that describes the beginning of life occurring in seven stages. This story provides a glimpse of how the Mi'kmaq may have understood their world and their society. In the beginning according to the legend, there was only one great spirit, *Gisoolg*. This spirit created the sun, which is the giver of life, of light, and of heat. The Creator then made the earth with its resources of animals and plants. Next, *Glooscap* (*kluskap* 'trickster') was created with a bolt of lightning. The Creator then gave *Glooscap* a grandmother from a rock, a nephew was created for him when the wind blew waves over some tall sweet grass, and in the final stage the Creator gave him a mother who came into the world from a leaf of a tree. *Glooscap* relied on his grandmother's wisdom, on his nephew's strength, and on his mother's love and care. His mother was told to keep a fire going, and after the passing of seven winters, seven sparks of this fire created seven men, and another seven sparks created seven women. They eventually formed seven families, and each one dispersed into an area that could provide them and their offspring with the resources they would need to subsist. Although the animals and plants in their districts were a means of sustaining and nourishing life, the legend instructs the Mi'kmaq people that these resources are their brothers and sisters (Pritchard, 1991; Augustine, 1992).

The majority of Mi'kmaq are Roman Catholics at least nominally. At the end of the sixteenth century, French missionaries who were determined to convert them to this faith began to make some inroads when Père Jessé Flèche baptized Grand Chief Membertou (Whitehead, 1991). By the end of the eighteenth century, most Mi'kmaq had been baptized. Traditional beliefs and practices seem to have been intertwined with their Roman Catholicism. Legends, symbols, and beliefs from the pre-European contact culture continued to play a role in their spirituality (Wallis and Wallis, 1974). Because these were transmitted orally, there may have been differences from one family or one community to another. Several ideas, however, appear to have had continuity in Mi'kmaq thought and appear to be widespread (Bock, 1991). These include a sense of the interconnectedness of the universe with life being everywhere, visible and invisible, beneath ground and under the sea; a belief in the equality of people and the notion that no one should put himself or herself above others; a valuing of balance, harmony, and moderation; a belief that some Mi'kmaq may receive special powers from supernatural sources; and a belief in the wisdom of their ancestors (Brock, 1991).

By 1950, traditional beliefs in magical power and non-Christian deities and symbols that were universally expressed in 1912 were virtually hidden because priests forbade their use (Wallis and Wallis, 1974). In the last couple of decades, this trend has been reversed, and there has been a resurgence of interest in traditional spirituality. Interest in Native beliefs varies, however: some Mi'kmaq give them priority, others combine them with Roman Catholicism, and still others are staunchly Catholic.

The sweat lodge is an example of a traditional healing ritual that has been revived. Based on the Mi'kmaq creation story, it is a purification ceremony in which participants are brought into contact with the elemental powers of the world, which include fire, stony earth, water, and air. Participants sit in a circle around a pit in the sweat lodge, where preheated rocks generate heat. There is chanting and meditating to restore or maintain health. The sweetgrass ceremony is another purification ritual whose symbolism is based on the creation story. It is used to open gatherings, start prayer circles, or initiate events. This ceremony is believed to create a sacred space, cleansing an area of negative energies and filling the space with positive energies. Sweetgrass placed in a stone pipe is lit and offered to the Creator, to the east, south, west, and north, to the Earth Mother, and lastly to Father Sky. The sweetgrass smoke is fanned around the area, and then each person present is smudged. Smudging means that the smoke is fanned to the heart, to the mind, and around the body.

Family roles and implications on the integrity of the family

During the 500 years of contact, Mi'kmaq culture has changed considerably but has continued to remain distinct. Rapid changes in the second half of the twentieth century, however, have been a formidable challenge to the Mi'kmaq's self-identity. A distinctive style of dress was utilized in the 1950s. More fundamentally, Mi'kmaq family and community values have deteriorated. In Nova Scotia, for example, a centralization policy during the late 1940s disrupted the community life of dozens of Mi'kwaq on small reserves by moving members to larger settlements (principally Shubenacadie and Eskasoni) (Wien, 1987). Attendance at the residential school in Shubenacadie stripped many Mi'kmaq children of their parent's values. Television has brought a barrage of non-Mi'kmaq perspectives into the reserves, and education off the reserve has exposed many young people to racism in the wider community. Involvement in the nonaboriginal society has also increased.

Level of education

The proportion of First Nation children remaining in school until grade 12 has more than doubled in Canada; from 31% in 1984-1985 to 73% in 1994-1995 (Indian and Northern Affairs, Canada, 1996). This national trend is reflected in the increased value given to education within Mi'kmaq communities (Davis, 1991). Despite educational gains, the level of education among the Mi'kmaq is still disproportionately lower compared to the general population. For example, statistics based on the 1992-1993 school year in New Brunswick indicated that aboriginal junior high school students have a dropout rate that is eight times higher compared with their nonaboriginal counterparts. In addition, the high school dropout rate for aboriginals is five times higher than the nonaboriginal rate (The New Brunswick Family Policy Secretariat, 1995).

In the past, a barrier to education for most First Nation people and the Mi'kmaq, who have not been an exception, has been the negative association with assimilation policies and the profound effect of racism. For example, Wallis and Wallis (1974) reported that early in the century, when schools were being built or expanded for Mi'kmaq children, as in 1912 and again in 1950, many Mi'kmaq considered schools to be a threat to community harmony. There was also a general distrust among nonaboriginals regarding Mi'kmaq who could read and write. Because education was devalued by some Mi'kmaq, school attendance was often sporadic among students and was not insisted on by their parents (Wallis and Wallis, 1974).

The residential school system also had a profound effect in the formulation of negative attitudes about education. Although the majority of Mi'kmaq children went to day schools, some attended the Shubenacadie Residential School, which opened in 1929 in Nova Scotia. It was part of a network of boarding schools across the country, established by the government as a means of assimilating the aboriginal population (Assembly of First Nations, 1994). The amendment of the Indian Act made school attendance compulsory for all First Nations children between 7 and 15 years of age. Compulsory attendance precipitated the act of children being forcibly taken from their families to boarding schools by priests, Indian agents, and Royal Commission of Mounted Police officers (Assembly of First Nations, 1994). The Royal Commission on Aboriginal Peoples (1996) reports that many aboriginal people submitted testimonies about physical deprivation, abuse, and humiliation at these schools. Davis (1971), a historian, has observed that "Shuby" lives on in infamy in the minds of many Mi'kmaq.

Level of income

First Nation people throughout Canada are economically disadvantaged compared with the general population, and the Mi'kmaq are no exception to this premise. Nonetheless, economic differences between the aboriginal and nonaboriginal population narrowed between 1986 and 1991 (Department of Indian and Northern Affairs, Canada, 1995). Between 1986 and 1991, a dramatic increase in income was evident, with an increase of 31% compared with 7% for nonaboriginal people. The average income level was slightly more than $12,000 for off-reserve registered Indians and $9000 for on-reserve registered Indians.

Unemployment

The age structure of Mi'kmaq communities has important social implications. It is believed that, in times of economic downturns, populations whose working-age cohort is still expanding are more likely to experience social displacements including higher levels of unemployment (Indian and Northern Affairs, Canada, 1995). The 1991 census indicated that unemployment for the population of registered Indians in Canada was 19% compared with 10% among the nonaboriginal population. The unemployment rate among the Mi'kmaq appears to reflect the national picture. For example, in Nova Scotia the unemployment rate for Mi'kmaq was 19.9%, in New Brunswick for Mi'kmaq and Maliseet 20.7%, and in Prince Edward Island 22.6%. The overall unemployment rate for aboriginal peoples has decreased to 23% in 1986, compared with virtually little change for their nonaboriginal counterparts. At present, the unemployment of the young on Mi'kmaq reserves is an issue of serious concern to members of these communities (Indian and Northern Affairs, Canada, 1995).

Implications for nursing care

Childrearing beliefs, attitudes toward elders, and the significance of the extended family have important implications for transcultural nursing care. It is essential for the nurse who counsels or cares for Mi'kmaq families to understand the significance of the value of noninterference. It is important to recognize that parents may not necessarily intervene in their children's lives to the same extent that would be typical among English Canadians or French Canadians. It is also important to understand that minimal intervention during childrearing is based on a moral system of values. When working with Mi'kmaq clients, the nurse should also recognize that the extended family is often a significant social unit. Many extended family members may wish to be involved in the health decisions concerning a client. When visitors are restricted to the immediate family as in the case of care in the intensive care units, it may be necessary to alter these rules to allow more relatives to be present because doing so is of value to the Mi'kmaq. The nurse needs to be sensitive to the dignity accorded to the elders among the Mi'kmaq and should take particular care to treat the elderly with respect.

TIME

A key cultural symbol is the circle, reflecting a cyclical view of life. The passage of time was traditionally viewed as a rhythmical rather than a linear phenomenon. Time seems conceptually to have been linked to the spatial dimension. For example, the word 'tomorrow', *sa-bow-nug* [*sapo'nuk*], literally means a place in the future (Pritchard, 1991). The Mi'kmaq calendar was based on natural cycles, and its units were nights, moons, and seasons, with 30 nights being a lunar month and the months being named to reflect seasonal changes. *Wikewiku's* corresponds to October and means 'animal-fattening moon', and *keptkewiku's* corresponds to November and means the 'river-freezing moon'.

Both the past and the future in this cyclical world view were symbolized by particular age groups, with children representing the future of the community and the elderly the past. The Mi'kmaq have tended to look to the wisdom and experience of their collective past to solve problems in the present and to discover the best path to the future. Traditional spiritual knowledge from elders, for example, is being applied to current problems of alcohol and suicide. Similarly, treaties from the past are being invoked to secure hunting and fishing rights for the future.

There is no word in the Mi'kmaq language that is equivalent to the word "time" (Pritchard, 1991). Western notions of linear clock time have been added to rather than derived from Mi'kmaq culture. Although both watches and the Gregorian calendar are part of their communities today, clock time appears to govern life less than it does among the surrounding nonaboriginal population. For example, events scheduled for a particular time start when people have arrived.

Time orientation and significance for nonadherence

Although there are individual differences regarding the degree that clock time has been internalized, typically it is treated somewhat differently depending on the time zone. This may create problems for individuals whose treatment regimen requires a strict adherence to a time schedule. It can also result in greater flexibility regarding appointment times, due dates, and so forth.

Implications for nursing care

When caring for a Mi'kmaq client, it is important for the nurse to assess to what extent an individual Mi'kmaq utilizes clock time. If a medication or treatment requires strict adherence to a time schedule and the person's orientation to time is flexible, the nurse can assist the client to determine culturally congruent indicators of the passage of time that correlate with the treatment schedule. It is also important to appreciate that Mi'kmaq clients find it helpful to look to their collective past to discover ways of dealing with current difficulties. It may be useful to also develop an appreciation for the significant role that the elders play in assisting others to maintain optimal wellness.

ENVIRONMENTAL CONTROL

Change tends to be viewed as cyclical or patterned rather than accidental (Augustine, 1992). There is also a tendency to believe that everything happens for a reason. It is common for the Mi'kmaq not to question the ways of the Creator. Another belief is the notion that each person has a purpose for being on this earth and has a responsibiility to discover that purpose. These ideas indicate that there may be less cultural emphasis on trying to control outcomes and more on finding and achieving harmony with a direction that is meant to be, and therefore there is a tendency for these persons to have an external locus of control (McMillan, 1988).

Folk beliefs and folk practices

The Mi'kmaq have remedies from their past that have been passed down within families. In addition, certain elders accumulate a store of information about traditional medicines, which are made from local plants, roots, and herbs and are used to treat ailments such as head colds, chest colds, and stomach upsets. Some of these herbs are also made into poultices for boils and skin infections (Lacey, 1993). One of the major roles of women is to maintain and store knowledge about medication. This is evident in the creation legend where *Glooscap* instructed his mother to collect and prepare seven medicines from the barks and roots of seven different kinds of plants (Pritchard, 1991). Information about remedies is transmitted orally from one generation to another, and thus it is a fragmented body of knowledge. Medicines were made and used in an underground fashion for several decades because the outside world disapproved of them (Lacy, 1993). In recent years, there has been a renewed and more open interest among Mi'kmaq in their traditional medicines.

Illness and wellness beliefs

The Mi'kmaq view of health is holistic and linked to the ideology of balance and the interconnectedness of the natural world. In the past, Mi'kmaq remedies were used to treat ailments considered to be relatively minor, whereas serious illnesses were addressed spiritually through a shaman (*puwowin*). Today, spirituality continues to be intrinsically linked to Mi'kmaq beliefs of health and wellness. Healing is associated with restoring harmony and connections. Ellingsen (1989) notes that, among Mi'kmaq women, health represented the creation of a unified self and this balance could be achieved only through spirituality. For the women studied, spirituality was perceived to be their fit with and connection to their culture, their family, and life itself (Ellingsen, 1989). For many of the women studied, creating a unified self required that they link the past with the present context in which unity or disunity was being experienced.

Traditional drumming, which is also being re-vived, represents the center of all life as if the drum were the heart providing life with its heart-beat. These notions are reflected in the medicine wheel. This symbol of good luck is made out of willow bark, sweetgrass, beads, and leather into the shape of a wheel with four cardinal points. The four points may represent the seasons, the stages of life, the cardinal directions, and so on. Some Mi'kmaq have adapted the medicine wheel for modern treatment programs by assigning emo-tions, thought, spirituality, and the physical self to the four quadrants and encouraging balance be-tween these quadrants.

Life expectancy

Living standards have improved among the Mi'-kmaq in the last 50 years, and the population is growing, and therefore one may assume with these quality indicators that although the life expectancy is lower compared with their nonaboriginal counter-parts it nonetheless has increased. In 1995, the life ex-pectancy for aboriginals was 69 years for men and 76 years for women. The infant mortality for registered Indians declined between 1981 and 1993 from 22 to 11 infant deaths per 1000 live births (Indian and Northern Affairs, Canada, 1996).

BIOLOGICAL VARIATIONS
Body structure

A high prevalence of obesity has been documented in many North American aboriginal groups (Waldram, Herring, and Young, 1995). This has been attributed to a metabolic pattern that rapidly con-verts an increased food intake to body fat. The pat-tern is believed to be a biological adaptation to an environment characterized by cycles of food avail-ability. When food was plentiful, it was quickly con-verted to fat to provide energy during periods of scarcity, and thus many Mi'kmaq were and are over-weight Harris et al., 1997; Young, 1994).

Visible physical characteristics

As typically found in the Asian population, body hair is scant, epicanthic folds are common, and hair is straight and black for most aboriginals. Many Mi'kmaq infants are born with mongolian spots, which is a point of concern for the nurse conducting physical assessments because these spots may be erroneously interpreted as a congeni-tal anomaly.

Enzymatic and genetic variations

Aboriginal Canadians are believed to have migrated from Asia and share some similiar genotypes and phenotypes with the Asian populations. However, after exposure to Europeans and the intermating and marriages of the races, the gene pool has been structurally altered.

Blood groups

The distribution of blood groups differs, however, from that in Asian populations. Blood group B, common among Asians, is absent among aboriginal Canadians. Their predominant blood group is group O. At the present time the distribution of group A varies between 1% to 35% among aboriginal peoples in Canada (Campbell, 1992).

Susceptibility to disease

Diabetes Being overweight has been linked to an increase in chronic illnesses among the aboriginal population and particularly to non-insulin depen-dent diabetes. This disease, almost nonexistent among them before the 1940s, is now significantly more prevalent than it is among the nonaboriginal population (Young et al., 1990; Waldram, Herring, and Young, 1995). The highest prevalence rate (8.7%) has been found among the aboriginal popu-lation of Atlantic Canada (Young et al., 1994).

Hypertension An increase in hypertension and heart disease has also been linked to the problem of being overweight and of obesity among aboriginal groups in Canada (Waldram, Herring, and Young, 1995).

Infectious diseases Regarding infectious diseases, recent osteological analyses have discredited the view that the aboriginals had no experience with in-fectious diseases before contact. Apparently, bacte-ria, fungi, and parasites caused diseases among them. Acute infectious diseases from Europe, however, added to the load (Waldram, Herring, and Young, 1995). Smallpox, the scourge of the sixteenth to eighteenth centuries, was probably introduced by Europeans.

Tuberculosis   Tuberculosis afflicts aboriginal populations; however, it was present before contact. By the twentieth century, however, it had reached such epidemic proportions that a genetic susceptibility was widely presumed to be the cause. It is now generally accepted that these outbreaks were attributable to social circumstances, particularly the change from a nomadic to a settled life on reserves. There have been steep declines in tuberculosis among aboriginal Canadians since the 1950s because of vaccinations (Waldram, Herring, and Young, 1995).

Nutritional preferences   The traditional diet of the Mi'kmaq included naturally available foods such as fresh fish, eel, seal, moose, and wild rice. Today these foods are supplemented by canned goods and processed foods.

Psychological characteristics   Many Mi'kmaq relate confusion about cultural values to the serious problem of alcohol and drug use among the young members of the reserves (Assembly of First Nations, 1994). Although the higher prevalence of alcoholism than that in whites has have been accounted for in terms of a genetic vulnerability, these explanations have not been substantiated. The data about a biological basis for prevalence of alcoholism differs substantially in the literature (Young, 1994).

The Mi'kmaq also relate confusion about cultural values to an increase in suicides and attempted suicides in this age group. The Big Cove Reserve, where over 60% of the residents are under 25 years of age and where unemployment is high, has been particularly affected by suicides. During a 6-week period in 1992, four young men took their lives. By the time the inquest was held, three more had killed themselves, and some 75 young people were estimated to have made a suicide attempt (Assembly of First Nations, 1994).

Many Mi'kmaq have looked to traditional customs for solutions to the problems of suicide and substance abuse among the young. After the epidemic of suicides at Big Cove, for example, the grand council and grand chief came to this reserve with scores of relatives and friends from other Mi'kmaq communities. Traditional sunrise ceremonies were conducted in the mornings, and at night there were drumming, dancing, and pipe ceremonies (Saint John Telegraph, February 15, 1995). Alcohol and drug programs that combine elements of Native spirituality with modern treatment approaches have also been set up.

Implications for nursing care

At the present time, diseases among the Mi'kmaq are believed to be primarily linked to social conditions and to lifestyle factors, though this does not negate the premise that susceptibility to certain diseases may also have a biological predisposition. The nurse, therefore, needs to be aware that the combination of a metabolic predisposition and changes in lifestyle have increased the risk for obesity, diabetes, and hypertension among the Mi'kmaq. In the counseling of Mi'kmaq clients about nutrition, it may be helpful to explore the availability of traditional foods such as fresh fish and include them in any proposed diet regimen. Although alcoholism and alcohol-related diseases are prevalent, the nurse must exercise caution to avoid overgeneralizing and assuming that alcohol is an overriding medical concern for all Mi'kmaq. Besides the negative emotional effect that stereotypes can have, there is also a danger of inaccurately confusing signs of serious conditions such as insulin reactions or an impending diabetic coma with drunkenness.

SUMMARY

The Mi'kmaq have adapted to a multitude of changes in the natural, economic, and political environment throughout half a millennium since their initial contact with Europeans. Despite many changes after exposure to Westernization, the Mi'kmaq still see themselves as a people and have a distinct cultural heritage. It is important that nurses caring for Mi'kmaq clients are sensitive to and respectful of this heritage.

Case Study

Mary is a 20-year-old Mi'kmaw who is pregnant and is 5 months into the pregnancy. This is her first pregnancy. She has been diagnosed with NIDDM. She is 5 feet 4 inches tall and weighs 245 lb. She is married, and her husband John and she live on the reserve. Upon admission, the nurse notes that Mary's blood pressure is 140/92, her temperature is 98.8° F, her pulse is 102, and her tongue appears coated. The laboratory test done at Mary's last clinic visit 1 week ago revealed that her fasting serum glucose was 160 mg/dL.

CARE PLAN

 Nursing diagnosis   Health maintenance, altered, related to a high-risk pregnancy.

Client Outcomes

1. Client and family will verbalize a desire to learn more about high-risk pregnancies, diabetes, gestational diabetes, and appropriate techniques to reduce symptoms.
2. Client and family will verbalize a willingness to comply with a medical therapeutic regimen to control diabetes.

Nursing Interventions

1. Identify with client and family sociocultural factors that influence health- seeking behaviors.

2. Determine client's and family's knowledge level about diabetes, and implications for high-risk pregnancies.

STUDY QUESTIONS

1. Identify ways nurses can increase mutual understanding when communicating with Mi'kmaq clients.
2. Describe how the Mi'kmaq traditionally view their relationship to life and to the world.
3. Identify ways the traditional Mi'kmaq understanding of time differs from how nurses tend to think about it.
4. Describe the significance of the circle to the Mi'kmaq culture.
5. Describe ways the circle is related to ideas about healing and health among some Mi'kmaq.
6. Relate why it is important for many Mi'kmaq to have family members present with them when hospitalized.
7. Describe the role of elders among the Mi'kmaq community.

References

Assembly of First Nations. (1994). *Breaking the silence.* Ottawa: First Nations Health Commission.

Augustine, S. (1992). *The early history of Big Cove: a Micmac perspective.* (Unpublished paper).

Baker, C., & Cormier Daigle, M. (1996). Hospitalization experiences of members of the Big Cove Reserve. Paper presented at Spring Research Conference, University of New Brunswick, Faculty of Nursing, Fredericton.

Bock, P. (1966). The Micmac Indians of Restigouche. History and contemporary description. *National Museum of Canada, Bulletin No. 213.* Ottawa.

Davis, C.M. (1991). Living with the past. Native people of Atlantic Canada. 1950-1980.*The Oracle.* National Museum of Man, National Museums of Canada.

DeBlois, A.D. (1996). *Micmac dictionary.* Mercury Series, Canadian Ethnology Service, Paper 131. Hull, Quebec: Canadian Museum of Civilization.

Ellingsen, R. (1989). Factors influencing the perceptions of health among Micmac Indian women: creating a unified self. Unpublished master's thesis, Dalhousie University, Halifax, Nova Scotia.

Francis, Bernard (1998, Feb. 19). Personal communication, Sidney, Nova Scotia.

Gilpin, B. (1974). Indians of Nova Scotia. In McGee, H. (Ed.), *The native people of Atlantic Canada.* Toronto: McClelland & Stewart.

Gold, S. (1992). Mental health and illness in Vietnamese refugees. *The Western Journal of Medicine, 157*(3), 290-294.

Gray, V. (1976). A visit with Mildred Milliea of Big Cove, New Brunswick. *Tawow, 5*(2), 47-49 (published by Indian and Northern Affairs, Canada).

Harris, S., Gittelson, J., Hanley, A., Barne, A., Wolever, T., Gao, J., Logan, A., & Zinman, B. (1997). The prevalence of NIDDM and associated risk factors in Native Canadians. *Diabetes Care, 20*(2), 185-187.

Indian and Northern Affairs, Canada. (1992). *Schedule of Indian bands, reserves and settlements.* Ottawa: Minister of Government Services, Canada. Catalogue No. R31-5/1992.

Indian and Northern Affairs, Canada. (1995). *Highlights of aboriginal conditions, 1991, 1986. Demographic and economic characteristics.* Ottawa: Minister of Public Works and Government Services, Canada. R32-154/1-1986E.

Indian and Northern Affairs, Canada. (1996). *Facts from Stats.* Issue No. 11, March-April. Ottawa: Information Quality and Research Directorate.

Irwin, R. (1995). *Aboriginal self-government.* Ottawa: Minister of Public Works and Government Services, Canada.

Lacey, L. (1993). *Micmac medicines.* Halifax: Nimbus.

McMillan, A. (1988). *Native peoples and cultures of Canada. Vancouver: Douglas & McIntyre.*

Miller, V. (1989). The Micmac: a maritime woodland group. In Morrison, R., & Wilson, C. (Eds.), *Native peoples: the Canadian experience* (pp. 324-352). Toronto: McClelland & Stewart.

Pritchard, E. (1991). *Introductory guide to Micmac words and phrases.* Beacon, N.Y.: Resonance Communication.

Royal Commission on Aboriginal Peoples. (1996). *Report of the royal commission on aboriginal peoples.* Ottawa: Minister of Indian Affairs and Northern Development.

The New Brunswick Family Policy Secretariat. (1995). *Foundations for the future.* Fredericton: The Secretariat.

Waldram, J., Herring, D., & Young, T. (1995). *Aboriginal health in Canada.* Toronto: University of Toronto Press.

Wallis, W., & Wallis, R. (1974). Culture loss and culture change among the Micmac of the Canadian maritime provinces. In McGee, H. (Ed.), *The native peoples of Atlantic Canada.* Toronto: McClelland & Stewart.

Whitehead, R. (1991). *The old man told us.* Halifax: Nimbus.

Wien, F. (1987). *Rebuilding the economic base of Indian communities: the Micmac in Nova Scotia* (2nd printing). Halifax: The Institute for Research on Public Policy.

Wien, F. (1991). *The role of social policy in economic restructuring.* Halifax: The Institute for Research on Public Policy.

Young, T. (1994). *The health of Native Americans.* Oxford: Oxford University Press.

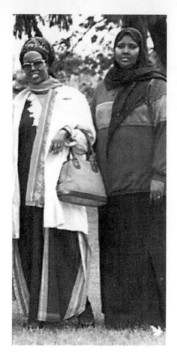

CHAPTER 18

Somalis in Canada

Katherine Jones

BEHAVIORAL OBJECTIVES

After reading this chapter, the nurse will be able to:

1. Identify communication styles that may be utilized by persons of Somalian origin.
2. Appreciate the value Somalian people place on outdoor life.
3. Discuss the role of clans and their influence on Somalian life.
4. Recognize the dissonance of role expectations and family responsibilities between traditional Somalian life and that in Canada.
5. Develop a sensitivity for and understanding of the stressors of assimilation and acculturation for resettled Somalis.
6. Respond appropriately to the present orientation evidenced by many Somalian clients.
7. Identify ways in which the Somalian culture influences health-seeking behaviors and practices.
8. Develop a sensitivity for and understanding of the psychological phenomena that influence the functioning of a Somali when providing nursing care.

OVERVIEW OF SOMALIA

Located on the Horn of Africa (the easternmost portion of Africa), the Somali Republic was formed in 1960 by the union of the two former colonies, British Somaliland Protectorate in northern Somalia and Italian Somaliland in southern Somalia. The country consists of 1,036,000 square kilometers of arid savannah grassland with an estimated population of 6 to 7 million (World Almanac, 1997). Somalia shares boundaries with Kenya to the south, Ethiopia to the northwest, and the republic of Djibouti to the north (Johnson, 1997). The northeast boundary of Somalia is the Red Sea and to the east is the Indian Ocean (Lewis 1988; Simons, 1976).

The capital of Somalia is Mogadishu (Muqdisho), which is located in the southern part of the country. Other important southern cities include Galkayu, Kismayo, Merka, and Baidoa. Significant cities identified in the north include Hargesia, Berbera, Burao, and Boorama (Samatar, 1988). Less than a third of the country's population are located in the cities with the majority spread across the land engaged in pastoral activities raising livestock such as camels, cattle, sheep, and goats for export to the Arab world, principally Saudi Arabia. As a result of famine and ongoing civil wars, the economy of the country is highly unstable, and many refugees have been displaced internally and to neighboring African countries or have emigrated fearing torture, persecution, and ethnic cleansing within their own country (Samatar, 1991). According to both the United Nations and current media reports, power struggles, tribalism, factionism, and civil wars are continuing in the country, and although there is some indication of reduction of fighting and terrorism in the north, facilitating repatriation of some refugees, some peacekeeping forces have been withdrawn, and political disruption is ongoing.

The people

Somalians as a people are racially, linguistically, and religiously homogeneous (Chiswick and Miller, 1996; Liberson, 1970). Somalis believe that they are all descended from two mystical brothers, Samaale and Saab. From these two brothers, six major clan families evolved, and from these further subclans developed (Chiswick and Miller, 1996). The six clan families, sometimes called "tribes" are Darood, Hawiye, Isaaq, Dir, Digil, and Rahanway. The first four of these clans constitute over 75% of the population, and it is the Majeerteen subclan of the Darood clan family who are considered to be Somalia's mandarin class, accustomed to wielding political power. Lineage is based on paternity, which is taken very seriously, and clan history follows genealogical lines tracing ancestry for 200 or more years (Stoffman, 1995). Because of the nature of the nomadic and pastoral life, following the rain and herding their animals to food and water, the clans or tribes maintained strong ties to identify where support and assistance lay. A nomad or herder finding members of his or her own clan had a place to stay, to pitch a tent, or to share a meal. Only recently had the concept of clan been used to define individuals in relation to a group a person belongs to as opposed to an enemy (Stoffman, 1995).

The clan-family system is the basis of Somali society; it acts as a source of internal solidarity and external division. On the surface, the Somali clan system appears to be an unstable, fragile system, characterized at all levels by shifting allegiances. In reality, however, it is resilient, having survived centuries of colonialism, centralized state administration, and other forms of Western influence that are based on individualism rather than communalism (Mohamed, 1994).

A Somalian's full name is composed of a given name and the father's and the paternal grandfather's name. Because each family member had a different grandfather, family surnames differ even within the nuclear family. Kinship ties are extensive and reference to families includes the extended family as well as the nuclear family. The term "cousin" or "uncle" is applied to those other than brothers who share a recognized common descent. These terms are also used as polite terms when speaking to an unrelated stranger.

Linguistically the common language throughout the country is Somali. In addition, with acknowledgment to the colonial influences, English and Italian were also studied and spoken, especially by those who attended school before 1972. Arabic is the second language of many Somalis and is taught in schools as part of their Islamic instruction (Opoku-Dapaah, 1995).

Over 95% of Somalis are Sunni Muslims who preserve the five pillars of Islam as well as Muslim special days. Islam plays an important role in most families. Children are taught the Koran (*Qur'an*) from a very early age before starting formal schooling. In schools, Islam and Arabic are compulsory subjects, and most of the cultural events such as marriages and funerals have their roots in the Islamic religion (Mohamed, 1992). Mohamed (1992) describes ways in which Somalis have modified Islamic requirements to suit their traditional social organization and ecology, such as not requiring women to wear the veil or to be confined indoors.

Within the past four decades, girls and boys have been allowed to attend school for up to 6 years. This primary education is compulsory for all Somali males and a privilege for females. Secondary education is noncompulsory and lasts for 4 years. Students proceeding through postsecondary education often do so in other African or Arab countries or those where there is a strong Islamic focus.

Immigration to Canada

In the mid-1980s, the first Somalis to immigrate settled in and around the Montreal area, where their flights brought them from their native Somalia or the refugee camps of neighboring states (Loescher and Scanlan, 1986). The majority of Somalis who have immigrated are refugees. The very nature of the circumstances for immigration have forced families to separate with women bringing young children but leaving older sons, brothers, husbands, and fathers as prisoners, combatants, or tortured and murdered victims of the ongoing civil wars (Loescher and Scanlan, 1986). Although printed statistics are not available, the Somali Immigrant Aid Organization of Toronto reports that of the approximately 100,000 Somalis who have immigrated or are in the process of obtaining landed status in Canada only 20% are males, 40% are women, and the remainder are all children.

The trickle of Somalis began as early as 1981, with the first large wave arriving in 1986, the second in 1991, and the third in 1995. Both the United States and Canada have now modified their immigration policies. The United States discontinued eligibility for Ethiopians (from where most of the displaced Somalis emigrated) in 1991 (United Nations High Committee on Refugees, 1993; Clayton, 1996; Solomon, 1996). Canada, with more liberal immigration policies, has continued to allow immigration but has increased the waiting period for landed status to 5 years, thus providing a disincentive to those who were attempting to come from other countries that were not perceived as being so welcoming. In 1995, approximately 300,000 Somalis who had been internally displaced to neighboring countries began the repatriation process with the assistance of the United Nations (UNHCR, 1996). Estimates of the success of the repatriation process vary but are considered to be in the range of 200,000 with the majority of the unrepatriated remaining in Kenya. Although civil and political unrest remain a problem and land mines are still present in densely populated areas and food remains scarce, some emigrants are returning to help rebuild the country, and others are being involuntarily returned as refugee claims are increasingly denied (Nichols, 1996; Craig, 1996; Schreuder, 1996; Knox, 1996). The Somali Immigrant Aid Organization estimates that, of the 100,000 Somalis in Canada, between 50% and 75%

reside in the Province of Ontario, with the largest concentration in and around the greater Toronto area. Somalis are not found in the Maritime Provinces, and a group of Somalis continues to reside in and around the Montreal area of Quebec where the first strongholds were established. The only one of the Prairie Provinces to have Somalis is Alberta, with a group of Somalis in Edmonton. Some Somalis have also moved to the West coast and can be found in the greater Vancouver area of British Columbia. In Ontario, although the greatest concentrations of Somalis are in the Toronto area, others have moved to where they are more likely to find work (the border cities of Niagara Falls and Windsor) or where they can further their education (the university cities of Hamilton, Ottawa, and Waterloo) (UNHCR, 1996). Because of the relatively small number of Somalis in Canada, they are rarely mentioned in books describing Canada (Fodor's staff, 1988; Jepson, Lee, and Smith, 1995; Noble, 1992; Takaki, 1993; Baumgart and Larsen, 1988; Pederson, O'Neill, and Rootman, 1994).

The median age of Somalis in Canada is estimated to be 32. Women arriving in the mid-1980s with young children have seen them grow to late teens and young adults, and those arriving more recently have brought more young children with them. In some situations, men are being reunited with their families who had immigrated earlier, and more young children are part of the result of that reunification (UNHCR, 1996).

Most adult Somali Canadians have had at least 6 years of education, but statistics are not available for the breakdown of those with secondary and postsecondary education. For the most part, new immigrants, as refugees, receive government assistance with shelter and support. Those who are able to work and find jobs are often underemployed in menial jobs at minimum wages despite their educational qualifications or inherent abilities. It is probably safe to say that the majority of Somalis live in crowded or overcrowded housing conditions and are at or below the poverty line. Longitudinal studies (in process) of those who have been in the country for the longest periods of time indicate that the majority of Somalis are highly motivated and work hard to break out of the cycle of poverty, become accultur-ated, increase their academic credentials or other qualifications, and complete requirements for certi-fication in Canada or professional licensure (Statis-tics Canada, 1996).

COMMUNICATION
Language and dialect

Although Somali is the native tongue of all Soma-lians, the oral as opposed to written nature of Somali traditions facilitates learning the spoken word in new languages. Many adult Somalis enroll in English as a second language (ESL) classes, school-aged chil-dren acquire the language in the classroom, and younger siblings acquire some rudiments of the lan-guage through their older ones. Somalians are learn-ing English through the Peace Corps, American films and television, as well as from the blackboard (Campbell, 1996).

Spoken and, to some degree, written English are based primarily on what the Somalis have learned within their life context. However, to some degree, based on residential location within larger pre-dominantly African-Canadian communities, many Somalis, particularly youth, tend to use Black English as described in Cherry and Giger's chapter on African Americans (Chapter 8) in the second edition of *Transcultural Nursing*, where *th*, as in *the, these*, and *them*, may be pronounced as *d*, as in /de/, /des/, and /dem/. There is also the tendency to drop the final *r* or *g* from words; thus *father* or *mother* becomes /fatha/ or /motha/. The words *laughing, talking*, and *going* are pronounced /laughin/, /talkin/, and /goin/. Speakers of Black English may also place more emphasis on one syllable as opposed to another; for example, *brother* may be pronounced /bro-tha/.

Copula deletion of the verb *to be* is a common omission with significance in some environments; for example, for a short-term situation, the speaker of Black English might say, "He walking" or "She at work" in contrast to standard English, "He is walk-ing" or "She is at work." Black English speakers may also use for a long-term situation the unconjugated form of the verb *to be* where standard English speak-ers would use the conjugated form. An example of this is, "He be working," in contrast to the standard English, "He is (always) working."

The speech of some African Americans is very colorful and dynamic. For these persons, communi-cation also involves body movement (kinesics). Some African Americans tend to use a wide range of body movements, such as facial gestures, hand and arm movements, expressive stances, handshakes, and hand signals, along with verbal interaction. This rep-ertoire of body movements can also be seen in sports and in dance, which is the highest communi-cative form of body language (Giger and Davidhizar, 1995). Somali women tend to be soft spoken and to avoid eye contact in keeping with their Islamic back-ground and traditions. In fact, many Somali women follow Islamic traditions more closely in Canada than in Somalia. Women have been noted to adopt the veil (uncommon in Somalia) and follow more traditional Islamic rituals, particularly in relation to eye contact, dating behaviors, and the selection of clothing and makeup.

The nomadic and verbal nature of Somali life with songs and dances at encampments relating his-tory and traditions has led many Somalis to con-tinue incorporating such body language in daily life; however, the women who have become more strict in Islamic traditions have tended to limit the use of body language to a great degree. The animated form of communication, often speaking in what may be perceived as a loud and aggressive fashion, is com-mon among Somalis and should not be interpreted as a form of intimidation.

Implications for transcultural nursing care

Because of the diversity of cultural differences within the same ethnic population, it is difficult to generalize or provide overall guidelines for commu-nication and transcultural nursing. Nurses must take their cues from the client and validate perceptions before formulating diagnoses. For example, the length of time the client has actually been in Canada, the nature of education or other resources accessed, and the number, ages, and disposition of children all have a significant effect on the client's ability to articulate and communicate his or her health needs. Even then, because of the phenomenon of Black English and inherent idioms in the dialect, the nurse must work within the context of a practice that still communicates respect for the client, clarifies values, and recognizes diversity in a nonjudgmental manner (Guruge and Donner, 1996; Grypma, 1993). Somali women relied on males as the head of house to communicate with and provide direction for strangers. Women faced with these responsibilities may be very reluctant to discuss health concerns or problems with male nurses or physicians. Health centers with female nurse practitioners are the setting of choice for health-seeking behaviors, and public health nurses as representatives of an official agency (interpreted as "government") are viewed with suspicion and distrust. Public health nurses working with this population on health promotion programs, under the Ontario Mandatory Programs and Services Guidelines (currently under revision), have identified more success through training volunteers to run the programs than through direct delivery of service (Ottawa Health Department, 1989; Anderson, 1985; Dobson, 1991).

Somalis are not accustomed to dealing with paperwork. Most daily transactions are oral and do not usually involve receipts, invoices, contracts, or any other business documents. Somalis therefore often hesitate to complete questionnaires, fill out health history forms, or comprehend the need to sign consent forms, which can sometimes cause misunderstandings or result in delays of service or the withholding of treatment.

SPACE

Somalis love and are accustomed to an outdoor life. This stems from their background as a nomadic people and a climate that made it uncomfortable to be indoors much of the time. Meeting and chatting in a courtyard is not only normal, but also enjoyable. It is part of the Somali custom to constantly socialize, frequently visiting without prior notice. It is also common for small groups to meet and exchange views, ideas, information, or just rumors. Socializing reduces stress and enhances the collective spirit. In a country such as Canada with its colder climate, outdoor socializing is often difficult for at least 4 months of the year. Somalis tend to live in high-rise

apartment complexes where other Somalis live. Somalis also tend to provide shelter for relatives or extended family who have none of their own or are newly arrived. Because of the high cost of shelter and limited income, families may tend to live together to save expenses. In such situations, as many as 10 or 12 individuals, including children, may live in an apartment designed to accommodate a family of three or four.

Such population density produces early wear and deterioration of facilities and equipment, raises property maintenance, repair, utility, and security costs, and decreases the quality of life. In the Kingsview Village on Dixon Road in the City of Etobicoke (on Toronto's western boundary), 4000 people lived in 1800 units in six high-rise apartment units in 1971. In 1995, 8500 people, 4000 of them Somalis, lived in the same complex. Although they make up almost half the Dixon population, Somalis occupy only one third of the units (Stoffman, 1995). Tension has increased with the other tenants and condominium owners, who have now been accused of being racist. The most recent wave of immigrants were the well-educated and influential individuals who have been using the tactics that caused so much strife in Somalia to force Somalis currently in the country to obey their dictates. Funding from three levels of government that had been allocated for education and recreation programs for youth to reduce the crime and violence resulting from overcrowding has not been reflected by the development of those programs but diverted to employing educated and multilingual Somalis to develop training manuals and run programs to increase cultural sensitization. Twenty-three different organizations have developed in the greater Toronto area alone to help deal with many of the issues resulting from overcrowding and resettlement of Somali immigrants (Opoku-Dapaah, 1995).

Implications for nursing care

The nurse should be aware that Somalis often do not identify the need for personal space and accept the realities of living conditions that are considered less than ideal by North American standards. Limitations of personal space and possessions are part of the Somali way of life and are accepted as such. Somalis are highly involved and polychronic in nature as described by Cherry and Giger (1995) in relation to African Americans.

The nurse should also be cognizant of the fact that Somali people, who are polychronic, may maintain several projects simultaneously, almost like jugglers (Giger and Davidhizar, 1995). The nurse who works with polychronic, highly involved individuals must be prepared to review and clarify personal values within the context of practice. The context of religious value and meaning must be included in the overall context of care. The call to prayer five times daily and the rituals of washing and focusing on personal religious health and other traditions may conflict with the priorities set by the health care professional. The priorities of the recipient of care may also produce dissonance with those of the health care provider. Institutions that limit the exposure of health-challenged individuals may have difficulty coping with the numbers and frequency of visitors who don't understand or value the standards that have been set. One goal of nursing intervention should be to help the client structure activities in a ranked order that will produce maximal benefits for the client (Giger and Davidhizar, 1995).

Finally, the nurse should appreciate that there may be an intense level of involvement between Somali-Canadian people. This is particularly true when individuals live in proximity to one another. However, it is important for the nurse to assess each person as an individual because behaviors vary not only between but within ethnic groups (Barkauskas, 1994; Orque, 1983; Rosenbaum, 1991).

SOCIAL ORGANIZATION

The concept of the nuclear childbearing family does not exist within the context of the Somali culture. Women take responsibility for bearing and providing the necessities of life for all children under 10 years of age. Maternal-infant bonding, so highly valued in North American society, does not often occur to the same degree in the Somali culture. Children are valued, nurtured, and cared for by not only the birth mother, but also women of the extended family. Infants are traditionally breast fed, but the very

nature of the harsh life from which these women have come with famine, starvation, and drought limits the degree to which the birth mother can make an emotional commitment to a newborn infant until it is clear that the infant is healthy and able to thrive. All children are valued equally, but a mother, having to make difficult decisions about the welfare of her offspring, will give preference to those who have the greatest chance of survival.

The extended family, subclan, or clan are the units of Somali society. The senior man, traditionally the dominant factor in nondomestic Somali society, is absent in 80% of the Somali-Canadian experience. Women accustomed to making decisions related to home, family, and childrearing are having to cope with the realities of dealing with government officials, financial officers, planning, investing, and supporting and educating children with little support except from the women of the extended family, friends, and neighbors. Single women as heads of households must make decisions and deal with many issues that would normally have been the elder man's responsibility. The traditions of naming the individual with a given name and the surnames of his or her father and grandfather mean that members of the same nuclear family may have different last names, which may raise questions related to their relationships when the context of the family and its dependents are examined within government guidelines.

When young men reach 10 years of age, older men undertake the responsibility for their training in Somali tradition and culture if the father is not present and able to do so. Where the father or an older brother is present, the responsibility is assumed within the family but usually includes considerable socialization with other men and boys. Men who came to Canada with their families or have since been able to join them find themselves unemployed or underemployed. University-educated, multilingual men find themselves working as taxi drivers, security guards, and parking lot attendants for minimum wage. Women seem to manage to find some better-paying jobs, and such a tendency often undermines the husband's self-esteem because he is not able to be the responsible provider. Women may also find themselves in situations of minimal job security, contract work, and layoffs because much of their employment is also in the low-paying service sectors (Murialdo, 1997).

Most Somali-Canadian immigrants adhere to their Islamic faith, and some practice more strictly than in their homeland, with women adopting the veil and the *abaye* (loose, long-sleeved light robe to cover the body). Young women, who remained at home and did not date and for whom marriages were arranged, are rejecting the constraints of their religion and family expectations by wishing to socialize with Canadian friends and acquaintances and to date and select potential partners without the intervention of parents and marriage brokers.

Implications for nursing care

The nurse should be aware that for Somalis who have immigrated to Canada childbirth is often considered a woman's issue, attended by a midwife or other women. In Somalia, with less than 400 physicians to serve a population in excess of 7 million, perinatal mortality and morbidity rank very low on the list of health care priorities. In Canada, with universal accessibility to health care services, physicians practicing family medicine, and specialists in obstetrics and gynecology, few Somali women seek prenatal care even though the majority are considered to be an at-risk population (Canadian Public Health Association, 1991), living below the poverty line and in some cases delivering low-birth-weight or premature infants.

Family practitioners have indicated an increase in the number of Somalis seeking prenatal and perinatal care in their practices only within the past few years. As Somali women learn more about the Canadian health care delivery system and seek immunizations and other treatment for their children, they are gradually beginning to accept and seek more health services for themselves. The practice of midwifery received professional recognition only with the passage of the Regulated Health Professions Legislation in 1994, and, with the College of Midwives now established in the Province of Ontario, professional licensure and regulation is in the preliminary stages. Although

there are internationally trained midwives practicing in Ontario and many aboriginal and immigrant midwives as well, the profession has only recently become self-regulating, and experienced midwives dealing with a variety of different ethnic origins are only just beginning to meet the standards of certified practice that will enable them to obtain professional licensure in Ontario.

Health care professionals working with handicapped, low-birth-weight or premature infants and their parents may have difficulty accepting the lack of male attendance and the perceived decreased motivation of mothers who do not appear to bond well with their infants. Such circumstances, though required by law, necessitate referral to child protection agencies and may result in negative outcomes because of prevailing cultural values and a general lack of trust and experience with official agencies and the Canadian health care delivery system.

The nurse should also be aware that the practice of circumcision for prepubescent females, common in many Islamic countries but not based on religious teachings or tenets, used to be highly valued in Somali society (Davies, 1996). Somalia is one of six countries including Egypt, Ethiopia, Kenya, Nigeria, and Sudan that account for three fourths of the world's cases of female genital mutilation, a practice traditionally designed to preserve virginity, ensure marriageability, and contain sexuality (Stackhouse, 1996). However, it has also been related to childbirth deaths (Stackhouse, 1996). Nevertheless, Somalian mothers are often disappointed when health care practitioners counsel and advise against it. Surgeons asked to perform such procedures tell women it is against the law, but girls under 10 years of age are still circumcised by a midwife or female members of the extended family, often using a razor blade or piece of broken glass, without an anesthetic and not necessarily in the cleanest of conditions. The procedure can range from simple clitorectomy to complete infibulation ('buckling together') with excision of the labia minora and suturing of the labia majora to leave only a small opening for the passage of urine and menstrual flow. Although the procedure is still valued and performed without the child's consent, efforts to educate Somali immigrant families has met with some success, and professionals working with this population indicate that they are seeing a steady decrease in the frequency of the procedure (Baya, 1997). The Ontario Association of Obstetricians and Gynecologists has reported an increase in requests for reconstructive surgery or repair after childbirth or to relieve complications of recurrent yeast and urinary tract infections. Informal estimates from a recent conference (April 1966) indicate that values are changing both in North America and in the countries of origin. Legislation is being passed, and although the World Health Organization's goal of Healthy People 2,000 will not be met, there is optimism that the practice will be discontinued within the next two or three generations.

Nurses working with the Somali population need to clarify their own values in order to provide culturally sensitive care. However, it is important to know that women of childbearing age who have been circumcised are at risk for perinatal complications or subsequent genital and urinary tract infections (Stackhouse, 1996).

TIME

Most Somalis, like other African Canadians, react to the present situation with little attention to the future. The nomadic nature of Somali life was such that the passing of the seasons and the availability of food and water for their herds guided their lifestyle and activities. Because literacy levels were so low with less than 25% of the population able to read, storytelling and history were related to past experiences and past time and present-time orientation. Somalis describe a sense of hopelessness related to the future attributable to previous negative experiences. Those Somalis who have most successfully become acculturated are demonstrating tendencies to value punctuality and to plan for the future to a greater degree. These individuals keep scheduled appointments and are compliant with medication regimes to a much greater degree than the majority of individuals who may appear up to 3 hours late if at all and may choose when and whether they take prescribed medications (Morrison, 1997).

Implications for nursing care

Nurses working with members of the Somali population need to clarify the meaning of time to the client. Different practitioners have developed their own assessment tools to determine client commitment to a specific treatment regime. The development of client contracts has also been a successful tool. Once the contract has been developed with the client and the client has made a verbal commitment, that commitment is usually honored. Compliance with treatment regimes is most effectively established within the daily prayer cycle. The nurse who is familiar with this cycle can often develop a plan that will work within this context. Visiting nurses will find their clients more likely to remember and keep appointments if they are scheduled for the same time each day and coincide with the completion of a prayer cycle or precede it by at least a half an hour.

ENVIRONMENTAL CONTROL

Most Somalis identify an external locus of control dependent on their environment and on family and religious expectations. The strong religious influence of Islam, which views illness as disharmony between the body and the soul, considered an inseparable unit, often results in consultation with spiritual leaders and teachers before approaching healers. Elders in the community (usually women) who may have greater knowledge of healing activities are often consulted, and the entire family are involved in prayer and treatment to resolve the disharmony. Folk practices, spells, and herbal remedies are used, and the services of a physician are rarely sought. Somalis identify nurses and naturopaths as their principal sources of professional assistance in Canada and will usually seek the services of a physician when required by law (as for immunizations) or when they need to obtain prescriptions.

Illness may also be perceived as either a natural process or as a punishment for some misdeed. A deformed infant may be perceived as a punishment for the sins of a parent, and therefore it may be hidden away from others and kept segregated from the extended family if possible. Somalis having immigrated to Canada only in the past two decades and acculturated to a different climate, environment, language, and circumstances of living do not have a sufficient history to document common health problems or reasons for accessing the health care delivery system. Limited health care facilities in Somalia and the paucity of physicians in that population have provided limited records and no studies of the determinants of health. Somalia does not test or screen for many diseases because it has no resources to treat them. The World Health Organization (WHO), the United Nations International Children's Emergency Fund (UNICEF), and the International Red Cross have provided resources to help with specific problems such as famine and starvation and provided some immunizations for children as well as working on hygiene and nutrition in the refugee camps. The life expectancy for women in Somalia is 57 years, 1 year more than that for men. Somalis in Canada are unable to define morbidity and mortality parameters or to identify common health problems within the country of origin. The relatively young age of the new Somali Canadians and lack of use of the health care delivery system precludes generalized assumptions regarding the determinants of health, mortality, and morbidity.

Implications for nursing care

Nurses who must work with Somali clients should assess which folk practices have been used and determine whether these are harmful (such as bloodletting or trephining to let out evil spirits), neutral (placing a knife under the mattress of a person to cut the pain), or harmless (the use of herbal decoctions to promote relaxation and control pain in childbirth). Where traditional practices are not considered harmful to the client, they should be ignored or allowed to continue (Leininger, 1991; Andrews and Boyle, 1994; Giger and Davidhizar, 1995; Spector, 1996). However those practices that are potentially harmful or counteract prevailing scientific practice should be discouraged.

BIOLOGICAL VARIATIONS
Body structure and skin color

Because the mean birth weights of African-American and White infants in the United States dif-

fer, with African-American infants weighing approximately 240 g less than White infants, this is likely to be true for babies whose families have immigrated from Somalia living in Canada. African-American infants are 2 cm shorter and 0.7 cm smaller in circumference (Giger and Davidhizar, 1995). The gestational period for African Americans tends to be 9 days shorter than that for Whites, and a slowing down of gestational growth occurs in African-American infants after 35 weeks. Before 35 weeks of gestation, African-American infants are usually larger than White infants (Giger and Davidhizar, 1995).

African-American children tend to mature faster than White children. They are more mature at birth in both the musculoskeletal and neurological systems. Neurologically, African-American children tend to be more advanced until 2 or 3 years of age and in the musculoskeletal system tend to be more advanced until puberty. The differences in skeletal maturity are attributed to genetic and environmental factors (Giger and Davidhizar, 1995). Educators in the early childhood field describe similarities with African Canadians of Somali descent. Body proportion and weight issues described by Davidhizar and Giger (1995) have not been verified by Canadian health care practitioners who have not had the time period necessary to validate corresponding studies within the Canadian experience.

Somali skin color, similar to that of other Canadians of African origin, is darker pigmented because of the large concentration of melanocytes and may be lighter in areas covered by clothing except for skin folds in the groin, genitalia, and nipples, which are usually darker, whereas the palms of the hands and soles of the feet are lighter in color. The newborn color may range from dusky white to dark reddish brown, with the ears being the darkest portion of the infant's body at birth (Nadeau, 1996).

Irregular pigmentation, known as "mongolian spots," may be present on the lower back, buttocks, or thighs and may be interpreted as bruises to the uninformed. Pigmentation usually evens out, and the spots disappear by the time the child is 3 or 4 years of age (Nadeau, 1996).

Susceptibility to disease

Nurses working with Somali Canadians should be aware that common health problems such as atherosclerosis, hypertension, coronary artery disease, and diabetes are common health problems among Canadians and Americans of African descent (Giger and Davidhizar, 1995). Although these health problems are not documented as being specific to the Somali population, nurses with access to the Somali should be aware of the potential risks and, after careful assessment, consider the need for health promotion and education and primary prevention programs (Thompson and McDonald, 1989; Grossman, 1996). If possible, screening programs should also be considered. Somalis, like others of African descent, are also genetically at risk for the sickle cell trait with corresponding anemias and crises. Although statistics in Canada indicate that recent immigrants report fewer chronic health problems than individuals born in Canada as the length of residency in Canada increases, they also indicate a lowered incidence of sore joints, allergies, and hypertension (Canadian Press, 1996). Michael Rachlis, a Toronto health consultant, said that immigrants tend to be healthier than the general population because they have to be to survive or escape from a country like Somalia (Canadian Press, 1996).

Psychological characteristics

Because many Somalis have immigrated as refugees, having witnessed the atrocities of civil war, knowing that some family members were tortured and killed, and probably having waited long periods in refugee camps leaving behind husbands, sons, and fathers without knowing what has happened to them, there is a greater incidence of mental health problems such as depression and post-traumatic stress disorder. Some Somali women remain in mourning for prolonged periods of time after becoming widows but are unable to carry out the Islamic funeral rituals (Community Resource Consultants of Toronto, 1997).

Authorities in Canada have recently discovered that a substance called "khat," which does not differ much from cocaine or heroin in its social consequences, has been introduced into Canada and is being distributed freely in the marketplace. *Khat* was traditionally grown and marketed in Somalia, but it is now believed that as much as 24 to 32 tons of *khat* are airlifted each week to Toronto (Hirave, 1996). In the Somali culture *khat*-chewing habits are as socially acceptable as drinking Coca-Cola is in the West, and chewing *khat* often takes place in social gatherings. Selling *khat* in Canada is a source of revenue for tribal warlords in Somalia and has become a profitable new market (Hirave, 1996).

Although the Islamic faith specifically forbids the use of alcohol or other intoxicants, Somali youth, faced with the realities of poverty and overcrowding, are showing evidence of increased use of alcohol and drugs (Addiction Research Foundation, 1996). This problem has been identified in Canada as well. The city of Scarborough (on the eastern boundary of Toronto) has the second largest Somali population in Canada and the highest teenager suicide rate except for Canadian aboriginal and Inuit peoples. The correlation between drug and alcohol use and teenager suicide is currently under investigation, not necessarily related to the Somali population and undifferentiated to avoid violation of human rights legislation. However, the Somali community themselves have identified major concerns related to the needs of their youth for recreation and employment (Scarborough Department of Public Health, 1997). Rebellious youth, attempting to acculturate and be a part of their newly adopted Canadian life, are at risk for increased drug and alcohol abuse or dependency. Because religious traditions remain strong, the risk of HIV and other sexually transmitted diseases remains relatively low just as the risk of teen pregnancy does (Morrison, 1997).

Implications for nursing care

Although data are available on biological differences identified in African Americans, few data are available specifically on the Somalis living in Canada (Overfield, 1985; Giger and Davidhizar, 1995). Nevertheless, nurses working with the Somali population must recognize that there are many biological differences and that Somali children may be slower achieving or may fail to achieve some developmental milestones. Because nurses are not employed in schools and public health nurses working with at-risk populations may be unable to obtain adequate baseline assessments to determine developmental progress, all nurse practitioners and nurses working in physicians' offices or within health clinics, family practice settings, or group practices must be aware of the risks and issues. The child must also be assessed within the context of the family unit, particularly the mother, to assess parental impressions and compare development of siblings as well as other children of the same group. Assessment of each client from a unique cultural perspective is important to provide competent health care (Spector, 1996; Henderson and Primeaux, 1981; Tripp-Reimer, Brink, and Saunders, 1984).

SUMMARY

One of Canada's newest transcultural populations are the Somalis, who have come in increasingly large numbers over the past two decades and make up one of the largest proportions of new immigrants at the present time. Although their Canadian history and determinants of health are only recently being researched and documented, Somalis themselves and the organizations set up to serve them describe difficulties adjusting to relocation, poverty and financial hardship, and racism and blatant prejudice.

Nurses working with this population need to be aware of and sensitive to the variety of needs expressed and the effects on physical, psychological, emotional, and spiritual health. Some generalities can be drawn though work with other African-Canadian clients, but the Somali experience is differently articulated by different organizations, which disagree on many issues. Some Somalis are fighting to maintain their pride, culture, religion, and family values, whereas others are trying to acculturate themselves within their new environment and to be accepted.

Somali youth, taught to respect their elders, are becoming increasingly rebellious when placed under the constraints of traditional family and when faced with fewer religious constraints and more opportunities for a variety of experiences. With unemployment running at close to 25% for youth between 18 and 25 years of age and with fewer new jobs being created for this age group, Somali youths have few opportunities to find employment, and such a lack leads health care professionals to express concern for the mental health status and potential for substance abuse and violence among those youths. Frustrated, angry, and marginalized youths need programs and diversions to facilitate the acculturation process and develop a strong sense of self-worth.

Case Study

Myriam is a 38-year-old Somali woman who was admitted to the psychiatric hospital yesterday because she was no longer able to care for herself or her family. Her 17-year-old daughter Laronda became concerned when she noticed that her mother was sleeping all the time, was not eating, and talked about ending it all because life is just too difficult. Laronda stays with her mother during the interview.

During the assessment and admission interview Myriam states that she is the mother of three children whose husband disappeared at the time she was trying to make her way with the children to neighboring Kenya to find safety during fighting in her native Mogadishu. Laronda is attending community college part-time and works part-time as a cashier in a gas station. Laronda's older brother, Ben, works part-time washing dishes in a restaurant and is also a part-time student. The younger brother, Jesse, though just 15, has dropped out of school and was placed in a Board of Education delinquency program. Myriam's eyes fill with tears as she states that "that boy be out all hours, comes home wid money he cain't explain and won't lissen to me no mo. I done lost my part-time job cause I was worryin so much where he was at. My boss said I was makin too many mistakes. I cain't pray no moah and I just know I'm bein punished—nothin I do comes right."

CARE PLAN

 Nursing Diagnosis   Hopelessness related to long-term stress and loss of religious beliefs, evidenced by vegetative symptoms of depression and verbalization of despair.

Client Outcome

1. Client will convey reduction in suicidal ideation and verbalize feelings associated with depression.

Nursing Interventions

1. Monitor and assess suicidal ideation and initiate appropriate staff supervision.
2. Administer antidepressant medication as ordered.
3. Briefly discuss the meaning and significance of symptoms to the client.
4. Explain that the medication will take time to help relieve symptoms.
5. Spend short periods of time as tolerated by client exploring feelings and establishing trust.

 Nursing Diagnosis   Sleep-pattern disturbance related to expressed feelings of hopelessness evidenced by vegetative symptoms of depression.

Client Outcome

1. Client will report restful sleep and waking patterns.

Nursing Interventions

1. Assess client's normal sleep rest pattern and develop a schedule to move toward this pattern.
2. Assess client's need for *prn* medication to promote restful sleep and personal wishes in relation to their use.
3. Encourage client to request *prn* medication if desired for sleep.
4. Assess normal bedtime routines to promote restful sleep and encourage appropriate practices.

 Nursing Diagnosis   Potential for nutrition deficits—less than daily requirements related to vegetative state as described by daughter indicating failure to eat.

Client Outcome

1. Client will report a desire to eat.

Nursing Interventions

1. Assess previous normal eating patterns and preferred foods.
2. Assess for lactose intolerance and encourage nutritionally appropriate liquids.
3. Have daughter or other family friends bring in favorite or preferred foods.
4. Monitor nutritional intake; determine if client will keep a daily log.

 Nursing Diagnosis   Self-care deficit related to expressions of hopelessness as evidenced by vegetative symptoms of depression.

Client Outcome

1. Client will initiate self-grooming activities.

Nursing interventions

1. Assess client's normal practices for grooming.
2. Assist client to set goals for grooming and other self-care activities.
3. Offer genuine praise for client's efforts to meet goals for grooming and other self-care activities.
4. Encourage client to participate in groups and other activities that promote positive validation such as recreation therapy and possibly a grief group.

Nursing Diagnosis   Social isolation related to hospitalization, job loss, unfamiliar environment, and cultural mix.

Client Outcome

1. Client will identify activities and ways to reduce social isolation.

Nursing Interventions

1. Explore with the client the possibility of having visits from family and friends.
2. Encourage daughter to visit regularly.
3. Encourage client to socialize with others on the unit who might be appropriate or share common interests.
4. Explore with the client which acquaintances or support services or agencies she might feel comfortable contacting.
5. Develop with the client a plan for returning to the community after discharge.
6. Explore with the client the possibility of a family conference.

 Nursing Diagnosis   Low self-esteem related to long-standing history of minimal accomplishments and losses, evidenced by self-negating verbalizations and feelings of shame, guilt, and despair.

Client Outcome

1. Client will verbalize realistic statements about self and others.

Nursing Interventions

1. Avoid judgments or arguments if client makes negative statements.
2. Give positive affirmations when client is able to accept praise verbally or nonverbally.
3. Encourage client to be proactive and assertive, taking on leadership responsibilities when and as she is able.
4. Explore with client the potential resources for resuming religious practices.
5. Encourage client to set and meet at least one daily goal.
6. As the depression lifts, suggest client begin to set both daily and longer-term goals.
7. Encourage client to report or diarize accomplishments.

STUDY QUESTIONS

1. Describe reasons why it may be difficult to obtain a detailed health history from a Somali client.
2. Identify issues inherent to Somali youth attempting to acculturate in Canada.
3. Describes ways in which nurses may provide culturally sensitive care to Somali clients using folk traditions and health care practices.
4. Compare and contrast Canadian Somali population with African Canadians who have been in Canada and studied extensively in the United States for several decades.
5. Describe the reasons why Canadian Somalis may hesitate to seek health care services in Canada.
6. Describe adaptations to living accommodations made by Somali Canadians.
7. State the reasons why the majority of Somalis in Canada currently live below the poverty line.
8. Describe ways in which nurses can provide culturally sensitive care to Somalis with strong religious and value orientation that may be in conflict with current Canadian values and laws.

References

Addiction Research Foundation. (1996). 1996 Workshop on Youth and Addictions, Toronto.

Anderson, J.M. (1985). Perspectives on the health of immigrant women. A feminist analysis. *Advances in Nursing Science, 8*(1), 61-76.

Andrews, M.M., & Boyle, J.S. (1994). *Transcultural nursing.* Philadelphia: Lippincott-Raven.

Bailey, E., & Bailey, R. (1995). *Discover Canada.* Oxford: Berlitz Publishing Company.

Barkauskas. (1994). *Quick reference to cultural assessment.* St. Louis: Mosby.

Baumgart, A., & Larsen, J. (1988). *Canadian nursing faces the future.* St. Louis: Mosby.

Baya, K. (1997). *Female genital mutilation: values, issues and trends.* Unpublished manuscript, Toronto.

Campbell, K. (1996, September 4). The world rushes to speak and write American English; Britain's mother tongue takes a lickin from the Americanization of the emerging global average. *Christian Science Monitor,* p. 10.

Canadian Press. (1996, April 2). Immigrants suffer fewer health ailments. *Calgary Herald,* p. A9.

Canadian Public Health Association. (1991). Somalis in Canada. *Monograph for Health Care Professionals,* Ottawa.

Chiswick, B., & Miller, P. (1996). Language and earnings among immigrants in Canada: a survey. In Duleep, H., & Wunnava, P. (Eds.), *Immigrants and immigration policy: individual skills, family ties, and group identities.* London: JAI Press (Division of Johnson Associates, Inc.).

Clayton, M. (1996, November 13). Refugees to Canada slip to U.S. to Mohawk trail smuggler's alley. *Christian Science Monitor,* p. 1.

Community Resources Consultants of Toronto. (1997). *Making choices: a consumer/survivor's guide to adult mental health services and supports in metro Toronto,* Toronto.

Craig, T. (1996, October 9). Canadian military chief is latest casualty of scandal. *Los Angeles Times,* p. A4.

Davies, K. (1996, July 6). Female circumcision continues. *The Associated Press News Service,* p. 1.

Dobson, S. (1991). *Transcultural nursing: a contemporary imperative.* London: Scutari Press.

Fodor's staff. (1987). *Fodor's Canada, 1988.* New York: Fodor's Travel Publications.

Giger, J., & Davidhizar, R. (1995). *Transcultural nursing: assessment and intervention.* St. Louis: Mosby.

Grossman, D. (1996). Cultural dimensions in home health care nursing. *American Journal of Nursing, 96*(7), 33-36.

Grypma, S. (1993). Culture shock. *The Canadian Nurse, 89*(9), 33-37.

Gunderson, J. (1996). Progress in building communication links. *The Canadian Nurse, 92*(4), 9-10.

Guruge, S., & Donner, G. (1996). Transcultural nursing in Canada. *The Canadian Nurse, 92*(9), 34-39.

Henderson, G., & Primeaux, M. (1981). *Transcultural health care.* Don Mills, Ont.: Addison-Wesley Publishing Company.

Hirave, H. (1996, January 2). New drug finds a home in metro: potentially violent trade in khat arrived along with influx of Somali refugees. *Toronto Star,* p. A13.

Jepson, T., Lee, P., & Smith, T. (1996). *Canada.* London: The Rough Guides.

Johnson, O. (Ed.). (1997). *Information please almanac.* Boston & New York: Houghton Mifflin Company.

Knox, P. (1996, June 17). Foreign aid sending too few kids to school, report says. *Toronto Globe and Mail,* p. 7.

Leininger, M. (1991). *Culture care diversity and universality: a theory of nursing.* New York: National League for Nursing.

Lewis, I. (1988). *A modern history of Somalia: nation state in the horn of Africa.* Boulder, Colo.: Westview Press.

Liberson, S. (1970). *Language and ethnic relations in Canada.* New York: John Wiley.

Loescher, G., & Scanlan, J. (1986). *Calculated kindness.* New York: The Free Press.

Mohamed, A. (1994). Refugee exodus from Somalia: revisiting the causes. *Refuge, 14*(1).

Mohamed, S. (1992). The rise and fall of Somali nationalism. *Refuge, 12*(5).

Morrison, L. (1997). *What nurse practitioners should know about at-risk African-Canadian populations.* Unpublished manuscript, Toronto.

Murialdo, E. (1997). *Employment patterns for refugees in Ontario.* Unpublished manuscript, Toronto.

Nadeau, N. (1996). *Perinatal counseling and care of Ethiopian and Somali women.* Unpublished manuscript, Toronto.

Nichols, R. (1996, November 19). America's grain machine strains under huge demand. *The Philadelphia Inquirer,* p. 1.

Noble, A. (1992). *To build a new land.* London: Johns Hopkins University Press.

Opoku-Dapaah, E. (1995). *Somali refugees in Toronto: a profile.* Toronto: York Lanes Press.

Orque, M.S. (1983). Orque's ethnic/cultural system: a framework for ethnic nursing care. In Orque, M.S., Bloch, B., & Monrroy, L.S.A. (Eds.), *Ethnic nursing care: a multicultural approach.* St. Louis: Mosby.

Overfield, T. (1985). *Biologic variation in health and illness.* Reading, Mass.: Addison-Wesley.

Pederson, A., O'Neill, M., & Rootman, I. (1994). *Health promotion in Canada.* Toronto: W.B. Saunders.

Rosenbaum, J. (1991). A cultural assessment guide. *The Canadian Nurse, 87*(4), 32-33.

Samatar, A. (1988). *Socialist Somalia: rhetoric and reality.* London: Zed Books.

Samatar, S. (1991). *Somalia: a nation in turmoil. A minority rights report,* Washington, D.C.

Scarborough Department of Public Health. (1997).

Schreuder, C. (1996, September 9). Malaria frustrating best efforts of science. *Chicago Tribune,* p. 1.

Simons, B. (Ed.). (1976). *The volume library.* Nashville, Tenn.: The Southwestern Company.

Solomon, W. (1996, October 6). Immigration: are we closing the door? *York Daily Record,* p. 1.

Spector, R. (1996). *Cultural diversity in health care* (ed. 4). Stamford, Conn.: Appleton & Lange.

Stackhouse, J. (1996, June 11). Childbirth-related deaths most neglected tragedy of our times. *Toronto Globe and Mail.*

Statistics Canada. (1996). *Canada at a glance.* 1996 Communication Division of Statistics, Canada. Ottawa.

Stoffman, D. (1995, August). Dispatch from Dixon. *Toronto Life.*

Takaki, R. (1993). *A different mirror.* Toronto: Little, Brown & Co.

Thompson, P., & McDonald, J. (1989). Multicultural health education: responding to the challenge. *Health Promotion, 28*(2), 8-11.

Tripp-Reimer, T., Brink, P., & Saunders, J. (1984). Cultural assessment: content and process. *Nursing Outlook, 32*(2), 78-82.

United Nations High Commission on Refugees. (1996). Significant populations of internally displaced persons. *Refugees,* Geneva.

United Nations High Commission on Refugees. (1993). Repatriation costs of the internally displaced. *Refugees,* Geneva.

World Almanac. (1997). Mahwah, N.J.: World Almanac Books.

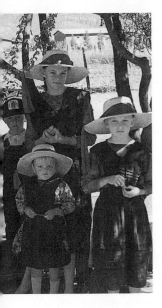

CHAPTER 19

Old Colony Mexican-Canadian Mennonites

Sandra C. DeLuca and Mary Anne Krahn

BEHAVIORAL OBJECTIVES

After reading this chapter, the nurse will be able to:

1. Appreciate the diversity across various Mennonite groups and within the Mexican-Canadian Mennonite group in particular.
2. Describe the influence that religious beliefs, family and social structure, and the cultural goals of conformity and separation have on the Mexican-Canadian Mennonite conception of health.
3. Understand the ways in which poverty has affected health, illness, and health-seeking behaviors of Mexican-Canadian Mennonite people.
4. Understand the perspectives of Mexican-Canadian Mennonite people toward education and the implications that educational views have for health teaching.
5. Understand the way in which endogamy and interrelatedness contribute to biological health risks among the Mexican-Canadian Mennonites.

OVERVIEW OF THE OLD COLONY MEXICAN MENNONITES

The Mennonites are a people of diversity. To understand and appreciate the nature and richness of this diversity, it is helpful to become familiar with the origins of the religion and culture and how beliefs have shaped the Mennonites' place in the world.

The authors would like to express their appreciation for the information, wisdom, and suggestions provided by the Mennonite Central Committees of Aylmer, Ontario, and of Winnipeg, Manitoba, Canada.

From the beginnings in Europe at the time of the Reformation, the constants that have remained the same across every Mennonite group are Anabaptist beliefs, namely, adult baptism, separation of church and state, and nonresistance. To be Mennonite involves more than belonging to a religious organization. For many Canadian Mennonites today, it is also a way of life.

There are many subgroups of Mennonites, each of which has culturally unique features. This often causes confusion for non-Mennonites (Regehr, 1996). Historically Mennonites have been a minority group and have been persecuted for their beliefs. Their migration patterns from central Europe to Prussia, Russia, and finally the Americas can be explained by their desire for freedom to live life according to their beliefs and to educate children in the ways of their church. To appreciate the differences between the various groups, it is necessary to understand their antecedent history and the dates and sequence in which they arrived in Canada (Regehr, 1996). This chapter is an attempt to describe one small group, commonly called "Old Colony Mexican-Canadian Mennonites." To illuminate this group, a brief overview of the history of the Mennonite people is provided, with specific focus on how the Mexican-Canadian Mennonites came to be. This chapter explains the influence of this minority group on the southwestern Ontario communities in which they live, how their beliefs shape their lifestyle, and the wide diversity even within this group.

THE OLD COLONY MEXICAN MENNONITE PEOPLE

Mexican Mennonite is the popular name for a group of people who left Canada during the 1920s in search of religious freedom. The largest group is the Old Colony Mennonite church, and a smaller group is the New Reinland Mennonite Church (Reimer, 1990). *Kanadier,* or Canadian Mennonite, is another name often associated with those Mennonites who come from Mexico. Most have claims on Canadian citizenship (Mennonite Central Committee, 1996).

It is difficult to estimate the number of Old Colony Mennonites who live in Canada because of the seasonal migration of many families who are seeking work as farm laborers. Also, many who arrive in Canada are undocumented, and others claim no church membership (Reimer, 1990). Most Old Colony Mennonites who come to Canada arrive in the province of Ontario because of the longer growing season, with smaller numbers going to the provinces of Alberta and Manitoba (Mennonite Central Committee, 1996). Of those who come to Ontario, many are attracted to Elgin County, a rich agricultural area in the southwestern region of the province. Estimates of people of Mennonite origin in Elgin County range between 4000 to 7000 (Van Ryswyk, 1993), and around 20,000 have settled in Ontario since the mid-1970s (Mennonite Central Committee, 1996). The town of Aylmer, Ontario, has been the hub of the Old Colony community since the 1960s (Regehr, 1996).

Van Ryswyk (1993) states that "the value placed on education by the [Mexican] Mennonite people is different from that of Canadian society." In fact, resistance to public education has been one factor that has contributed to immigration patterns during the last hundred years. Education is controlled by the church leaders and is based on three premises that shape the personal, societal, and religious aspects of life (Van Ryswyk, 1993).

The first premise, held by some of these individuals, is a personal one, in that the more educated you become, the more at risk you are of becoming "lost" and the further away from God you will be. The second premise involves the church. The belief is that the more you know, the more God expects of you. The less you know, the less God expects of you. The less God expects of you, the less likely you are to displease God. . . . The less you know, the less likely . . . you will challenge the leadership of the church. . . . The final premise is a societal one, in that education must be functional if one is to be a servant of the church. This is a recognition that one may need a certain level of education to be useful in society but that education must serve some useful purpose . . . (Van Ryswyk, 1993).

These premises continue to have pivotal effects on the Old Colony way of life. The resulting school system is substandard when compared to the system in North America (Redekop, 1969; Sawatsky, 1971; Van Ryswyk, 1993). Significant numbers of these people are functionally illiterate (Woodhouse, 1993).

The education system in the Mennonite colonies in Mexico described by Van Ryswyk (1993) is almost identical to that depicted by Redekop (1969) and Sawatsky (1971) and has remained virtually unchanged since the beginning of the century. The schools continue to be controlled by the church leaders, who determine the school curricula and who hire teachers. Teachers do not receive any professional training and are usually men chosen for their commitment to Old Colony life, for their orthodoxy, and for their lack of skills or interest in farming. Subjects taught are reading, writing, and arithmetic.

The school year revolves around the agricultural cycle. Children begin school at 6 years of age, when most of the harvesting is complete. The school year ends when the planting season begins in the spring. Children attend school for about 6 years, with the girls often leaving earlier than the boys. Older children in families may leave earlier if their help is needed at home or in the fields (Redekop, 1969; Sawatsky, 1971; Van Ryswyk, 1993).

Adherence to the three premises has also stopped progress in the education of Old Colony Mennonites. The language of school is High German even though the students speak Low German *(Plautdietsch,* or *Plattdeutsch),* a language with no written expression (Edmunds, 1993), at home. Learning is by rote and memorization because they must learn to read and write a language that they do not speak (Van Ryswyk, 1993). In most schools, the only textbooks are the Bible, the catechism, a song book, and a German reader called a *Fibel* ('primer') (Mennonite Central Committee, 1996, April 30). Spanish, English, science, history, and geography are not taught.

Education does not seem to be a priority among these people. The hands of all family members are required to meet the physical requirements of day-to-day life. Education is sacrificed for farm labor. Intellectual stimulation is lacking (Redekop, 1969), and creativity is dampened by the control of the church leaders (Sawatsky, 1971). Parents who are functionally illiterate rarely find or take time to give educational stimulation to their children, and reading material and manipulative play materials are absent from most homes (Mennonite Central Committee, 1994). *Das Blatt,* a German magazine published for Old Colony children and designed to promote literacy, is welcomed in many homes, but many families cannot afford the 10-dollar (Canadian) subscription rate (Mennonite Central Committee, 1996, April 30).

When these families arrive in southwestern Ontario, education of their children is not seen as being of a priority. They are unaware of the law that mandates that children between 6 and 16 years of age must be registered in school. Absentee rates are high because children will stay at home if their help is needed. Especially problematic is attendance at high school because children perceive that they are finished with school at 12 to 14 years of age, and parents are fearful that more education will bring unwanted changes (Van Ryswyk, 1993). This fearfulness lessens with the length of residence in Canada.

Several programs have developed in Elgin County in response to the needs of the children. English-as-a-second-language programs are in place in most schools in eastern Elgin County. Attendance counselors track the children to try and keep them in school. The Elgin County Board of Education had developed the "Supervised Alternative Learning for Excused Pupils" (SALEP) program, which offers individualized alternative learning experiences outside of the high school setting that can be combined with work (Van Ryswyk, 1993).

Old Colony families have formed three private schools in the area that are affiliated with the church. Most of the children who attend are in the elementary grades; however the schools do offer up to grade 10. Parents are responsible for tuition fees and school transportation. For some parents, this is the education of choice because their children are with others of the same background (Van Ryswyk, 1993).

As the adults of the Old Colony Church have come to realize that they need basic literacy skills to be successful in Canada, classes in English as a second language have become more accepted. Separate programs have been developed for men and women; however, these programs are threatened by unstable funding (Van Ryswyk, 1993). Although the federal government funds such programs, many Mennonites from Mexico are ineligible because they are not Canadian citizens. These people face many other barriers to literacy education. Woodhouse (1993) believes that illiteracy contributes to many families being forced to live in a survivalist lifestyle, extensive poverty, and less than optimal health of all family members.

HISTORICAL ORIGINS OF THE OLD COLONY MEXICAN MENNONITES

The Anabaptist movement in sixteenth-century Europe began during the time of the Reformation. In response to the social, cultural, and religious conditions, the movement developed into two streams (Fretz, 1989). The first stream started in 1525 in Zürich, Switzerland, in protest against the Reformation movements, which followers believed did not go far enough. The first congregations were formed in January of that year, and adherents rejected all the sacraments of the medieval church except baptism and communion (Fretz, 1989). Infant baptism was rejected because no biblical basis could be found and because faith was perceived as a personal response that an infant was incapable of making (Dyck, 1981).

Anabaptism spread north along the Rhine valley, and the second stream of the movement developed. Menno Simons, a Dutch Catholic priest, became a convert, was rebaptized, and became the leader of the movement in the Netherlands. His followers became known as "Mennonites." Migration east to Danzig and Elbing was spurred by the severe persecution Anabaptists were experiencing. They were tolerated as citizens because of their expertise in dike building and farming (Fretz, 1989). It is from this stream that the Old Colony Mennonites have developed.

As the eighteenth century approached, Prussian rule over the Danzig region was increasing the restrictions on the Mennonites. They were seen as a threat to the Lutheran church (Sawatsky, 1971) and were not allowed to acquire any land to accommodate for growth in the community (Redekop, 1969). Church leaders began to look elsewhere for land, and eventually Mennonites were invited to southern Russia by Tsarina Catherine II. She granted special privileges, which included free land, "perpetual exemption from military and civil service, freedom of religion, the right to control their schools and churches, and the right and obligation of agricultural colonies to be locally anonymous" (Sawatsky, 1971). The Mennonites settled in the southern Ukraine on lands vacated by the Turks (Epp, 1962). The first colony founded in 1789 was called "Chor-

titza" and was followed by the colony of Molotschna in 1804, and by 1910 almost 2 million acres of land had been acquired (Fretz, 1989). The colonies thrived and were maintained in an atmosphere of relative freedom and peace.

By the 1870s the autonomy of the Mennonite colonies was threatened by the mounting pressure to integrate into Russian society. Tsar Alexander II issued a document that abolished the privileges and isolation. All colonies were to be integrated into the Russian government. When the Russian government threatened to reject the Mennonites' exemption from military service, church leaders began to investigate emigration once again (Sawatsky, 1971). An agreement in which Mennonite men could serve for 3 years with the Forestry Department in lieu of military service was negotiated. Other problems that contributed to the desire to emigrate faced the colonies. They were unable to acquire more land and lacked economic opportunities. Many were unwilling to accept that they would have equal status with the rest of the Russians.

In 1874, the first groups of Russian Mennonites arrived in Manitoba. Sawatsky (1971) states that these groups were "among the most conservative and economically least well-endowed of the migrants." The Mennonites who emigrated from the Chortitza settlement became known as the "Old Colony" (Redekop, 1969). In Manitoba, they tried to mimic life as it had been in Russia. However, when municipal governments were started in 1880, many felt threatened by interference from outside (Sawatsky, 1971). In 1890, the Manitoba Schools Act was passed, legislating English as the language of instruction in schools. Since attendance was not compulsory, children continued to attend private schools. Once again, the most conservative in the settlement began to consider moving. Between 1895 and 1905, several groups moved to the province of Saskatchewan (Redekop, 1969).

During the early years of the twentieth century, the pressures on these conservative Mennonite groups to conform to the public school system was increasing. In 1918, all rural private schools in Manitoba were condemned (Sawatsky, 1971). In Saskatchewan, parents were fined for not sending their children to public schools. When parents were unable to pay the fines, livestock was seized, and even auctions were held (Ens, 1980).

As the school crisis intensified, Old Colony members considered leaving Canada. In 1921, delegates to Mexico were able to negotiate the *Privilegium,* which allowed, for men, an exemption from military service and exemptions from making oaths and provided total autonomy in organizing and administering their churches, schools, and properties (Sawatsky, 1971). This was acceptable to the majority of church members. Land was purchased in northern Mexico, and approximately half of the Old Colony population of Manitoba and Saskatchewan relocated in the regions of Chihuahua and Durango (Redekop, 1969).

Life has not always been easy for the Old Colony Mennonites in Mexico. Initially, lack of knowledge about the climate and appropriate crops for the land led to hunger and poverty. Drought and crop failures have been common. Once again, Old Colony Mennonites are faced with land shortages and few economic resources. The church continues to dictate that members live the conservative orthodox lifestyle (Van Ryswyk, 1993). Many families find themselves landless with no means of income to support large and growing families.

Economic hardship has spurred the latest migration trends in this group. In the late 1950s families have been finding their way to southwestern Ontario, lured by labor-intensive seasonal crops, which provide many well-paying jobs. Van Ryswyk (1993) identifies the following reasons cited for the move to Canada: wanted work, didn't enjoy farm work in Mexico, no longer wanting to be poor, family in Canada, and problems with the church. Many of the returnees are, or have the potential to become, Canadian citizens. A resource center has been established in Aylmer, Ontario, to assist Old Colony people in becoming Canadian citizens and accessing social services. Although it is difficult to ascertain exact numbers of Old Colony people arriving in Canada each spring, it is estimated that several hundred families travel from Mexico to Canada each year (Mennonite Central Committee, 1996, July 12). Many return to Mexico in the fall to avoid the winter months, but the trend now seems to be to stay in Canada (Van Ryswyk, 1993).

COMMUNICATION
Language

The oral language of Old Colony Mennonites was based upon seventeenth-century West Prussian *Plattdeutsch,* or *Plautdietsch* (Edmunds, 1993). Plautdietsch is one of several Low German languages, which include Dutch, Flemish, Frisian, and English (Beckett, no date). Low German, in this context, refers to a geographical location of the lowlands of northern Europe that includes the Netherlands and northern Germany (Prussia). The language, which is a combination of Dutch, German, and Russian-Prussian, has been referred to as "a *muttasproak,* or mother-tongue, that has been common to Mennonites all over the world in the last two and a half centuries" (Van Ryswyk, 1993).

Low German is primarily a spoken language and differs from present-day German in that there was no written expression until the 1970s when Dr. Jack Thiessen published the first *Mennonite Low-German Dictionary* (Van Ryswyk, 1993). This publication was followed by a similar one, written by Herman Rempel in 1979 and subsequently updated in 1984, entitled *Kjenn jie noch Plautdietsch?* This Low German–to–English and English–to–Low German dictionary allows people of Mennonite origin, as well as others, access to a language rich in history (Van Ryswyk, 1993).

Plautdietsch is not the language of those peoples who have been educated in Mexico. Instead, the language that is used and written in schools and churches is German business language, or "High German." Because of the difference in the language of the Mexican Mennonite culture and the language of the institutions, the acquisition of literacy skills has been compromised. Children learned to speak one language at home and a different language once they entered the school system in Mexico. When they come to Canada as adults or children, "they need to learn oral and written English . . . that actually becomes a third or even fourth language depending [on whether] they learned Spanish while living in Mexico" (Van Ryswyk, 1993). In southwestern Ontario, the Old Colony Mennonite church founded a private school in 1990 that offered and taught classes in English, with prayers and hymns in German for grades 1 through 12 (Edmunds, 1993).

Despite some efforts by the schools and government to encourage the Old Colony Mennonites to improve English literacy skills, some Mennonites continue to resist the government's wish that children be taught English. There is evidence to indicate that literacy is a major problem within the community and that there are some Old Colony Mennonites who are not literate in any language, including their first language (Woodhouse, 1993). Poverty and the survivalist lifestyle are not conducive to increasing access to consistent educational sessions for literacy on a long-term basis.

There are implications of language issues for the provision of care as well as for health teaching. Translators who are trusted by the community or who are members of the community may be essential. Explanations should be given in clear and specific terms and may require a visual aid for clarification. The nurse must not assume that the adult or child who is speaking Plautdietsch is necessarily literate in the language.

Speech and kinesics

Although there is much diversity within the culture, many of the Old Colony Mennonites, women in particular, are soft-spoken and hesitant in their speech. A video produced by the Mennonite Central Committee—Canada (1995), entitled *Migration North: Mennonites from Mexico,* shows most of the conversation being conducted by the males of the community, whereas the females quietly stand back from the group with eyes averted. An outsider seldom sees a heated discussion among members of the group. Gestures are minimal. Instead, the speech and conversational tone of the Old Colony Mennonites are indicative of teachings of their church. The Old Colony Mennonites understand pride as a sin and humility as a virtue and are not accustomed to being asked for their opinion on issues of life, spirituality, or education. They are more accustomed to being told what to do (Van Ryswyk, 1993).

Implication for nursing care

The nurse working with Canadian Old Colony Mennonite people needs to be cognizant of the way in which their spiritual beliefs influence how they speak, discuss, and respond to questions. The absence of a verbalized opinion does not signify a lack of interest or resistance to a health-related question. On the other hand, the nurse must not assume compliance because of the absence of argument. Mexican Mennonite patients may often nod their heads in response to a doctor's comments. As well, "gestures of 'so-called' understanding do not necessarily reveal understanding by the patient" (Woodhouse, 1993). Therefore the client's lack of initiating asking questions of the nurse or physician is likely to be related to the client's perception of the health care worker, rather than a lack of English-language skill. The male physician may be perceived as "all-knowing" and in some cases likened to a "mind-reader" in regard to the patient's state of health (Woodhouse, 1993). Thus, Old Colony Mennonite clients may not volunteer information or ask questions.

Considering the prevalence of oral language as the sole language form, the nurse may expect that some Mexican Mennonites will attempt to memorize instructions or information. Clear, simple written instructions and verbal repetition of key points are important (Woodhouse, 1993).

It is important to realize that the lack of touch among adults does not necessarily signify a lack of caring for each other. Caring tends to be demonstrated by action rather than words. This may also be true of the way in which they interpret the care administered to them. Therefore the nurse caring for the Old Colony Mennonite client must be sure not only to speak of concern to help, but also to act upon the care intention.

SPACE

Public demonstration of touching, among the same sex or opposite sex, are minimal or absent among the Old Colony Mennonites. Instead, kinship is shown through activities, such as visiting and keeping in contact with relatives. Relatives are visited as often "as time and distance will allow" (Edmunds, 1993). Mutual aid within families is valued, and in times of adversity, Mexican Mennonites provide limited aid to other families.

The concepts of conformity and separation are understood as goals of Old Colony life. Conforming to Old Colony norms is one of the most important of all goals (Redekop, 1969). In the classic work of Redekop (1969), he notes that "conformity is a goal because it will preserve the Old Colony way of life and contribute to the quest for salvation." Deviance from the norms of the culture may precipitate the breakdown of solidarity and discipline. The maintenance of separation from the world supports the goal of conformity. Redekop (1969) points out that separation implies "not mixing with 'worldly' people and not adopting 'worldly' practices." The realization of this goal is addressed in religious worship, everyday conversations, and the architecture of meetinghouses. Redekop (1969) gives an example of the way in which the goal of separation is addressed by an Old Colony member in Mexico.

At this meeting many lay people got up and lamented the sad plight of the *Gemeent* [a Low German word meaning 'church'], how it had got worldly, how it had taken on more of the world's show, and how it was necessary to return to old truths. Some of the worldly things mentioned were rubber tires, wristwatches, ties, belts on trousers, and cars.

Yet, within the community, boundaries do not seem as foreboding and limiting as in the capitalist non-Old Colony world (Redekop, 1969). There is an absence of fences, which creates an atmosphere of open communal ecology.

From the outsider's perspective, conformity and separation may be understood as aloofness and a turning away from human contact outside of the community and the family. This distancing behavior should not be interpreted as rejection.

Implications for nursing care

The nurse who cares for an Old Colony Mennonite client must remember the close relationship between religious values and response to gestures that enter personal space. For example, the nurse may want to ask the Old Colony client if there is a family member who would like to perform activities such as mouth care or bathing. Old Colony Mennonites are quite modest about bodily functions, and matters pertaining to sexuality and reproduction are not discussed openly even within the family context. It may be more comfortable for a Mexican Mennonite women to have another woman from within the family structure present for childbearing because in many cases the father is uninvolved with the birthing process and early childhood nurture (Mennonite Central Committee, 1994).

SOCIAL ORGANIZATION
The Family

Family is the center of much of the Old Colony Mennonite way of life. The kinship structure is patrilineal and patriarchal with the father remaining the foundation of Old Colony structure (Edmunds, 1993). Fathers continue to provide for the family in material and spiritual ways, whereas mothers are responsible for the home and the children (Edmunds, 1993). Marriage is the ultimate goal in life, and true independence is not recognized until either the man or woman is married (Van Ryswyk, 1993). Marriage is understood as a lifelong commitment, and close interactions with others pertains mainly to the men, who interact in a closely knit fashion generally aiding one another with farm work. Women have less opportunity to interact with others, except through visiting (Edmunds, 1993; Redekop, 1969).

In the Old Colony family, there are usually many children. They are often seen as "an economic asset and as security for old age" (Van Ryswyk, 1993). The children share in the work of the family from a very young age, and it is expected that education within schools will supplement learning in the home. Formal education traditionally had the purpose of providing basic reading and writing skills and religious instruction in the German language (Epp, cited in Edmunds, 1993). Education within the Old Colony in Mexico was viewed with suspicion by the clergy, who had direct control over the schools. Perspectives on education are changing. In southwestern Ontario, the Old Colony Mennonite church founded a private school in 1990, which was seen as a positive development by the Old Colony community (Edmunds, 1993). This school offered a grade 1 through grade 12 education with classes taught in English and prayers and hymns in German (Edmunds, 1993).

Accompanying the expansion of education for children is an increasing tension within some families as children become more influenced by Canadian culture (Van Ryswyk, 1993). It becomes more difficult to exercise control of children and to maintain the separation from the outside influences of the dominant society. Some are concerned that as children become aware of the dress of others at public school traditional Old Colony Mennonite dress, which consists of modest and plain clothes, no jewelry or cosmetics, and head coverings for married women (Edmunds, 1993), may become an issue.

According to Van Ryswyk (1993), there is fear of education. It is believed that the more educated a person becomes, the more at risk that person is of moving further away from God and becoming lost to the church (Van Ryswyk, 1993). The less one knows, some Old Colony people believe, the less likely one is to displease God, and the less likely one might challenge the church leadership (Van Ryswyk, 1993). Acculturation for many of the Old Colony Mexican Mennonites is therefore controlled by educational views.

The social system

According to Redekop (1969), "the most inclusive social control resides in the Church's power over the total Old Colony life." The clergy guards religious and social norms as well as the behavior of the people. Yet, although in both Canada and Mexico smoking, drinking, and worldly dress are forbidden, there is not complete obedience (Redekop, 1969). In fact, alcohol and substance abuse are becoming an increasing problem (Mennonite Central Committee, 1994; Woodhouse, 1993). The actual power of the religious leaders to achieve the conformity in social patterns varies greatly (Redekop, 1969). It is important for the nurse to understand that there is significant variance and diversity in social patterns among

the Old Colony Mexican Mennonites in both Mexico and Canada.

A second sphere of social control by the church concerns village social structure (Redekop, 1969). Although the Old Colony Mexican-Canadian Mennonite church has permitted some loosening of social structure, as long as the people still live in a village or community setting, economic, social, and ecological processes are rigidly controlled (Redekop, 1969).

A third sphere of control is the power structure in the kinship system (Redekop, 1969). The father has power over sons and daughters (Redekop, 1969; Edmunds, 1993). Although decisions are made with the counsel of the wife and she has ultimate responsibility for the family, she yields little power (Redekop, 1969; Edmunds, 1993). The advice of grandparents is respected because of their knowledge gained from life experience (Edmunds, 1993).

A fourth area of power lies within the informal social structure (Redekop, 1969). Because of the *Gemeinschaft,* or 'community', characteristics of the Old Colony Mexican Mennonites, "power does not necessarily reside in institutionalized offices or in prescribed roles" (Redekop, 1969). Positive interpersonal relations and personableness can constitute a tremendous amount of influence over others. It is important for the nurse to have an understanding of the power structure within the Old Colony Mexican Mennonite community. The power structure will have significant effects upon decisions made related to health care and upon receptiveness to health education provided by the nurse.

Religious views

Old Colony Mexican-Canadian Mennonites generally hold the belief that they are God's chosen people (Redekop, 1969; Edmunds, 1993). They believe God will take care of those who are faithful and punish those who do not remain pure from the world (Edmunds, 1993; Redekop, 1969). The Old Colony Mexican-Canadian Mennonites view God as their personal benefactor and believe that God will take care of them in all aspects of life as long as they are faithful. If they are unfaithful, it is understood that God will punish them.

Church services assume a central role within community life. Ministers are elected by the congregation from male members and are then expected to preach from books of sermons that have been prepared by previous ministers (Edmunds, 1993). In some Old Colony churches of southwestern Ontario, men and women are seated on opposite sides of the church, whereas in others families may sit together for worship (Van Ryswyk, 1993). Churches now vary in whether music is offered and whether there is accompaniment with musical instruments. New congregations of Old Colony Mexican-Canadian Mennonites are forming in the southwestern Ontario area. Some Mexican Mennonite people do not attend church.

Implications for nursing care

Many Old Colony Mexican-Canadian Mennonites experience a survivalist lifestyle, with a significant number of employed individuals and their families who live below the poverty line (Van Ryswyk, 1993). Many have emigrated because they have been unable to generate enough income or yield enough produce to support their families in Mexico (Mennonite Central Committee, 1994). Large families, social control, illiteracy, and barriers to education influence the Old Colony Mennonites' perception of health and illness, as well as the reasons why they will seek health care.

Motivation to enhance literacy and understanding about the concept of health are related to health-related actions by Old Colony Mexican-Canadian Mennonites. In other words, many Old Colony Mexican-Canadian Mennonite people determine what education is needed and when they will need health care by their capabilities to complete the tasks set out for them by their role in the family and by the views of their roles held by the church. One is "healthy" and sufficiently "educated" if one is able to carry out one's daily responsibilities. Thus, if one is able to carry out daily responsibilities, there may be little interest in activities related to health promotion and prevention of illness (Woodhouse, 1993). Mental illness and emotional pain may not be fully acknowledged, understood, or addressed by Old Colony Mexican-Canadian Mennonites (Wood-

house, 1993). Old Colony children are often burdened, at a young age, with the stress and responsibility of being useful to their family. For example, because the mother tends to be so involved in all the household tasks and the father is frequently uninvolved, care of the younger children is frequently the responsibility of the older ones (Mennonite Central Committee, 1994). For the Old Colony Mexican-Canadian Mennonite child who tends to be quiet and obedient, self-esteem is very much affected by how helpful his or her family determines their child to be.

Definitions of abuse according to some of the Old Colony Mexican Mennonite population may differ significantly from that of Canadian society (Mennonite Central Committee, 1994; Woodhouse, 1993; East Elgin Community Development Steering Committee, 1989). The following was noted in the report from the Family and Educational Support Program project (Mennonite Central Committee, 1994):

> It is not unusual for a father to be charged with physical or sexual abuse against his children. Physical violence including severe beatings are often justified by the Old Testament principle: "Spare the rod, spoil the child." An interview with an adult who had been abused as a young child revealed that her father believed it to be his obligation as a parent to literally "beat" the truths of right and wrong behavior into his children.

The patriarchal principles of some Old Colony Mexican-Canadian Mennonites dictate that when the child is being punished by the father the mother does not interfere (Mennonite Central Committee, 1994). Thus the culturally determined role of passivity of women appears to contribute to emotional abuse experienced by many children (Mennonite Central Committee, 1994).

Deprivation may also be an issue for children in the Old Colony Mexican-Canadian Mennonite community. On the one hand, deprivation is physical. Children may not be equipped with adequate clothing upon emigration from Mexico to the harsher Canadian climate. Traditionally, shoes are worn instead of boots, and there may be the absence of a winter coat, hat, and mittens (Mennonite Central Committee, 1994). On the other hand, deprivation also occurs when educational knowledge and subsequent potential for future employment are limited (Mennonite Central Committee, 1994).

Religious beliefs and practices are powerful influences on the understanding of health and illness. Religion is a central force in Old Colony Mexican-Canadian Mennonite life, and it affects perspectives of health and illness as well as health-seeking behaviors. Issues surrounding pregnancy and gynecological problems are interwoven with family values, religion, and cultural expectations. Marriage and children are thought of as part of God's plan. Thus birth control is not generally sanctioned because children are a blessing from God, and any interference in their conception would be contrary to God's will (Edmunds, 1993).

TIME

In Redekop's (1969) classic work on the Old Colony Mexican-Canadian Mennonites the various goals of the community are identified. He identifies the highest goal as salvation. This is understood as acceptance by God as a faithful people rather than as individuals. Redekop (1969) says that it is important that there be "no deviants to spoil the chances of the whole group." In time perception, this description of the communal and religious goal might be seen as a future-oriented perspective. All that is accomplished now is judged for its contribution to the quest for salvation. Yet, on the other hand, the perception that they are God's chosen people and the reality of substandard economic conditions may superimpose a more immediate and present-oriented time perception.

There is no evidence of a desire to move up in the world (Redekop, 1969). Many Old Colony Mexican-Canadian Mennonites reject technological advances, higher education levels for self and children, health education, modern dress, and anything that may demonstrate an attempt to keep up with fast-paced Canadian society. The Old Colony Mexican-Canadian Mennonite way of life is ultimate, and for many there is no desire to mix with "worldly people" and adopt "worldly practices" (Redekop, 1969).

Edmunds (1993) refers to the Old Colony Mexican-Canadian Mennonite's world view as one of closeness and presence. A survivalist existence is one that is very focused on day-to-day needs. Both poverty and religious beliefs are significant determinants of health-seeking behavior. Because there is no central regulating authority or institution for all Old Colony Mexican-Canadian Mennonites, interpretation of the Bible may differ from one congregation to another (Edmunds, 1993). Because congregational decisions are biblically based, the way in which the Bible is understood influences choices concerning seeking help. It is important for the nurse to recognize then that there might be significant differences between the health-seeking behaviors of individual members of the Old Colony Mexican-Canadian Mennonites. Health education in areas such as prenatal care, dental care, nutrition, and the way in which medication and treatment regimes are followed will depend on how closely the Old Colony Mexican-Canadian Mennonite holds to the present-oriented perceptions and values of his or her religious and survivalist experience.

Implications for nursing care

Prenatal care is not a common practice for Old Colony Mexican-Canadian Mennonite women because it is customary for women to give birth every year, as enabled by God (Mennonite Central Committee, 1994). Outside advice is neither sought nor welcomed. The Old Colony community concerns itself to a greater extent with curative care (Mennonite Central Committee, 1994), or care that will enable them to carry out what is necessary at present to fulfill their responsibilities. Such preventive care as dental visits and immunizations tend to be given minimal attention. There is a general lack of knowledge of nutritious foods and thus an absence of vitamins and necessary nutrients in the diet (Mennonite Central Committee, 1994). Some immigrant families in southwestern Ontario Old Colony Mexican Mennonite communities are finding it more economical and convenient to buy prepackaged foods in bulk, as well as pastries, chips, and soda pop, and feel that they are doing their children a favor because the children enjoy it (Mennonite Central Committee, 1994). The nurse should be aware that the selection of food may be related to a lack of awareness of the nutritional value of foods and indifference concerning the effect of food on health.

Unless physician appointments are for a curative treatment activity, the Old Colony Mennonite may not see the relevance of keeping the designated appointment time. The nurse should be aware that preventive or educational activities might not be ranked as important within the responsibilities of any particular day, unless the activities have an immediate and understandable significance.

ENVIRONMENTAL CONTROL

The Old Colony Mexican-Canadian Mennonite highly values conformity to community norms as opposed to individual expressions of dissent or self-determination (Redekop, 1969). Salvation is seen as collective. God will take care of those who are faithful and will punish those who do not remain pure from the world (Redekop, 1969). The Old Colony Mexican-Canadian Mennonite's relational orientation is collateral in nature, with the good of the spiritual community and of family as the prime responsibility. To live the Old Colony way of life is to be in full fellowship with other Old Colony people (Redekop, 1969). God is a personal benefactor who will take care of every area of life of the faithful (Redekop, 1969).

Belief, which is collective, incorporates faith in the Old Colony as the people of God (Redekop, 1969). Although the individual member of the community believes that it is their personal and collective responsibility to adhere to the beliefs and practices of the Old Colony, the individual is always working for the collective, rather than for the self. Decisions are based upon that which is of most benefit to community norms and goals. Yet because of the prevalence of impoverished living situations and the need to rely on seasonal employment places and because of the fragmentation of some of the religious congregations, there are differing degrees of loyalty to the collective. It is not infrequent that scarce family fi-

nances are "inappropriately wasted on cigarettes, alcohol, and in some cases drugs" (Mennonite Central Committee, 1994).

Old colony perceptions of health and illness

While caring for a member of the Old Colony, the nurse may hear a somewhat fatalistic and subjective philosophy about life and illness. Health is understood in a very restricted way, and many Old Colony Mexican-Canadian Mennonites rely on fate or providence for their welfare (Woodhouse, 1993). Attitudinal and religious factors precipitate a resignation of one's health to uncontrollable factors (Woodhouse, 1993). Woodhouse also notes that service providers and Old Colony Mexican-Canadian Mennonites agreed on two points: "Health is the absence of illness," and "health is being able to work." Woodhouse (1993) noted that health definitions varied when new Old Colony Mexican Mennonite residents to Canada were compared with those who had been here for over 5 years. Still, many Old Colony Mennonites believe that health occurs "when a person engages in age and sex-related activities and leads their life as 'God would want' " (Edmunds, 1993). There are no formal rituals associated with puberty, pregnancy, or childbirth, because these are very private matters (Edmunds, 1993).

With increasing acculturation, some Old Colony Mexican-Canadian Mennonites have developed a broader view of health. Yet education, which has been identified as a determinant of health by the Premiere's Council on Health, or in this case, the lack of education, has also contributed to the poor health of the individual within this population. For example, the cultural belief that bearing numerous children secures them a place in heaven is a strong belief for the nurse to argue against (Woodhouse, 1993). Yet, it may seem obvious to the nurse educated within a Western medical value system that continuous childbearing will most likely place serious strain on a woman's body, not allowing the body to physically recuperate. When constant childbearing is combined with poor diet, these factors contribute to an increased risk of delivering infants with a low birth weight (Premier's Council on Health,

Well-being, and Social Justice, cited in Mennonite Central Committee, 1994).

Folk beliefs and practices

Edmunds (1993) found that because of educational values "there were no formally trained traditional Old Colony health practitioners." However, there does exist generic or health practices within the Old Colony community. Edmunds (1993) explains that in Mexico, lay pharmacists, chiropractors, and midwives were openly consulted. She quoted an informant as stating that "in Mexico, you can go to the pharmacist. You tell him what's wrong, and he will figure out what you need." Another informant in her study related, "My husband has the touch to set bones, just like his father and grandfather. . . . He knows by touch what to do" (Edmunds, 1993).

Some folklore views, however, increase the risk for the health of newborns. For example, the Mennonite Central Committee's Family Education and Support Project (1994) mentions that folklore has it that newborns whose heads may not have the "right" shape should be taken to the community chiropractor to have its head "made right." The community chiropractor may have no formal training but instead possess "the gift" (Mennonite Central Committee, 1994). Thus the baby may be in serious risk of skull damage, even though the chiropractor is quite well meaning. Midwives may be used to "reposition" the fetus during pregnancy to allow for an easier delivery (Edmunds, 1993).

Edmunds (1993) points out that access to professional health care in Mexico was based upon an ability to pay. Yet there may have been a negative experience with the quality of care within the system or a problem with accessing enough money to pay for the services that affect the frequency of usage. As well, the utilization of the physician for preventive health care or health promotion was practically nonexistent (Edmunds, 1993). Public health nursing services, as Edmunds (1993) writes, were often "limited to sporadic immunization programs." Thus, in Mexico, the Mennonite people relied heavily on home remedies, folk medicine, and the advice from family and friends (Van Ryswyk, 1993).

Implications for nursing care

Although the Canadian health care system may have drawn some Old Colony Mennonites to Canada, because of these past experiences in Mexico, the professional health care system in Canada may be reluctantly used (Edmunds, 1993). The nurse must be wary of interpreting this reluctance as a sign that little value has been placed by the Old Colony Mennonite on disease prevention and health promotion (Edmunds, 1993). Instead, the reluctance to access the health care system may be more related to the history and cultural context of the individual from the Old Colony community. Edmunds (1993) claims that many Canadians remain unaware of the reason why appointments, such as prenatal visits, have been missed and then may fall into the act of labeling the client as noncompliant.

Despite this, Old Colony Mexican-Canadian Mennonites do utilize the government-funded Canadian health care system. Edmunds (1993) comments on this as follows:

Public health nurses are accepted in their homes, and families are receptive to health teaching when it is done in a culturally sensitive way. Physicians are consulted and deliveries take place in hospitals. Alongside the professional system and largely unknown by it, the generic health system continues to exist.

Unfortunately, whereas treatment and technology that is used by the professional health care system has been accepted by some, other Old Colony Mexican-Canadian Mennonite families may be quite unaware of the "procedures, practices, and assumptions used by health professionals" (Edmunds, 1993). Distrust, experienced by the Old Colony community, of the care of some health professionals continues to be a problem.

BIOLOGICAL VARIATIONS

Endogamy (marriage within the community) and interrelatedness are contributing factors to the specific biological health risks with the Old Colony Mexican-Canadian Mennonite community (Edmunds, 1993; Redekop, 1969). According to Redekop (1969), the Old Colony Mexican-Canadian Mennonite people originated with about 30 families in

1890. Considering the fact that the present population stems from those families, it is relatively easy to trace the roots of an individual back to a particular family of origin. Few new genes have been introduced from outside, resulting in genetic interrelatedness (Redekop, 1969). The cultural goals of separateness from the outside world support the continuation of intermarriage, particularly marriages of second cousins. Redekop (1969) points out that this high ratio of interaction, along with cultural homogeneity, serves to support the Old Colony Mexican-Canadian Mennonite attitude toward each other that includes a feeling of identity, common purpose, and understanding. On the other hand, the possibility for biological consequences from interrelatedness, such as the increased risk of congenital anomalies, would most likely increase. Yet, there is a scarcity of documented information for the Old Colony community on this subject.

The East Elgin Community Development Steering Committee Proposal (1989) compares the special health risks of the Mexican Mennonite peoples to any population with poor housing, inadequate nutrition, lack of access to health care facilities, low socioeconomic status, and so on. In addition, this 1989 proposal for a Kanadier Mennonite Family Resource Centre alludes to the added risks of the female population, particularly reproductive health risks related to the lack of use of birth control, the cultural norm of large families, and the inadequate prenatal care. The following example, which was seen as illustrative of some of the basic health risks faced by the Mennonite population and not usually seen in present-day Canadian society, was given.

A recent migrant to the area was found to be 29 weeks pregnant with no history of prenatal care. A reproductive history revealed one live birth and a series of five stillbirths. Fortunately the public health nurse had also trained as a midwife and recognized possible Rhesus factor incompatibility (East Elgin Community Development Steering Committee, 1989).

The proposal (1989) also notes alcohol abuse, higher number of smokers, higher incidence of child and spousal abuse, and family breakdown as problems that some of the members of the Old Colony community face. Because female members of the population are held in lower esteem than males, they may also be at risk for problems related to self-esteem issues, such as depression. Adolescents may face mental health problems because they may experience value conflict between their peers in school and their parents at home (East Elgin Community Development Steering Committee, 1989).

Implications for nursing care

Van Ryswyk's study (1993) points to some of the differences in reports regarding health status of the Old Colony Mexican-Canadian Mennonite population as compiled by service providers versus the Mennonite population themselves. The service providers observed health concerns, which included poor nutrition, substance abuse, lack of health knowledge, obesity, dental problems, work-related injuries, heart problems, multiple closely spaced pregnancies and gynecological problems, mental health issues (such as depression, stress, and anxiety), widespread smoking, and eyesight and hearing problems (Van Ryswyk, 1993). The Mennonite community, in contrast, described primarily medical conditions such as heart and weight problems, kidney stones, cancer, arthritis, gallstones, stomach problems, and lung and breathing problems (Van Ryswyk, 1993). Van Ryswyk (1993) also makes note of the fact that many of the people interviewed discussed the issue of "bad nerves," although not all the people interviewed regard this issue as a health problem or understand the way in which it can affect their physical health.

Many of the health issues of the Old Colony Mennonites could be addressed with health education. However, it is important for the nurse to be aware of the strong cultural heritage of some of the practices of the Old Colony Mexican-Canadian Mennonites. For example, weight problems may be linked to food myths that have originated from past generations. Many people believe that eating fish and milk in the same meal will make a person violently ill (Van Ryswyk, 1993). Some Old Colony Mexican-Canadian Mennonite women believe that the solution to weight problems is to exclude bread and potatoes from the diet because they are fattening, yet these same woman used a large amount of cream in the preparation of soups, sauces, and cookies (Van Ryswyk, 1993). The following explains how the diet of a Mexican Mennonite family is influenced by the history of the people.

The eastern European influence brings the *pierogi* type of dishes, the rich sauces, and the hearty soups called "borshch." Other staples such as beans, tortillas, and tacos were introduced from the Mexican diet. Almost all women bake their own bread, but wanting their children to fit in socially at public school, they will buy bread for children's lunches (Van Ryswyk, 1993).

It is important for the nurse involved in health education to modify teaching related to proper diet and healthful food to encompass the reality of the economic conditions of the family and the importance of some of the food choices in relation to cultural heritage.

There are few studies of biological variation, no studies of the effects of genetic interrelatedness, and no special studies of disease burden considerations for the Old Colony Mexican-Canadian Mennonite population. Therefore it is imperative that the nurse utilize acute observational skills, as well as culturally sensitive communication skills that respect the family-oriented and religiously based cultural norms and values, when working with each individual member of the Old Colony Mexican-Canadian Mennonite community.

SUMMARY

It is important for nurse to remember that every person is a product of past experiences. As such, every person is culturally unique. Therefore it is essential that the nurse consider cultural values, beliefs, and traditions as important to the care of the individual. In this regard Mexican Mennonites are no exception to this premise. It is also essential that the nurse remember that both the family and its religious orientation are integral to the holistic functioning of this group of individuals.

Case Study

Because of the extreme diversity of the Old Colony Mexican Mennonite population and out of respect for the privacy and wishes of individuals with whom we have collaborated on this project, rather than providing a specific case study, we include considerations for care based on the possible health problems arising from poverty, limited education, religious beliefs, and interrelatedness, which are widespread among the Old Colony peoples. Along with possible nursing diagnoses, we consider the challenges that may arise and require attention when a nurse is caring for each individual (based upon the research of the Mennonite Central Committee, 1994; Woodhouse, 1993). They may be further developed and individualized by the nurse who is working with a Mexican Mennonite patient.

CARE PLAN

 Nursing Diagnosis   Low birth weight of infants related to inadequate nutrition of the mother, lack of understanding of the health implications of repeated pregnancies, and smoking during pregnancy.

Client Outcomes

1. Client will adhere to a balanced diet capable of sustaining self and fetus.

Nursing Interventions

1. Encourage client to adhere to a balanced diet, whereby she consumes three balanced meals a day.
2. Encourage client to eliminate diet high in fats and sugars, and low in vitamins and important nutrients.

2. Client will verbalize an understanding of risks associated with repeated pregnancy.
3. Client will maintain regularly scheduled visits to physicians.

3. Encourage family to provide protein-rich foods, which are reserved for the men and working children and to the expectant mother, and encourage other children to increase nutrient value.
4. Discuss the value of milk, which may be rationed in large families because it is expensive.
5. Explain the risks associated with lack of adequate nutrition and smoking during pregnancy.
6. Encourage client to keep regularly scheduled physician appointments.

 Nursing Diagnosis   Potential health risks related to misuse of drugs, inability to read prescriptions and instructions from a physician, minimal health-seeking behaviors, cultural norms, and interrelatedness.

Client Outcomes

1. Client and family will view health in a holistic manner.

Nursing Interventions

1. Encourage family to examine health beliefs and develop more efficacious health care practices.

STUDY QUESTIONS

1. Discuss the ways in which poverty and interrelatedness may affect the overall health of the Mexican Mennonite people.
2. List several contributing factors related to the low birth weight of many of the Mexican Mennonite children.
3. Describe the social and family structure of the Mexican Mennonite people and the effect this structure may have on decisions regarding health care and treatment.

4. Identify factors related to religious belief that affect the health-seeking behaviors of many of the Mexican Mennonite people.
5. Identify factors related to literacy and education that may contribute to the health risks of the Mexican Mennonite community.
6. List several common folk practices that may have an effect on the health of Mexican Mennonite infants.

References

Beckett, A. (n.d.). *A brief history of the Mennonite people of Southwestern Ontario.* Unpublished manuscript.

Dyck, C.J. (1981). *An introduction to Mennonite history.* Scottdale, Pa.: Herald Press.

East Elgin Community Development Steering Committee (Unincorporated). (1989). *East Elgin Community Development Steering Committee Proposal.* Draft document prepared as a proposal for a Kanadier Family Resource Centre in Elgin County, Ontario.

Edmunds, K. (1993). Old Colony Mennonites in a school context. In Parker, M.E. (Ed). *Patterns of nursing theories in practice* (pp. 122-141). New York: National League for Nursing Press.

Ens, A. (1980). The public school crisis among Mennonites in Saskatchewan 1916-1925. In Loewen, H. (Ed.). *Mennonite images.* Winnipeg: Hyperion Press Ltd.

Epp, F.H. (1962). *Mennonite exodus.* Altona, Manitoba: Canadian Mennonite Relief and Immigration Council.

Fretz, J.W. (1989). *The Waterloo Mennonites: a community in paradox.* Waterloo, Ont.: Wilfred Laurier Press.

Mennonite Central Committee. (1994, March 7). *A family education and support program for low German families settling in southwestern Ontario.* Kitchener, Ont.

Mennonite Central Committee (Producer). (1995). *Migration north: mennonites for Mexico* [Videotape]. (Available from Mennonite Central Committee—Canada, 134 Plaza Drive, Winnepeg, MB R3T 5K9.)

Mennonite Central Committee. (1996). *Mennonites in Canada, 1996: Colony Mennonites from Mexico.* [on-line]. (Available from http://portal.mbnet.mb.ca/mcc/menno-guide/mexico.html)

Mennonite Central Committee (1996, April 30). *Magazine promotes literacy, broadens horizons for Mennonite Children in Latin America.* [on-line]. (Available from http://portal.mbnet.mb.ca/mcc/pr/1996/04-30/10.html)

Mennonite Central Committee (1996, July 12). *Economic woes erode lives of Kanadier Mennonites in Mexico.* [on-line]. (Available from http://portal.mbet.mb.ca/mcc/pr/1996/07-12/5.html

Redekop, C.W. (1969). *The Old Colony Mennonites: dilemma of ethnic minority life.* Baltimore, Md.: The Johns Hopkins Press.

Regehr, T.D. (1996). *Mennonites in Canada, 1939-1970: a people transformed* (volume 3 of *Mennonites in Canada*). Toronto: University of Toronto Press.

Reimer, M.L. (1990). *One quilt many pieces: a reference guide to Mennonite groups in Canada* (ed. 3). Waterloo, Ont.: Mennonite Publishing Service.

Sawatsky, H. L. (1971). *They sought a country: Mennonite colonization in Mexico.* Berkley, Calif.: University of California Press.

Van Ryswyk, J. (1993). *A profile of the Mennonite community in Elgin County.* St. Thomas, Ont.: Elgin-St. Thomas Health Unit.

Woodhouse, W. (1993). *Directions in rural literacy and health concerns.* Tillsonburg, Ont.: Tillsonburg and District Multi-Service Centre.

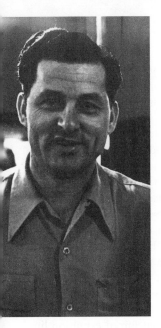

CHAPTER 20
The Greek Canadians

Josefina Estéban Richard and Geraldine T. Thomas

BEHAVIORAL OBJECTIVES

After reading this chapter the nurse will be able to:

1. Appreciate the cultural value that some Greek Canadians place on preserving the Greek language.
2. Recognize the cultural value Greek Canadians place on privacy in personal and social space.
3. Explain the unique historical and cultural heritage of the Greek people who have immigrated to Canada.
4. Describe the social organization of the Greek-Canadian family related to marriage and family roles, gender roles, religion, and adolescent behaviors.
5. Understand the past-present-future orientation of many Greek Canadians.
6. Identify traditional folk beliefs and folk practices among Greek Canadians.
7. Describe biological variations that may be present among Greek Canadians.

HISTORICAL ORIGIN
OF THE GREEK CANADIANS

Greece is well known to North Americans as one of the principal sources for Western civilization. This country and its people have roots that go back 4000 years (The World Book Encyclopedia, 1991). Situated in eastern Europe, Greece, or *Ellas* (anciently *Hellas*), as its own people call it, is surrounded by three seas. The southern part of the country, or the Peloponnese, is itself a peninsula narrowly connected to the north at the Isthmus of Corinth. Numerous islands belonging to Greece dot the Aegean sea up to the Turkish coast and south into the Mediterranean. The island of Cyprus off the coast of Lebanon is divided into two political entities, one Greek and one Turkish, but despite many cultural and linguistic ties with Greece, Greek Cyprus is an independent state.

Compared to Canada, Greece is a small country of just over 50,000 square miles, or 132,000 square kilometers, and is home today to about 10 million people (The World Book Encyclopedia, 1991). In the northeast and across the Aegean, Greece shares a frontier with Turkey. The north of Greece proper borders on Bulgaria, Albania, and what used to be Yugoslavia. Almost two thirds of Greece is mountainous. In fact, the whole country is a mountainous headland broken across the middle into two parts and with its whole eastern side split into fragments. The mountains continue out into the sea, breaking out again on the island of Crete to the south. Greece is also prone to earthquakes, and in recent years earth tremors have caused major damage in the northeast and on the island of Thera. Rich crops of grain, fruit, vegetables, and tobacco grow in the plains of Boeotia and Thessaly, in eastern Macedonia, and in the Peloponnese, while all over Greece grapes and olives grow in abundance.

The Greek climate is typically Mediterranean. Spring comes as early as February with the blooming of the almond trees, and by May the hills are blazing with multicolored wild flowers. With the onset of July, intense heat, where temperatures hover between 30° and 45° C, blasts the countryside. Although the heat decreases gradually through September and October, little rain arrives until November. Winters are cool and wet, with very little snow except in the mountains.

A characteristic feature of Greek geography is the changing light as it strikes the water or the hills. Given the striking beauty of the landscape, the attraction of a warm, sunny climate for much of the year, and the ability to live life so much in the outdoors, it is not surprising that most Greeks in North America, including those who are now in the second and third generation of those who came from Greece, maintain a deep love for the Greek homeland and a constant yearning to see it again and again.

Canadians of Greek descent are often students of their ancient past. These students are keenly aware that Greece gave the world its first democracy and that art, philosophy, literature, and drama flourished in Greece as early as the sixth and fifth centuries B.C. To a modern Greek, Alexander the Great (Alexander II), who conquered much of the known world in the fourth century B.C., is as familiar as the latest rock star. Greece has faced many wars and invasions, and over the centuries the population has been mixed with Albanians, Slavs, Turks, and western Europeans. Nevertheless, to the modern Greek and their relatives in North America, the Greek War of Independence against the Turks, which began in 1821, is very significant for their sense of identity as a united,

free people. The celebration of the conclusion of that war, which is commemorated on March 25, Greek Independence Day, is an important, annual celebration in many Greek-Canadian communities. In modern times the liberation of various places from "alien" rule has tended to be more important than the welfare of individual Greek citizens. Into the 1920s Greeks were still fighting to reacquire territory once held by their ancestors. Fighting between Greece and Turkey in the 1920s existed because substantial Greek and Turkish minorities were present in one another's countries. In an attempt to end the friction the Treaty of Lausanne in 1923 designed an exchange of populations in which 40,000 Turks left Greece and over 1 million Greeks were forced to leave Turkey. However, this did not end feelings of ill will. Bitterness caused by that forced expulsion lingers on in the late twentieth century both in Greece and in the hearts of the Greek emigrant families.

Immigration to the United States and Canada

In the 1880s and 1890s widespread poverty in Greece produced by a complex mixture of crop failures, hostilities with Turkey, the strain of dowering unmarried women, and conscription into the Turkish army caused a large number of Greek men to leave for a permanent life abroad, usually in the United States (Patterson, 1976). As immigrant quotas in the United States stiffened, Greek emmigrants turned their eyes north to Canada, where some Greeks had already immigrated and where some had relatives. Canadian census figures compiled by Lambrou (1975) show 3200 Greeks living in Canada in 1911, with the largest numbers in Montreal and Toronto. By 1931 the numbers had swelled to about 9500, half of whom were Canadian born. Although the number of Greeks in Canada gradually increased as the twentieth century proceeded, a flood of immigrants arrived after World War II and the subsequent civil wars in Greece (Petras, 1988; Loescher and Scanlan, 1986; Archdeacon, 1993). During these wars Greeks suffered from poverty, disease, and cruel treatment. Many endured punishment and even death trying to hide members of the Western allied forces who had slipped into Greece to lead the resistance. The farmlands were devastated, and lines of communication all over the country lay in ruins (Ferenczi, 1992).

In the years after 1950 hundreds of Greeks left to seek new lives abroad in Australia, the United States, and Canada. Continuing poverty in Greece and a series of repressive governments, particularly the military dictatorship between 1967 and 1974, caused still more Greeks to emigrate. Since that time the flood of permanent emigrants has largely stopped as Greece gradually increased its prosperity and democratically elected governments gained power. Although problems associated with inflation and chronic unemployment continue to plague certain parts of Greece, today only a few Greeks are coming to North America to work, study, or marry. In fact, the reverse is sometimes seen in the 1990s as some Greek Canadians are returning to Greece with hopes of finding employment and sometimes staying for an extended period of time (Rosenbaum, 1990; Takaki, 1993; Noble, 1992; Moskos, 1980). Some come to America temporarily to earn money and then return to Greece to live.

The fact that so many Greeks left Greece, usually from the villages, in the 1950s and early 1960s is important in understanding these individuals and their families in Canada today. That world of the Greek villages in the 1950s and 1960s was in many ways much more conservative than the cities like Athens. The values of the communities in Greece that existed at the time of the emigrants' leaving shaped the personal relations, the work ethics, attitudes to education, and the importance of the church and religion for many Greek Canadians today. The values and ideology that the immigrants brought to Canada in many cases are very different from those that exist in Greece today. Today young Greek Canadians are amused and sometimes annoyed when their parents or grandparents, visiting Greece, react with horror at the freedom allowed Greek teenagers in Greece, especially around the question of dating. Even when the older Greek Canadians are well aware that Greece has changed and that attitudes there have changed as well, they are hesitant to relax the standards they grew up with in rural Greece.

Some 151,150 Canadians claim Greek descent (Statistics Canada, 1997). The greatest concentrations of Greek people are in Quebec (almost 50,000), Ontario (85,000), and British Columbia (8500) with most Greek Canadians in those provinces living in large cities like Montreal (almost 50,000), Toronto (almost 65,000), and Vancouver (6500). Of the industrial Ontario cities such as Hamilton, London, and Windsor, each has a Greek population close to or in excess of 3000 people. Manitoba, Saskatchewan, and Alberta together have more than 6000 Greek Canadians, almost half of whom are in or near Edmonton. Atlantic Canada has about 1800 people of Greek origin, 1280 of whom are in Nova Scotia. The Yukon has only about 40 persons of Greek origin, and the Northwest Territories 30 persons of Greek origin. *Statistics Canada* lists no people of Greek descent on Prince Edward Island.

In the 1950s studies in the United States indicated that Greek immigrants scored poorly on IQ tests and were similar to disadvantaged groups today such as Blacks and Hispanics (Sowell, 1978). In fact, many of the Greeks who came to Canada in the 1950s and 1960s arrived having a very limited education because of the environment from which they had fled. Lacking English or French, they turned to jobs as unskilled laborers from which to make an immediate living. Gradually, as the family was able to save money, small businesses and restaurants in which the whole family worked were opened. As well as emphasizing hard work, many Greek-Canadian families made obtaining a good education for their children a priority. Today, most Greek-Canadian families will make every effort to provide personal financing for college for their children and rarely rely on educational loans (Chimbos, 1972; Chimbos, 1980).

Of the number of people who indicated in 1990 that they were of Greek descent over 15 years of age, 43.5% had less than a high school certificate (71,125) and 24.7% had less than a grade 9 education (40,385), compared to only 12.1% who had actually completed high school (19,720). Those with completed trade or other sorts of certificates make up another 12.1% of the population (19,730). The remaining 32.3% of the Greek-Canadian people have some university or trade school education with 12.6% (20,600) holding a university degree (Statistics Canada, 1991).

In 1991, among Greek-Canadian men, the average annual income was $25,421, compared to $15,793 for Greek-Canadian women (Statistics Canada, 1991). When these statistics are used, it is important to note that those statistics report income for everyone from 15 years of age or greater, thus driving the average income down. More significant than average incomes are the incomes for the largest groups of men and women. In 1991 the largest group of Greek-Canadian men (9925) reported incomes between $30,000 and $40,000, the second largest group reported incomes between $10,000 and $14,999 (9040 men), and the third largest group reported incomes between $15,000 and $19,999 (7640 men). Of the men, 7595 reported incomes over $50,000 per annum. The average annual income for all women reported in 1991 was $15,793. The largest group of women reported incomes between $10,000 and $14,999 (11,590), the second largest group reported incomes between $15,000 and $19,999 (7535 women), and the third largest group reported incomes between $20,000 and $24,999 (6290 women). Of the women, 1550 reported incomes in excess of $50,000.

Communication

Although there are very obvious regional differences in the spoken Greek language—a mainland Greek can immediately recognize the special intonations, for example, of a Greek from Crete—a regular form of Greek called *Dhimotiki* (Demotic) is now spoken and taught all over Greece and in Greek communities beyond Greece (Chitiri and Willows, 1993).

In the modern Greek language noun inflections give information about the gender (masculine, feminine, neuter), the number (singular, plural), and the case (nominative, genitive, accusative, vocative). Greek has a verb infection for mood (indicative, subjunctive, imperative); aspect (perfective, imperfective); voice (active, middle, passive); tense (present, past); person (first, second, third), and number (singular, plural) (modified from The New Enclopaedia Britannica, 1993). Greek words are

typically polysyllabic (Mirambel, 1959). Two-syllable words are most common. Stressed syllables are somewhat louder and longer than unstressed syllables, though the difference is not so pronounced as in English.

Many older, educated Greeks continue to retain an affection for *Katharevusa,* the formal written Greek language, which they themselves learned as children. The differences between the two forms of the language are gradually becoming obsolete, ever since the Greek Parliament in 1976 made *Dhimotiki* the official written form of the national language (The Encyclopedia Americana International Edition, 1992).

The determination to preserve the Greek language in North America and to pass it onto the next generation is one of the most characteristic features of life among the Greek people on this continent. The first North American Greek school, suitably called "Plato," was organized in 1910 in Montreal. As Greek immigrants to Canada increased after World War II, professional teachers and lay people with some training in Greece were hired to teach in afternoon schools run by the Greek communities in Toronto and Montreal. Like many other cities with Greek communities in Canada, Halifax has had a Greek school since the 1960s. Funding for the Greek school comes from the fees paid by the parents and from fund-raising activities organized by the school boards and communities. Along with language instruction comes a strong measure of Greek religion, history, and traditions. Like many other Greek schools, the one in Halifax operates an evening program, which means the children attending it must go after a regular school day. The timing of the classes and the stress it puts on parents to provide transportation have caused a decline in the number of children attending the Halifax Greek school in recent years. On the other hand, many young Greek Canadians say that they feel special having knowledge of a language their "Canadian" friends cannot understand. It helps set them apart in a way they like and bonds them more closely to one another and to their Greek heritage.

Because the Greek language is so important to the Greek identity in North America, most large Canadian cities also offer Greek language classes to adults through the universities or through the Greek community centers. The adults taking such classes may be drawn by an admiration for Greek culture and history, or they may be contemplating marriage to a Greek spouse. To feel comfortable in a strong Greek-Canadian family a non-Greek spouse knows that some familiarity with the Greek language is essential. However, outsiders often find the unfamiliar alphabet and complicated Greek syntax difficult to learn.

Young Greek Canadians are usually fluent in both Greek and either English or French. Many of them have added the second, official Canadian language through the Canadian school system. A problem for many older, first-generation Greeks, especially women, who did not receive any education in Canada, is a lack of any real fluency in English or French. Having received very little formal education in Greece, because of World War II and poverty conditions, these women remained mostly in their homes, wrapped up in their families, church, and Greek community. They were fearful of moving much beyond that world and the large Greek-speaking communities of Toronto and Montreal except for things like medical appointments. On the other hand, their male counterparts tended to learn basic English or French in the stores and businesses they operated. Today, even in less populated areas like Nova Scotia, some Greek-Canadian women remain cut off from the rest of Canadian society by the language barrier. On a recent (summer 1997) visit to Toronto the second author (G.T.T) found that in the "Greektown" area of Danforth Street, older Greek women whom she met could speak little or no English. However, Greek women under 50 years of age were perfectly fluent in English, as were all the men to whom she talked.

Kinesics

When Greek people meet one another, they routinely kiss one another on both cheeks or otherwise greet one another in a warm, affectionate style. That kiss and affectionate warmth may well be extended to non-Greek friends whom they know understand their customs. Speaking together often involves ex-

pressive movements of the hands and head. On the other side, a volatile argument can easily arise between two Greeks over some rather minor point. Those on the sidelines join in to support one or the other of the principals in the argument. The non-Greek bystander may assume that immediate, physical violence is about to erupt, but such is rarely the case, and the former combatants move off to other passing interests. When speaking to non-Greeks whom they do not know or know only slightly, some Greek Canadians tend to be quite formal, rather stilted in their behavior, and quite shy, especially if they perceive a difference in social status. This has much to do with the enormous respect Greek Canadians tend to have for educated and professional people from all backgrounds. It is important to note that the head motions for "yes" and "no" are opposite to those used in the United States and Canada.

Implications for nursing care

The nurse should be cognizant that the written Greek language uses a different alphabet and syntactic characteristics from that of the English language. Because Greek is an inflected language, whereas English is a word-order, or analytic, language, it is also possible that syntax might influence word-recognition patterns in the two languages (Chitiri and Willows, 1993).

The nurse should be aware that, although young Greek Canadians of the second or third generation are usually fluent in both Greek and either English or French, many older first-generation Greeks or those who are new to Canada may not be fluent in English or French. It is necessary to be sensitive to the feelings of insecurity and the special needs of people who lack basic language skills in English or French. According to Lynam (1991) the problem of caring for persons who do not speak English can be considered from a broader perspective—that of the right of clients. Such rights include informed consent, equitable and accessible level of care, and the rights to confidentiality. Most health care institutions or agencies keep a resource list of staff and interpreters who speak a variety of languages and dialects. However, these persons are not always around when needed, and it is important for the nurse to make an effort to rectify language barriers and to seek out interpreters when they are needed. Another issue raised in relation to using interpreters from the ethnic community of the client is confidentiality. Greek Canadians are often intensely conscious of being watched by others in the community. Many Greek Canadians want to maintain their own family's privacy and to protect the family's reputation. Health care professionals may also find some of their Greek-Canadian clients wanting to change doctors, not because of any dislike of the doctor concerned, but because they are trying to remove themselves from waiting-room situations where they are likely to run into another Greek client and thus start the inevitable round of talk about their own condition. Unless the interpreters are health professionals, it is essential that they be appropriately trained in linguistic and cultural interpretation in the health care setting. One example of the enormity of providing appropriately trained interpreters is the Montreal Children's Hospital, which in the 1992-1993 fiscal year was able to provide 873 interpreters for a total of 36 languages and dialects (Clarke, 1993).

Although there were some initiatives to implement the use of trained interpreters in a few provinces, the use of these resources is not maximized as a result of the lack of funding because these services may not be covered under the provincial health insurance. Health professionals should ensure that any Greek client who is not fluent in English or French actually understands how and when medications are to be taken. If there is any concern about such understanding, it is important to provide an explanation to a family member who has a good command of English or French.

SPACE

Greek families often take part in social engagements as a family unit and to surround themselves with other Greek family members in the Greek community. In times of stress it is common to find several members of a family supporting one another with their physical presence.

Greek families have prospered through their hard work and are "upwardly mobile" as far as housing is concerned. Many have moved to large homes in the suburbs of Canadian cities, out from the inner cities

where their parents once lived close to their small shops and restaurants (Thomas, 1988b). A survey conducted in Halifax in the 1980s found that although three, four, or five Greek-Canadian families may be known to live not far from one another (it is especially common to find two or three closely related households in one neighborhood), the Greek people interviewed had no desire to see the number of Greeks in the neighborhood to whom they were not related increase (Thomas, 1988b). Greek Canadians have sometimes reported that they would consider moving "if any more Greeks move into this area" (Thomas, 1988b). This indicates that although Greek-Canadian families are generally gregarious they also tend to be intensely private and most unwilling to have their personal lives become the subject of talk among other Greeks in the community who do not belong to the family (Thomas, 1988b).

Implications for nursing care.

The nurse should be aware of the value Greek Canadians place on personal space but in relation to their own family. When placing clients in hospital rooms, the nurse would not necessarily be wise in placing unrelated Greek Canadians together because such proximity may be seen as an invasion of their privacy. Placing a Greek client with someone that client does not know and who is not Greek may increase the client's comfort level.

The nurse should be aware that bridging the interpersonal space between individuals and building trust with a Greek client who sees the nurse as a stranger may take time. Encouraging clients to talk about themselves, encouraging the client to share experiences about their family, and sharing a sample of Greek food can facilitate the development of a relationship and reduce interpersonal distance. The need to focus on the building of a therapeutic relationship is especially true in a home visit where the nurse is intruding on the client's personal family space.

SOCIAL ORGANIZATION
Marriage and family roles

Most Greek Canadians are married. *Statistics Canada* figures for 1991 give 57.6% of all Greek Canadians as married, 4.1% widowed, 34.9% single, and 3.4% divorced. The high percentage of single persons can be explained by the fact that many Greek Canadians do not marry until well along into their twenties and sometimes into their thirties, and *Statistics Canada* figures are for everyone from 15 years of age and up. An unmarried Greek adult, especially a woman, feels strong pressure from her family and from her own sense of her cultural background to marry and start a family (Lambert, Mermigis, and Taylor, 1986). A variety of studies indicates that Greek Canadians prefer people from their own background as the most suitable marriage partners (Lambert, Mermigis, and Taylor, 1986; Fitzgerald and Rouvalis, 1995). This type of comment reported from a 15-year-old, second-generation Greek-Canadian girl in Halifax is common: "I couldn't see myself marrying a 100% Greek man. Greek men are chauvinistic. I would not want to live or work all the time in Greece. It would be easier to communicate with a Greek Canadian. It would make my parents happier and would make life easier all around" (Fitzgerald and Rouvalis, 1995). Fitzgerald and Rouvalis also note that "increasingly, the youths have come to see their parents' beliefs and practices as efforts to preserve their culture in all its components and to provide for the safety and well-being of their children's futures."

However, even given such preferences for endogamy, many Greek Canadians have already married outside their ethnic group. In Canadian society, which has a limited number of persons of Greek background, inevitably more marriages between Greeks and non-Greeks will occur. A study in Nova Scotia noted that 66% of young Greeks interviewed in the province reported that they have just as many good friends among non-Greeks as they do among the Greeks (Kayal, 1979). The marriage between a Greek Orthodox person and a non-Greek usually takes place in the local Greek church, the non-Orthodox partner often becomes a convert, and the children of the marriage are almost always raised as Orthodox communicants (Kayal, 1979).

In Greece, the traditional patriarchal or extended family, that is, the cohabitation of three generations—grandparents, children, and grandchildren—has begun to change its form and become more and more a nuclear family of parents and children (Tep-

eroglou, 1980; Raya, 1989). This is true in Canada as well. When it was possible, Greek immigrants to Canada lived in extended-family situations, but because society is changing and becoming more mobile, this also is changing. Adult children are moving away to find work, and when unable to care for themselves, the elderly may be placed in nursing homes.

Young Greek Canadians

Young adult Greek Canadians who have finished their education and are now working are also considering their heritage and trying to adapt it to their lives in a way that lets them live both as "Canadian" and as Greek. Although some remain living with their families until marriage, others are moving to their own apartments, despite some parental disapproval. Similarly, they simply do not talk to their parents about dating habits they know their parents would dislike. That is not to say that they have fully accepted the extent of sexual freedom in contemporary North America. Some young women have come to see marriage—any marriage—as the opportunity to get away from parental rules and interference in their lives. Although they want to maintain their Greek history and culture, they also want to be able to have many different friends, to go to dances, to have a boyfriend whom they will not necessarily marry, and to go out on casual, social occasions without strong parental reaction (Rouvalis, 1990).

Although girls may want more freedom, they do not necessarily "buy into" the current mores of North American life. Some young Greek-Canadian women dislike that their parents regard a university education as absolutely essential for their sons, who will be the breadwinners in their future families, but only of passing interest for the girls, as something to take up their time until they marry.

Young Greek males have considerable freedom in their lives and in many ways are the pampered darlings of their households. They are the particular favorites of their mothers and are seen by their fathers as the ones who will carry the family into the future. They are not expected to take much of a share in household responsibilities, and often their sisters have to clean up after them.

Young married Greek Canadians are more likely to fit back into the existing Greek communities with some degree of comfort. Some volunteer for church and community projects, teach in Sunday school or Greek school, and become involved in organizations like the women's Philoptochos ('befriending beggars'; a combination church-charity organization) and AHEPA (a Greek men's community and charity club).

Many young Greeks are making a significant effort to maintain the Greek language and heritage, which is crucial in the survival of their communities. With the decline, almost the elimination of large-scale Greek immigration to Canada, the future of the Greek-Canadian communities depends on the young. Many young Greek Canadians want the Greek community in their area to survive and are willing to put personal effort into its survival. They study and speak Greek, have Greek friends, and remain close to their Greek families. They may continue to associate themselves with the Greek church, even if not particularly interested in religion or if they feel dissatisfied with the church, because the Greek church is a major part of their Greek heritage. Rouvalis (1990) quotes a young Greek-Canadian woman: "Sometimes I think we've lost a bit of morality in the Canadian society today; we've really gone too far, and in that respect I fall back on my parents' values." Young Greek-Canadian women are finding the Greek church restrictive, particularly in its attitude to women, and some consider the church unsuited to helping them with their personal problems. Many attend church only under family pressure or on the occasion of major church festivals like Easter. They can have a real sense of alienation, of being caught between two worlds—one Greek and one "Canadian"—and not fitting truly in either.

One other group of young Greek Canadians deserves some notice. They are the individuals who are the children of one Greek parent and one non-Greek parent. Despite their Greek surnames, some of these people have no knowledge of the Greek language and little or no knowledge of Greek culture or heritage other than an occasional desire for some Greek food. They can be discounted as in any way representative of the Greek communities. More interesting are those children of mixed background who maintain a strong sense of the Greek part of them. With the encouragement of the one Greek parent and usually with the active support of the parent who is not Greek, these young people have studied Greek, probably have visited Greece, and understand a great deal about Greek history and customs. They move very easily between the Greek and non-Greek worlds and are able to draw on the strengths of the Greek part of themselves, without feeling bound by its restrictive side. It will be interesting to see whether they care to keep alive their Greek side, since in many cases they are almost certain to marry non-Greeks and probably will spend most of their lives in a non-Greek environment. Recent studies in the United States indicate that although ethnic identification is often weakened from the first to the second generation of the original immigrants, it often strengthens again in the third and subsequent generations. Greek Americans are now more recognizable and more eager to be recognized as an identifiable ethnic group than was the case with their parents (Moskos, 1980; Kourvetaris, 1990).

Role of women

It is perceived to be particularly the woman's role to provide moral and physical support for family members. In many Greek-Canadian families a daughter-in-law is expected to be the chief caregiver for aging parents of her husband, even if she does not get along with those parents-in-law particularly well. That stress may increase if, for example, an aged mother-in-law arrives from Greece to be cared for by the daughter-in-law who hardly knows her husband's mother and who may find her mother-in-law's ideas about family life inconsistent with the style of the Greek-Canadian family. Or the Greek-Canadian daughter-in-law may be pressed by her husband to spend weeks or months in Greece caring for his aging parents.

Whether working outside the home or not, a Greek wife is expected to be a fine cook both of the traditional and time-consuming foods like *moussaka, galaktoburiko,* and *baklava* and of "Canadian" foods that her family has come to know and like. Some young Greek-Canadian women feel tension between traditional gender roles for Greek women and the endless possibilities open to non-Greek Canadian women, especially if they have attended a university and wish to pursue a career (Rouvalis, 1990).

Childcare has typically been the role of the Greek woman. The first wave of Greek immigrants looked after their own children. Even a few years ago it was so unusual for anyone outside the family to look after the children that there is no Greek equivalent for the term "babysitter." Today many Greek children go to day care centers and nurseries. The preferred ones are those where the staff can provide some instruction in the Greek language and where the children can mix with others of a similar Greek background.

Role of men

Traditionally, Greek men have been socialized by their mothers not to share in household responsibilities. The man's role is delineated to be that of the breadwinner. Although there is a fairly defined gender roles for the husband and wife within the family, Greek-Canadian marriages often reveal that the married couple shares a strong sense of partnership. Once the children are beyond the infant years the husband and wife work closely together bringing up the children and often making personal and financial sacrifices for their education and well-being.

Religion and the Greek Orthodox church

With only a few exceptions, Greeks belong to the Greek Orthodox church. Even Greek people who attend church only on very rare occasions will identify themselves as Greek Orthodox, and some give substantial sums of money to help the financial operations of the Greek church in Canada. In many Greek communities the parish priest is the most important individual in the life of the whole community. He is not only the spiritual leader to the whole community, but often a source of personal support to Greek families in times of stress, sickness, and death. The priest will come to the hospital to administer Holy Communion and, when required, the last rites of the church. The individual Greek churches in Canada are under the general direction of the church's Canadian bishop, who lives in Montreal. The Greek Or-

thodox Church takes great pride in tracing its roots, its theology, and its practices back to the first Christian centuries. The continuity of the traditions across the centuries gives the Greek people, whether in Greece or in Canada, a strong identification with their origins and a pride in the antiquity of their religion.

Although the church services, rituals, and the calendar year for the Greek church in Canada are those of the Greek homeland, the life of the church in North America differs in certain important ways from that in Greece. For example, in Greece since the 1960s the priests have been paid by the state and are civil servants. The church of Greece is the state church, and most maintenance payments for the church buildings come from the government. In Canada there are no regular, direct grants for churches. Clergy salaries and the maintenance of the church buildings are the responsibility of the individual congregations. In many Greek-Canadian communities much of the people's time, energy, and money is consumed by the need to do fund raising to maintain the life of their particular church.

The Greek church in Greece is not the social center of the Greek community that it can be for an immigrant population in a new and ethnically diverse country (Thomas, 1988a). For example, in Nova Scotia Greek people of all ages look to St. George's Church in Halifax to provide many of their social activities and to foster a Greek identity and spirit. Greek dances, parties, and bazaars not only raise money, but also provide a place where the whole community can come together and participate in the familiar ways of the homeland. In larger cities with big Greek populations like Toronto, Montreal, and Vancouver there is more separation of community and church. Greek social activities in those cities often take place in community centers or through various organizations and clubs. Studies in 1975 and 1976 found that the church, now situated in the Kitsilano area, had only about 600 families as formal, or *kinotis,* members out of a total Greek population of over 7000 people (Lambrou, 1975; Patterson, 1976).

Undoubtably the church strengthens the life of an individual Greek community; however, there are some features of church life that may cause stress for individual parishioners or cause some families to ignore the church. Membership in the Greek church is dependent on the payment of set, annual fees. Nagata (1969) found that many of the working-class Greeks in Toronto whom she interviewed paid the fees only when they had a family function like a wedding or baptism, which required the church's services.

Implications for nursing care

Because of the family-centered values of Greeks, it is essential to include all the family members in the assessment, planning, and implementation of nursing care to facilitate the success of the treatment and care. Love, companionship, and protection are reciprocated between wives and husbands as patterned relationships. Since husbands and wives provide illness care for each other, it will be helpful for the nurse to inquire how they provide care for one another (Rosenbaum, 1990). Strong, familial values and respect for elders mitigate against nursing homes for the aged. If they are unwilling to consider nursing homes for family members who need special care, Greek-Canadian families may encounter conflicts or dilemmas on how to care for their aging parents. This is particularly true of first-generation parents whose children are born and raised here in Canada. Grown children will particularly make sacrifices to assist their widowed mothers. This is to reciprocate their mother's love and care (Rosenbaum, 1990). It is important to note that in the caring for Greek-Canadian widows there is an expectation from the mother that the children will take care of their mothers and the mothers will be involved in decision making about their care.

The nurse should be familiar with the traditional gender roles existing in many Greek-Canadian households. The nurse may need to assist the families in developing strategies on how to meet their needs particularly when the ill person is the primary caregiver and is accustomed to being in charge of the household. The nurse may also need to mention nursing home facilities that are available in a community. In larger cities such as Toronto, Greek nursing homes are now available,

and some smaller cities may have nursing homes with a few Greek staff.

The Greek family traditions have important implications on discharge planning, since Greek Canadians depend heavily on the family. The nurse can help maximize these relationships and ascertain when help from the church and communities are needed. Since Greek people are accustomed to having family and close friends around them, they will expect and need that support when visiting medical personnel or while in hospital. Where possible, there should be some relaxation of normal visitation policies to accommodate that Greek need for closeness in times of stress.

It is essential that the nurse incorporate a cultural assessment in a family with a marriage of a Greek and a non-Greek. The nurse must know the culture that they subscribe to and become sensitive to their needs. Nurses should watch for signs of stress and tension in Greek-Canadian women weighed down with family responsibilities, which may well go beyond the needs of the usual nuclear family. Careful and sensitive questions may (or may not) reveal the family obligations a Greek-Canadian woman has taken on, especially with regard to her husband's parents.

It is important for the nurse to remember that because religion is an important aspect of the Greek culture, it must be incorporated in the planning and delivery of nursing care. Because the parish priest has a very important role, the nurse must assess if the patient wishes to seek support and counseling or receive sacraments for the sick from the parish priest of the Orthodox church. The nurse must also be cognizant of the strain that the church places on the individual members of the community because of its expectation of financial support from its members. It is essential that the nurse become aware of the role of the Orthodox church in illness and after death so that she can incorporate this knowledge in her delivery of nursing care.

TIME

Greek Canadians tend to have a combination of past, present, and future time orientation. In cultural traditions the past is considered of great importance.

However, the Greeks in Canada have worked hard in their present situation in Canada to make a stable and prosperous life for themselves and their families. They strive for the future, ensuring, as much as they can, good education for their children and solid careers. In some situations Greek parents have placed extraordinary burdens on themselves and their children in their desire to keep a small business or restaurant operating almost 24 hours a day, 7 days a week to make it a success both in the present and for the future benefits this requirement can bring for the family.

Greek Canadians have adapted extremely well to the North American style of time organization and precision with time. They generally do not have difficulty in keeping important appointments or remembering the proper time for things like medications.

Implications for nursing care

It is important for the nurse to assess each patient individually to identify personal ethnocentric attitudes. The nurse may need to assist clients and their families to develop strategies that will help them understand the implications of past and present behavior on future health-promotion behaviors. The nurse must maximize the client's future-time orientation by encouraging them to do preventive screening for illness.

ENVIRONMENTAL CONTROL
Folk beliefs and folk practices

Sick care practices among Greeks may involve both biomedical and magicoreligious areas (Geissler, 1994). In general, the Greeks regard the doctor with a great esteem and have a high expectation as a healer. However, paradoxically the trust of the doctor is low (Patterson, 1976). This traditional attitude is reflected in the findings of Patterson that Greek Canadians, because of their insecurity related to the diagnosis of their ailment, may consult not only with several different doctors but also with nonprofessional members of the community.

The most prevalent health attitude of Greeks is focused on the concept of medical ailment in relation to illness. Many Greek Canadians maintain a disease-oriented approach to medical care, particularly centered on consulting the doctors for physical symptoms they believe themselves to have. Their visits to doctors are founded on a specific complaint and are symptom oriented. They seldom consult their physicians for checkups. According to Patterson, many Greek Canadians have difficulty accepting the concept of psychosomatic medicine, in that there is a relationship between physical manifestation and psychological strain.

Although Greek Canadians seek and receive the existing medical care for the mainstream population, research has shown (Patterson, 1976; Tripp-Reimer, 1983; Rosenbaum, 1991a) that certain folk practices do exist among members of this ethnic community. The most pervasive folk illness among Greeks is called the "evil eye," *matiasma,* or simply *mati* (the 'eye'). The evil eye *(matiasma)* is the result of a harmful infection of a sender who may be envious of or admirer of the victim. The people who possess *mati* power are often believed to be women who are spinsters or those with blue eyes. The eye was believed to be able to harm not only humans, but also animals and inanimate objects such as vases or plants. Persons may be susceptible to *matiasma* because of their beauty, happiness, or personal excellence. Although the Greeks consider the *matiasma* to be very threatening, there was no consensus on the seriousness of its effects. Some of the common symptoms resulting from *matiasma* include headaches, fever, chills, and stomachaches. Protection from this folk illness included blue beads or blue stones (occasionally with black spots) called "eye beads" to reflect the eye. They also use *phylactoi,* or amulets, made of wood from a saint's statue or a monastery, religious medals or crosses, garlic (worn or placed in the kitchen), and teeth from a dead person (Tripp-Reimer, 1983).

According to Zola (1972) 70% to 90% of all self-recognized episodes of folk illness are managed outside of the health care system. Greeks do not seek professional health care for diagnosis or treatment of *matiasma.* One of the fears of Greek parents is the exposure of their newborn to an evil eye. They attempt to prevent this by spitting three times on the ground and repeating various phrases to keep the evil eye away from the child when visitors come to see their newborn and give compliment.

Another folk belief is that a woman may not leave the house for 40 days after a baby is born. According to Patterson there are some Greek folk remedies identified in his study of this ethnic group in Kitsilano, British Columbia. These are:

a. *Cupping glass (Ventosa;* Greek *ventouza, venduza).* This procedure is to relieve common cold, pleurisy, or pneumonia. It consists in applying heated glasses on the back of the afflicted person to create a suction effect, hence sucking out the cold.

b. *Headache.* To ease a headache, one must fix fresh coffee grounds with slices of potatoes, form a compress, and apply it to the forehead.

c. *Ear infection.* To heal an infection of the ear in women with a pierced ear, one should place sticks of oregano (wild marjoram) in the earring holes until they are healed.

d. *Diarrhea.* The person is given tea first and then rice mash made by boiling plain rice until the starch flavor is out of it and it has turned into gruel.

e. *Skin blemishes.* Drinking boiled dandelion leaves gathered and prepared by the afflicted will clear the skin.

f. *Skin rashes.* Camomile is boiled until the liquid is reduced, strained, and used as a compress and cleansing liquid. This is repeated with mallow *(moloche)* leaves and washed with soap. The rashes should be cured in 2 days.

g. *Nervous tension and high blood pressure.* Herbal decoctions made from cinnamon, oregano, camomile, wild mint, sage, and *himerokissei** are used for high blood pressure.

h. *Cuts and wounds.* Tomato paste is applied over a cut to promote healing. Cigarette ash is placed in the wound to stop the bleeding. Castor oil is used as a drink to clean bowels. Olive oil drops are used for relief of earaches, with rubbing to pro-

mote healing. Honey and lemon for treating sore throat. Quinine for reducing pain and fever.

Grief and death

The death rituals of rural Greece were studied by Danforth and Tsiaras (1982). Danforth and Tsiaras (1982) found that death-related practices such as memorial services, wearing special funeral clothes, eating special foods and displaying the body, help the grieving person face the reality of the death and help organize the Greek community about the gieving family. Many Canadian Greeks also practice these death rituals. Rosenbaum (1991b) notes that two major themes regarding grief were evident in interviews with Greek-Canadian widows: (1) meanings and expressions of grief focused on beliefs about the endurance of the life spirit and an integral part of the widow's cultural care lifeways, and (2) transition from wife to widow means resignation to the husband's death based on the belief that "life goes on," with the active remembrance of the husband's care values and lifeways.

Rituals that are observed by Greek Canadians at the time of a death include singing mourning songs or lament dirges. A *Trisayios* ('thrice-holy') prayer service may be conducted at the funeral home and church by the priest to pray for forgiveness of sins. At the ceremony, after services at both the funeral home and the church, more prayers are said in Greek. The priest places a cross marked by olive oil on the flower-covered casket. The family then sprinkles earth on the casket (Rosenbaum, 1991b). Ladies who are not menstruating or who have not participated recently in sexual intercourse and are therefore "clean" bake *prosphora* ('what is fitting': special bread baked on the day of the funeral) for everyone to eat. A large attendance at the funeral is a sign of honor toward the dead person.

Rosenbaum (1990) noted that, when their husbands died, Greek widows in Ontario reported receiving support from family, neighbors, friends, and members of the Greek community. Neighbors from a variety of cultures came to the assistance of the Greek widows at the time of the death. Continuing care was provided by friends, family, and members of the Greek community. The widows related that

---

*This word corresponding to two possible spelling forms does not occur in any Greek encyclopedia or dictionary or dialect dictionary and cannot be equaled to any plant, unless it is the *hemerokalles* 'day lily'.

these persons brought in food, took them out, invited them to their homes, provided hospitality, and gave companionship. The widows also reported the value of cultural cohesiveness, which was described as "sticking together" and "helping each other," which was reinforced by in-group marriages, visits to Greece, and use of the Greek language (Rosenbaum, 1990). Rosenbaum (1990) also noted that widows reported that they received much comfort from prayer as care from God. Additionally, comfort was experienced by seeing people who had not been seen for a long time (Rosenbaum, 1990).

Prayer for the deceased after the funeral serves as symbolic care by offering to the deceased's soul forgiveness from then on. *Mnimosina* ('memorials') are services that are also conducted the fortieth day after the death, in recognition of the Ascension of Jesus, as an additional way to protect the soul of the dead. In addition, *Mnimosina* are conducted afterwards at 3 months, 6 months, 9 months, 1 year, and 3 years. Thereafter, the major prayers for the dead are said during Soul Saturdays in church. Sweetened boiled wheat, kóliva, is distributed on these occasions. The wheat in kóliva is symbolic of death and resurrection; wheat must be buried for it to grow just as people must die to be resurrected (Rosenbaum, 1991b). In Greece at the end of the 3-year period the body is exhumed, and the bones are laid to rest in the village ossuary (Danforth and Tsiaras, 1982). In Canada, the practice of secondary burial is not performed. Thus the resolution of grief at the end of 3 years may be less complete by Greek women oriented to expect this transition period.

Rosenbaum (1991b) noted that remarriage by a Greek-Canadian widow is uncommon. Rather, widows reported the desire to carry on their husband's lifeways and values. Solace is felt by the belief that the husband's spiritual presence lives on. Ongoing support is received from the church and family.

Implications for nursing care

The practice of traditional rituals in relation to death is very important for Greeks even though they may live in Canada. It is especially important for the nurse to encourage a Greek widow to express widowhood lifeways with a trusted Greek Orthodox priest or with staff at a Greek community social service agency. The type of counseling that is appropriate may vary depending on whether the widow is of the first generation or the second generation. Second-generation widows may accept support from group counseling and self-help groups for widows (Rosenbaum, 1991b). It is important for the nurse to avoid assessing the Greek widow as having abnormal grief when waves of grief are experienced over the years because this is a practice based on cultural tradition and is thus a normal pattern of grieving.

It is important for nurses caring for Greek Canadians to include, in their assessments, the identification of traditional folk beliefs held by this ethnic group. The nurse should know to what extent clients subscribe to these folk medicines before or in conjunction with the scientific health practices. Nurses must recognize that traditional health behaviors may not be retained, even in individuals with strong ethnic affiliation. Nurses must be careful not to overgeneralize or stereotype the client as a member of a particular ethnic group but rather develop an individualized plan of care.

Nurses in a variety of settings should be sensitive to and respectful of Greeks believing in *matiasma*. For example, mothers in the newborn unit or the pediatric unit may wish for their children to keep the protective blue stone, or *phylacto*, while in the hospital. By the same token, the school nurses may also encounter these protective charms among school children. Health professionals should be aware that people who believe in the *matiasma* are not paranoid. However practice of folk medicine may delay entry to the health care system. Identification and assessment of the client's folk health practices will assist the nurse in the planning and delivery of nursing care to Greek Canadians. It is important for the nurse to remember that there are several other factors that may influence the Greek Canadians in their attitudes and utilization of health care services such as individual background, education, socioeconomic status, birthplace (Greece or Canada, rural or urban), length of stay in Canada, and the degree of assimilation. Because the Greeks focused on physical ailments and symptoms, the nurse must be cognizant of the underlying psychological origins of these physical symptoms. The nurse must assist the patient in identifying strategies for prevention as well.

BIOLOGICAL VARIATIONS
Skin color

Because people of Greek origin are part of the White race, they blend in well with other White North Americans. Although some have very dark skin tones, typical of eastern Mediterranean people in general, they are unlikely to be confused with African Canadians or to face much discrimination based only on physiognomy.

Enzymatic and genetic variations

Greeks have been found to have enzymatic and genetic variations. Studies of a population of Greek and French individuals indicate that great consumption of monounsaturated fat and olive oil by Greeks and other environmental and genetic factors involving them may contribute to differences in some sphingoid bases (sphingomyelins), fatty acids, and ceramides in the Greek population (Katsikas and Wolf, 1995). Genetically Greeks are also unique in their frequencies of HLA-DQA1*2 and *4 and THO1*8 (Robinson et al., 1996). Both Israeli Jews and Greeks of non-Jewish origin suffering from primary Sjögren's syndrome were found to carry either DRB1*1101 or DRB1*1104 alleles that are in linkage disequilibrium with DQB1*0301 and DQA1*0501 (Roitberg-Tambur et al., 1993).

In a study by Mitchell et al. (1994) of Greeks and Italians, Greek females were found to have a significantly higher high-density lipoprotein (HDL) cholesterol than Greek males, whereas Italian females had a significantly higher low-density lipoprotein (LDL), HDL, and total cholesterol than Italian males. The genetic polymorphism of two salivary enzymes (esterase and alpha-amylase) has been studied in Greeks as well as in persons from other European countries. There was no intrapopulation heterogeneity, but there was a sigificant difference between the Greeks and the other populations (Petalopoulos et al., 1993).

A particular health problem that is found among Greek Canadians is a form of inherited blood disorder that is a persistent form of anemia called "thalassemia minor." It is defined as a chronic familial hemolytic anemia occurring in a population from countries bordering on the Mediterranean Sea and in the South Sea (Bare and Smeltzer, 1992). There are two major groups of thalassemias: alpha-thalassemia and beta-thalassemia. Beta-thalassemia, which is the most prevalent among the Greeks, is further classified into three types: thalassemia minor, intermedia, and major. The minor type is usually asymptomatic, though significant anemia may occur during pregnancy requiring blood transfusions. The intermedia type has a life expectancy of about 3 to 4 decades. Symptoms include chronic fatigue syndrome, debilitating bone pain, cardiac disease, and hypersplenism (or hepatosplenomegaly).

Another medical condition that affects up to 50% of male Greeks is called "glucose-6-phosphate dehydrogenase deficiency (Bare and Smeltzer, 1992). It is an inherited enzyme defect that causes chronic hemolytic anemia. Hemolysis results when the red blood cells are stressed by the presence of certain triggers such as fever or certain drugs. The drugs that are hemolytic for persons with G-6-PD include antimalarial drugs, sulfanomides, nitrofurantoin, common coal-tar analgesics including aspirin, thiazide diuretics, oral hypoglycemic agents, chloramphenicol, para-aminosalicylic acid, and vitamin K and for individuals subject to favism. Favism is one of the most severe forms of G-6-PD resulting from the ingesting of the fava bean, a dietary staple in Mediterranean countries such as Greece. The worst type is the Mediterranean G-6-PD.

The patients are asymptomatic with normal hemoglobin until they are exposed to offending drugs. Several days after exposure the patient may experience pallor, jaundice, hemoglobinuria, and an increase in the number of reticulocytes. Usually hemolysis lasts for a week, and then the count is spontaneously improved because the new red blood cells are resistant to lysis (such resistance not occur in the Mediterranean type).

Susceptibility to disease

Thromboembolic disease Venous thrombosis is related to the presence of factor V Leiden. Rees, Cox, and Clegg (1995) found European Greeks to have the highest allele prevalence, 7%, compared to 4.4% among other Europeans studied and suggested this as a cause of the high incidence of thromboembolic disease. This high prevalence is suggestive that screening for this mutation should be considered in some circumstances (Rees, Cox, and Clegg 1995).

Rheumatoid arthritis In northern Europeans, rheumatoid arthritis (RA) is strongly associated with a relatively conserved pentapeptide sequence of HLA-DR-beta found notably in the HLA-DR4 subtypes Dw4 and Dw14 and in DR1. In a study by Boki et al. (1992) of Greek clients with RA, 57% of the Greek clients lacked the putative HLA-DR-beta motif, and such a lack is suggestive that considerable immunogenetic heterogeneity underlies disease susceptibility among Greeks.

Nutritional preferences Traditionally, Greeks eat more lamb than any other meat, but they also enjoy a variety of fish and other seafood. Greeks almost always cook in olive oil and often use olive oil for flavoring. Popular Greek dishes include *soupa avgholemono* (lemon-flavored chicken soup), *dholmadhes* (vine leaves filled with rice and ground meat), *moussaka* (layers of eggplant and ground meat), and *souvlaki* (meat cooked on a long skewer, usually with onions and tomatoes). Also popular are feta cheese (a cheese made from sheep or goat milk), olives, *ouzo* (a licorice-flavored liquor), and *retsina* (a white wine flavored with pine resin). In Canada most Greek families will eat a blend of Greek and Canadian food, but the traditional Greek foods will certainly appear at all major festivals or important days in the families' lives (The World Book Encyclopedia, 1991).

Psychological characteristics Anderson (1985) noted that Greek-Canadian immigrant women reported feelings of loneliness and depression. In contrast to Southeast Asian Canadians, who did not discuss their feelings, Greek women were willing to share feelings with health professionals. Searl, Hughes, and Majumdar (1985) also noted that elderly Greek women often outlive their husbands and report feelings of depression.

Implications for nursing care

It is important that the nurse caring for Greek Canadians incorporate in her assessments their genetic predisposition to G-6-PD and thalassemias. The nurse must educate and assist patients to identify and avoid substances that precipitate hemolytic disorders.

SUMMARY

The nurse who cares for Greek-Canadian clients should be aware of the unique cultural heritage of this group of Canadians. Care should be designed with an appreciation of the traditions and customs that these Canadians may practice being kept in mind. The nurse should also appreciate that some Greek Canadians identify feelings of discrimination and prejudice from other Canadians because of their Greek background (Thomas, 1988a). Some parents report that they have placed their children in other schools to get away from constant taunting of other children because they are different. Greeks often have long last names, very difficult to pronounce by awkward Canadian tongues, and their first names (such as "Panagiotos" and "Anastasia") may seem peculiar in a culture used to short names like "Sean" and "Lisa." In the past Canadian immigration officials sometimes shortened long Greek surnames, and their descendants now live with the results. Cruel school-ground taunts about their names have reduced many Greek children to tears. Greek Canadians come from homes and from a culture with different social, moral, and religious traditions, and they may seem uptight and old fashioned to those non-Greeks who consider themselves the standard for contemporary Canadian life (Psomiades and Scourby, 1982). Older, well-educated Greek Canadians sometimes complain that their non-Greek counterparts believe that all Greeks are essentially peasants, interesting for their foods and dances but basically unsophisticated and somehow alien to normal Canadian life (Chimbos, 1974; Gavaki, 1991).

Case Study

A 20-year-old Greek-Canadian woman is admitted to the hospital with a diagnosis of G-6-PD. She has only recently immigrated to Canada and speaks only Greek. Although a Greek-speaking interpreter has been brought in, there is still some difficulty in assisting the client to understand the nature of the condition and ways to reduce the chronicity of the condition.

CARE PLAN

 Nursing Diagnosis   Health maintenance: altered, related to knowledge deficit about thalassemia and G-6-PD.

Client Outcomes

1. Verbalize understanding of the nature of the diseases.

2. Assess patient's level of knowledge related to the disease process, hemolytic episodes, signs, symptoms, prevention, and treatment.
3. Verbalize willingness to comply with preventive teachings to reduce symptoms and treatment regime.

Nursing Interventions

1. Determine patient's willingness to learn and note sociocultural factors that affect learning process.
2. Identify the substances and situations related to the disease process and treatment regime.

3. Explain the disease process, prevention reduction of symptoms, and treatment regime.
4. Assess patients level and stage of adaptation to the illness.
5. Explain through the use of appropriate visual aids the necessity of blood transfusions for thalassemias and G-6-PD.

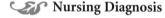 **Nursing Diagnosis**   Communication: impaired, verbal, related to foreign-language barrier.

Client Outcomes

1. Patient will be able to communicate basic health needs to health care professionals.
2. Patient will verbalize feelings of acceptance and reduced feelings of frustrations.

Nursing Interventions

1. Assess patient's ability to read, write, and comprehend English or the dominant language.
2. Speak clearly, facing the client and using simple words.
3. Use gestures or actions instead of words to communicate information.
4. Use visual aids such as pictures or drawings that will help convey to patient the necessary procedure to be done.
5. Convey attitude of acceptance and warmth.
6. Make flash cards that translate words or phrases.
7. Be cognizant of possible cultural barriers to communication such as the appropriateness of touching and discussion of personal matters.
8. Use a fluent interpreter when discussing matters of importance (such as taking a health history or signing an operation permit). If possible, allow the interpreter to spend as much time as the person wishes (be flexible with visitor's rules and regulations). If an interpreter is not available, try to plan a daily visit from someone who has some knowledge of the person's language (many hospitals and social welfare offices keep a language bank with names and phone numbers of people who are willing to interpret and translate).

STUDY QUESTIONS

1. Identify some strategies that will assist the nurse in communicating effectively with the Greek-Canadian patients and their families.

2. Explain the influence of traditional family values and culture of Greek Canadians in the caring of the elders.

3. Describe the folk beliefs and practices of the Greeks and the implications for nursing care.

4. Identify why favism is common among Greeks and other Mediterranean groups.

5. List substances and situations that can precipitate a G-6-P deficiency episode.

6. Describe some of the factors that can cause conflicts among Greek-Canadian adolescents.

7. Explain some of the stresses that may affect Greek-Canadian women.

References

Anderson, J. (1985). Perspectives on the health of immigrant women: a feminist analysis. *Advances in Nursing Science, 8*(1), 61-76.

Archdeacon, T. (1993). *Becoming American.* New York: The Free Press

Bare, B., & Smeltzer, S. (1992). *Medical surgical nursing,* (Ed. 7). (p. 797). Philadelphia: J.B. Lippincott Co.

Boki, K., Panayi, G., Vaughan, R., Drosos, A., Moutsopoulos, H., & Lanchbury, J. (1992). LHA class II sequence polymorphisms and susceptibility to rheumatoid arthritis in Greeks. The HLA-DR beta shared-epitope hypothesis accounts for the disease in only a minority of Greek patients. *Arthritis and Rheumatism, 35*(7), 749-755.

Chimbos, P.D. (1972). A comparison of the social adaptation of Dutch, Greek, and Slovak immigrants in a Canadian community. *International Migration Review, 6,* 230-244.

Chimbos, P.D. (1974). Ethnicity and occupational mobility: a comparative study of Greek and Slovak immigrants in Ontario City. *International Migration Review, 15,* 57-67.

Chimbos, P.D. (1980). *The Canadian odyssey: the Greek experience in Canada.* Toronto: McClelland & Stewart Ltd.

Chitiri, H., & Willows, D. (1993). Word recognition in two languages and orthographies: English and Greek. *Memory and Cognition, 22*(3), 313-325.

Clarke, H. (1993). The Montreal Childrens Hospital: a hospital response to cultural diversity. In Masi, R., Mensah, L, & McLeod, K. (Eds.), *Health and cultures.* San Bernardino, Calif.: Borgo Press (and Miami Beach, Fla.: Mosiac).

Danforth, L., & Tsiaras, A. (1982). *The death rituals of rural Greece.* Princeton: Princeton University Press.

Ferenczi, I. (1992). *International migrations.* Vol I: *Statistics.* New York: National Bureau of Economic Research.

Fitzgerald, M., & Rouvalis, M. (1995). Greek Canadian youths: cultural and familiar influences. *Journal of Child and Youth Care, 10*(3), 43-53.

Gavaki, E. (1991). Greek immigration to Quebec: the process and the settlement, *Journal of the Hellenic Diaspora, 1*(1, March), 68-89.

Geissler, E. (1994). *Cultural assessment* (pp. 85-87). St. Louis: Mosby.

Giger, J., & Davidhizar, R. (1991). *Transcultural nursing* (p. 137-138). Toronto: Mosby.

Kayal, P. (1979). Eastern Orthodoxy exogamy and triple melting pot theory: Herberg revisited. *Sociological Abstracts.*

Katsikas, H., & Wolf, C. (1995). Blood sphingomyelins from two European countries. *Biochimica et Biophysica Acta, 1258*(2), 95-100.

Kourvetaris, G. (1990). Conflicts and identity crises among Greek Americans and Greeks of the Diaspora, *International Journal of contemporary Sociology, 27*(3-4), 137-153.

Lambert, W.C., Mermigis, L., & Taylor, D. (1986). Greek-Canadian attitudes towards own group and other Canadian ethnic groups: a test of the multicultural hypothesis. *Canadian Journal Of Behavioral Science, 18*(1), 33-51.

Lambrou, Y. (1975). *The Greek community of Vancouver.* Unpublished M.A. thesis, University of British Columbia, Vancouver, B.C.

Loescher, G., & Scanlan, J. (1986). *Calculated kindness.* New York: The Free Press.

Lynam, J. (1991). Taking culture into account: a challenging prospect for cardiovascular nursing. *Canadian Journal of Cardiovascular Nursing, 2*(3), 10-15.

Mirambel, A. (1959). *La langue grecque.* Paris: Librairie C. Klincksieck.

Mitchell, R., Earl, L., Williams, J., Bisucci, T., & Gasiasmis, H. (1994). Polymorphisms of the gene coding for the cholesteryl ester transfer protein and plasma lipid levels in Italian and Greek migrants to Australia. *Human Biology, 66*(1), 13-25.

Moskos, C. (l980). *Greek Americans.* Englewood Cliffs, N.J.: Prentice-Hall, Inc.

Nagata, J. (1969). Adaptation and integration of Greek working class immigrants in the city of Toronto, Canada: a situational approach. *International Migration Review, 4,* 44-70

Noble, A. (1992). *To build in a new land.* Baltimore, Md.: Johns Hopkins University Press.

Patterson, J.G. (1976). *The Greeks of Vancouver: a study in the preservation of ethnicity.* Ottawa: National Museum of Man, Canadian Centre for Folk Culture Studies.

Petalopoulos, A., Fousteri, M., Kouvatsi, A., Triantaphyllidis, C. (1993). Polymorphism of salivary esterase and alpha-amylase in the Greek population. *Human Heredity, 43*(6), 375-379.

Petras, E.M. (1988). Returning migrant characteristics and labor market demands in Greece, *International Migration Review, 22*(4), 586-608.

Psomiades, H., & Scourby, A. (eds.) (1982). *The Greek American community in transition.* New York: Pella Publishing Company.

Raya, A. (1989). Family care of the elderly in Greece: culture and research. *Recent Advances in Nursing, 23,* 72-81.

Rees, D., Cox, M., & Clegg, J. (1995). World distribution of factor V Leiden. *The Lancet, 346,* 1133-1134.

Robinson, S., Gutowski, S., van Oorschot, R., Fripp, Y., & Mitchell, J. (1996). Genetic diversity among selected ethnic subpopulations of Australia: evidence from three highly polymorphic DNA loci. *Human Biology, 68*(4), 489-508.

Rosenbaum, J. (1990). Cultural care of older Greek Canadian widows within Leininger's theory of culture care. *Journal of Transcultural Nursing, 2*(1), 37-47.

Rosenbaum, J. (1991a). The health meanings of older Greek Canadian widows. *Journal of Advanced Nursing, 16,* 1320-1327.

Rosenbaum, J. (1991b). Widowhood grief: a cultural perspective. *The Canadian Journal of Nursing Resarch, 23*(2), 61-76.

Roitberg-Tambur, A., Friedmann, A., Safirman, C., et al. (1993). Molecular analysis of HLA class II genes in primary Sjögren's syndrome: a study of Israeli Jewish and Greek non-Jewish patients. *Human Immunology, 36*(4), 235-242.

Rouvalis, M. (1990). *Women, education, and gender-role expectation: a Greek Canadian perspective.* Unpublished M.A. thesis, Dalhousie University, Halifax, N.S.

Searl, S., Hughes, J., & Majumdar, B. (1985). The health status of Canadians. In Stewart, M., Innes, J., Searl, S., & Smillie, C. (Eds.), *Community Health Nursing in Canada* (pp. 129-141). Toronto: Gage.

Sowell, T. (1978). Race and IQ reconsidered. In Sowell, T. (Ed.), *Essays and data on American ethnic groups.* Washington, D.C.: The Urban Institute.

Statistics Canada (1991). Cat. No. 93-315.

Takaki, R. (1993). *A different mirror.* Boston: Little, Brown & Co.

Teperoglou, A. (1980). Open care for the elderly—Greece. In Amann, A. (Ed.), *Open care for the elderly in seven European countries.* Exeter: Pergamon Press.

The encyclopedia Americana international edition. (1992). Canbury, Conn.: Grolier Incorporated.

The new encyclopaedia Britannica. (1993). Vol. 5. Chicago: Encylopaedia Britannica, Inc.

The world book encyclopedia (1991). Vol. 8. Chicago: World Book, Inc.

Thomas, G.T. (1988a). The role of the Greek Orthodox church in the Hellenic community of Nova Scotia. In Moore, D., & Morrison, J. (Eds.), *Work, ethnicity and oral history,* pp. 177-186.

Thomas, G.T. (1988b). Women in the Greek Community of Nova Scotia. *Canadian Ethnic Studies, 3,* 84-93.

Thomas, G.T. (1966). Personal conversations in a Greek community.

Tripp-Reimer, T. (1983). Retention of a folk-healing practice *(matiasma)* among four generations of urban Greek immigrants. *Nursing Research, 32*(2), 97-101.

Vlassis, G. (1953). *The Greeks in Canada.* Ottawa: Leclerc Printers.

Zola, I. (1972). Studying the decision to see the doctor. *Advances in Psychosomatic Medicine, 8,* 216-236.

INDEX

A

Aboriginal Nurses Association of Canada, 63
Aboriginal people, 4
  family violence, 145
  language, 23-24
Abuse
  domestic, 144-145
    Mexican Mennonites, 351
    Ojibwa, 206-207
  drug
    Quebeckers, 169
    sickle cell anemia and, 137
    Somalis, 337
Accident
  Hutterites, 241
  Quebeckers, 167
Acculturation, 183
Acetaldehyde dehydrogenase, 128-129
Acquired immunodeficiency syndrome, 138-139
  Quebeckers, 168, 169-170
Activity orientation, 110
Adapters in movement therapy, 55
ADH; *see* Alcohol dehydrogenase
Adolescents
  French Canadians of Quebec origin, 162
  Greek Canadians, 365-366
Adoption among Nunavut Inuit, 267, 268
Affect displays in movement therapy, 55
African-American population
  cultural behaviors relevant to health assessment, 16
  growth and development, 336
  hypertension, 133-134, 135
  language, 331
  sickle cell anemia, 136-137
African population, cultural phenomena impacting on nursing care, 15
Age-standard mortality, 225
Aging; *see* Elderly
AIDS; *see* Acquired immunodeficiency syndrome
Air pollution in Quebec province, 166
Albinism, 240
Alcohol
  metabolism, 128-130
    Kwa-kwa'ka-wakw, 224
    Ojibwa, 207

Alcohol—cont'd
  use and abuse
    Cree, 191
    Finnish Canadians, 306-307, 307
    Kwa-kwa'ka-wakw, 224
    Mi'kmaq, 325
    Ojibwa, 208-209
    Quebeckers, 169
    Somalis, 337
    Ukrainian Canadians, 289
Alcohol dehydrogenase, 128-129, 224
Aldehyde dehydrogenase, 224
ALDH; *see* Acetaldehyde dehydrogenase
Algonquians, 5, 181
Allergy, 167
Alopecia, 138
Alprazolam, 129
Alternative family, 67
Alternative therapy, 115-116
  Quebeckers, 164
Alzheimer's disease, 190
American Eskimos, cultural behaviors relevant to health assessment, 16
Americans, cultural behaviors relevant to health assessment, 16
Amish, 116
Anabaptist movement, 346
ANAC; *see* Aboriginal Nurses Association of Canada
Anemia
  glucose-6-phosphate dehydrogenase deficiency and, 142
  sickle cell, 136-137
Anfechtung, 238
Angiotensin-converting enzyme inhibitors metabolism, 129
Anishinaabe, 197
Anopheles mosquito, 136
Antigen D, 132
Antihypertensives, metabolism of, 129
Apolipoprotein E4, 190
Appalachians, 16
Arctic, nutritional preferences in, 140
Arthritis
  Greek Canadians, 373
  systemic lupus erythematosus and, 138
Asians, 15

To help us publish the most useful materials for students, we would appreciate your comments on this book. Please take a few moments to complete the form below, then tear it out and mail it back to us. Thank you in advance for your input!

Book Title: _____
Author Name: _____

1. Did the content of this textbook help you meet the requirements for passing this course? Explain: _____
_____
_____

2. What do you like most about this product? _____
_____

   What do you like least? _____
_____
_____

3. Which chapters were most helpful? Which were least helpful? _____
_____
_____

4. If you could change one thing about this book, what would it be? _____
_____
_____

5. If applicable, did you purchase/use the student learning guide accompanying the text? If so, did you purchase the student learning guide on your own or at the direction of the instructor? _____
_____
_____

6. Was the book a good value for the price? _____
_____
_____

7. Are you planning to keep this text? Why or why not? _____
_____
_____

Are you interested in doing in-depth reviews of our nursing textbooks? If so, please fill out the information below:

Name: _____ Telephone: _____
Address: _____

Thank you!

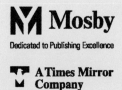

Mosby
Dedicated to Publishing Excellence

A Times Mirror Company

fold here -

NO POSTAGE
NECESSARY
IF MAILED
IN THE
UNITED STATES

BUSINESS REPLY MAIL
FIRST-CLASS MAIL   PERMIT NO. 135   SAINT LOUIS MO

POSTAGE WILL BE PAID BY ADDRESSEE

**JANET BLANNER
NURSING MARKETING
MOSBY INC
11830 WESTLINE INDUSTRIAL DR
SAINT LOUIS MO 63146-9987**

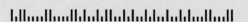

fold here -